AF682747

A Resource for Nurse Anesthesia Educators

Second edition

Bernadette Henrichs, PhD, CRNA, CCRN
Judy Thompson, DNAP, APRN, CRNA

Published by
American Association of Nurse Anesthetists

American Association of Nurse Anesthetists
222 South Prospect Avenue
Park Ridge, IL 60068-4001

Copyright © 2017 American Association of Nurse Anesthetists

All rights reserved. This book is protected by copyright. No part of it may be reproduced, stored in a retrieval system, or transmitted in any form or by any means, electronic, mechanical, photocopying, recording, or otherwise without written permission from the publisher.

Printed in the United States of America.

Last digit indicates print number: 10 9 8 7 6 5 4 3 2 1

The authors and publisher have done everything possible to make this book accurate, up to date, and in accord with accepted standards at the time of publication. The authors, editors, and publisher are not responsible for errors or omissions or for consequences from application of the book, and make no warranty, expressed or implied, in regard to the contents of this book. Any practice is this book should be applied in accordance with professional standards of care used in regard to the unique circumstances that may apply in each situation.

Library of Congress Cataloging-in-Publication Data

Names: Henrichs, Bernadette, 1960- editor. | Thompson, Judy, 1948- editor. | American Association of Nurse Anesthetists, issuing body.

Title: A resource for nurse anesthesia educators / edited by Bernadette Henrichs and Judy Thompson.

Description: Second edition. | Park Ridge, IL : American Association of Nurse Anesthetists, [2017] | Includes bibliographical references and index.

Identifiers: LCCN 2017026615 | ISBN 9780982991251

Subjects: | MESH: Nurse Anesthetists--education | Anesthesia--nursing | Education, Nursing

Classification: LCC RD80.3 | NLM WY 18 | DDC 617.9/60711--dc23 LC record available at https://lccn.loc.gov/2017026615

Foreword

If you could be a fly on the wall of an operating room, unnoticed and beyond the reach of the circulating nurse, how long would it take you to confidently say if the person at the head of the OR table is a Certified Registered Nurse Anesthetist (CRNA)?

Every one of the many CRNAs who I have interviewed (I am a history writer) says it would take "only a few minutes." Some even say it would take "no time at all." These leaders of our profession, many of whom are educators, believe that CRNAs exhibit unique observable traits.

Yet these same leaders struggle to describe CRNA traits. They say a CRNA keeps an orderly workspace, and may touch the patient. But these features could apply to any clinician. They leave us wondering: What really sets CRNAs apart from other clinicians? The answer to that question can be found in the history of nurse anesthesia education.

In the 1890s, anesthesia was dangerous because it was poorly administered. Alice Magaw and her colleagues at the St Mary's Hospital in Rochester, Minnesota perfected the use of ether. Before long surgeons sent nurses to Magaw to learn safe anesthesia. Magaw and her colleagues recognized that each student gained proficiency at her own pace, and they allowed students to train for 2 or 3 months. Magaw also carefully supervised trainees before sending them home to practice alone. Magaw's careful methods were entirely new and made anesthesia safe for the first time ever.

Subsequent nurse anesthetist educators built on Magaw's work. Alice McGee introduced the teaching of anatomy, physiology, pharmacology, and case management in 1912 at the St Vincent's Hospital in Portland, Oregon. In 1915, Agatha Hodgins, at the Lakeside Hospital in Cleveland, gave students a 6-month didactic curriculum and, for the first time, a variety of rotations at different hospitals. The evidence that these efforts improved anesthesia is that by 1948 they were widely accepted. Fifty-four schools of anesthesia around the country replicated the Lakeside model. And graduates of these programs provided anesthesia at more than 75% of our nation's hospitals.

Dedication to improving education endured. Agatha Hodgins formed the American Association of Nurse Anesthetists (AANA) in 1931 specifically to improve education; Hodgins together with Helen Lamb, Gertrude Fife, and others agitated for better nationwide curriculum standards, inspection and accreditation of schools, and certification of graduates by examination. In the second half of the 20th century, new teaching methods were developed and refined, continuing education was implemented, and teacher education was developed. In the 21st century the influence of American nurse anesthetist educators expanded globally when the International Federation of Nurse Anesthetists adopted an Anesthesia Program Approval Process. The continuous effort to guarantee a quality education for nurses in anesthesia is a hallmark of nurse anesthesia culture.

That culture is reflected in the pages of this text. Magaw's flexible approach to individualized learning can be seen in the chapters on different learning styles and the modern emphasis on mentorship throughout the novice-to-expert transition. The didactic training begun by McGee and Hodgins morphed into today's evidence-based thinking and the promotion of scholarship. Hodgins' effort to provide students a varied clinical experience is reflected in today's teaching of psychomotor skills and simulation labs.

Notably, throughout these changes, two aspects of CRNA culture have not changed. One-to-one supervision of nurse anesthesia students, a practice that began with Alice Magaw remains. In consideration of patient safety a student is never left to fend for herself. A seasoned CRNA mind is always immediately available.

The second unchanged feature of CRNA culture is the desire among nurse anesthetists for acceptance within the academy. In 1936 Helen Lamb wrote that nurse anesthesia schools should "strive to secure the benefits which universities have extended to other professional groups." With the advent of doctoral education, nurse anesthesia now seems poised to gain the benefits that Lamb envisioned 80 years ago.

A Resource for Nurse Anesthesia Educators sums up what makes a CRNA unique. Each chapter tells us a part of what we want our students to understand, to do, and to become. Here you will find the means for teaching adult learners to think for themselves, develop skills, and solve the myriad problems associated with nurse anesthesia.

Evan Koch, MSN, CRNA
Spirit Lake, Idaho

Authors

Brian Benham, DNP, CRNA

Chuck Biddle, PhD, CRNA

Madeline K. Chalenor, DNP, MHS, CRNA

Shawn Collins, DNP, PhD, CRNA

Vicki Coopmans, PhD, CRNA

Michael D. Fallacaro, DNS, CRNA, FAAN

Francis Gerbasi, PhD, CRNA

Richard E. Haas, PhD, CRNA, PHRN

James R. Halliburton, DNSc, CRNA, APRN

Adrienne G. Hartgerink, DNP, CRNA

William Hartland Jr., PhD, CRNA

Bernadette Henrichs, PhD, CRNA, CCRN

Betty J. Horton, PhD, CRNA, FAAN

Anne Marie Hranchook, DNP, CRNA

Karita Käck, DNAP, CRNA

Rachel C. Lerner, MSLS

Lilia Loriz, PhD, ARNP, BC

Kiran Macha, MBBS, MPH

Mary Jeanette Mannino, JD, CRNA

Maura McAuliffe, PhD, CRNA, FAAN

John P. McDonough, EdD, CRNA, ARNP

Marlene R. McDowell, MA

Authors (continued)

John J. McFadden, PhD, CRNA

Lisa Mileto, DNP, CRNA

Meghan Niemczyk, MPH

John M. O'Donnell, DrPH, MSN, CRNA

Paul E. Phrampus, MD, FACEP, FSSH

John C. Preston, DNSc, CRNA, FNAP, APN

Charles A. Reese, PhD, CRNA

Kelli J. Scott, MS, CDM

Elizabeth Seibert, PhD, CRNA

Judy Thompson, DNAP, APRN, CRNA

Sandra K. Tunajek, DNP, CRNA

Celeste G. Villanueva, EdD, CRNA, FNAP

Brenda Wands, PhD, CRNA

Kathy Wren, PhD, CRNA

Timothy Wren, DNP, RN

Contents

CHAPTER 1

The Socratic Method and Its Use in Teaching Student Nurse Anesthetists

Richard E. Haas, PhD, CRNA, PHRN

Keywords: Individual, instruction, questioning, Socratic method.

Key Concepts

- The use of Socratic instruction is pivotal in determining the depth of knowledge of nurse anesthesia students.
- A tone of openness to dialogue and the importance of questioning concepts must be set for Socratic instruction to succeed.
- Good Socratic instructors know that after any question is asked, one must have the necessary background to know a correct answer and evaluate the extent to which the student's response is correct.
- Although Socratic instruction usually is associated with one-to-one clinical instruction, it may be modified easily for use in small groups.

An Open Letter to the Clinical or Didactic Faculty Member (Second Edition)

Dear fellow teacher:

I still know you, in fact, even better than the last time.

You aren't a "facilitator" or a "guide." You are a teacher. Some of you have been around for a while, and others are entering this amazing, frustrating, rewarding, agonizing, awe-inspiring world of teaching our next generation of nurse anesthetists. Each of you knows your profession and knows it well. It is more than your vocation, it is your passion. You take your specialized clinical skills, a vast knowledge base, and finely honed intuitive abilities, and pass them along to the next generation of nurse anesthetists. This chapter is designed to help you become a more effective teacher, in the classroom and in the operating room. So, first things first, thank you! Teaching student nurse anesthetists is a demanding and frequently unpaid "benefit" of your position. Oh, sometimes you get a title (like "Preceptor" or "Clinical faculty" or "Adjunct lecturer") and free run of the medical library (not to mention a really impressive line on your resume), but usually that is it. Yet, few people in health care make as great a contribution to the future successes of our profession as do you. Socrates, the father of instruction in just about everything, would have been proud of you, because he made it a point to never take payment for his teaching.[1] The general public doesn't know who you are, much less the value of your teaching skills, but your colleagues in nurse anesthesia education circles do. We have seen you there in the trenches. You are watching, teaching, cajoling, praising, yes, and even sometimes growling at the students assigned to you. We have seen you, because we have been there with you.

Well, friends and colleagues, it is time to let the "cat out of the bag." There is a way to do this job that is enjoyable, fun, exciting, and stimulating for both you and your students. The technique has been around for thousands of years, and was indirectly referred to earlier. You have probably been exposed to it yourself, if you think back over your own education and look for fond memories. It is Socratic instruction.

OK, now stop sighing and rolling your eyes! Breathe deeply, in and out…there, feel better? This is not about philosophy, amateur or otherwise. This is both a "how-to" chapter describing a technique that you can use to be an effective teacher as well as a partial explanation of why this works so well. And here is the payoff: not only will you be an effective teacher, but you'll be a popular teacher as well. Most nurse anesthesia students love this technique. They love it in spite of the fact that it makes them work harder than ever. Most love it because of this fact! This type of teaching results in a deep and profound understanding of the material presented. You get to experience the joy every teacher seeks, that of seeing students really engaged with their studies.

The good news is that this style of teaching works much better with small groups, and works best with individuals, precisely the way we teach in the operating room. Socrates saw himself in the "two-on-a-log" model: a log with a student on one end and a teacher on the other. The final payoff comes in the form of a quote from the statesman Seneca, "*docendo discimus*": "When we teach, we learn."[2]

Please join me as we probe the secrets of the Socratic method; you'll be glad you did, and so will your students!

—Rich

Introduction

This chapter is divided into three parts. The first concerns background and basics, focusing briefly on Socrates and the nature of his breakthrough in instruction that has formed the cornerstone of education for 2,500 hundred years. It will also show you the importance of "setting the tone" for Socratic instruction, and provide some suggestions for dealing with small groups. The second part discusses the instruction itself, a kind of "how-to-do-it" manual. It also includes some concrete examples of how the Socratic teacher takes "what everyone knows" and guides the students through the perilous waters of truth. Part-three discusses the perceived drawbacks of the Socratic method, and seeks to alleviate these concerns which teachers may associate with its use.

Part 1: The Background and the Basics

Socrates for the Uninterested; Who He Was and Why this Works

"For there is far greater peril in buying knowledge than in buying meat and drink... you cannot buy the wares of knowledge and carry them away in another vessel; when you have paid for them you must receive them into your soul and go your way, either greatly harmed or greatly benefited."[2]

Ah yes, the voices of the skeptics. I can hear their questions. Who was this Socrates guy anyway, and what could he possibly say to me in the 21st century? I mean really, the guy has been dead for 2,300 years; he didn't have the Internet, a computer, television, smartphone, or students with a 30-second attention span. Can he possibly be germane to teaching ultrasound guided nerve blocks? Those, as Socrates might have said, are excellent questions! In fact, let's begin by doing as Socrates would have done, and break this question into its component parts and carefully examine each part.

Who was Socrates? Born in 470 BC, this questioner after truth was the son of a sculptor, Sophroniscus. He lived in the era that immediately followed the retreat of Xerxes, a Persian ruler, and the end of the war against the Persians in which Socrates served as a Greek hoplite (an armored foot soldier carrying a heavy shield and sword). In short, his times, like ours, were filled with change, chaos, and upheaval. His biggest concern was the teaching of virtuous behavior to a civilization of Greeks, whom he felt were beginning the downfall of their existence. Socrates wrote nothing himself;[2] his existence and dialogues depend upon his faithful reporters Plato and Xenophon, among others. In this "publish or perish" age of higher education, Socrates might never have received tenure. In Socrates' time, he constantly skirmished (intellectually) with a group known as the Sophists. They are described by Hurst as "traveling wise men" with "spectacular" presentations; yet Socrates thought they were "poor teachers," while they found him a "dangerous eccentric."[3] In short, they followed the "Sage on a Stage" model which Socrates and others like him abhorred. Hurst speaks to this when he says, "True teaching is more than simply announcing information at lectures."[3(p.1,606)]

What we know about Socrates comes to us primarily from Plato. Plato was Socrates' student, and knew him for about 10 years before Socrates was put to death.[1]

Students in Socrates' time frequently lived with or near their teachers, and spent untold hours in conversations, lessons, and simply living together day in and day out. If any of our own students were to be with us day and night for 10 years, they would have our every statement tattooed in their memory. They would also know each and every quirk, smirk, smile, and grimace, every gesture and platitude. They would undoubtedly write things about us we would never write about ourselves. This is what makes Plato a particularly good source of information about how Socrates taught, and how we might go about teaching as Socrates did.

There is a great deal more to the "who" Socrates was, but this section is primarily about how he taught. If you want more details on the life of Socrates, almost any computer-based search engine can reveal as much as you'd like to read. Let's move on to the "what" part of the question.

The question under discussion was the degree of importance of Socrates and his techniques here in the 21st century. Indeed, the importance is the same as in the 20th century, 19th, 18th, and so on. To begin with, numerous authors have cited and continue to cite the utility of Socratic technique in teaching.[3–8] The techniques Socrates authored and used do not have an expiration date. They are just as useful today in our technology driven age as they were when first used. Indeed, I would make the case they are more useful. Students today live in "factoid land." Hurst best describes this when he says, "Unfortunately, however, the brains of many of students have already been programmed to act as sponges that hold on to information just long enough for the student to make an A on an examination...."[3] They want a one-word answer to complex questions which can be regurgitated upon demand to satisfy (they think) the requirements of a robust education in anesthesia. Students soon find, however, the most frequently used response is, "It depends." This is why Socratic technique is priceless. You see, Socrates was a seeker: a seeker after information, a seeker after truth, and a seeker after virtue. He found answers by asking questions. He also developed word pictures and insights. He was fond of taking a statement made by a classical Greek author (such as Homer) and then expanding upon it. The expansion was based on the application of the statement to some common occurrence in life, and then following the precept of the statement out to its logical end. His technique was referred to (far later in history) as the Socratic method.

There are two technical terms used to describe this type of learning: *elenchus* and *aporia*.[10] Elenchus can be thought of in terms of a series of questions, designed to challenge a concept or idea. They are usually thought of as "why" questions: Why does this happen? What is the nature of this phenomenon? What is the underlying goal of this action? These questions should be open in nature. Dichotomous "yes or no," "true or false" questions are less useful in this type of instruction, but they may be helpful in pinning down terms associated with the question. The aporia is generally thought of as a state of confusion or consternation: students are required to come to grips with their statements and deal with the logical results of their answers. Although confusion is often thought of as something bad, confusion can be positive when it precipitates further thought on the part of the student. As Green and Rose point out, this type of intellectual probing turns education into, "...an active process and not a passive spectator sport."[11] This technique of probing questions followed by answers leading to more questions was referred to (far later in history) as the Socratic method. Actually, the Socratic method, as we use it in modern education, came from the former dean of Harvard Law School, Christopher Columbus Langdell, who began to use it in 1870.[12]

Despite the fact that most of us are not in the habit of teaching virtue, this technique can easily be transformed to fit nearly all of the health sciences. Why? Because it fits the nature of the knowledge we are required to possess. Further, as Tucker[13] points out, the Socratic method is particularly effective for instruction in professions that are self-governing. This refers to professions that understand the technical vagaries of their work better than the general public or a governmental bureau. This sounds obtuse, but think for a moment. Anesthetists know that a simple list of memorized rote data is insufficient to care for the patient, despite the fact that in other trades or skills this is all that is needed (or more reliance is based on this aspect than the critical thinking required in anesthesia). Data are the bricks from which concepts are constructed. But all bricks and no mortar make a shaky house indeed. The mortar is the defining concept of anesthesia practice, allowing us to take myriad data points, look at them logically, and "construct" the best anesthetic for the patient.

People who have tried to convert the art and science of patient care to an interactive computer program have rapidly found the failings in this technique. For example, a frequent complaint about patient simulation, no matter how good, is that it is not sufficiently complex to mimic the living, breathing patient. The nurse anesthetist must understand complex relationships and the concepts that undergird the clinical decisions they make. A clinical anesthesia example helps clear this up (by the way, Socrates used examples called "thought experiments" like these all the time in his instruction).

A patient is hypoxic. Insertion of an endotracheal tube and manually ventilating the patient may not work to treat the hypoxia. Why not? Because the anesthetist does not know if the cause of the patient's hypoxia is an absent heartbeat, a tumor occluding the bottom part of the trachea, or because a toxin is preventing the attachment of oxygen molecules to the hemoglobin. The complex relationships between cardiovascular function and pulmonary function must be understood before therapy can be initiated. Note that this example is in the form of questions that could be asked of the seeker after knowledge (ie, your student). This example shows that there is knowledge beyond the simple recall of data that the student must have. The teacher's ability to discern the level of the student's knowledge and then to build on that level is the strength of Socratic instruction. Socrates showed that one is able to establish the deep understanding of complex relationships. In this manner, the use of Socrates' technique makes one a more efficient, focused, and interesting teacher.

Neither teachers nor students exist in a vacuum. Rather, they flourish (or perish) within an educational environment designed to support (or kill) academic endeavors. The next part of the chapter deals with setting the proper tone for the use of the Socratic method.

Part 2: Setting the Tone

Demolishing Ineffective Habits

This is the part of the instruction that no one, least of all myself, cares for. The Oracle at Delphi, someone with whom Socrates was intimately familiar, said that a key aspect of human development was to "know thyself." The hallmark of Socratic instruction is that of a teacher guiding a student through skillful questioning to a deeper understanding of the concepts needed to administer anesthesia. This is in distinct contrast to "pimping," which is designed only to reinforce a hierarchy of the "wise" teacher over the "inept" student (see **Table 1.1**).[4] More will be said on this later, when we investigate the proposed "weaknesses" of the Socratic method. But for now, all of us know that it is tough to undo the habits that make one an inefficient or ineffective teacher. Consider this: some of you may have come from programs that had one or more instructors whose favorite "teaching" technique was to criticize and berate you for every perceived shortcoming. What did you learn from these individuals? You learned how to respond in such a fashion that prevented further offense. In other words, you learned a great deal about how not to get criticized and very little about how to do anesthesia. In educational parlance, this is a classic error in validity. Your desire, as a good Socratic instructor, is to teach all about anesthesia.

Socratic instruction, however, requires an atmosphere that makes the student answer questions, and allows the student to make mistakes. These mistakes, obviously, can never come at the expense of the care rendered to the patient; that is, after all, why you as the instructor are present. Students, however, will discuss decisions relating to care with you throughout the case, and these decisions can enlighten or demolish the student's learning for the day. How does one set the proper tone each day? Let's take it one step at a time.

Step 1: **Understand that most students want to learn**, particularly nurse anesthesia students who have competed assiduously for the privilege simply to sit in the class. We are indeed fortunate that, on the whole, we have some of the most dedicated and curious learners in graduate education.

Step 2: **Know that you have a repository of specific and esoteric knowledge locked up inside your head**; your actions in the operating room have become such second nature that you would have to take a moment to stop and explain why you are doing what you are doing. Do not be dismayed by this; it is actually the hallmark of the expert practitioner.[9] Socratic instruction requires that you *first* unlock this data source in your own head. In other words, you, as the teacher, need to go back and rethink why you do what you do. This is harder than it first appears; you'll find you have in fact forgotten why you do some of the things you do (other than the fact they work!). Do not let this discourage you; Socrates frequently said the only thing he knew for sure was that he didn't really know anything.[1]

Step 3: **Set a workplace tone of encouragement.** This is frequently one of the hardest things to do in a fast-paced, production-centered operating room. The operating room is far too often not the place where such a tone occurs. In too many ORs, everyone is barking at everyone else. With the advent of crew resource management, many facilities are overcoming this problem, and the overall tone is beginning to change, but there is still much work to be done. Your abilities may not extend to creating a cultural sea change for an entire department. It is possible, though, to modify and enhance your interactions with the student. You must break this pattern where your conversations with your student are concerned. The student needs to know two important things: (1) The student can present even the most ridiculous idea at minimal personal risk. Saying that an idea is ridiculous is fair game; saying that the person is ridiculous is not. You have far more power than does your student, and the student's perception of your power may be exaggerated. Student nurse anesthetists frequently feel as if they are constantly "on the bubble" or that they are one mediocre evaluation away from dismissal. These self-defeating attitudes must be reined in by the Socratic teacher. (2) The student is responsible for his or her answers and knowledge. Although in a learner role, their learning cannot be passive; it must be active. The job of the student is to come equipped with basic knowledge and intellectual curiosity, which increases in complexity throughout the course of their studies. The active portion comes when the teacher requires them to use this bank of knowledge and make inferential voyages into the complexities of administering an anesthetic. Rigorous instruction, however, is not hostile instruction.

Step 4: **Have a plan for the events of the day (or class) and patiently stick to it.** Good teaching happens when you ask a student open-ended questions, and require that student to answer. You must prepare for your period of instruction, whether in the classroom or in the operating room. The Socratic method is easy if you thoroughly understand the topic you are teaching. Poor Socratic instructors, however, err in thinking that it is enough to simply ask question after question. In fact, after the question is asked, you must have the necessary background both to know a correct answer and to evaluate the extent to which the student's response is correct. Your depth of knowledge about your subject is crucial to successful instruction. If some of your knowledge is dated or uncertain, it is important to review the subject matter before instruction.

Also, students respond differently to questions. Sometimes you'll have to wait for the answer. Sometimes you can wait (if you are talking during morning report), and sometimes you cannot (you are aggressively resuscitating the patient). Try this experiment. Ask yourself aloud, "How could I use Socratic instruction with my students?" Look at your watch or phone, and wait 30 seconds in silence, as though you were waiting for an answer. This is a lot longer than it seems, but it will become more comfortable as you practice.

To sum up, the tone of your instruction, as well as the environment in which it takes place, is important for you to succeed. We'll move on to specific techniques in the next section, but without an open environment, the Socratic method is reduced to students parroting your whims and desires, some of which may not be correct.

Part 3: The Technique

"Teaching is the only major occupation of man for which we have not yet developed tools that make an average person capable of competence and performance. In teaching we rely on the 'naturals,' the ones who somehow know how to teach."[11]

—Peter F. Drucker

Talking and Listening

What do you think would happen if you, the teacher, were to try to teach the average nurse anesthesia student everything you know about the conduct of an anesthetic on the very first day of their very first clinical rotation? One would not be surprised to see the student collapse in a gibbering, scrub-suit-covered mass in the corner of the operating room. The reason for the collapse is that there is too much information compressed into too short a time. Indeed, some of the information would not relate at all to the case at hand. Yet, interestingly enough, clinical instructors make a mistake similar to this each day.

The mistake is *a lack of focus*: trying to be "a mile wide and an inch deep." When you read Plato and Socrates' interactions with his students, you find that Socrates was frequently an "inch wide and a mile deep." Depth of understanding was his goal, because students so equipped could take these principles and apply them to many aspects of life. Let's take this whole idea one step at a time.

As you teach future anesthetists, you need to remember how you learned things about your science and craft. Richard Feynman, perhaps the greatest theoretical physicist since Newton, advised his students in this fashion: "You start at the beginning and read as far as you can get until you are lost. Then you start at the beginning again and keep working through until you can understand the whole book."[12–16] Note that Feynman did *not* say, "Understand the whole book today!" Grasping complex principles and inter-relationships takes time (reflected, at least partially, by the fact that nurse anesthesia programs keep increasing in length and in requirements for ever more advanced terminal degrees).

So how did Socrates do it? What was his secret? Samples[17] stresses some of the more important aspects of Socrates' technique. First, Samples tells us that Socrates began from skepticism. Note the term is skepticism and not cynicism. In setting a proper tone, cynicism must be banished. Skepticism implies that a truth can be known; we just don't know it yet. In fact, I prefer to call this an attitude of "intellectual curiosity." Contrariwise, cynicism implies that nothing is correct or true. Socrates refused to believe the things that "Everyone knows" (at our institution, this crazy guy "Everyone" seems to know a lot!).

Let's try an example. You have heard things like, "Everyone knows cardiovascular depression after propofol is due to the release of histamine." When a student says something like that, the Socratic instructor responds with a question such as, "Really? How do you know that?" or "Who says that?" or "What is the evidence for your statement?" Sound familiar? It should, because this is the driving precept behind evidence-based practice. Who would have thought Socrates might be involved in that? But let's return to the topic at hand.

Note that the veracity of the student's statement, at this point in your instruction, is immaterial. "But," you reply, "I thought we were searching for truth." Yes, that is the pursuit of both you and your student. The point of the exercise is for you, the teacher, to determine the depth of your student's knowledge and, if possible, give the student the tools to add to this depth. The use of the mystery person "everyone" may reflect the student's discomfiture or lack of knowledge about the given statement. Your skepticism (actual or assumed) drives the first part of this type of teaching. If "Everyone" already knows something, well then there is no sense in trying to learn about it. In the practice of anesthesia, assuming nothing about the student and his or her abilities is the start of a good, solid teaching plan.

Next, as Samples further describes, Socrates spoke with people. He didn't pass the time of day engaging in mere pleasantries; he really wanted to figure out why they knew what they knew. Good students want the instructor to engage them, and students on their way to becoming good need the instructor to engage them. In the operating room, your conversations with the students can go on throughout the day.[1]

Finally, Samples tell us Socrates' method is both inductive (applying general knowledge to a specific instance to see if it works each time) and deductive (seeks clues to a thing by determining consequences). The problem is always converting these concepts into practice. One of the best initial ways to learn things is to watch others model the technique you are attempting to learn. I would like you to imagine Sam Student, a mid-level student nurse anesthetist having a clinical conversation with his teacher for the day, Izzy Instructor. They are preparing for their first case of the day.

Let's listen in on their conversation.

Sam Student:	"Uh-oh, I just saw this patient in the holding area and she has red hair; that means trouble!"
Izzy Instructor:	"Really? What do you mean by that?" (*A properly skeptical Socratic response*)
Sam Student:	"Everyone knows redheads have trouble with anesthesia."
Izzy Instructor:	"OK, but what do you mean by 'trouble'?"
Sam Student:	"You know (*eyes now rolling*)...trouble."
Izzy Instructor:	"No I don't know. Tell me what you mean."
Sam Student:	"Well, I'm not sure, but somebody told me that everyone knows that redheads have trouble with anesthesia."
Izzy Instructor:	"I am still not sure what trouble means. Help me understand."
Sam Student:	"I don't know exactly, and I couldn't find anything in the chart during my workup. Can you help me out?"
Izzy Instructor:	"OK, so we don't know what happens or what trouble may occur. Let's start at the beginning. Have you read anything about this?"

What just happened in this encounter with a student? The mysterious "Everyone," accompanied by his willing assistant "Somebody," has told the student an aphorism which, after an uneasy night's sleep, has grown, developed, and reached the status of incontrovertible fact. The instructor knows, however, that hearing someone say something does not necessarily mean that the statement is true. It is up to Izzy to make the student rethink his paradigm. This is the *elenchus*. It has had the decided effect of creating *aporia* within the student. Note that Izzy has not had to rant and rave or impugn the student's intelligence. He is creating an opportunity for the student to gain more knowledge (or dispel faulty hearsay) and then report back. Izzy has ensured

1 Warning, some surgeons need silence more than they need air. These are not good rooms to spend the day in Socratic dialogue. Even though Socrates drank hemlock for telling the truth, there is no need for you to do so. Who will be the Socratic teacher if you are gone?

that the student does not change techniques or agents based on questionable data; the student is forced to think through the problem and develop an answer. In our current educational and clinical environment, this is called "evidence-based practice." Socrates would have wildly applauded this idea, as actions should be based on the best knowledge we have at any given time.

Here is another example: Let's assume you are the staff anesthetist teaching a student in the operating room. You have only one student for the entire day. One good idea is for the Socratic teacher to sit down with the student in advance (particularly the new student) and ask the following question, "What one thing do you want to learn well today?" (And it is an even better question if asked the night before the case, allowing you time to plan). You are now allowing the student the freedom to select something with which he or she is unfamiliar, and then taking on the task of teaching that subject. Note that if you haven't set the tone (see Part 1) this cannot occur. In the absence of the correct tone, you might hear, "I don't know, what do *you* think is important?" This may be a translation of the student thinking the following: "I wonder what my staff thinks is important and how I can answer the question to meet their expectations?" That defeats the effort toward making the student be self-directed.

Assume the student comes up with a critical concept they wish to evaluate. The skeptical clinician now has two thoughts: 1) What if they pick some topic or technique they already know, and 2) how can only one thing be made to last the whole day? The answer to the first question is that it is your responsibility as the teacher to see if the student is trying to "game the system." There will be more on that in later sections, so I'll answer the second question first.

One key topic can make a whole day of instruction, provided you key into the deeper aspects of the topic. Asking questions does this; moreover, starting questions always lead to more follow-up questions. The best part of teaching anesthesia is that there are usually occasions during the case where there is time for the give and take of instruction while still watching the patient. An example may be instructive here. Let's listen in once again. Here is a dialogue between another student (Kelly) and her instructor (Pat).

Pat: (surveying the operating room and checking the schedule): Good morning, Kelly. It looks like we are all set up and ready for a big surgical day. What is the one area you want to focus on today?

Kelly: "Today I want to focus on how to correctly mask a patient as part of airway management."

Pat: "Great idea, what do you think are the key aspects of this?"

Kelly: "Correctly fitting the mask, using the oral airway, pressure on the bag...."

Pat: "Anything else?"

Kelly: "Uh...." (*long pause*)

Pat: (*after waiting 30 seconds*): "How about when the technique can be used? For example, which patients are good candidates for mask anesthesia?"

Kelly: "Well, they can be used for...."

And so on. The student, while learning the psychomotor skill associated with using an anesthesia mask, also has to look at complex relationships related to the skill itself. This is two-for-the-price-of-one teaching: efficient and effective.

Note that this conversation can be had while actually administering the anesthetic. If, for example, the student is having difficulty maintaining a seal, the Socratic instructor asks, "Why do you think you are having difficulty?" as they make the necessary adjustments to secure the airway. The non-Socratic instructor tells the student, "Put your fingers here and here and hold this until I tell you to stop."

You may still have to show the student the correct technique, but it should always be accompanied with the "why" explanation, eg, "I use a mask strap because my hands are too small to get around this patient's mandible." You are taking the student to a depth that he or she never anticipated when they said they wanted to "mask a patient better." They thought in terms of psychomotor skill acquisition. You, the Socratic teacher, taught that and more.

Making Simple Diagrams Work

Socrates used spoken pictures called metaphors (drawn in the mind's eye) to make his audience understand concepts and issues. The audience of ancient Greece was very much a culture of verbal interaction and narrative tradition. Students of today are from the visual and sound bite generation: give me a factoid and give it to me now. This cultural aspect is often thought to stand between today's learner and the Socratic method. Nothing could be further from the truth. Indeed, one author describes our newest millennial students as wanting "frequent, focused, positive feedback from their mentors."[8] This sounds like Socrates at his best!

The Socratic teacher always has a tool at his or her side to battle ignorance each time it shows up. It is the pencil and the sheet of scratch paper.[II] "The pen is mightier than the sword," said English novelist and dramatist Edward George Earle Lytton Bulwer-Lytton, and it is certainly mightier than most questions. How does one draw anesthesia? Well, one doesn't, but things like neurons, synapses, charts, and graphs that describe anesthesia are relatively easy to draw. Let's look at some examples.

Let us assume the student comes to you and states that she has read an article describing the effect of the alpha-2 (α_2) adrenoreceptor agonist dexmedetomidine on blood pressure, and that it seems to also be an excellent anesthetic. She now wants to know why a blood pressure medicine could make the patient sleepier. You know that stimulation of these receptors decrease neurotransmitter release from the presynaptic neuron, but that verbal explanation seems a little unclear. How could the Socratic instructor describe this more graphically?

Try this. Here is a picture of a neuron (**Figure 1.1**, next page). This doesn't exactly look like the polished picture from the expensive textbook, but the simple schematic does the job. It is easy to understand. Let's go back to our hypothetical student's question about the α_2 receptor. We've already discussed the correct answer; here is the illustration of the phenomenon in an easy format (**Figure 1.2**, next page). We take the neuron, remove the dendrites, and add a box, some dots, two arrows, and a minus sign (inside the

II For those of you more technologically driven, computer applications such as Notability or other drawing programs may fit the bill, with the added benefit of being able to email your diagram to the student. I prefer folding the paper in half and handing it to the student.

left box). We can now see that the release of neurotransmitters (dots) from the presynaptic neuron stimulates the α_2 receptor (the "α_2" box) and provides negative feedback to decrease neurotransmitter release from that same presynaptic neuron. The decreased neurotransmitter release is shown by placing an "x" inside a down arrow on of the dots. This entire complex discussion was facilitated with lines, dots, arrows, and boxes. When combined with your explanation of how things work (along, of course, with your Socratic questions) you have made a difficult process understandable and memorable.

Figure 1.1 Simple Neuron

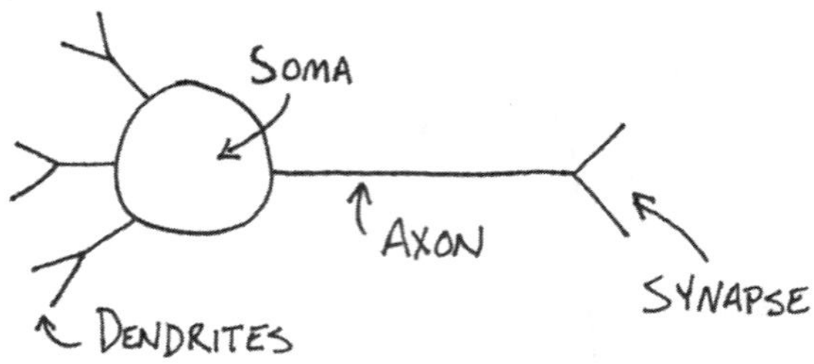

Figure 1.2 α_2 Receptor Explanation

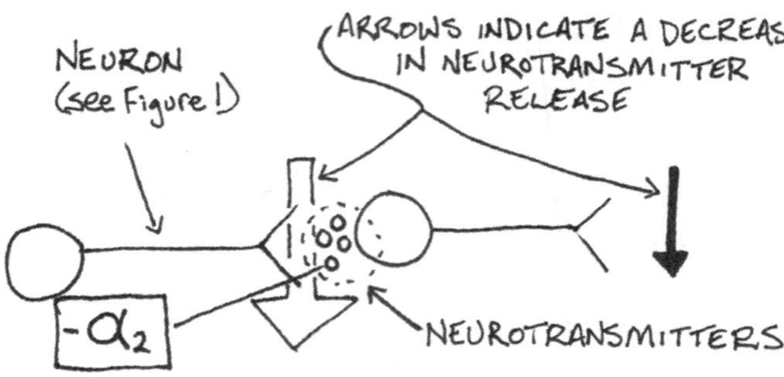

Relationships can also be drawn, but here is a strict caveat. The drawing of the relationship reinforces the Socratic instruction; it does not replace it. Let's imagine you are explaining the baroreceptor response. An easy way of explaining it would look something like this (**Figure 1.3**). The problem with this approach is that it is very easy to forget which arrows go which way, particularly if you are trying to recall this in the heat of an anesthesia battle (say, for example, when your patient's blood pressure is 180/100 and the heart rate is 35).

Figure 1.3 Baroreceptor Response: Part 1

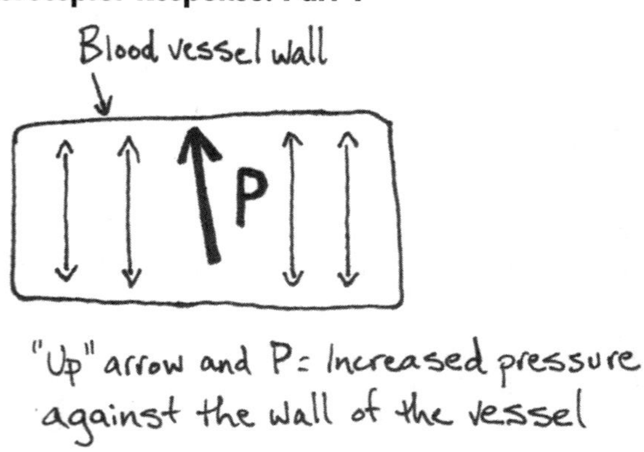

Figure 1.4 Baroreceptor Response: Part 2

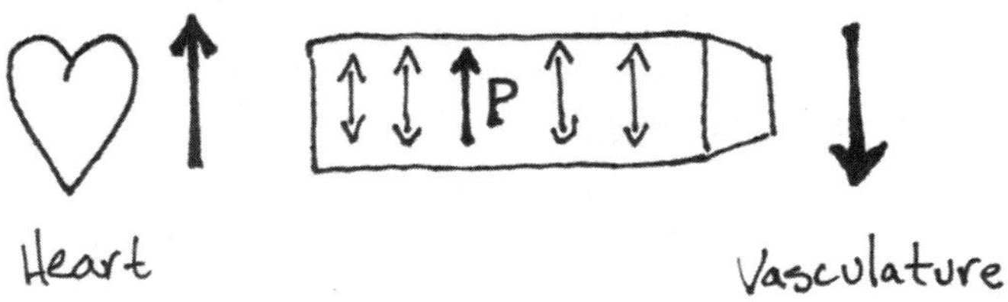

Figure 1.5 Baroreceptor Response: Part 3

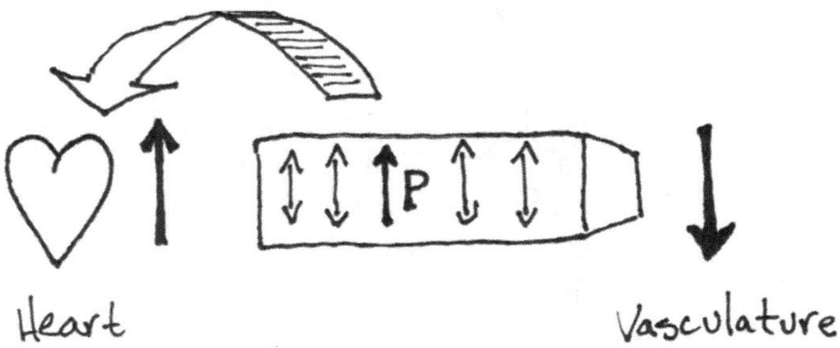

The teacher knows that the baroreceptor is a small neural sense organ that responds via a complex process to changes in blood pressure. As blood pressure rises, the body senses that the pressure against the vessels and organs is too great. It compensates by decreasing cardiac output (CO). One way of doing this is decreasing heart rate (HR), since CO = HR × Stroke Volume (SV). Providing the formula above is simple and efficient. Unfortunately, the harried student will soon forget this quick explanation, losing it in myriad up and down arrows in an ever-changing list of crucial physiologic relationships.

The Socratic instructor might try something like the following to keep the student focused and enhance their understanding of this reflex. Let's begin by assuming the multiple pictures you see in **Figures 1.3** to **1.5** are just one picture, and that the subsequent diagrams show how objects are added to the original as the discussion goes on. The instructor begins by asking the student a simple and open question: If the pressure inside your blood vessel is too high, can bad things happen to the body, and, if so, what bad things?

The student responds (correctly) that vessels could rupture in the brain, or elsewhere in the body. Question 2: What creates high blood pressure? Answer 2: Cardiac output (heart picture) goes up and/or systemic vascular resistance increases (vessels squeeze down).

Question 3: If baroreceptors fire when the blood pressure is high, what do you think their purpose is? Answer 3: To reduce blood pressure. Follow-up question 3A: Do they affect the blood vessels or the heart? Follow-up answer 3A: The heart.

Final point: If you were the brain, and you wanted to make the body's blood pressure go down, and you couldn't make the vessels bigger, what could you do to the heart? Final answer: Make it go slower.

This entire explanation has taken 5 to 10 minutes, but the student has had to work through the problem. The oral and recitation work are accompanied by visual and cognitive work. Pathways are laid down in the brain, and memories are more readily formed than with a 15-second explanation. Further, you can, at later points, require the student to reproduce this drawing, creating a more solid memory pattern upon which to build. In short, hearing something, then reading it, then explaining it, and then reproducing it builds the memories required for the competent CRNA.

Part 4: Possible Concerns Regarding the Use of the Socratic Method

By now the discerning teacher is asking the question, "Is there any possible downside to this type of instruction?" The advocate wants to say, "Of course not!" but the Socratic method is not without its critics. Many of the critics of Socratic method are unfamiliar with its use, or have seen it used poorly.[18,19] At its extremes, the Socratic method has been used cruelly, to embarrass and humiliate students in front of their peers as the instructor engages in a lively game of what one author calls, "hide the ball."[18] The television program, "The Paper Chase," shows the downside quite clearly in the quote with which the mythical law professor Kingsfield opens each episode: "The study of law is something new and unfamiliar to most of you—unlike any other schooling you've ever known before. You teach yourselves the law, but I train your minds. You come in here with a skull full of mush, and, if you survive, you leave thinking like a lawyer."[19] Gordon has gone so far as to ask the question, "Is the Socratic method illegal?"[20] He asks the reader an interesting question: In the day and age in which interest in the students' emotional needs seems to trump rigorous instruction, how can one use the Socratic method? Does not the very nature of this technique and its dependence on the creation of aporia in the student strike at the heart of students' need for self-esteem? Other authors have also related the problems that may accompany the Socratic method, including the ideas that women and minorities are unfairly treated by the process.[12,13,20]

The answer to these objections is relatively simple to state, albeit more difficult to accomplish. Rigor is simply not to be confused with cruelty. Education is not initiation, a hazing process through which students might go. True education is teaching students to critically examine the facts before them, and come to a solution based on the knowledge they have. The teacher helps form that knowledge, recognizing the students' gaps therein.[9] Regrettably, there are still many areas in clinical education in which the instructors feel students must first be "torn down" before they can be correctly educated.[18,19] Kost and Chen are particularly poignant in their description of the worst aspects of "pimping" (a practice which is not to be confused with Socratic method):

> *"One medical student published a poem specifically describing his unpleasant experiences with pimping, using the words "indignity" to describe his emotions and "worthless" to describe the perception his teacher held of him.[23] Collectively, these pieces all highlight the negative learning environment that results from the practice of pimping."*[18]

The author who asked if the Socratic method was illegal relates his own experience in this regard as a novice learner.[20] Some clinical instructors are of the opinion that since they were made to suffer at the hands of their teachers, so must new students now experience that same level of suffering. This attitude not only flies in the face of current clinical practice, with its emphasis on both the just culture and culture of safety, but it also would comprise a chapter all its own were it to be discussed thoroughly. Table 1.1, previously cited, expands further on the difference between Socratic method and "pimping."

Table 1.1 Socratic method versus "Pimping": *Abusus non tollit usum*[III]

Socratic method	Pimping
Teachers ask students probing questions designed to increase the student's knowledge.	Teachers ask students trivial questions designed to show the student "who is boss."[21]
Teachers assume students have a desire to learn, and will provide their best efforts.	Teachers assume students will not prepare unless sufficiently goaded by the possibility of looking ridiculous in front of their peers.[21]
Teachers set an environment that invites respectful dialogue in learning, viewing student weaknesses as ripe areas for instruction.[22]	Teachers set an environment in which students speak when spoken to, and view student weakness as an opportunity to sharpen an attack.
Ad hominem attacks are seen as unacceptable deviations from true teaching, rendering instruction inefficient and ineffective, not to mention cruel.	Ad hominem attacks are par for the course, and invite the sharks to circle; found to be much funnier on television doctor shows than in real life (ie, "Hawkeye Pierce" isn't as entertaining when he is in your operating room).
Teaching is evidence-based, rigorous, interactive, and challenging.	Teaching *may* be evidence-based, is rigorous, one-way, and defeating in the absence of knowing the precise answer the instructor wants to hear.[21,22]
"The true teacher knows his or her students' and is able to identify their strengths or weaknesses"[4(p.1,606)]	The teacher knows little about the students, and cares little for their strengths (presumably none) and weaknesses (a proxy measure for stupidity).
To think, at the end of the day, "What a great bunch of students, we're lucky to have them."	To think, at the end of the day, "What a great teacher am I, they are lucky to have me."

Let's just agree for the moment that intimidation is inefficient and lacks validity. Your goal is to teach the student how to safely administer an anesthetic. Intimidation teaches the student how not to be yelled at. Making cultural changes in the clinical environment to decrease these behaviors will not be easy, though enormous strides are being made, even since the previous edition of this text. Since our time in instruction is necessarily limited, and the amount to be learned so great, is it not in all of our best interests

III "The abuse of a thing does not preclude its use" (eg, people drive drunk, but we do not outlaw cars).

to be efficient in our instruction? Students may need remediation, remonstration, and, unfortunately in some cases, removal from the program. Intentional cruelty masquerading as instruction does not assist the faculty member in accomplishing this; indeed, it weakens the ability of nurse anesthesia educational programs to engage in any of these functions, and it ought not to be confused with rigorous but fair Socratic instruction.

In the first part of the chapter, the concept of establishing a tone for education was discussed and overcoming objections to the Socratic method, as discussed, rests extensively on classroom and clinical culture. Students need to understand the following:

1. They are students as well as professional registered nurses. If they already knew everything about anesthesia, there would be no need to come to class.
2. They will make mistakes during their classroom and clinical recitations that are based on the Socratic method. The mistakes they make are designed to be used to further their education and do not mark them as stupid. (The evaluation of students is discussed extensively in chapter 17 of this text. Socratic method is about instruction, not evaluation.)
3. They ought not to be embarrassed to speak in front of their peers, and denigration of the students by their peers in the classroom will not be tolerated by the Socratic method instructor.
4. Their only goal as students in the classroom is the acquisition of knowledge, skills, and judgment that will make them excellent clinicians better able to care for their patients.
5. Their only goal in clinical instruction is the use of knowledge and judgment and the honing of skills that result in excellent care of the anesthetized patient.

The program faculty members need to emphasize repeatedly and, more importantly, model and follow through on these precepts. It is critical that these preceptors continuously engage the students during instruction, didactic, or clinical.

The final perceived downside is that the Socratic method is a lot of work for the teacher. In this, there can be no argument. It is far less onerous to be the "sage on the stage," pouring data into the heads of our students. The problem is we really cannot be sure what they heard and responded to. Engagement with students using the Socratic method provides the teacher with almost instantaneous feedback regarding the level of knowledge that students have.

Summary

The Socratic method is an extraordinary way of teaching your students how to think for themselves, respond to questions regarding their practice, and explain their rationale behind the clinical decisions they make. It is equally demanding for the instructor and the student, yet filled with rewards for both. The student is engaged with the teacher, self-directed, and growing in confidence with each passing day. The instructor gets to make a palpable difference in the lives of his or her students, while continuously monitoring their progression through a demanding program of study. Very few ideas have been subjected to 2,400 years of modification, trial, feedback, and use. The Socratic method is efficient, effective, and fun for the teacher and learner, so get out there and ask some questions!

References

1. Kreeft P. *Philosophy 101 by Socrates.* San Francisco, CA: Ignatius Press; 2002.
2. Holper L, Goldin AP, Shalom DE, Battro AM, Wolf M, Sigman M. The teaching and the learning brain: A cortical hemodynamic marker of teacher-student interactions in the Socratic Dialog. *Int J Educ Res.* 2013;59:1–10.
3. Buchanan S. *The Portable Plato.* New York, NY: The Viking Press; 1948.
4. Hurst JW. The overlecturing and underteaching of clinical medicine. *Arch Intern Med.* 2004;164(15):1605–1608.
5. Carr D. Professional and personal values and virtues in education and teaching. *Oxf Rev Edu.* 2006;32(2):171–183.
6. Brezis M, Cohen R. Interactive Learning in medicine: Socrates in electronic clothes. *QJM.* 2004;97(1):47–51.
7. Elkind DH, Sweet F. The Socratic approach to character education. *Educ Leadersh.* 1997;54(8):56–59.
8. Mohr N, Moreno-Walton L, Mills A, Brunett P, Promes S. Generational influences in academic emergency medicine: Teaching and learning, mentoring, and technology. *Acad Emerg Med.* 2011;18(2):190–199.
9. Oyler DR, Romanelli F. The fact of ignorance: revisiting the Socratic method as a tool for teaching critical thinking. *Am J Pharm Educ.* 2014;78(7):1–9.
10. Paraskevas A, Wickens E. Andragogy and the Socratic method: The adult learner perspective. *JoHLSTE.* 2003;2(2):4–14.
11. Green A, Rose W. The professor's dream: getting students to talk and read intelligently. *PS Polit Sci Polit.* 1996;29(4):687–690.
12. Pedersen AM. In defense of the oft-maligned Socratic method. *Natl Law J.* 2006;9:2.
13. Tucker AA. Leadership by the Socratic method. *ASPJ.* 2007;21(2):80–88.
14. Dreyfus HL, Dreyfus SE. *Mind over Machine.* New York, NY: Free Press; 1986.
15. Drucker PF. *The Age of Discontinuity: Guidelines to Our Changing Society.* London, England: William Heinemann LTD.; 1969.
16. Satinover J. *The Quantum Brain:The search for freedom and the next generation of man.* New York, NY: John Wiley and Sons; 2001.
17. Samples K. The Socratic Method. Stand to Reason.http://www.str.org. Accessed 2015.
18. Areeda PE. The Socratic Method. *Harv Law Rev.* 1996;109:911–930.
19. *The Paper Chase.* New York, NY: Columbia Broadcasting System Television Network; 1978.
20. Gordon LA. Is the Socratic method legal? *Am Surg.* 2003;69(2):181–182.

21. Tredway L. Socratic seminars: engaging students in intellectual discourse. *Educ Leadersh.* 1995;53(1):26–29.

22. Cavalcanti RB, Detsky AS. The education and training of future physicians: why coaches can't be judges. *JAMA.* 2011;306(9):993–994.

CHAPTER 2

A Conceptual Model for Nurse Anesthesia Education

Maura McAuliffe, PhD, CRNA, FAAN

Keywords: Case-based instruction, clinical education, conceptual model advanced practice nursing, metacognition, skill acquisition.

Key Concepts

- This chapter presents a conceptual model for nurse anesthesia education. The model includes the required declarative, procedural, and conditional knowledge components of advanced knowledge acquisition.
- The model suggests that acquisition and integration of knowledge bases are best accomplished using metacognitive strategies with case-based instruction.
- Patient-centered strategic thinking evolves in the learner as a result of real-world practice applying theory and principles with a large number and wide variety of cases.
- Learning to be cognitively flexible and to adaptively reconstruct one's knowledge to new situations also requires guidance from expert mentors. Mentors can assist the student to progress through the stages of learning by aiming instruction at the student's zone of proximal development.
- Many teaching strategies such as cognitive modeling, scaffolded instruction, and reflection in action can be employed in the clinical area; however, in assisting the student to become an independent problem-solver, dialogue between the student and the teacher is essential.
- Evaluations of student progress should be actionable and performance-based. They are most useful when coupled with opportunities for follow-up.
- The conceptual model can be used by students and faculty as an organizing framework to maximize student learning during clinical experiences. It can also serve as a conceptual framework for educational research and curricular development.

Introduction

Excellence in nurse anesthesia education is indeed firmly established. Today's nurse anesthesia educational programs are often viewed by nurse educators as premier graduate-level nursing programs. Given the multitude of operating rooms and clinical sites used by nurse anesthesia programs in the United States today, practicing nurse anesthetists find that they are often involved in clinical teaching. In this chapter, an educational conceptual framework is presented in order to provide a vocabulary and principles of clinical instruction to assist nurse anesthesia educators to do what they do even better.

It is often said that theory guides practice and practice informs theory. In this chapter, principles to guide case-based nurse anesthesia education are presented within a conceptual model. The model shows how student registered nurse anesthetists, with the aid of expert mentors and using metacognitive strategies, gradually integrate the three essential knowledge bases (declarative, procedural, and conditional) as they become competent and proficient nurse anesthetists. Full integration, however, requires case-based instruction in the clinical area, which aids learners to view the conceptual terrain from multiple perspectives as they learn to think strategically and provide the best solutions to patient anesthetic challenges. The model can be used by learners, but it also shows faculty how to assist learners as they progress through the stages of learning. The model can also serve as a diagnostic tool for identifying problems when student progress is not as anticipated. The model has been tested and used as a conceptual framework in research and curriculum development.[1]

Background

The conceptual model of nurse anesthesia education is guided by constructivist ideology. Constructivism is a collection of theories and ideas about issues in pedagogy and is informed by a range of philosophical and epistemological outlooks, each adding a different dimension, but all complementing each other. Learning theories within the constructivist paradigm view all learning as inherently situated, that is embedded in social and physical environments that reflect real world complexity. Learning is also viewed as based on a learner's prior knowledge, which means that learners construct understanding by integrating newly acquired knowledge into their existing knowledge and skills. Meaning and understanding are built through processes that depend on the students' foundational knowledge, the cognitive strategies they use, and the learning activities they engage in. Experiences are first filtered through learners personal knowledge constructs before a shift in thinking assimilates the new learning into their existing conceptual frameworks and modifies these mental frameworks. Traditional teaching models have been criticized for producing learners who cannot recall, use, or transfer skills to novel situations.[2] When learning is approached from a constructivist perspective, teachers understand that all learning begins with what the student already "knows," and this inert knowledge is not always transferable because it is frequently memorized devoid of context. Teachers can assist learners in making linkages and facilitate the students' transformation of knowledge, but they cannot transmit knowledge directly. Learning requires active student engagement.[3] Teachers can facilitate student learning by (1) identifying misconceptions in their knowledge and (2) assisting them to avoid the tendency to oversimplify (reductive bias) when they encounter new problems.[2] This constructivist philosophy often undergirds the teaching modalities employed in the professions and basic sciences. Although variations in educational curricula exist among and within professions, professional education usually includes three types of experiences: (1) courses in the basic arts or basic sciences; (2) courses addressing the profession's typical problems and activities taught in a classroom setting; and (3) the professional initiation—apprenticeship or internship experience. Instruction in each area is essential for students to learn to think as professionals.[4]

Thomas Kuhn, who is known for coining the term "paradigm shift" to indicate how knowledge in science is understood, described the change in thinking that occurs when a physics student (novice) learns to think as a physicist (professional): "Looking at a bubble-chamber photograph, the student sees confused and broken lines, the physicist, a record of familiar subnuclear events. Only after a number of transformations of vision does the student become an inhabitant of the scientist's world, seeing what the scientist sees and responding as the scientist does."[5] The transformation of vision that Kuhn refers to results from theory-based instruction coupled with real life experience. Unfortunately, in many professions, there has been little systematic inquiry into adult educational means and ends.[4] One reason for the lack of empirical studies is that professional education suffers from a lack of two theories. First, there is no theory of action for the profession to guide educational research.[6] Second, there is little general educational theory of action for instruction. The conceptual model for nurse anesthesia education described in this chapter (**Figure 2.1**) can serve as an organizing framework for development, refinement, and research in nurse anesthesia educational programs. The six stages in the model, which are discussed later in the chapter, are based upon the original framework for skill acquisition developed by Dreyfus and Dreyfus.[7,8]

Figure 2.1 The Conceptual Model of Nurse Anesthesia Education

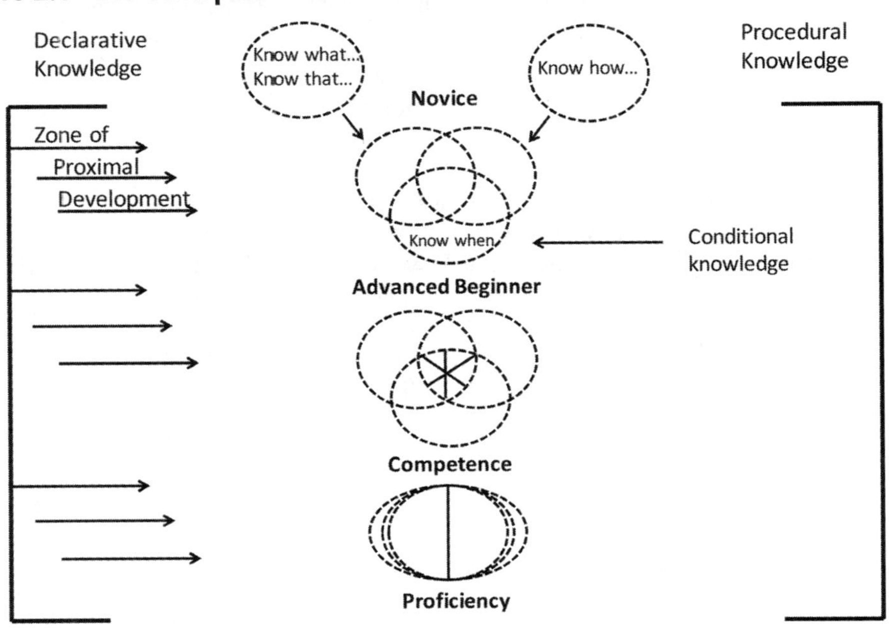

Skill Acquisition and Piloting an Aircraft

In the 1970s, when the United States Air Force required a theoretical framework to provide an educational structure for training pilots, they turned to Dreyfus and Dreyfus, who developed the theory of skill acquisition.[7,8] The skill acquisition that occurs in learning to fly aircraft is particularly relevant to nurse anesthesia because piloting an aircraft and administering an anesthetic are often seen as analogous. The takeoff of the aircraft is similar to the induction of anesthesia, and the landing to the emergence from anesthesia, while the time during anesthetic maintenance is like cruising.

Piloting an aircraft and administering an anesthetic demand continuous processing of information. The pilot's monitoring and scanning of gauges and dials is analogous to the anesthetist's vigilant monitoring of patients while scanning dials and gauges on the anesthesia equipment.[9] The Dreyfus model for skill acquisition, developed to assist in pilot training can inform the conceptual model of nurse anesthesia education.

Dreyfus and Dreyfus were pioneers in advocating the use of computer-assisted instruction in teaching advanced skill acquisition. Their model of instruction had its beginnings in interactive desktop personal computer programs. In the aviation industry, it evolved into the development and use of flight simulators to train pilots. Today, both desktop computer programs and high-fidelity simulators are used in many anesthesia training programs, and simulated instruction in anesthesia and anesthesia crisis management have become widespread. Simulated training can provide an interactive learning environment where students can apply theoretical principles, coupled with practical skills and critical thinking, in a risk-free environment.

The Dreyfus model of skill acquisition has six stages: novice, advanced beginner, competent, proficient, expert, and master (**Table 2.1**). The Dreyfus model suggests that skill acquisition occurs systematically as students progress through each stage of learning.[10] The *novice* follows rules and is unable to appreciate the unique situational aspects of an experience. The *advanced beginner* has gained some experience, and based on this, begins to recognize situational elements. The *competent* performer uses plans and begins to incorporate his or her point of view into the plans. The *proficient* performer has gained more experience and has a deeper, more involved understanding. The *expert* performer has mastered analytical decision making and has developed intuitive knowledge. In each stage, learners' sophistication in thinking and monitoring of their thinking increases.

Table 2.1 Components of Skill Acquisition

Skill Level	Components	Perspective	Decision	Commitment
Novice	Context-free	None	Analytical	Detached
Advanced Beginner	Context-free & situational	None	Analytical	Detached
Competent	Context-free & situational	Chosen	Analytical	Detached understanding & deciding involved in outcome
Proficient	Context-free & situational	Experienced	Analytical	Involved understanding, detached deciding
Expert	Context-free & situational	Experienced	Intuitive	Involved

Metacognition

An essential element in skill acquisition is monitoring one's thinking. John H. Flavel coined the term *metacognition* to define this concept.[11] Metacognition, or monitoring one's thinking, is essential to learning in all education. It enables learners to draw on various thinking strategies and then to accurately assess their understanding of a situation in light of those strategies. Using metacognitive strategies, learners become aware that they are developing new skills as problem solvers. The development of these new thinking skills requires real-world and/or realistic-world (simulated) experiences.

The conceptual model of nurse anesthesia education is grounded in the work of Dreyfus and Dreyfus, and informed by the work of other constructivists and learning theorists. Effective learning requires the cognitive and control strategies of skill, will, and control (**Figure 2.2**). Skill includes declarative knowledge (knowing what to do) and procedural knowledge (knowing how to do it); however, while both knowledge bases are important, they are not sufficient for effective learning. Even conditional or strategic knowledge (knowing when to do it) is not sufficient. Learners must also have the *will* to learn, that is, they must possess the desire and motivation to learn.[12]

Figure 2.2 Components of Succesful Learning

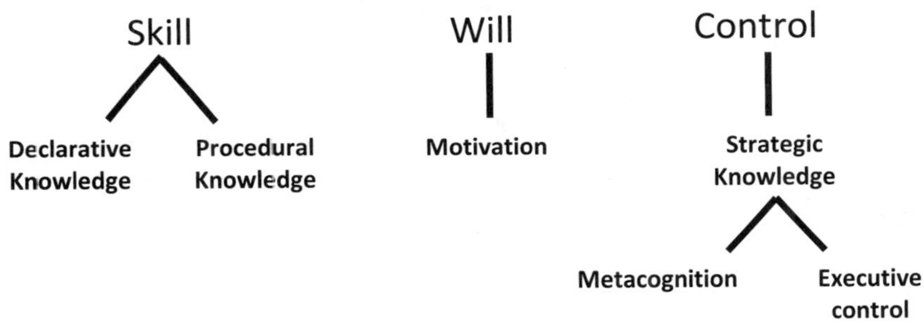

The components of skill, will, and control are interdependent variables, and the extent to which each contributes to successful learning may vary from student to student. Prior success with effective learning strategies assists learners with subsequent learning; however, student motivation is also essential. With motivation, the student who possesses less sophisticated learning strategies may overcome this obstacle and become a successful learner; conversely, a highly skilled learner who lacks the motivation to learn may be unsuccessful despite that advantage.

Declarative, Procedural, and Conditional Knowledge

In the conceptual model for nurse anesthesia education, the overlapping circles represent the interdependence of declarative, procedural, and conditional knowledge essential to learning.[13] Declarative knowledge (domain knowledge) is also referred to as systems knowledge.[14] It includes information about task structure and goals, as well as beliefs about one's ability in relation to the ability to achieve those goals." In nurse anesthesia, declarative knowledge includes knowledge of basic sciences such as pharmacology and physiology and knowledge of applied sciences such as the principles of nurse anesthesia practice. Much, but not all of declarative knowledge, is taught in the classroom, and it is frequently referred to as didactic education.

Procedural knowledge includes information about the execution of various actions. It is a repertoire of behaviors available to learners who select particular behaviors to attain particular goals. It includes knowledge of how to perform a procedure—for example, intubating the trachea or administering a spinal anesthetic—as well as algorithmic-type knowledge such as knowledge of the American Society of Anesthesiologists' difficult airway algorithm. Procedural knowledge is acquired through direct instruction in conjunction with repeated experience.[13]

Declarative and procedural knowledge differ from conditional knowledge; one must select or execute an action. Conditional knowledge describes the circumstances of the application of procedures. It refers to knowing when and *why* to take various actions, and how to adjust behavior to changing task demands.[13] Conditional knowledge provides the rationale for various actions and for choosing, planning, and evaluating a selected course of action. Conditional knowledge (also referred to as strategic knowledge) includes metacognitive knowledge.[14]

Metacognitive Aspects of Learning

Being aware of being conscious is the defining feature of metacognitive knowledge. The term means "cognition about cognition." Monitoring one's thinking is essential for successful learning—especially in areas that require complex problem solving.[11] One is apt to engage in a lot of cognition when there is an explicit demand for it. For example, nurse anesthesia requires one to think up and evaluate alternative courses of action and solve complex problems. In general, "there is apt to be more ideation, and more monitoring of that ideation (metacognition), when one is faced with risky decisions, especially if one believes that risk might be reduced by engaging in careful and sustained thought."[11]

Metacognitive knowledge evolves in learners as a result of planned, real-world practice with strategic thinking and technical skills. When the frequency and quality of experiences are enhanced, student insights into learning and metacognitive understanding evolve. Teachers frequently focus on domain knowledge (facts, procedures, and concepts) and heuristic strategies (tricks of the trade); however, if learners are to become proficient practitioners in complex domains such as anesthesia, teachers must also focus on metacognitive processes. This involves student instruction about how to generate alternative courses of action, evaluation of those who will make more progress toward a solution, and the use of strategies for acquiring new information when the knowledge available is not adequate for the problem at hand.

Complex forms of metacognition place heavy demands on attention and occupy considerable space in working memory.[15] Consequently, student registered nurse anesthetists are more likely to have these types of experiences when attention and memory permit, that is, when they have sufficient time to think about their thinking and are not in a highly emotional state. A student who is involved in a complex case with a critically ill patient may be in a highly emotional state. It is common in this type of situation for the student to be unable to answer simple questions posed by the instructor or to remember the instructor's explanations for decision-making. In such instances, the instructor might best assist the student by asking a specific question after the situation has ended. The teacher could also use a post-case conference or student journaling to help the student to reflect and learn from the clinical experience.

Many learning theorists suggest that learners have a central processor, or executive controller, that allows them to perform intelligent evaluations of their own thinking.[16] Student registered nurse anesthetists should be instructed not only in the use of cognitive strategies, but also be instructed in how to use executive control. For example, the students could be instructed on how to employ, monitor, check, and evaluate their thinking strategies.[16,17] A common example of teaching a cognitive strategy is instructing students in the use of differential diagnosis. Students are typically taught, for example, how to think about and respond to intraoperative hypotension by using differential diagnoses for hypotension (the etiology may be hypovolemia or vagal stimulation) as well as the use of executive control (providing the patient with a fluid bolus and then reevaluating the situation). Over time, the inculcation of these thinking processes will improve students' abilities to marshal the required knowledge and construct solutions tailored to the needs of problem-solving situations in the future.

How can anesthesia instructors best assist students to develop and use self-regulatory executive control in their thinking? It has been shown in real-life situations that interactive learning experiences result in the passing of executive control from teacher to student or master craftsman to apprentice.[18] In this process, teachers are viewed as the supportive other, acting first as models and later, as interrogators. This leads students toward strategic thinking. Eventually, during the interactive process, self-regulatory control becomes internalized by the student and the teacher relinquishes control.

Ill-Structured Domains and Learning

Anesthesia knowledge is considered an ill-structured domain. Domains of knowledge are considered to be ill-structured when required thinking and problem-solving do not have predetermined algorithms. In ill-structured domains, expert mentorship and experience with a wide variety of cases are required for students to develop cognitively flexible processing skills. A learning environment that permits knowledge to be learned in various ways and for various purposes is also required.[19–24]

Although students progress incrementally through the six stages of learning in the conceptual model for nurse anesthesia education, the teaching and learning that occur in each stage are not always linear and orderly. This is true of the learning that occurs in all ill-structured domains. In these domains, practitioners must construct the actions that are most appropriate and efficient for the task at hand.[19–24] Learning in these disciplines is best accomplished through case-based instruction with the goal of fostering cognitive flexibility.

Cognitive Flexibility

In ill-structured domains such as anesthesia, the goals of learning shift from the attainment of superficial understanding of facts to mastery of important aspects of conceptual complexity, and from knowledge reproduction to knowledge use, which is the ability to apply what was taught in new and varying contexts.[19–24] The ill-structuredness (combination of breadth, complexity, and irregularity of content) and goals of advanced knowledge acquisition can, in combination, be challenging for teachers and students if they use simple strategies to present and learn complex subject matter.[2] Spiro and his colleagues found that medical students had difficulty transferring knowledge learned in one context, such as medical school coursework, to new situations such as clinical problem solving. Thus, they developed Cognitive Flexibility Theory as a means to understand and teach the complexity and multidimensionality of the content required in ill-structured domains.[19–24] Cognitive flexibility theory provided conceptual perspectives for instructional strategies in teacher education, medicine,[25–27] advanced practice nursing,[1] law,[25] social work,[28] physical therapy,[29] computer science,[2] interdisciplinary science,[30] and public administration.[31]

In most undergraduate learning (introductory learning), the goal is exposure to subject content or general orientation to a field of study, and learning assessment usually involves simple recognition or recall; however, in advanced knowledge acquisition, the student must attain a deeper understanding of content, reason with it, and apply it flexibly in diverse situations.[19–24]

The best way to learn and instruct others to achieve cognitive flexibility for future application is nonlinear and using case-based instruction.[19–24] Although student registered nurse anesthetists can initially learn basic concepts in a linear context, eventually the emphasis must be shifted from retrieval of intact knowledge structures. An example would be the recitation of a mnemonic for construction of new understandings. The goal is case-specific knowledge assembly drawn from multiple sources to address the problem-solving needs of the current situation. Adapting one's knowledge to tasks involving new situations requires metacognitive executive control strategies (predicting, planning, checking, evaluating, and revising) and flexible knowledge structures.[19–24] A major goal of instruction in nurse anesthesia is to assist students in the development of cognitive flexibility.

To foster development of cognitive flexibility, cases must be studied as they occur in their natural, complex situations. By focusing a student's learning at the level of individual cases and providing experience with a large number of cases, student performance will be enhanced.[19–24]

Seven themes constitute the facets of cognitive flexibility. In the conceptual model of nurse anesthesia education (Figure 2.1), these themes are represented by the crisscrossed lines in the middle of the overlapping circles (knowledge domains).

Theme 1: Avoidance of Oversimplification and Overregularization

In advanced knowledge acquisition, educators must emphasize that knowledge is not as simple and orderly as it might at first seem. In other words, instruction must include measures to demonstrate complexity and to show how the superficially similar can be dissimilar. The problem is that oversimplification can lead to reductive bias. For example, when conceptual elements that are highly interrelated are treated in isolation, the learner may miss important aspects of their interaction.[19–24]

Teachers are often inclined to oversimplify in an attempt to increase the novice's initial understanding of a concept. The problem with this is that it can instill habits of mind that are later hard to break. It is actually better to introduce complexity early, though in a manageable manner. In a discussion about the lower acceptable limits of mean arterial blood pressure for deliberate hypotension, one instructor may simply teach that the safe lower limit is 55 to 60 mm Hg (the lower limit of cerebral autoregulation). Another might initiate a discussion with the student about variables that influence decision-making such as patient positioning, blood pressure measurement site relative to the brain, and the patient's underlying diseases, such as sickle cell anemia. Still another, introducing more complexity, might initiate dialogue based upon physiological models correlating blood pressure with organ blood flow (BP = SVR × CO). With the use of these models, students may better appreciate that while blood "pressure" may increase following administration of vasopressors, the increased vascular resistance may not necessarily result in increased blood flow to target organs.

Another example of avoiding oversimplification can be found in the clinical assignment of anesthesia cases. It is common to see beginning students assigned to the less complex or "bread and butter" cases; however, by occasionally assigning them more complicated cases, the instructor will expose them to complexity early, and they will understand that cases may not be as simple as they initially appear. In these instances, instructors are responsible for case management while keeping students engaged by giving them tasks they are able to accomplish.

This will not be a wasted experience for the student. Although the student may not understand all the components, the learning that occurs will be within the context of the complexity of the case.

Avoiding initial oversimplification allows students to gain an appreciation of complexities in cases and increases the likelihood that they will take into account more factors when confronted with similar situations in the future.

Theme 2: Multiple Representation

In ill-structured domains such as nurse anesthesia, if cases are treated narrowly in the educational process, the ability to process future cases will be limited. Students will assume that cases are simpler than they are, and their analysis of new cases will conclude prematurely.[19–24] Also, the learner's reasoning based on precedent cases will result in truncated decision-making after only partial analysis of the problem.

Narrowly treating cases (prematurely ending an assessment or overlooking relevant information) is more likely to occur when learners have inadequate exposure to multiple cases that upon initial assessment appear similar, but with deeper investigation, are found to be dissimilar. This can contribute to a cognitive error frequently seen in beginners called premature closure, that is, accepting the first plausible diagnosis before it is verified. The more similar situations appear to precedent cases; the sooner a beginner will assume a case is similar even though it may be very different. Students need to be taught to guard against this tendency by consciously searching for information that goes against their personal assumptions. For example, an etiology of tachycardia can be an inadequate level of anesthesia, and beginning students often observe this during the induction of anesthesia. A student who does not have experience with many cases might reflexively (truncated decision-making) increase the concentration of volatile agent when a patient's heart rate suddenly increases. In this case, the student is not considering the many other things that could be the cause of the tachycardia. In another example, a student may make an assumption that bronchospasm is anaphylaxis, because the student recently witnessed such a case. Some refer to this cognitive error as availability bias.[32,33]

A related error that is common with beginning students when encountering a problem is failure to consider reasonable alternatives. For example, based upon limited exposure to cases, a student may assume that hypotension in the trauma patient is due to bleeding and miss the fact that it may be due to a pneumothorax causing an obstruction to cardiac output. Practitioners who have experience with a wider variety of cases would have considered other possibilities. Another example can be seen in the novices who repeatedly cycle and change the location of an arterial pressure cuff because they do not believe a low reading. In this instance, they are seeking confirmatory evidence to support a diagnosis that discounts disconfirming evidence (confirmation bias).[32,33] Also, feedback errors occur when students misinterpret "no feedback" as positive feedback. An example might be students who believe they have never had a patient suffer from perioperative kidney injury simply because they have not been made aware of or received a complaint about it. While these cognitive errors frequently occur with students, there is research demonstrating that they can occur in seasoned providers as well. Anchoring is the most common cognitive error, followed by availability bias, premature closure and feedback bias.[32,33] While these errors do not necessarily reflect deficits in didactic knowledge, they do indicate deficits in strategic utilization of the knowledge. This can be addressed by ensuring that learners have experiences with many cases during which appropriate control (metacognitive strategies) are taught and utilized.

Theme 3: Centrality of Cases

The more ill-structured the domain, the poorer the guidance for knowledge application from top-down structures. Application of knowledge in ill-structured domains cannot be prescribed in advance by general principles, because cases vary greatly with respect to which conceptual elements are relevant and in what combinations. Overreliance on precompiled knowledge structures, such as fixed protocols, is a teaching and learning error.[17–23] Certain combinations of drugs work well for typical cases, and beginning students feel more comfortable when given "recipes" for case management; however, experienced nurse anesthetists know that they must always make adjustments to their anesthetic plan and titrate to effect. Students' future decision-making and practice skills benefit more when instructors teach them to titrate drugs and tailor anesthetics based on patients' needs instead of giving them prescribed recipes for anesthetic management.

Overreliance on protocols can actually lead to serious cognitive and clinical errors. For example, a protocol may specify that the fraction of inspired oxygen (FiO_2) be decreased when the surgeon is using cautery in/near the airway, but unless the practitioner continuously assesses the risk of endotracheal tube fire throughout non-airway cases, patients may be placed in danger. Another example might be the tendency of the new student to follow a protocol of using end-tidal concentration of carbon dioxide ($ETCO_2$) as confirmation of successful tracheal placement of the endotracheal tube (ETT); however, when confronted with a case of bronchospasm (correctly placed ETT but no $ETCO_2$ waveform), the student may incorrectly diagnose an esophageal intubation. In this case, the information received (no $ETCO_2$ waveform) fits the protocol, but the protocol does not fit the larger clinical picture.

Theme 4: Conceptual Knowledge Is Knowledge in Use

In ill-structured domains, the meanings of concepts are connected to their patterns of use. When a concept has a complex and irregular distribution, prepackaged prescriptions for proper activation of the concept cannot be provided.[19–24] A concept has many different uses in cases, and each concept must be tailored to the context of its application. A student may know a fact, but may not be able to apply it to a particular case. For example, a student may understand the concept of the carbon dioxide response curve and accurately draw the curve indicating the effect that volatile agents and opioids have on it; however, at the end of a case, when the student gives a patient a small amount of opioid for postoperative pain control and the patient's respiratory rate declines, the student may not be able to understand the application of that concept without assistance. This is where preceptors can help students make links between the facts and procedures learned in didactic courses and their clinical applications. For example, when discussing a patient's oxygen saturation a clinical preceptor can help students apply basic science principles by discussing the oxygen-hemoglobin dissociation curve and its correlation with SPO_2. Some preceptors might take the lesson further by reviewing concepts of ventilation/perfusion inequalities or diffusion impairment, and use the patient's data to calculate the alveolar gas equation, A-a gradient, arterial O_2 content, O_2 consumption, or the Bohr equation for dead space fraction. Within these discussions, preceptors, using good questioning techniques, can help students recall their prior knowledge and then activate it in the clinical setting. Through this spiral curricular approach, the basic science foundations of practice can be reinforced and misunderstandings brought to light where they can be addressed and corrected.

Theme 5: Schema Assembly (From Rigidity to Flexibility)

In ill-structured domains, the goal is to teach students to assemble knowledge from different theoretical and precedent case sources and adaptively fit it to the situation at hand. Knowledge in nurse anesthesia is used in far too many ways to be all anticipated in advance. There must be a shift in learning from retrieval of intact knowledge structures to situation-specific problem-solving.[19–24] We sometimes hear students say "We weren't taught that," meaning "We weren't taught exactly that." One learning goal is to foster students' abilities to think for themselves and use their knowledge in new ways. It is important for them, as well as their instructors, to understand and work toward this goal. Schema assembly should be addressed early in didactic courses, and students should be given opportunities to demonstrate comprehension with test questions written at analysis/synthesis levels. Questions that require students to combine two or more pieces of information, much as they will have to do in the clinical setting, will help them understand that the goal is not simple recall but assembly of knowledge in order to arrive at solutions. Central to this process is the notion that students must take responsibility for their learning: They must abandon passivity and the idea that they should be handed or "spoon-fed" answers to all classroom and clinical problems they will encounter. Instead, they must learn to adopt an active approach to learning that draws upon several points in the lecture and outside readings in order to arrive at the best answer to test questions.

Knowledge assembly is an essential component of clinical practice, so students need to appreciate that they will be required to combine knowledge in unique ways to solve clinical problems. To prepare them for this, faculty should require that they construct unique, patient-centered anesthetic plans using information from multiple sources. This will reinforce the notion that practitioners must anticipate each patient's anesthetic challenges and construct individualized anesthetic plans that best meet those needs.

Theme 6: Noncompartmentalization of Concepts (Multiple Interconnectedness)

Because of the irregular way in which various features weave through cases in ill-structured domains, knowledge cannot be neatly compartmentalized. A student strategy frequently encountered in didactic education is relegation of knowledge into separate compartments. For example, students learn anatomy in one course and pharmacology in another, often making lists or using mnemonics as study aids to pass examinations. The problem is that students often miss the interconnectedness of concepts and their applications along multiple conceptual and clinical dimensions.[19–24] This retards the development of advanced knowledge acquisition because students begin to rely on single explanations rather than search for more complete and interconnected ones.

One way clinical instructors can assist students with interconnectedness is by initiating case-based discussions that include several principles that, when combined, produce a complex clinical picture. Instructors can then demonstrate how simple linear thinking in these cases may be insufficient or misleading. This type of instruction can highlight important instructional relationships between aspects of one case with aspects of another case. Understanding what to do in a given case usually requires reference to more than one prototype—the case will be "kind of like this earlier one, kind of like that one." Reviewing students reflective journals and concept mappings, and also engaging in post-case conferences are additional strategies instructors can use to assist students to appreciate gaps in their knowledge and relational aspects between cases.[34] Identifying common denominators among a series of cases is a common teaching strategy. But it is also important to highlight aspects of cases that are different. For example, patients' differing underlying disease processes, pain tolerance, or body habitus, and the ways these differing aspects may influence case management should be highlighted. Students frequently suggest anesthetic plans in which they have observed being successful in similar cases. This provides an opportunity to ask students to step back and identify those aspects of the case at hand that are different from the last, and how those might influence their plans.

It is not uncommon for beginning students to focus on one often minor aspect of a clinical problem at the expense of understanding the whole situation. For example, beginning students might be so focused on inserting a second intravenous catheter or arterial line during a large case that they are unaware of the patient's sudden blood loss and hypotension. This type of compartmentalization, known as anchoring or fixation error, is a common cognitive error of beginners and must be brought to their attention if they are to begin to appreciate the problem and engage in metacognitive strategies (thinking about their thinking) to overcome the tendency.

Theme 7: Active Participation

Knowledge cannot simply be handed to student registered nurse anesthetists. There must be active learner involvement in knowledge acquisition, accompanied by guidance and commentary from expert mentors to help students derive maximum benefit from their experiences. When instructors aim for cognitive flexibility, they can build integrated knowledge structures that permit greater flexibility in the ways knowledge can be assembled and used or transferred to different situations. In contrast, overreliance on automation processes can lead to performance errors. One such error is the continuation of a course of action or strategy when it would be rational to change to an alternative course because conditions have changed (cognitive blockade). Another error might be seen in a person who, lacking cognitive flexibility, adheres to a decision when it has been demonstrated to be a mistake or who persists in a false diagnosis when new information suggests otherwise. A lack of cognitive flexibility can lead a student to consider only part of a problem because he or she is putting information into precompiled knowledge structures that do not fit the situation at hand. To help avoid these types of errors, it is important to teach students to be cognitively flexible so they can adapt their behaviors appropriately to changing situations. Clinical preceptors can assist students by encouraging them to use cognitive self-monitoring strategies (questioning their hypothesis, searching for information that does *not* fit their diagnosis, specifically addressing their personal cognitive biases) as a part of their clinical decision-making process. Preceptors should routinely ask students about specific strategies they are selecting to combat potential cognitive errors in the clinical setting. Universities typically have processes in place to assist students in recognizing cognitive errors that interfere with successful didactic learning and test taking; in a similar manner, instructors should provide remediation of cognitive errors observed in the clinical setting.

Cognitive Apprenticeship: Thinking Out Loud and Gradually Ceding Control

Learning in the clinical area is characterized as situated learning, because students learn in an environment that reflects the multiple ways in which their knowledge structures will be put to use in professional practice. It is important to keep in the forefront the main goal of clinical instruction: to provide opportunities for students to develop flexible, declarative, procedural, and conditional knowledge structures with cases containing complexity, so they can master conceptual complexity and apply what is taught in new and varying contexts. With this in mind, clinical preceptors must select appropriate instructional techniques for the situation at hand, so students gain the most from their experiences.

A framework for clinical preceptors should incorporate several instructional techniques. One such framework is the cognitive apprenticeship model, which comprises six teaching tools: modeling, coaching, scaffolding, articulation, reflection, and exploration. This provides an organizing framework and practical application tools that can be used for teaching, evaluation, feedback, and self-assessment in the clinical area.[35, 36]

Learning to think as a professional takes time because the learner's process of internalization occurs gradually. Initially, teachers control and guide students' activities. Later, they share control over problem-solving functions with the students taking initiatives and teachers correcting and guiding them when they make mistakes. Finally, the teacher cedes control to the student and functions primarily as a supportive and sympathetic audience. This implies phases of transition from external guidance (from the preceptor) through shared guidance (by the student together with the preceptor) to internal guidance (by the student alone).[37] This type of instruction is not unique to nurse anesthesia. Teachers, tutors, and master craftsmen in traditional apprenticeship situations all function as promoters of self-regulation (executive control) by nurturing the emergence of self-control while gradually ceding external control. Within these transitional phases, the major components of declarative and procedural knowledge (content), as well as the affective and metacognitive aspects (thinking about one's thinking), must be addressed. For example, an instructor confronted with a problem during an anesthetic could model the thought processes used in decision-making by thinking out loud. After allowing the student to observe several examples of this strategic thinking, the instructor could give the student an opportunity to demonstrate problem-solving strategies while he or she uses coaching and scaffolding techniques. After several successful demonstrations, the instructor could begin to cede control of the problem-solving to the student. For example, an instructor could think out loud (modeling) while managing the patient undergoing an abdominal aortic aneurysm repair, during which fluid management can be extremely challenging. The decisions about fluid management, blood volume, and vasoactive therapy are complex and there are no reliable formulas to guide therapy. The aorta is typically cross-clamped for surgical repair. To prevent early cardiovascular strain and subsequent hypotension upon aortic cross-clamp removal, the vascular space is dilated and filled with intravenous fluid so that maximum cardiac output can be achieved. The vasodilator is stopped before unclamping while rapid volume administration is often initiated. These decisions for perioperative management are made to balance the need for blood pressure control with the risk of fluid overload. Modeling one's professional reasoning in the midst of clinical decision-making allows learners to see how skilled practitioners think through cases and wrestle with uncertainty. By being reflective and articulating their thinking process, skilled anesthetists can help novices learn to appreciate their approach to problems.[38]

Scaffolded Instruction

Scaffolded instruction describes the assistance teachers can offer learners so they can accomplish tasks they would not be able to perform on their own. The instructor provides initial support, or scaffolding, until the student is ready to be more independent, and then the instructor removes the scaffold when the student is ready. In successful scaffolding, the instructor initially ascertains the student's prior knowledge so that it can be connected to the new knowledge and made relevant to the learner. There are many ways that an instructor can use scaffolding in student learning. Instructors break tasks into smaller, more manageable parts; verbalize their thinking process when completing tasks; and use questioning, coaching, and modeling to reinforce the learning of concepts. Other methods include the activation of background knowledge by providing tips, strategies, and cues.

Nurse anesthesia preceptors frequently use a "think-out-loud" strategy when they require students to give the rationale for their answers to specific questions and to produce the evidence/clinical data they used to arrive at their conclusions. By providing support and encouragement as the student thinks out loud, preceptors foster the development of clinical reasoning skills. It is a useful technique with all levels of learners, but especially beginning students, because it requires them to verbalize their thoughts in an effort to support their decisions.[39] Another strategy is for the preceptor to provide verbal cues as the student moves through a technical procedure, initially using more explicit directives, followed by less explicit ones the next time the student needs assistance. The intent is to assist students as they develop skills and master steps that may not yet be automatic in nature.

Regardless of the specific technique used, scaffolding should be removed gradually and then completely when the student demonstrates mastery of the task. Preceptors should attempt to aim their instruction at the appropriate level for the student. Skills or tasks too far out of reach or too simple can lead to student frustration.

The Zone of Proximal Development

Dialogue between teacher and student is central to using scaffolded instruction to assist students to become independent problem-solvers. The purpose of dialogue is to provide students with just enough support and guidance to achieve goals that are beyond their unassisted efforts. In accomplishing this, teachers must appreciate the zone of proximal development. This zone is depicted by the arrows to the side in the conceptual model for nurse anesthesia education (Figure 2.1). Vygotsky, who developed the concept, defines this as the distance between the learners' actual developmental level (determined by independent problem-solving) and the level of their potential development (as determined through problem-solving with the guidance of mentors).[40–41] Once the student has increased knowledge, the level of development expands and the zone of proximal development shifts. Thus, the zone is always changing as the student gains knowledge, and instructors using scaffolded instruction must constantly individualize their interactions with students in response to the changing zone of proximal development.

It is important that the instructor appropriately assess the zone of proximal development. Misjudging the zone can lead to under instruction and boredom or instruction beyond the student's abilities and frustration. Scaffolded instruction includes the following components:

- Recruitment: The instructor must recruit the student's interest.
- Reduction in degrees of freedom: The instructor must reduce the size of the task to a level where the student can fit the task requirements.
- Direction maintenance: The instructor must keep the student in pursuit of the task.
- Marking critical features: The instructor must accentuate the features of the task.
- Frustration control: The instructor must help reduce stress to make the situation less stressful than if the tutor had not been present.
- Demonstration: The instructor must demonstrate idealization of the task by completing the task or explicating a solution that is beyond the learner's current ability.

Planning and the use of instructional strategies such as scaffolded instruction when engaging in clinical teaching will result in more productive student learning experience and a smoother progression through the stages of learning.

Since all learning begins with the experience of the learner (what the student already knows), it is important to ascertain the student's current knowledge level. In anesthesia, students are experienced critical care nurses who have a wealth of knowledge and experience; however, the first step may be clarifying learned misconceptions.

In all cases, students will gain maximally from scaffolded instruction when they have experiences that are accompanied by reflective activities guided by instructors (**Figure 2.3**, next page).[42] Nurse anesthesia instructors can best assist students' learning by providing them with experiences (real-world and simulated cases) that require deliberation and action. One method of assisting them in analyzing situations is the use of reflection.[43,44] Schön describes this process as reflection in action.[43,44]

Figure 2.3 Experience as the Driving Force for Reflection and Learning

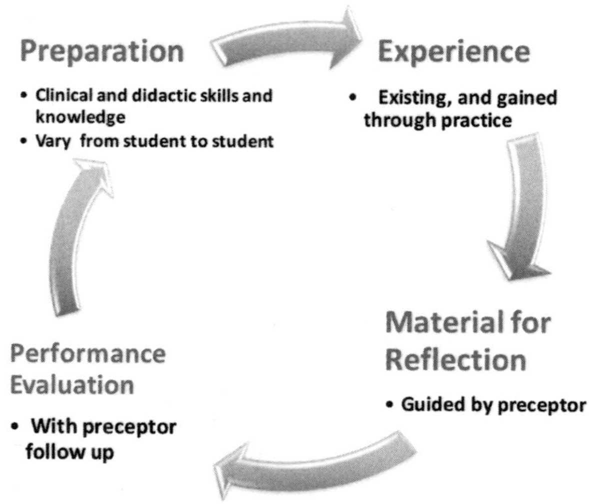

Reflection in Action

Practitioners first make sense of new situations by imposing a structure, which often comes through analogy to other previously encountered situations. Through these experiences, they build a repertoire of examples, images, understandings, and actions. When they encounter a new situation similar to something already present in their repertoire, they bring past experience to bear on the case, which enables them to see an unfamiliar situation as a familiar one. Schön also describes a method of assisting students by reflecting their thinking back to them so that they better understand their own deliberations.[32,33] The notion of zones of development is recast by Schön as zones of mastery.[43,44] By having learners engage in reflecting, instructors teach them how to be metacognitively aware of their own thinking processes.

Dialogue: The Art of Questioning

Direct questioning by preceptors helps foster students' clinical thinking.[45,46] Questions such as "What do you think?" help determine the depth of students' declarative, procedural, and conditional knowledge. Asking "How do you know?" "How sure are you?" or "Is this an area where you need more information?" helps monitor the *quality* of their ideas and encourages metacognitive development. The challenge is to stimulate student thinking by asking students to commit to hypotheses and share their rationale without offering clues to one's personal opinion; however, questioning will not be effective in achieving this goal when it is perceived as "grilling."[39]

One approach to effective questioning is the "Five-Step Microskill Model," also known as the "One Minute Preceptor Technique" described by Neher, Gordon, Meyer, and Stevens.[47] (This strategy requires the preceptor to first get a commitment from the student about what the student thinks is going on in a particular case. The preceptor then challenges the student to provide supporting evidence for the assessment. This enables the student to draw from declarative and procedural knowledge bases as well as from previous clinical experiences (conditional knowledge). The preceptor then gives immediate feedback about what was correct: This helps the student recognize that he or she has constructed an appropriate solution to the clinical problem and has appropriately demonstrated the use of metacognitive strategies (**Table 2.2**).

Table 2.2 The One-Minute Preceptor Technique

Learning Goal	Potential Questions	Rationale
1. Get a Commitment Students must make a commitment about a clinical decision	"What do you think"	• This gives the preceptor a starting point for the subsequent conversation
2. Probe for Supporting Evidence	• What led you to that conclusion?" • "Did you consider any alternative diagnoses/actions?" • "What other things were in your differential diagnosis?" "Why did you rule them out ?" • "Did you look for evidence that did not support your diagnosis?"	• This assists the preceptor in determining students' knowledge base • Assesses knowledge depth (declarative, procedural, conditional) and integration; identifies misunderstandings • Identifies good and poor assessment /reasoning skills
3. Review with students what was correct in their conclusion, and as importantly, in their thinking (cognition and metacognition)	• "You were correct to get a blood gas to inform your thinking" • "Your assessment included the important points" • "It was wise to recheck those calculations before you treated the hypovolemia"	• It is important to reinforce what was done well
4. Correct Mistakes	• "You did not adequately perform the preop or introp assessment" • "You seem to have missed important lab values" • "Your interpretation of the patient's hemodynamic data is incorrect"	• It is important to correct misunderstandings in knowledge (declarative, procedural, conditional) and ineffective cognitive or metacognitive strategies
5. Teach General Principles	• "Don't jump to a conclusion because you had a similar case" • "The lack of ETCO2 does not always indicate esophageal intubation; it may be due to bronchospasm" • "The decrease in SPO2 does not always indicate hypoxia; it may be a reflection of poor perfusion (BP cuff inflation, cold extremity) or poor waveform (probe malposition, cautery, dyes, etc) • "Not every instance of hypotension should be treated with phenylephrine"	• Point out key ideas and cognitive strategies • "Try this approach to interpreting ABGs" • "Using Stroke Volume Variation is another approach to managing hypotension"

Adapted with permission from Nehr, Gordon, Meyer & Stevens, 1991.

Evaluation

The assessment-evaluation process is an essential component of clinical education.[48] The intent is to provide students information about their performance for the purpose of improving their performance. Feedback gives students a clearer idea of areas where they need to improve and sets the stage for remediation of problems. Useful feedback is specific, measurable, based upon what is observed (behaviors, actions, decisions), relevant, timely, and achievable. Providing hollow praise such as "You did great" or "Great day today" and simply chronicling the day's activities are not effective techniques. It is important to identify learning needs by correctly diagnosing the processes that drive the students' clinical actions. In order to assess their ability to integrate multidimensional aspects of practice, evaluation must include assessment of students' cognitive understanding as well as the metacognitive processes used.[29] Misdiagnosis of either one wastes time and may diminish students' faith in the value of the instruction and evaluation.[48]

Brown, Hodges, and Wakefield[49] developed a six-stage model for quality assessment-evaluation that provides a framework for targeted and actionable performance feedback. The steps are

1. Observe students' behaviors/work. It is important to document direct observations.
2. Ask students for their self-assessments. Inquire about how they integrated didactic content and what cognitive/metacognitive strategies they employed in their decision-making.
3. Compare students' behavior with the desired behavior. Are they meeting the stated educational objectives of the course (criterion referenced assessment)? These criteria become more sophisticated as students progress through the program, advancing from novice to competent and, finally, to proficient practice.
4. Ensure that students understand the gap between their current and desired behaviors.
5. Develop a plan with students to close the gap.
6. Then, follow up to evaluate any improvement.

Evaluation of students' clinical performances should occur in a private setting using a respectful, nonjudgmental, and nonthreatening approach. Preceptors should focus on students' behaviors, not the person, and tailor the amount of feedback to what students can constructively use without overloading them. Techniques to help reduce anxiety and make students more receptive to feedback should be employed. Some preceptors prefer the "sandwiching" technique of providing negative feedback between positive comments. This can help reduce anxiety, but when overused, students may begin to discount the positive feedback as simply a lead-in to the critical message. Follow-up between the preceptor and student is an essential aspect of the evaluation process. It is important that students have an opportunity to demonstrate to their preceptors that they have made progress in closing the identified gaps between their current and desired behaviors.

Summary

Nurse anesthesia is a complex domain that requires mastery of a broad range of components that together reflect the real-world complexity of the field. Prepackaged prescriptions for action do not exist in nurse anesthesia because all possible scenarios are impossible to anticipate. The goal of education is for students to acquire a mastery of experiences with a broad range of cases that reflect the complexity of anesthesia practice. To accomplish this, learners must assimilate knowledge from a variety of sources to construct solutions that suit the needs of the situation at hand. To achieve a level of successful performance as entry-level providers, student registered nurse anesthetists need experience in applying theory and principles to a large number and variety of cases.

Understanding the stages through which skillful performance develops is important in designing educational programs and materials. This information will help instructors facilitate the students' acquisition of advanced knowledge and development of cognitive flexibility.[50] To assist the learners as they progress through the stages of learning in case-based instruction, it is essential to identify at each stage which capacities the learners have acquired and which ones they may be in a position to attain. The role of the teacher is that of an expert mentor who guides students' learning through reflective deliberations and facilitates their acquisition of higher-order skills. Through this process of using appropriate applications of anesthesia and educational theory, expert mentors can assist learners to develop the sophisticated, integrated knowledge structures required for adaptation of behavior to rapidly changing situations.

On completion of an educational program, graduate nurse anesthetists will have successfully progressed through the first four stages of learning. On completion of the proficiency stage, graduates can safely and independently administer anesthesia as entry-level nurse anesthetists after passing the national certification examination. Some graduates will be content to practice proficiently and will not attempt to progress further. A few will even regress to the stage of competence, still able to safely administer an anesthetic, but requiring much direction. Those content to practice at the competent stage will not keep themselves informed of advances in the field. Graduates who continue to learn about the art and science of nurse anesthesia can develop into expert nurse anesthetists who are confident and secure in their practice, because they have excellent clinical and critical thinking skills. Through continued study, expert nurse anesthetists maintain up-to-date declarative, procedural, and conditional knowledge.

Some nurse anesthetists will continue their professional growth and achieve the sixth stage, *master.* Those functioning at this level formally or informally deepen their understanding of nurse anesthesia, usually through intensive study in a specific area. These anesthetists are often the ones who advance the science of the profession through teaching, writing, managing, or conducting research.

In the educational setting, it is important for both learners and instructors to be aware that instructors advance through the stages of a parallel educational model as they progress from novice to master teacher. Master teachers value learners' expertise and encourage them to take responsibility for their own educational needs.[45] Learners can enrich an educator's experience in ways that may inform the instructor's practice. Those who reflect on their teaching and evaluation competencies can become more capable of adjusting their approaches to meet students' needs and learning styles. Master teachers value learners' expertise and encourage them to take responsibility for their own educational needs. This eventually leads to a sense of empowerment that is important for lifelong learning and professional development.

References

1. McAuliffe MS. Case-Based Instruction: an analysis of clinical instruction in nurse anesthesiology. Ann Arbor, MI: University of Michigan Dissertation Services; 1993:1–156.

2. Heath S, Higgs, J, Ambruso DR. Evidence of knowledge acquisition in a cognitive flexibility-based computer learning environment. *Med Educ Online*. 2008;13:16.

3. Dennick R. Twelve tips for incorporating educational theory into teaching practices. *Med Teach*. 2012;34(8):618–624.

4. Dinham SM, Stritter FT. Research on Professional Education. In: Wittrock M. *Handbook of Research on Teaching*. 3rd ed. New York, NY: Macmillan; 1986:952–969.

5. Kuhn TS. *The Structure of Scientific Revolutions*. Chicago, IL: University of Chicago Press; 1970:111.

6. Argyris C, Schön DA. *Theory in Practice: Increasing Professional Effectiveness*. San Francisco, CA: Jossey-Bass; 1974:173–196.

7. Dreyfus SE, Dreyfus HL. A five-stage model of mental activities involved in directed skill acquisition. Unpublished report supported by the Air Force Office of Scientific Research (AFSC), USAF (Contract F49620-79-C-0063). University of California at Berkeley: 1980.

8. Dreyfus SE. The five-stage model of adult skill acquisition. *B Sci Technol Soc*. 2004;24(3):177–181.

9. Friedrich MJ. Practice makes perfect: risk-free medical training with patient simulators. *JAMA*. 2002; 288(22):2808–2812.

10. Dreyfus HL, Dreyfus SE. *Mind Over machine*. New York, NY: Free Press; 1986:122–157.

11. Flavel JH. Speculations about the nature and development of metacognition. In: Weinert F, Klewe R, eds. *Metacognition, Motivation, and Understanding*. Hillsdale, NJ: Lawrence Erlbaum; 1987:21–29.

12. Weinstein CE, Husman J, Dierking, DR, et al. Self-regulation interventions with a focus on learning strategies. In: Boekaerts M, Pintrich PR, Ziedner M, eds, *Handbook of Self-Regulation*. San Diego, CA: Academic Press; 2000:727–747.

13. Paris SG, Lipson MY, Wixson KK. Becoming a strategic reader. *Contemp Educ Psychol*. 1983;8(3):293–316.

14. Gott SP. Apprenticeship instruction for real world tasks: the coordination on procedures, mental models, and strategies. In: Rothkopf, EZ, ed. *Review of Research in Education*. Washington, DC: American Educational Research Association; 1988:97–169.

15. Flavel JH. Cognitive monitoring. In: Dickson WP, ed. *Children's Oral Communication Skills*. New York, NY: Academic Press; 1981:35–60.

16. Brown AL, Bransford JD, Ferrara RA, et al. Learning, remembering and understanding. In: Mussen PH. *Carmichael's Manual of Child Psychology.* Vol 1. Hoboken, NJ: John Wiley & Sons; 1983:77–166.

17. Brown AL, Campione JC, Day JD. Learning to learn: on training students to learn from texts. *Educ Res.* 1981;10:14–21.

18. Baker L, Brown AL. Metacognitive skills and reading. In: Kamil M, Mosenthal P, Pearson D, Barr R, eds. *Handbook of Reading Research.* New York, NY: Longman; 1984:353–394.

19. Spiro RJ, Jehng JC. Cognitive flexibility and hypertext. In: Spiro R, Nix D, eds. *Cognition, Education and Multimedia.* Hillsdale, NJ: Lawrence Erlbaum; 1990:163–205.

20. Spiro RJ, Feltovich PJ, Jacobson MJ, et al. Cognitive flexibility, constructivism and hypertext: random access instruction for advanced knowledge acquisition in ill-structured domains. In: Duffy T, Jonassen D, eds. *Constructivism and the Technology of Instruction.* Hillsdale, NJ: Lawrence Erlbaum; 1992:57–166.

21. Spiro RJ, Vispoel WL, Schmitz JG, et al. Knowledge acquisition for application: cognitive flexibility and transfer in complex content domains. In: Britton BK, Glynn SM, eds. *Executive Control Processes.* Hillsdale, NJ: Lawrence Erlbaum; 1987.

22. Spiro RJ, Coulson RL, Feltovich PJ, et al. Cognitive flexibility theory: advanced knowledge acquisition in ill-structured domains. In: Ruddel RB, ed. *Proceedings of the 10th Annual Conference of the Cognitive Science Society.* Hillsdale, NJ: Lawrence Erlbaum; 2004:602–616.

23. Jonassen D, Ambruso D, Olesen J. Designing hypertext on transfusion medicine using cognitive flexibilty theory. *J Educ Multimedia Hypermedia.* 1992;1(3):309–322.

24. Spiro RJ, Feltovich PJ, Jacobson MI, Coulson RI. Cognitive flexibility, constructivism and hypertext: random access instruction for advanced knowledge acquisition in ill-structured domains. In: Duffy T, Jonassen D, eds. *Constructivism and the Technology of Instruction.* Hillsdale, NJ: Lawrence Erlbaum; 1992:57–75.

25. Williams SM. Putting case-based instruction into context: examples from legal and medical education. *J Learn Sci.* 1992;2(4):367–427.

26. Coulson RL, Feltovich PJ, Spiro RJ. Cognitive flexibility in medicine: an application to the recognition and understanding of hypertension. *Adv Health Sci Educ.* 1997;2(2):141–161.

27. Coleson RL, Feltovich PJ, Spiro RJ. Cognitive flexibility in medicine: an application in the recognition and understanding of hypertension. Advances in Health Sciences Education. 1997;2:141–161

28. Tucker TM. *Predictors of critical thinking as a component of an outcomes assessment in a graduate level school of social work* [dissertation]. Louisville: University of Louisville; 2008.

29. Greene R, Rogers GL. Justifying core faculty assessment of students' clinical performance using cognitive flexibility theory: a case example. *The Internet Journal of Allied Health Sciences and Practice.* 2006;4(3):1–5.

30. Fiore SM, Hoffman RR, Salas E. Learning and performance across disciplines: an epilogue for moving multidisciplinary research toward an interdisciplinary science of expertise. *Mil Psychol.* 2008;20(Suppl 1):S155–S170.

31. Newswander LK, Newswander CB. Encouraging cognitive flexibility and interdisciplinarity in public administration programs. *Admin Soc.* 2012;44(3):285–309.

32. Stiegler, MP, Neelankavil JP, Canales, C, et al. Cognitive errors detected in anesthesiology: a literature review and pilot study. *Br J Anaesth.* 2012;108:229–235.

33. Stiegler, MP, Ruskin KJ. Decision-making and safety in anesthesiology. *Curr Opin in Anaesthesiol.* 2012;25(6):724–729.

34. Houben KW, van den Hombergh CLM, Stalmeijer, RE. New training strategies for anaesthesia residents. *Curr Opin in Anaesthesiol.* 2011;24(6):682–688.

35. Stalmeijer RE, Dolmans DHJ, Wolfhagen IHA, Scherpbier AJJ. Cognitive apprenticeship in clinical practice: can it stimulate learning in the opinion of students? *Adv in Health Sci Educ.* 2009;14(4):535–546.

36. Stalmeijer RE, Dolmans DHJ, Snellen-Balendong HAM, et al. Clinical teaching based on principles of cognitive apprenticeship: Views of experienced clinical teachers. *Acad Med.* 2013;88(6):861–865.

37. ten Cate O, Snell L, Mann K, Vermunt J. Orienting teaching toward the learn ng process. *Acad Med.* 2004;79(3):219–228.

38. Irby DM. Three exemplary models of case-based teaching. *Acad Med.* 1994;69(12):947–953.

39. Burns C, Beauchesne M, Ryan-Krause P, Sawin, K. Mastering the preceptor role: challenges of clinical teaching. *Jour Pediatr Health Car.* 2006;20(3):172–183.

40. Vygotsky LS, Cole M, John-Steiner V, Scribner S, Souberman E. *Mind in Society: Development of Higher Psychological Processes.* Cambridge, MA: Harvard University Press; 1978:76.

41. Vygotsky LS, Kozulin A. *Thought and Language.* Cambridge, MA: The MIT Press; 1986:210–256.

42. Spencer J. Learning and teaching in the clinical environment. *BMJ.* 2003;326(7389):591–594.

43. Schön DA. *Educating the Reflective Practitioner.* San Francisco, CA: Jossey-Bass; 1990.

44. Schön DA. *The Reflective Practitioner: How Professionals Think in Action.* New York, NY: Basic Books; 1983:128–168.

45. Newman P, Peile E. Valuing learners' experience and supporting further growth: educational models to help experienced adult learners in medicine. *BMJ.* 2002;325(7357):200–202.

46. Peile EB, Easton GP. Johnson N. The year in a training practice: what has lasting value? Grounded theoretical categories and dimensions from a pilot study. *Med Teach.* 2001;23(2):205–211.

47. Neher J Gordon, K, Meyer B, Stevens N. A five-step "microskills" model of clinical teaching. *J Am Board Fam Pract.* 1992;5(4):419–424.

48. Rudolph J, Raemer D, Shapiro J. We know what they did wrong, but not why: the case for "frame-based" feedback. *Clin Teach.* 2013;10(3):186–189.

49. Brown M, Hodges B, Wakefield J. Chapter 1.3. Points for giving effective feedback. In: Norman G, ed. *Evaluation Methods: A resource handbook.* Ontario, Canada: McMaster University; 1995.

50. Coulson RW, Feltovich PJ, Spiro RJ. *Foundations of a Misunderstanding of the Ultra Structural Basis for Myocardial Failure: A Reciprocating Network of Over-Simplifications (Tech. Rep. No. 1).* Springfield, IL: Southern Illinois University School of Medicine, Conceptual Knowledge Research Project; 1986.

CHAPTER 3

Health and Wellness in Nurse Anesthesia Education

Adrienne G. Hartgerink, DNP, CRNA
Sandra K. Tunajek, DNP, CRNA

Keywords: Coping, critical incident management, nurse anesthesia education, peer support, stress management, student registered nurse anesthetist, substance use disorder, wellness, wellness curriculum.

Key Concepts

- Instruction on health and wellness topics is a Council on Accreditation of Nurse Anesthesia Programs (COA) required teaching component for nurse anesthesia educational programs and needs to be a part of the planned curriculum.
- Although it is impossible to change the stress that is inherent to the anesthesia profession, it is possible to identify factors that contribute to workplace or educational stress, improve knowledge on how to adaptively cope with the stress, and avoid maladaptive behaviors through education about wellness and stress management.
- The educational preparation of nurse anesthetists is a highly stressful experience for both faculty and students. Psychological burnout may inhibit the ability of faculty to effectively manage periods of change. For student registered nurse anesthetists, academic information overload and fear of clinical error are the highest stressors.
- Research shows that stress is a major influence affecting performance and interpersonal relationships among faculty and students. Stress may compromise health and well-being in pronounced ways.
- Academic and clinical faculty must understand the stress and anxiety that students experience in order to devise the best techniques to help students cope with daily stressors. The characteristics of stress and burnout may impede effective teaching and learning, and they are likely to intensify unless faculty members devise and implement specific interventions.
- Substance use disorder, also known as chemical dependency or addiction, is a risk for the anesthesia professional and can affect both nurse anesthesia educators and students.
- Faculty and students need to be aware of the resources at their disposal related to health and wellness issues.

Introduction

The explosion of the health and wellness movement across the country has ignited the health care arena to truly embrace these initiatives. Stressful health care work environments and individual well-being can impact patient safety and are factors that must be taken seriously. Many health care institutions now have processes for evaluating professional competence and individual fitness for duty. Further, largely in response to productivity and regulatory concerns, many facilities, including teaching institutions, are highlighting the importance of stress management and personal wellness with a myriad of wellness-related programs and resources.

The focus on wellness for health care workers has slowly been gaining momentum over the last few decades with the American Association of Nurse Anesthetists (AANA) as the trendsetter in peer assistance and wellness initiatives in health care organizations. The AANA Peer Assistance Advisors Committee was formed in 1983 in response to concerns about the high number of substance use-related deaths in the nurse anesthesia profession. Dedicated peer advisor volunteers across the country provide confidential assistance, informational support, and referral resources to addicted nurse anesthetists, their families, and supervisors.[1] The committee also educates the nurse anesthesia community on the dangers of substance misuse.[1,2]

The AANA Wellness Program was officially launched in February 2004 after a call from the membership to broaden the initiatives of the Peer Assistance Program to include other workplace wellness issues.[1] Now called the AANA Health and Wellness program, it covers all aspects of member wellness. The program provides resources to help the Certified Registered Nurse Anesthetist (CRNA) and student registered nurse anesthetist (SRNA) identify and cope with occupational and educational stressors.[3]

The profession has taken great strides in recent years to increase member awareness by adding more wellness educational offerings at state and national meetings; publishing health and wellness articles in the AANA *NewsBulletin* and *Journal*; discussing current health and wellness issues through social media pages for students and CRNAs; and providing a warehouse of educational materials available to faculty and students on the AANA website. A broad range of overall fitness and health topics geared toward the nurse anesthesia community are discussed in these resources including addiction concerns, stress, fatigue, coping mechanisms, critical incident management, peer support, and more.

In the not too distant past, the inclusion of wellness education for nurse anesthesia students was something that only a few passionate individuals embraced. In a 2010 nurse anesthesia program director's survey, 13.3% stated their program did not teach wellness or chemical dependency topics and 30% said they discussed chemical dependency but no other wellness topics.[4] Today, the picture is much different with 100% of the 82 programs responding to a recent Health and Wellness Committee survey stating they teach wellness topics in addition to substance use risk.[5] The Council on Accreditation for Nurse Anesthesia Educational Programs (COA) has required nurse anesthesia programs teach content related to wellness and chemical dependency (now referred to as substance use disorder) in the anesthesia profession since January 2013.[3,6] Although no specific content or hour requirement is currently attached to this criterion, it is the responsibility of individual programs to demonstrate that an evidence-based program of study on this information is being taught and that knowledge related to these content areas is demonstrated.

Students start their anesthesia program with the expectation that faculty will show concern for their health and wellness and provide resources to keep them well throughout their academic journey.[6,7] This phenomenon is a fairly recent one. Informal discussions with nurse anesthesia program faculty provided common concerns surrounding health and wellness topics specific to nurse anesthesia education, including stress and stress management; impact of stress on learning; student and faculty coping; resiliency; substance use and monitoring; critical incident management; peer support; and available resources. This chapter will focus on these health and wellness issues as they relate to nurse anesthesia faculty and students.

Stress and Education

Health and wellness discussions in the educational arena often focus on stress management, and for good reason. Regardless of specialty, simply being enrolled in an educational program is a stressor. Stress is a response to change from the norm, whether it is from a positive or negative event. It is a necessary and unavoidable parallel of daily living and can be beneficial in helping us to be motivated to perform necessary tasks. Too much stress, however, can deplete coping mechanisms and can be harmful to overall wellness. Stress is often difficult to define because individuals react to it differently. Situations that are stressful for one person may not be for another. Further, individuals vary widely in their ability to cope effectively with stress.

Learning how to effectively manage stress is a key component in keeping us well. It is not uncommon for graduate students to experience stressful situations, coping issues, and other problems during their academic careers. There is ample evidence that students in health professional educational programs experience varying levels of stress; for many, it is significant and is associated with poor academic performance.[1,8–13]

Studies in medical specialties have found that stress during residency training affects efficiency, productivity, error rates, and physician burnout.[9,10] The studies related to the anesthesia student experience[12,14,15] suggest the major sources of stressors are similar to those in other types of graduate educational programs; however, there is a significant added concern for making clinical errors that may harm patients. For most students, the ability to cope was related to the sequencing of clinical time and the year in school, but was also impacted by their ability to effect change in their learning environment and the availability of support systems.[7,14–17]

In the nurse anesthesia-related studies, a common theme for both students and faculty is the lack of resources,[12,18,19] suggesting an influence on the individual's ability to cope. Further, some teaching environments may not recognize or encourage the need for supportive resources. More important, students may be reluctant to access resources or seek assistance for fear of appearing weak, less capable of achievement, or fear of retaliation.[12,13]

In addition to these educational stressors, nurse anesthesia students and faculty are exposed to occupational risks in the clinical setting such as workplace bullying, fatigue, substance use, critical incidents, and adverse events.

Faculty Stress

Research in the medical, dental, and nursing literature indicates that considerable stress is a factor for graduate level faculty.[9,20] Of the three functions performed by faculty in higher education—teaching, research, and administrative activities—teaching was designated as the most stressful.[9,21] Most of the stressors appear to relate directly to time management and access to resources. The areas causing the most stress for faculty appeared to be excessively high self-expectations; securing financial support for educational programs; having insufficient time and being continually overloaded with work; receiving low pay for work done; lack of time for individual research; interference of work with personal activities; and interruptions and meetings.[18,20,22]

Educators also reported experiencing role ambiguity, intellectual fatigue, physical exhaustion, and loss of morale. Demands to generate revenues, the accelerating competition for grant funding, and the explosion of new technology and emerging biomedical knowledge also contribute to the challenges.[18,21]

Studies that have investigated nurse anesthesia faculty indicate that high levels of stress are directly related to job dissatisfaction, heavy workload, multiple demands on time, and perceptions of lack of authority and control.[18,19,23] Furthermore, the supply of excellent role models and mentors is dwindling as current nurse anesthesia faculty members approach retirement.[19] This compares with similar concerns for faculty in other disciplines of graduate education.

Program director turnover is high within nurse anesthesia programs, which adds to faculty stress.[19] Faculty have to deal with frequent new administrators or perhaps step into the position themselves. Faculty also report dealing with difficult or struggling students and student failures as major stressors. At least 20% of faculty reported major depressive symptoms[24] as well as other signs of stress such as agitation, cravings, headaches, hypertension, and inability to concentrate.[1] Faculty not only need to recognize and cope with their own stressors, but are also faced with the challenge of recognizing stress and meeting the learning needs of students even when they also may be feeling overwhelmed.

Student Stress

Student stress in anesthesia training has been well documented in nurse anesthesia literature.[1,14,17,26–29] Nurse anesthesia students must adapt to unpredictable workloads; the use of new, advanced technology; long working hours; altered sleep and eating patterns; and the juggling of academic and clinical hours. For many, there is a need for immediate modification in financial status, relocation, long-distance family relationships, and loss of personal time. Further, the student is expected to master large amounts of complex material in a short amount of time; perform complex assessments of patient health problems; develop independent, critical reading, listening, and thinking abilities; and, to clearly articulate problem-solving solutions in a professional, confident manner.[17,25]

Although a certain amount of stress has been identified as enhancing learning, little is known about how much is motivational and how much is detrimental.[14,25] Models that are useful in understanding stress among students are based on the concept that the individual perceives stressful events as challenging or threatening.[30] When students consider their education as a challenge, stress can bring them a sense of competence and an increased capacity to learn. Competence is the internal drive to be effective and master the environment and is associated with academic performance. However, when education is seen as a threat, stress can elicit feelings of helplessness, self-doubt, and a foreboding sense of failure.[14,30,31]

Adult students entering graduate education can experience a reaction similar to shock as they attempt to adjust to the multiplicity of new responsibilities while organizing their time and dealing with changes in their relationships at home.[31,32] Evidence from several studies suggests that academic performance is the most critical concern of students, especially first-year students, and that the problems perceived to be the most intense source of stress are examinations and grades, financial concerns, and fear of failure on specific assignments.

Among student registered nurse anesthetists, academic information overload, fear of clinical error, and lack of control are the highest stressors.[7,15] A comparison study between graduate nurse anesthetists and general nursing graduates found student registered nurse anesthetists to have significantly higher scores on excitement seeking and addictive tendency ($P = .002$).[4,5] Excitement seeking, by definition, describes an individual's preference for quantity and intensity of interpersonal relationships and is a facet of extraverted personalities. Because the neurochemistry is not well understood, ongoing research in drug and alcohol abuse is investigating the association between personality, excitement seeking, and addiction tendency.[33]

Another process in nurse anesthesia schools that also can cause stress is the subtle, but pervasive, process of being socialized into a profession. Adding to the occupational stressors, the student must deal with an identity shift from a competent registered nurse to a novice student anesthetist, often experiencing a perceived loss of control and professional recognition. Students take the new skills they are learning, absorb these skills as fundamental parts of their personalities, and undergo a transformation in their sense of identity. The transformation of a nurse into a CRNA is an adjustment to a new role, which, if successful, creates the new status of belonging to a unique social group.[24] Peer expectations and adherence to these high standards of professional conduct during the educational process are additional stressors.

Neumann et al[34] found that emotional exhaustion greatly influences student performance and affects personal commitment. The degree to which the student experiences emotional fatigue depends on individual flexibility, engagement in learning, student-faculty contact, and the perception of stress. Regarding the latter, one study indicated a considerable mismatch between faculty and students in their perceptions of students' stressors and reactions to stressors.[16] The faculty members perceived the students to experience a higher level of stress and to display reactions to stressors more frequently than the students actually perceived they were experiencing stress; however, both groups identified work overload and variability in faculty expectations as the major perceived stressors.

Nurse anesthetist students are highly motivated, achievement-oriented individuals with high expectations. Upon graduation, they will enter one of the most stressful occupations in health care. An attitude of self-reliance, a driven personality, and tendencies to overachieve contribute to a cycle that leads to burnout, and which further exacerbates stressful circumstances.[35] Finally, students may not be aware of the significant impact these pressures can exert on physical and mental health, and they may not be aware of resources available to assist students in coping with these new, stressful experiences.[4,12,14]

It is the responsibility of faculty to make sure students are aware of the resources available to them. The Council on Accreditation of Nurse Anesthesia Educational Programs' standards require accountability of the schools in regard to the students, including fair and equitable processes, nondiscrimination, and limits on workload.[36] Policies must include a mechanism to address complaints, grievances, and student concerns. Students should be informed of the program's policies and processes.

Stress, Fatigue, and Burnout

Burnout is a distinctive kind of job-related stress that inhibits the person's capacity to function effectively.[13] Research indicates that individuals engaged in the helping professions or human services are especially susceptible to burnout and nurse anesthesia is no exception. A Stress and Burnout survey of CRNAs and SRNAs by Chipas and McKenna[1] found nurse anesthesia students to be the most stressed followed by nurse anesthesia faculty. Sustained stress levels over time can lead to burnout. Although burnout, with its accompanying emotional exhaustion and dissatisfaction, has prompted much study as it relates to management and business, it is just beginning to be documented in the anesthesia literature.

Educational processes for health care professionals, which have historically accepted fatigue as a condition of teaching and learning, are slowly recognizing that fatigue contributes to burnout for both students and faculty.

Fatigue is an inherent part of life as an anesthesia provider and can have grave consequences if not managed properly. Getting enough sleep is often one of the most difficult goals for the anesthesia professional to achieve. Early mornings, late nights, and long hours on call, all contribute to interrupted normal sleep patterns. Sleep deprivation has been shown to mimic acute alcohol intoxication and can lead to poor decision-making, careless performance, and slowed reaction times that jeopardize personal as well as patient safety.[37–39]

Sleep deprivation is a relative concept. Small amounts of sleep loss have subtle cognitive costs, which appear to go unrecognized by the individual experiencing the sleep loss. More severe restriction of sleep, for example, over a week leads to profound cognitive deficits similar to those seen in some stroke patients. These symptoms also appear to go unrecognized by the individual. The lack of recognition of the effects of sleep deprivation equals a setup for all kinds of errors to occur. The reality is humans can make mistakes and sleep-deprived individuals are more likely to make more mistakes.[40] The AANA Position Statement 2.17 Patient Safety: Fatigue, Sleep, and Work Schedule Effects[39] states, "CRNAs are ethically responsible for adhering to the AANA *Code of Ethics for the Certified Registered Nurse Anesthetists*[41] by assuring they are well rested and fit for duty." Nurse anesthesia faculty should be familiar with these guidelines including ensuring students are not overcommitted. Providing anesthesia patient care for more than 16 consecutive hours without adequate breaks for meals and rest is not recommended.[37,39] **Table 3.1** highlights some of the major symptoms of fatigue.

Table 3.1 Fatigue Signs and Symptoms[37–40]

- Conducting multiple rechecks of completed tasks
- Tiredness during the day
- Vague symptoms such as a headache
- Drooping eyelids or red eyes
- Nodding off while awake
- Diminished reaction time
- Increased restlessness, lethargy, irritability, and/or anxiety
- Impaired concentration or memory
- Diminished reflexes
- Impaired decision-making
- Increased snoring
- Difficulty awakening after adequate sleep
- Unawareness of surroundings
- Indecisiveness
- Decreased situational awareness

Burnout is not just a temporary condition, but an unhealthy situation that can make productive, enthusiastic workers a detriment to their profession, their colleagues, and themselves. Burnout usually affects the most together individuals; those who are the most competent and committed, feel the most strongly about the value of what they do, and set high expectations for themselves.

Some stress is to be expected in education and has been found to be motivational. Yet, how much stress is productive and where the counterproductive line begins is not clear. What is clear is that burnout and stress among students affects academic performance and can impact retention and, therefore, attrition rates.[42]

Burnout among faculty inhibits the ability to effectively lead programs, particularly during periods of change. Teaching can generate a high level of stress and fatigue and can lead to burnout. Academic demands, financial difficulties, family problems, and the relationships between students and faculty advisers were cited as the biggest contributors to stress and burnout.[20] Factors contributing to overall faculty stress are noted in **Table 3.2** on the next page.

Table 3.2 Faculty Stressors

- Heavy workload (combined clinical and classroom teaching)
- Retaining failing students or dealing with difficult students
- Meeting research requirements
- Providing individual clinical supervision
- Dealing with learning disabilities and attention deficit disorders
- Use of new technologies
- Increasing diversification of expertise
- Campus politics and meeting the economic necessities of the institution
- Changes in administrative demands or administrative leadership
- Lack of financial and personnel support
- Time pressures and deadlines
- Dealing with inequities and inequalities

One of the greatest challenges in education is effectively managing teaching loads and schedules. This includes time for family, friends, personal endeavors, and nourishing the soul, and time for reflection, renewal, and reinvigoration. Demands are increasing with more work, more students, and less free time. The increased demands and workloads result in teachers having less time for preparation, teaching, and interaction with students. Unfortunately, student interaction may be one of the first things that overworked instructors decrease, affecting the attitudes, self-esteem, and motivation of both faculty and students. If unable to fulfill all expected activities, faculty may feel increased pressure, experiencing greater stress. Regrettably, the prevalence of stress and burnout syndromes reported among practitioners, residents, and students in nursing and medicine studies show that stress is associated with depression, alcohol and drug use, relationship difficulties, anxiety, and even suicide.[7,10,33]

Personality Type and Stress

Stress is connected with major changes in personal life or work-related environments. In general, adverse physical and emotional consequences usually result from the way an individual perceives particular events or conditions. Too many changes at one time, either positive or negative, can overload an individual's capacity to adapt successfully and may result in a variety of illnesses. Stress depends on the individual's perception of the situation. What may be perceived as distressful to one person may be excitingly challenging and positively stressful to another. Even to the same person, the same event can be distressful at one time and stimulating or not stressful at another time. How someone responds to stress depends on the environment, the magnitude of the stressor, the person's self-perceived ability to handle the stressor, the person's physical condition, and more often, the habitual response.[43] Sapolsky[43] recommends prevention by learning to recognize the signs of stress and what situations trigger it.

Stress can be self-imposed by setting standards too high or having unrealistic expectations regarding one's abilities. Situational stressors include time constraints, lack of resources, threats to emotional or physical well-being, challenges beyond one's ability to respond, or conflicts between one's personal values and the values of others. Additionally, those individuals with Type A personalities, who exhibit a high degree of self-control, impatience, competitiveness, inability to relax, orientation to achievement, and denial of failure, appear to be more prone to stressful reactions.[9,43–45]

There are many personality frameworks that offer insights into differences among people. One of the most researched theories is the Myers-Briggs typology assessment, which refines personality into 16 types. This theory holds that people take in information and make decisions differently, which are two key processes in education. These variations in behavior are quite orderly and consistent. More and more career counselors, educators, and academic centers are using personality testing to determine specialty choice for medical professions.[46] Emotional intelligence exams are also gaining traction with nurse anesthesia programs to try to predict which applicants may be best-suited to adapt to the role of a nurse anesthetist.

Impact of Stress on Learning

The influences of behavioral, individual, cognitive, and environmental factors determine how people interact and learn from each other.[47] The effects of stress on learning and memory, both facilitating and impairing influences, are well-described in the literature,[43] and authors note that good stress can be invigorating and empowering. With good stress, energy peaks, memory sharpens, chemicals producing pleasure increase in the brain, and senses are heightened. Sustained stress can damage the hippocampus, the area of the brain critical to learning and memory. The body makes no distinction between immediate, pleasurable, or acutely threatening stress and chronic physical and psychological stress. Additionally, an individual's personality or frame of mind when encountering stress may influence the health effects of stress.

The brain interprets what is potentially threatening and, therefore, stressful, and determines the individual's behavioral and physiological responses. Behavioral responses may include the fight or flight response, overeating, smoking, drinking to excess, and losing sleep at night. Thus, lifestyle and behavior are key contributors to "being stressed out."

The literature documents that both increased and decreased stress responses can profoundly affect cognition and behavior.[48] The amygdala and hippocampus portions of the brain interpret what is stressful, then regulate appropriate responses by controlling the release of glucocorticoids and activating the sympathetic nervous system. Uncontrollable stress impedes hippocampal memory, and stress-induced alterations contribute to memory impairments.[48,49] Increased glucocorticoid levels also impair memory function, disrupt problem-solving, and weaken spatial recognition memory. The response to stress involves the active release of hormones and other mediators that produce adaptation to acute stress. Subsequent pathophysiology results when the same mediators are deregulated over long time periods.

In the hippocampus and prefrontal cortex—the center of emotion—repeated stress causes dendrites to shrink and spine synapses to decrease in number. In the basolateral amygdala, stress causes increased dendritic branching and synapse density, essentially leading to a constant state of fear. As remodeling of neural circuitry occurs, mediators are under repeated stress, leading to impaired memory, increased anxiety, aggression, and impaired attention. The body further reacts by compromising the immune system and the cardiovascular system, resulting in long-term health effects.[43]

Stress affects cognition in a number of ways, acting rapidly via catecholamines and more slowly via glucocorticoids. The activation or arousal of the stress systems leads to a cluster of behavioral and physiological changes that are consistent and predictable, including increased alertness, vigilance, improved cognition, and focused attention.[50]

The relationship between changes in arousal and motivation is often expressed as an Inverted-U function (also known as the Yerkes-Dodson law). The basic concept is that as arousal level increases, performance improves, but only to a point beyond which the increases in arousal lead to deterioration in performance (See **Figure 3.1**).[48,50]

Anxiety involves cognitive and somatic components. Cognitive anxiety (worry) is characterized by negative expectations, lack of concentration, and images of failure, whereas somatic anxiety refers to physical symptoms such as nervousness and tension.

Coping consists of adaptive resources to meet the demands and cognitive and behavioral efforts to manage the demands. This theory has been enhanced by the role that control plays in the appraisal, in which perception of control tends to reduce the negative emotional responses. This concept involves three components: cognitive, physiological, and overt behavioral and is the basis for recognizing, preventing, and coping interventions.

Figure 3.1 Relationship Between Changes in Arousal and Motivation

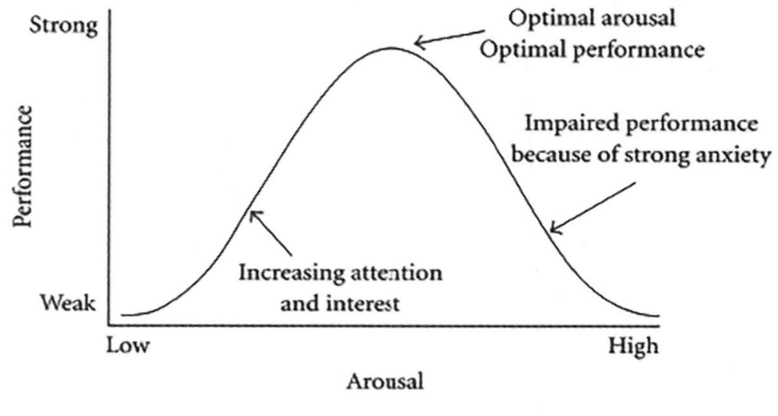

Wellness and Resiliency

Most of the studies regarding stressors in anesthesia deal with the increased risk of substance use disorder and not as much about what keeps us well.[51] Wellness is described by the AANA Health and Wellness Committee as "a positive state of the mind, body and spirit reflecting a balance of effective adaption, resilience, and coping mechanisms in personal and professional environments that enhance quality of life."[3]

There is growing evidence that concentrating on wellness issues such as improved diet, getting enough sleep, exercise, meditation, and strengthening support systems can improve coping mechanisms and increase general well-being.[3,51] The literature supports a wide range of practices to encourage self-care and enhance balance. They all emphasize the need to individualize these practices;one size does not fit all. Faculty should ensure they discuss the benefits of self-care with their students. There are many strategies for reducing both personal and workplace stress. Some of these strategies seem simple but really work, such as deep breathing exercises and meditation. Although there is not much time for fun and relaxation during anesthesia school, finding adaptive coping skills is an essential part of managing stress and staying well. Eric Swanlund II, student representative to the AANA Health and Wellness Committee, maintains the SRNA health and wellness Facebook page and also submits articles focusing on nurse anesthesia student health and wellness. He suggests it is important for students to not fall away from those activities that keep them balanced and to find what works for them.[6] Swanlund discussed exercise, sleep, nutrition, and support of classmates, friends, and family as his most effective coping strategies.[6,52] The plethora of wellness books and informational websites now available has increased the popularity of this initiative in the general population and lends credibility to the importance of wellness as part of the anesthesia provider's stress management plan. Many nurse anesthesia programs are now offering routine wellness events as well as stress reduction options as shown in **Table 3.3.**[3,53] Professional codes of ethics include very specific expectations for professionals to engage in self-care practices to ensure patient safety.

Table 3.3 Wellness Support Activities

- Gym facility or group exercise opportunities
- Counseling center services
- Group activities for social support
- Wellness events/guest speakers on wellness
- Stress reduction options, yoga or meditation
- Reduced prices on supportive resources (gym, healthy food alternatives)
- Critical incident stress management training
- Student-led support group

Another concept discussed in the literature related to wellness is resiliency. Resiliency is the ability to bounce back and adapt well when faced with traumatic, tragic, adverse, or significantly stressful situations.[52,54,55] This is an important area to explore, especially as it relates to nurse anesthesia students. Students' ability to manage stress varies by individual coping ability, support systems, and resiliency.[14,25] The literature has discussed at length the connection between resiliency and the ability to cope effectively with stressful situations. Questions related to resiliency include: Why do some students deal well with stress while others turn to maladaptive behaviors to cope? What makes some students more resilient than others? What can educators do to identify the patterns of resilience, cultivate the positive, and diminish the negative to increase resilience? These questions are fascinating and the answers would certainly make the job of successfully shepherding nurse anesthesia students through to graduation much easier.

The concept of resilience is an extremely relevant one in nursing. Nurses in all specialties are concerned with how their patients move through adversity and how they, as nurses, can help them through this process. Resilience has been studied often but seems to take on different meanings depending on the author and the context. Noting the importance of the concept of resilience to nursing and the inconsistencies in the literature on what constitutes resilience, the middle-range theory on resilience was developed in 1997 by Laura Polk.[56] She felt the inconsistencies suggested that further theoretical delineation of resilience was needed in order to clarify the confusion.[56]

Polk built on the previous work by Newman and Rogers and the concept that human beings change with the environment and have continuously intermingling human and environmental energy fields identified by a pattern.[56] Her middle range resilience theory is based on four constructs described as patterns and include:

- the dispositional pattern (sense of self, genetic factors);
- relational pattern (close relationships, social network);
- situational pattern (approach to stress, problem solving); and
- the philosophical pattern (personal beliefs, self-knowledge).

Although only a few examples are noted for each pattern here, Polk included a more detailed list of all the characteristics that constitute each of these identified patterns in the appendix of her original work. The synergistic relationship of these four constructs across the lifespan together manifest into a larger underlying pattern recognized as "resilience."[56,57]

The theory lends itself to many specialties, both inside and outside of nursing, to assist in recognizing effective and ineffective coping skills and building resilience. Resilience is vital for adaptation in demanding environments of all kinds. Polk's middle range theory helps to tie the pieces of what makes up resilience together and hopefully provides insight that can be utilized to improve the care given to nurse anesthesia students and to their patients.

No matter what theory or definition is used, the consensus seems to be that people are born with some level of inherent resilience (genetic) and are impacted along the way by their environment, but that education and effective self-care can improve resiliency behavior, the ability to cope, and overall sense of well-being.[58] An adapted model for combining these concepts is shown in **Figure 3.2**. Teaching these concepts in nurse anesthesia educational programs can help improve resiliency behavior and lay the foundation for both personal and professional wellness.

Figure 3.2 Well-Being and Resiliency Behavior Conceptual Model

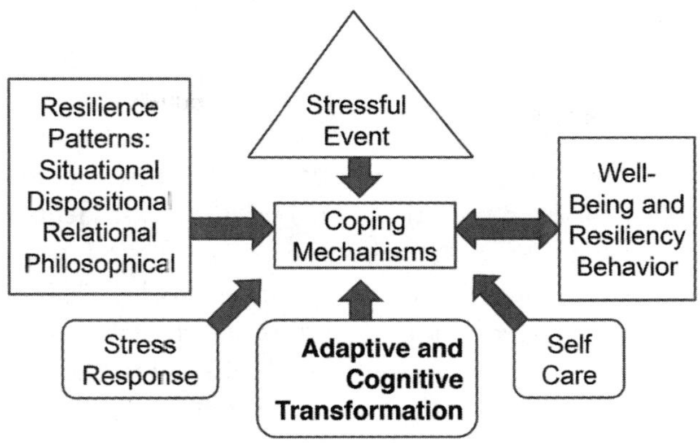

Adapted from : Grafton, E., Gillespie, B., & Henderson, S. 2010. Resilience: The power within. *Oncol Nurs Forum,* 35 (6), 698–705.

Polk, L.V. 1997. Toward a middle-range theory of resilience. *Advan Nurs Science,* 19(3), 1–13.

Distance Education Factors

As advances in technology change the face of education, a growing number of faculty are moving into a teaching environment that is geographically independent of both students and colleagues, especially as programs transition to doctoral education. The separation by distance of student and teacher removes a vital link of communication between these two parties. Isolated students experience anticipatory stress related to a perceived lack of support and technical assistance.[59] The isolation may have an impact on behavioral issues and academic achievement. Students need access to faculty for feedback on academic courses as well as contact with instructors to serve as a support system if stress becomes a problem.[34]

The distance aspect of distance learning takes away much of the social interaction that would be present in traditional learning environments. Geographical isolation has been identified as one of the major problems for distance students.[59,60] This may lead to feelings of inadequacy and insecurity and a lack of confidence in their own abilities.[59,60] The use of technology in education is increasing every day and faculty are certainly becoming more adept at distance or at least some sort of hybrid technology platform. Of particular importance is that, although the demand for transition to more technology use has increased, there is still a lack of staff training in course development, technology, and redesign of existing materials for distance students.[19] Perhaps the biggest problem for distance programs is the change in teaching styles from face-to-face instruction to that of an online mentor, tutor, and facilitator.

It is critical that the support needs of these faculty and students be identified and addressed. Although becoming more prevalent, the literature still offers little evidence of research into the experiences of the distance educator. Although there is general recognition that managing students is a demanding and often stressful aspect of conducting a distance course, faculty support is most often limited to technical and instructional design support.[21,61] There is little or no attention given to the totality of the experience of teaching at a distance and what the impact is on a social or personal level from the faculty perspective. McLean[21] also found a secondary factor that can directly influence the stress levels and job satisfaction of clinical faculty operating exclusively at a distance: the question of what is the scope of teaching in this environment.

Increasingly, nurse anesthesia education is heavily involved in distance education, and clinical rotations have created an organizational structure that unbundles both the student and instructor from their traditional roles. Both student and instructor stress is connected to workload and to self-imposed expectations about performance and achievement. Distance education is an around-the-clock endeavor. It is important for program administrators to recognize this stress and to realize that if faculty members are unable to temper it themselves, burnout is likely. The challenges faced by faculty teaching exclusively at a distance are not entirely different from those of their on-campus counterparts, but the form those challenges take and the avenues by which they are managed are necessarily changed in distance learning.[21]

It is even more difficult for faculty to identify students who are having difficulty coping when they are not seeing them face-to-face. It is critical that distance courses involve providing resources that are available for struggling students, whether academically or emotionally. If students try recommended strategies for coping and still experience the negative aspects of stress, then faculty should encourage students to contact the facility employment assistance program if one exists, or seek other professional assistance.

Coping Strategies

Faculty and staff are often the first to recognize students who are in trouble. Awareness of the potential effects of stress on students and faculty is critical to dealing with the potential ineffective and often unmanageable coping mechanisms that may contribute to inappropriate behaviors and the resulting bad consequences. It is prudent to look for a cluster of signs or signals that appear within a similar time frame. Recognizable indicators that students may be experiencing more stress than they can cope with are listed in **Table 3.4**.

Table 3.4 Ineffective Student Coping Signs

- Student states he or she needs assistance/help
- Inconsistent changes in academic or clinical performance
- Physical symptoms of exhaustion, loss of/increased appetite, headaches, crying, sleeplessness, and oversleeping
- Behavioral changes exhibited by withdrawal, sudden crying, unexplained anger, or unusual irritability
- Inappropriate behavior patterns exhibited by use of alcohol, drugs, or other compulsive behavior
- Reference to suicide (Do not leave alone and seek help immediately.)
- Concerns related to racial and ethnic identity and affectional preferences
- Marked change in personal lives, eg, death of a family member or close friend, termination of an important relationship, divorce, changes in family responsibilities

Larsson and Sanner[62] describe what the individual anesthetist can do to improve well-being at work and emphasize that although stress remains an inevitable aspect of anesthesia, adaptive coping, and reframing the way the provider looks at an event can make a huge difference. They point out that student anesthetists would especially benefit from these coping strategies. Effective coping skills are especially important for the student registered nurse anesthetist as excessive, unmanaged stress is counter-productive to learning and can affect success as well as patient safety.[14,25]

Student registered nurse anesthetists are adult learners who must acquire extensive critical knowledge, experiences, and personal growth to become competent professionals. Much of that knowledge is gained through anxiety-producing situations where the consequences can have a substantial impact on patients. It is beneficial for the faculty to be aware of the traits and anxiety tendencies of individual students in order to devise the best techniques to help students cope with the day-to-day stressors. Identification of stressors, unmanaged stress symptoms, and coping strategies should be reviewed with students often throughout the curriculum and individualized as needed. Research indicates that SRNAs and CRNAs develop multiple mechanisms to deal with daily stress.[12,14,15] The type of strategies that students use to cope with their problems will affect their well-being as well as influence their academic performance. These mechanisms can be adaptive or maladaptive in nature.

Adaptive Coping

Adaptive or positive coping strategies are characterized by a kind of behavior that allows the individual to change an unconstructive or disruptive behavior to something more constructive.[4] These coping strategies consist of family support, social support, religion, exercise, spirituality, mentoring, and talking to friends. Specific coping skills may include:

- establishing good study habits
- managing time wisely
- learning positive self-talk

- learning how to relax
- following a healthy lifestyle
- using humor
- forming or joining a peer support group[5,55,63]

There are many resources to help faculty learn simple techniques to facilitate adaptive coping mechanisms. Incorporating some of these techniques not only benefits the students, but the faculty as well.

Establishing Good Study Habits, Managing Time Wisely

Stress is necessary to challenge students to learn, but too much stress can be a detriment to effective learning. Individuals under low and high levels of stress learn the least, and those under moderate stress learn the most. Solutions suggested for reducing distress in students include instruction in recognizing learning styles,[64] informing students in advance of the difficulties they might face, and encouraging them to develop their own strategies to achieve personal goals. Negative aspects of stress that decrease students' learning and performance need to be reduced so that effective learning can take place. The key to reducing distress is providing students with a feeling of control over their education, giving them information about what to expect, and providing feedback to improve their performance. Self-efficacy is related to one's beliefs that objectives can be accomplished.[42,44] Students who do not feel helpless will adopt their own coping strategies.[32]

The ability to plan has been shown to be an effective adaptive coping mechanism.[63] Giving students as much information as possible related to schedules and expectations helps them to plan and therefore reduce stress. Unnecessary changes in schedules should be minimized and, if necessary, explained. Some students may need assistance in blocking their time and guidance on organizing study priorities. Nurse anesthesia school is notorious for the vast amount of information that must be learned in a short amount of time. Orientation to the program can include examples of time management, development of study groups, and effective study habits. Introducing these concepts early can often foster positive coping behavior. Struggling students should be brought in for counseling early before ineffective habits are out of control.

Positive Self-Talk

Positive self-talk is a key part of effective stress management. Self-talk is the endless stream of unspoken automatic thoughts that run through your head, and they can be positive or negative. Thinking the best will happen instead of the worst is positive self-talk. Some self-talk comes from logic and reason and some may arise from misconceptions created because of lack of information. Positive self-talk first starts with positive thinking. Positive thinking is a way to approach unpleasant situations in a more positive and productive way.

The effects of positive thinking and optimism on health continue to be explored. Positive thinking may provide health benefits such as an increased life span, lower rates of depression and distress, fewer illnesses, increased psychological and physical well-being, reduced risk of death from cardiovascular disease, and superior coping skills during hardship and times of stress.[65] It's unclear why people who engage in positive thinking experience these health benefits. One theory is that a positive outlook enables improved coping in stressful situations, which reduces the harmful health effects of stress on one's body.

Faculty should encourage students to be gentle with themselves and encourage them not to say anything to themselves that they would not say to anyone else. Most student registered nurse anesthetists are overachievers with high expectations of how they will perform, especially in the clinical area. It is easy for them to revert to negative self-talk if they miss an intubation or don't perform how they think they should on an exam. One suggestion is that when a negative thought occurs, to evaluate it rationally and put a positive spin on it. For example, instead of "I am horrible at intubations," think "I am improving my airway skills every day."

Negative people can impact the ability to carry out positive self-talk and to manage stress in healthy ways. Although students cannot control everyone they come in contact with in their professional lives, faculty should attempt to be positive, supportive role models that students can depend on to give helpful advice and feedback.[65]

Learning How to Relax

Learning how to relax is a key component to effective stress management and adaptive coping. Everyone relaxes differently. Not all students or faculty will embrace meditation or yoga, but there are many simple interventions that can help both student and faculty develop effective relaxation techniques. Things like listening to music, using laughter, taking a nature walk, doing hobbies and crafts, and taking a digital break from social media have all been shown to be effective relaxation techniques.[55] There are also some easy interventions that faculty can teach students and practice themselves to foster relaxation in both the classroom and in the clinical area.

Exercises such as having students practice regular, mindful breathing can be calming to the overworked mind.[55,66] Exaggerating exhalation in a slow steady manner can instantaneously decrease stress by triggering the parasympathetic nervous system activity and reducing the sympathetic influence.[55] Faculty should consider teaching students to do this simple exercise: Inhale over 3–4 seconds; hold the breath for 7 seconds and then exhale over 8 seconds while thinking about blowing out all the tension and pressure in the body. Students can practice this simple exercise before exams, in the clinical area, and in other stressful situations. Likewise, faculty can use this simple exercise to decrease their own stress.[55,67]

Mindfulness is intentionally paying attention with a curious and nonjudgmental attitude.[68] Mindfulness-based stress reduction (MBSR) has been shown as an efficient form of self-care. One of the underlying tenets of MBSR is that through mindfulness practice, one can reduce self-focused thoughts and emotions that lead to negative and unhealthy mood states. This program has been shown to reduce levels of distress and enhance well-being in individuals with myriad psychological and medical conditions as well as individuals in the health care field.[69,70]

Recently, mechanisms for stress reduction through the use of meditation, particularly for control of pain, have been introduced to patients with positive results. These techniques are being adopted by the health care institutions, introducing processes to support coping strategies among employees. Furthermore, these innovations are now emerging in medical schools and the nursing education communities as support for students and residents.[10,71]

Mindful meditation builds on the mindfulness attribute by incorporating quiet time with becoming a calm observer of one's own thoughts and feelings.[55] It can decrease stress, cortisol levels, blood pressure, and the risk of heart attack as well as help improve resilience and decrease inflammation. Mindful meditation stimulates the parasympathetic nervous system and quiets the frantic neurological activity in the amygdala.[72] Over time, this shift begins to strengthen new neural pathways transiting the brain away from a reactive state and toward a calming one.[66]

There are many resources in the literature on how to meditate but it doesn't need to be difficult.[55,68–70] Think of it as a time-out. Simply having students close their eyes, focus on their breathing and clear their thoughts can be relaxing and rejuvenating.

Healthy Lifestyles

Eating right, getting plenty of sleep, and making time for exercise are critical for the body to effectively combat stress, and yet they are often the first things that get thrown to the wayside when individuals get stressed out. Reminders of these basic tenets seem rudimentary but are an important part of the student's ability to learn and the faculty's ability to be effective.

Following a healthy diet will fuel the mind and body. A body that is nutritionally sound is a resilient body and is far better equipped to deal with and recover from stress.[55] A healthy diet also supports cognitive function, immunity, and energy levels. The goals should be to avoid excessive consumption of high carbohydrate, high fat, and processed foods, and instead concentrate on fruits, vegetables, healthy fats, and proteins. These healthy foods will keep blood sugar at an equilibrium and avoid wild swings. Healthy nutritional choices support positive mental energy, clarity, and mood stability.[73]

Exercise is crucial to effectively cope with stress and is one of the most important human functions. Forty percent of adults in America don't participate in any leisure time physical activity. Less than one-third of adults exercise at least 30 minutes most days. Physical activity at least three times a week will positively affect mood and reduce stress by increasing endorphins and serotonin and breaking down cortisol in the blood stream.[74] Exercise improves immune functions and contributes to psychological and emotional wellness.[55]

Sleep is vital to cognitive function and performance as previously discussed. Quality of sleep impacts moods. Sleep deprivation causes greater feelings of fatigue, anger, and hostility, and also impairs decision-making and alertness.[5,37,39] Most sources state at least 7-8 hours of sleep a night is necessary for adequate restoration. Consistent lack of sleep can decrease the ability to adapt to stressful situations.

Although all of these adaptive coping mechanisms are important to overall wellness, studies show that, for students, a sense of humor and a support system are probably the best stress reducers for dealing with new situations.[75,76]

Humor

Studies have shown the health benefit of humor.[75] A good hearty laugh can help to reduce stress, lower blood pressure, elevate mood, boost the immune system, improve brain functioning, protect the heart, make people feel closer to others, and foster instant relaxation. Humor is cathartic, can reduce fear and anxiety, offer alternative perspectives, and simply make people feel good. Research has shown that laughter decreases stress hormones and increases infection-fighting antibodies. Humor has been recognized by nurse researchers as a therapeutic intervention known to have positive psychological and physiological outcomes for patients.[76] Although sometimes overlooked, humor may be useful to the graduate student for mediating stress. It can facilitate moving into new roles, promote insight, help bring new situations into perspective, and promote more effective coping.

Despite the fact that humor and laughter have tremendous clinical potential, little attention has been given to the subject of using humor in graduate and postgraduate education. Wanzer and colleagues[77] noted that the inclusion of humor does not ensure that learning will occur. However, the appropriate and timely use of humor can augment teaching by increasing students' interest and attention and by reducing anxiety about subjects such as statistics and research methods. Humor reduces stress; increases motivation; improves morale, enjoyment, comprehension, interest, and rapport; and facilitates the transfer of knowledge and socialization into the profession.

The role of humor in education continues to be debated, and empirical studies have mixed results. Sapolsky[43] asserts that humor is vital to encourage critical thinking in students. Furthermore, humor has the potential to be a powerful method of motivating students and increasing cognitive ability. Studies of brain activity show that people who engage in humor exhibit similar brain activity as people who are engaged in divergent thinking.[75] Laughter has also been theorized as serving as a social function to help people identify with a group. Humor is an acceptable way of releasing tension and nervous energy.

Peer Support

Among protective resources that build positive coping strategies are social support relationships. Social support has been associated with beneficial outcomes for both mental and physical health. Support comes from a number of places, but peer support is the single, most effective mechanism for both faculty and students. Students seek out the support of their significant others, families, advisors, and mentors, but the largest number of students—over 80%—turn to their peers. The students' satisfaction levels for graduate student groups and peer support groups (where available) are among the highest valued resources.[12] Due to the time-consuming nature of anesthesia school, students often rely heavily on their classmates for support.[6,7,42]

A peer support program can take several forms. It might consist of a formal group of volunteer graduate students who meet regularly with students and work with department faculty as well. An informal "big buddy" mentorship program that partners every first-year graduate student with an experienced upperclassman also exists at many institutions. Many students are using social media as well as official and unofficial online SRNA/CRNA groups as their main source of peer support. As a first contact, the peer is often able to direct the student to a more knowledgeable faculty member or other individual resource and provide the student with the encouragement needed to seek help. All of these programs rely on the fact that students feel much more comfortable discussing their concerns with a peer they trust than they do with faculty, administrators, or mental health providers. Even more valuable, however, is that these programs allow students to get support without having to explicitly ask for it.[78,79]

Peer credibility tends to be based on firsthand knowledge and expertise. The strength of peer support groups lies in enhancing the effectiveness of existing counseling systems and providing a supporting link for successful self-care and improved health and wellness.[26]

Peer support programs by definition involve student-student interactions; however, the creation and success of these programs will require a great deal of faculty support, including seeking out interested clinical instructors and recent graduate students. Students must know that their advisors and their department both support participation and involvement in peer support programs. In a national study on the lifestyles of graduate students, most students placed a high value on good relationships that enable students to learn from the perceptions, experiences, and challenges of their comrades.[13] These relationships also provided an emotional release from academic intensity.

Program directors should keep in mind that the goal is not to eliminate all stress but to help students develop a variety of skills to cope with the negative aspects of stress. **Table 3.5** lists some specific student coping strategies.

Table 3.5 Student Coping Strategies

- Ask faculty members to help you set academic priorities.
- Break the work into pieces by setting small goals.
- Study in groups to prevent burnout and feeling isolated.
- Use relaxation techniques, eg, meditation and deep-breathing exercises.
- Manage time wisely.
- Join a student support group.
- Learn positive self-talk.
- Take care of yourself by eating right, getting enough sleep, and exercising.
- Ask for help.

Regrettably, even when the resources are available, not everyone copes effectively. If students try strategies for coping and still experience the negative aspects of stress, faculty should encourage students to seek professional counseling or therapy. This suggestion will more likely be received and acted on if a good relationship between the teacher and student already exists. Students should be made aware of professional counseling availability during orientation and periodically as needed.

A preventive approach involves giving people realistic warnings, recommendations, and reassurances. There is little research in the field of higher education that describes how best to inform students about the challenges. More research is needed to identify why and how teacher-student relationships deteriorate and to help faculty construct more successful relationships. Conversely, students should make efforts to behave respectfully toward faculty, staff, and peers and should willingly take responsibility for their behavior.

Maladaptive Coping

Maladaptive or negative coping strategies help to perpetuate problem situations. The inappropriate behavior may reduce distress immediately but is dysfunctional and can have profound lifelong implications and also become addictive. For example, avoiding situations because of unrealistic fears may initially reduce anxiety, but it is non-productive in alleviating the actual problem long term. These habits are difficult to change. Maladaptive coping methods include:

- isolation
- binge eating or undereating
- workaholic tendencies
- violent behavior
- angry intimidation of others
- use of drugs or alcohol
- other types of self-destructive behavior like cutting or attempting suicide

The ability to recognize these maladaptive behaviors is fundamental to seeking healthier alternative solutions. Using these types of ineffective coping mechanisms to deal with stress can put the anesthesia provider at both personal and professional risk, including potentially harming a patient, loved one, or self.

Isolation

According to Freud, isolation involves a mental gap or barrier between some threatening cognition and other thoughts and feelings.[80] Isolation is a maladaptive defense that does not actually remove the threatening idea but minimizes its impact by repressing it. Students suffering from this maladaptive coping technique may seem disengaged or aloof. They often deal with threatening situations in a minimal, rushed, or superficial fashion seemingly unphased by their stressful situation. A student presenting with this maladaptive coping style can be extremely frustrating for faculty as they seem unconcerned with their mistakes or performance. This coping style can be the undoing of a student as poor evaluations and a seemingly nonchalant attitude do not put them in a positive light. Faculty need to be aware of this coping mechanism and address unusual responses to stressful situations early.

Binge Eating or Undereating

A healthy diet is necessary for optimal performance of mind and body. Unfortunately, when under stress, overeating or undereating are frequent maladaptive behaviors. Although moderate weight gain or loss during a rigorous nurse anesthesia program is often expected, extreme changes in weight should be addressed and professional counseling offered, if necessary.

Workaholic Tendencies

Nurse anesthesia is a rigorous program of study and faculty want and need students to work hard. However, when students are working continuously because of fear of failure and become too unbalanced, this tendency can actually increase stress and decrease productivity. There is evidence in the literature that supports a range of practices such as setting limits and developing healthy habits that encourage self-care and enhance balance.[25,52,55] Ignoring self-care and other responsibilities increase problems in personal relationships and, therefore, stress. Working continuously can lead to difficulty in sleeping and fatigue, which can lead to using alcohol, drugs, or chemicals in order to get needed rest and relaxation. Once drugs become habitual to relax at night, opposing drugs are often needed to elevate the mood or wake up to go to class or the clinical area. This behavior can result in problematic social behavior such as withdrawal, aggression, and possible addiction. With this cycle of behavior, the ability to quickly develop a reasonable solution to problems is progressively affected and when constructive or critical criticism is given regarding a poor decision, the response is overreaction. The ability to recognize that one is making poor decisions is not easily recognized and leads to greater difficulty with coping.[81] Discussion about the importance of balance with students is imperative to their well-being. Faculty should also examine their life-work balance and make adjustments as necessary.

Anger and Violence

Anger is often a symptom of stress and a maladaptive coping mechanism. Hanging on to anger, road rage, and lashing out at a classmate, colleague, or patient are examples of this ineffective coping skill. This behavior not only endangers the individual, but it can also lead to dismissal or getting fired. If signs of violence are brought to the attention of faculty, immediate professional intervention is necessary. Basic ways to improve angry behavior include daily exercise, taking time out to cool off before reacting, and talking it out with loved ones and friends. Anger and violence are not effective coping mechanisms, and if simple interventions are not effective, referring the individual to anger management classes or professional counseling may be necessary.

Substance Use

Alcohol and substance misuse are very common maladaptive behaviors. How often do people say after a stressful day, "I need a drink"? The anesthesia profession and the life of an anesthesia student are filled with stressful days. Larsson et al[62] described the stress and difficult working environment of anesthesia students as "considerable" with many of the trainees describing feelings of insufficiency, inadequacy, and having difficulty adjusting to the professional role. To complicate the situation even further, high performance demands, perception of poor performance, decreased time with family, and the chronic fatigue and lack of control that come with being a student can lead to low self-esteem, overwhelming stress, and physical and psychological symptoms like illness or depression that can potentially increase the risk of substance abuse. Although stress in itself does not cause substance abuse, the literature suggests it can increase the risk.[1,62] Substance abuse has long been recognized as the primary occupational hazard for anesthesia providers and CRNA faculty and SRNAs need to be aware of the risk and potential consequences.[26,82] Multiple studies have shown that stress can lead to drug misuse in vulnerable individuals and increase drug craving and relapse for the drug seeker.[26,83–86]

It is estimated that 10% to as high as 15% of all health care professionals will misuse drugs or alcohol at some time during their careers in an attempt to deal with stress. Specialties such as anesthesia, emergency medicine, and psychiatry appear to have higher rates of substance abuse, most likely related to baseline provider personalities and functioning in a highly stressful, risk-prone environment with easy access to drugs.[33,87] The concepts of substance misuse and addiction are not new to the medical and nursing communities. It is considered the most common occupational hazard for anesthesia practice.[26] The nurse anesthesia profession has addressed the problem since the early 1980s, offering educational resources, peer support, and more recently the AANA Health and Wellness Program to assist CRNAs and students.[26,84] Substance abuse and chemical dependency among Certified Registered Nurse Anesthetists have been reported in the literature at the rate of 10%,[36] and perhaps as high as 23%.[88]

Colleagues are often the first to recognize an impaired practitioner and the last to address the concern. Often, they will make excuses, overlook obvious symptoms, and cover up for mistakes. This attitude and enabling behavior by coworkers is prevalent throughout the profession and contribute to the ongoing concerns for professional well-being. The substance abuse problem among nurse anesthesia professionals, along with prevention recommendations and treatment modalities, is extensively documented by Quinlan[26] in *A Professional Study and Resource Guide for the CRNA*. An analysis of the addictive disease process, behaviors, consequences of abuse, and recommendations for implementing educational programs, interventional policies, and tools to deal with the impaired professional can be found in the highly recommended text, *Substance Abuse Policies for Anesthesia,* by Higgins Roche.[50] Resource articles and information are also abundantly available under the peer assistance section of the AANA website, www.aana.com.

Complaints in the past have been that, despite the increased educational efforts, prevention, and awareness initiatives, there were not consistent mechanisms to address intervention, treatment, and reentry into the workforce.[87] In response, the literature on this topic has been exploding and the AANA Peer Assistance webpage has consolidated resources to assist clinical CRNAs as well as educators and students. A new AANA position statement has been published on Addressing Substance Use Disorder in the Anesthesia Profession. Guidelines for developing a facility program can be found at www.aana.com/SUDWorkplaceResources. The website includes resources on drug diversion, prevention, drug testing, educational resources, sample contracts and policies, safe intervention, treatment, reporting, and reentry to clinical practice. Established policies and procedures are important and should be understood and adhered to if students and Certified Registered Nurse Anesthetists are to recognize the problem and take necessary action in assisting themselves and their colleagues. For example, many nurse anesthesia programs are now requiring mandatory drug screens on their students. Brozimowski, et al[54] surveyed nurse anesthesia programs regarding the five-year period of 2008–2012. They found that 48.94% of responding programs performed drug testing for cause during their program and 14.89% did random drug testing during the program.[54] This trend is definitely increasing. In a recent survey of nurse anesthesia program directors, 53% reported toxicology screening on students prior to acceptance into the program, 37.3% reported random screening during the clinical phase, and 72.3% reported toxicology screening policies in place for cause.[5] A policy and student signed consent form for drug screening should be a part of the nurse anesthesia program orientation process.

Successful reentry to anesthesia practice or anesthesia training is possible with support, an established department policy, and a well-formed reentry plan.[89,90] It is important that the profession put public safety first with the removal of addicted providers until their safe return can be assured.[90] Anesthesia providers have a relapse rate of 25%-56%, which is similar to other health care specialties,[82] so it is imperative that a safe and well-documented plan be followed. Hamza and Monroe[90] discussed components that are frequently cited in the pro-reentry literature as necessary for success: a solid foundation in a 12-step program; participation in the state's monitoring program (if applicable); attendance at Health Care Professional's Caduceus support group meetings; a work-site monitor; random drug screens; a back-to-work contract; naltrexone use; and no overtime.

In response to a request for easy-to-find information on this topic, the AANA Peer Assistance Advisors have published reentry recommendations for anesthesia professionals or students on www.aanaPeerAssistance.com.[91-109] They have also published information wallet cards with the hotline phone number as well as warning signs of substance use disorder. These cards are available for nurse anesthesia programs to request for their students and faculty.

Advanced practice nurses have a high incidence of disciplinary action by regulatory boards, and impaired Certified Registered Nurse Anesthetists are at risk for loss of their licenses and ability to practice. Moreover, institutional, state, and federal guidelines to address impaired professionals often include conflicting ethical and legal components. Although many states have alternative disciplinary programs that address the impaired professional,[33,84,90] there is great variability in these models. Health care professionals face the stigma and prejudices associated with addiction, as well as loss of license, careers, and, all too often, their lives. It is imperative that faculty, students, and professional colleagues understand the stressors, risks, and coping mechanisms related to working in the nurse anesthesia profession.

Suicide

Suicide is a tragic and highly complex health issue which is usually the result of a combination of risk factors such as personal history, stressors, disrupted social network, judgment factors, and access to lethal means.[91] Nurses are four times more likely to commit suicide compared with people working outside medicine, and doctors are twice as likely to kill themselves compared with people working in other professions.[33] Chipas et al[7] reported 47% of student registered nurse anesthetists reported depression and 21% reported suicidal ideations. In a 2015 survey by the Health and Wellness Committee,[5] nurse anesthesia program directors reported 15% of SRNAs had suicide ideations with 20 deaths of SRNAs, CRNAs, or recent graduates over the last five years.

The problem is real and faculty need to be on the lookout for at-risk students. Events causing shame, guilt, and loss of status, feelings of rejection/abandonment, feelings of hopelessness, and patterns of increased alcohol or drug use all have been shown to contribute to depression and potentially suicidal ideation.[91] The Substance Abuse and Mental Health Services Administration (www.samhsa.gov) has excellent resource information for faculty and students. The Mental and Emotional Well-Being section on the AANA wellness page also has resource information including recognizing warning signs and how to get help.[110] Regardless of the circumstances, any reference to suicide should be taken seriously. These students should not be left alone and be referred to appropriate mental health professionals.

Active and Reactive Coping

Coping strategies can be either active or reactive. Active coping (dealing with the actual stressful situations or events) can be strengthened by providing students with clear expectations, early success, and positive support.[30] Authoritarian behavior of the instructor has an important influence on student motivation and autonomy and must be balanced with support and caring. Both are interrelated with student satisfaction.

Reactive coping (dealing with one's own thoughts and feelings) can be facilitated by offering accessible professional and peer counseling, student support groups, and adequate faculty advising. Faculty should attempt to challenge students, but not so much that they lose their motivation, spontaneity, and initiative. The following suggestions can help minimize sources of student stress: communicate explicit expectations and responsibilities for students; develop a positive interactive relationship with students; allow students to have at least a modicum sense of control over their student roles; treat students as individuals rather than as a generalized whole; and assist students to learn stress-coping strategies.

Although institutions of higher education have recognized the varied needs for support that must be provided to undergraduates, there is often a lack for support of graduate students who face issues that are different, but are no less complex or challenging. Similarly, there are few graduate educator support systems available to address faculty distress.[9] Methods of coping commonly used by faculty may be classified into two major categories: primarily preventive strategies and primarily combative strategies, as shown in **Table 3.6.**

Table 3.6 Faculty Coping Methods

Preventive	Combative
• Avoid stressors: develop more nurturing relationships, find a more suitable job, attempt to create a more rewarding work environment • Manage the self-imposed expectations and demands • Change stress-inducing ways and recognize unproductive behaviors • Augment personal coping resources	• Monitor stress: be aware of stress-related symptoms • Marshall personal resources • Take action to reduce the stressor: be assertive, refuse inappropriate requests for additional responsibilities • Develop tolerance for unavoidable stress; cognitively restructure the situation • Lower stress-arousal stressor or block it out

Preventive and combative strategies are active coping mechanisms. There are many healthy ways to manage and cope with stress. Many strategies focus on changing the situation or changing the individual's reaction. Preventive strategies concentrate on maintaining realistic self-expectations, recognizing unproductive stress-inducing ways of behaving, and learning to monitor stress-related symptoms and triggering events.

Combative strategies are active measures that promote assertive approaches to reducing stress. Positive actions to assist in managing stress include cognitive restructuring techniques; development of personal resources, positive attitudes and resilience; and actively finding alternative ways of responding to stressful situations.

Critical Incident Stress Management

Although occupational stress exists in all work situations, the intensity and emotional demands of the health care environment place exceptionally high performance expectations and stress on health care providers, including students. Stress associated with dramatic, emotionally overwhelming situations, known as critical incidents, have the potential to exhaust professionals' normal coping mechanisms. A critical incident is any event that causes an unusually intense stress reaction. In health care, it is typically related to a breakdown in a system or process, instead of negligence of one individual.[92–94] Critical incidents and adverse events are often discussed together. An adverse event is a complication, unintended injury, or patient harm that results in a prolonged hospital stay, disability, or death.[94] These events are typically caused by an overlap of system and human error rather than by the patient's underlying disease process.[92] Regardless of the cause, the distress that people experience after such events limits their ability to cope, impairs their ability to adjust, and negatively affects the work or learning environment. Examples of traumatic or adverse events that produce such reactions include the loss of a patient, a coworker's or student's death or serious illness, suicide, or a violent or threatening incident in the work setting.

Anesthesia programs spend a tremendous amount of time throughout their curriculum teaching students how to avoid a crisis and how to manage one if it occurs, but spend very little time discussing how to handle the aftermath of adverse events[95,96] Recent studies [95,96] have shown that an extremely high percentage of anesthesia providers have been involved in at least one unanticipated death or serious injury of a perioperative patient over their career.[95,96] Most providers in these studies experienced guilt, anxiety, sleeplessness, depression, and reliving of the event. They required time to recover emotionally with many acknowledging they never fully recovered and considered a career change. Although respondents believed their ability to provide patient care was compromised in the immediate hours after the event, very few were given time off.[96]

It is important for the wellness of both nurse anesthesia students and faculty to have a plan in place to deal with these types of events when they occur. Critical incident stress management (CISM) consists of a range of crisis intervention services that usually address preparing for an incident, the reactions that immediately follow, and the possible long-term effects from experiencing a critical incident.[94,97] Critical incident stress management aims to reduce the intensity of an individual's emotional, mental, physical, and behavioral reactions to a crisis (**Table 3.7**). It also helps individuals return to their level of functioning before the crisis, develop new coping skills, and eliminate ineffective, inappropriate ways of coping, such as social withdrawal, isolation, and substance abuse.

Table 3.7 Common Reactions to Traumatic Events

Type of Reaction	Common Reactions
Emotional/Psychological	Fear, anger, guilt, grief, drug or alcohol abuse, loss of trust, irritability, anxiety
Mental/Cognitive	Difficulty concentrating, confusion, nightmares, feeling distracted
Physical	Headaches, dizziness, fatigue, stomach problems
Behavioral	Sleep problems, loss of/increased appetite, isolation, restlessness, drug or alcohol abuse

Adapted with permission from MITSS (Medically Induced Trauma Support Services), www.mitss.org.

Critical incident stress debriefing (CISD) is probably the best known component of CISM.[97,98] Professionally conducted debriefings help people cope with and recover from the aftereffects of a critical incident. Not only does CISD enable participants to understand that they are not alone in their reactions to a distressing event, it also provides them with an opportunity to discuss their thoughts and feelings in a controlled, safe environment. Optimally, CISD should occur within 24 to 72 hours of a critical incident.

Psychological recovery from critical incidents often takes weeks or months and is severely hampered by lack of support.[95,99] Encouraging students to express their feelings is critical and will be more likely if a good relationship between teacher and student already exists. Having students express their feelings will also be more likely if teachers understand what stress is and the ramifications of their dealing poorly with a student's inability to cope.

Ensuring that student registered nurse anesthetists have the resources to effectively cope after these events is paramount to their success. There are multiple resources available to assist providers, faculty, and students dealing with critical incidents. European anesthesiologists published guidelines for dealing with the aftermath of anesthetic catastrophes and advise against underestimating the psychological impact on staff following the death or serious injury of an operative patient.[95] Medically Induced Trauma Support Services (MITSS) is a nonprofit organization whose mission is to support healing and restore hope to patients, families, and clinicians impacted by medical errors and adverse medical events at http://www.mitsstools.org.[100] The Adverse Event Protocol available on The Anesthesia Patient Safety Foundation website suggests a series of steps to minimize patient injury and identify the cause of an adverse anesthesia event after it occurs.[100] The AANA has also published guidelines and information cards for adverse events/critical incident stress management to support those anesthesia providers or students impacted by critical incidents in their career. These guidelines are available on the AANA website as AANA Adverse Medical Events/Critical Incidents-How to Cope. They can also be accessed without signing in at www.aana.com/AdverseEvents.

Education on how to handle the aftermath of critical incidents and adverse events, including formal support structures, should be provided to students at all levels of training.[95] In addition, faculty should be on the lookout for students who may need professional intervention and encourage open communication after any critical incident.

Health and Wellness Curriculum Resources

The number of health and wellness resources available to CRNAs and SRNAs increases daily. One of the goals of the AANA Health and Wellness Committee is to consolidate resources for CRNAs and SRNAs on these topics. The main pages for wellness and peer assistance can be accessed directly at www.aanaWellness.com[3] and www.aanaPeerAssistance.com.[109] There are so many resources now on these pages that the AANA Health and Wellness Committee has created a series of short URLs for quick access.[101] A few of the most commonly used ones are listed in **Table 3.8**.

Table 3.8 Shortcut URLs for Anesthesia Wellness and Peer Assistance Resources

Below is a list of short URLs for quick access:
• www.aanaWellness.com (main page, quick links to topics)
• www.aana.com/Physical
• www.aana.com/MentalWellbeing
• www.aanacom/WorkplaceWellness
• www.aana.com/Stress
• www.aana.com/AdverseEvents
• www.aana.com/bullying
• www.aana.com/domesticviolence
• www.aanaPeerAssistance.com (main page, quick links to topics)
• www.aana.com/sudworkplaceresources
• www.aana.com/addressingsud
•www.aana.com/SignsandBehaviors
•www.aana.com/GettingHelp
• www.aana.com/SUD
• www.aana.com/Intervention
• www.aana.com/Treatment
• www.aana.com/Reentry
• www.aana.com/AIR (Anesthetists in Recovery online support group)

Source: Rice J, Uranga T. Reflections on health and wellness. *AANA NewsBulletin*. November 2015:24–25.

On the main AANA website www.aana.com under the resources tab, there is a robust health and wellness section that includes peer assistance, information on how to get help, state health and wellness resources, student wellness, and wellness milestones. There is also an extensive "favorite finds" list which includes links to research articles and published resources, CRNA Speakers on Wellness and Substance Use Disorder, Getting Peer Assistance Help for Yourself and Others, Jan Stewart Memorial Wellness Lecture Series, Stress and Nurse Anesthesia Professionals, Student Wellness Connection, Workplace Wellness, and much more.[3] The Wearing Masks series can also be found in this section under favorite finds or by accessing www.aana.com/WearingMasks. This series highlights the dangers of substance use disorders from the perspective of actual anesthesia providers and families who have endured its consequences.[81] The series was originally distributed in a complimentary DVD format but is now available online, courtesy of the University of Minnesota School of Nursing, nurse anesthesia area of study. It is also available to download on a university learning platform such as BlackBoard. The Wearing Masks series was produced over a 13-year period with a total of 11 video segments and over three hours of content. Each segment is relatively short so faculty can assign viewing sessions for self-study with return to the classroom for discussion. A syllabus that faculty can individualize to their specific needs is also provided.[3] Another resource available on the website is the video Making Lemonade: One CRNA's story of Addiction and Recovery by Anita Bertrand, CRNA. This video can be played in class for students or as a homework assignment with follow-up discussion.

The literature supports the fact that education has been proven effective in substance abuse prevention[102–104] with many others stating it is a key component in prevention.[28,45,105–107] A January 2010 program director (PD) survey found that 89% of PDs would incorporate a standardized wellness and chemical dependency curriculum that "included all instructional, reading, media, and testing materials if it was provided."[83] However, comments in this survey from individual PDs indicated there was still significant resistance to making this curriculum a mandatory requirement. The Wellness and Chemical Dependency Task force was formed in 2010 by then AANA board of directors to examine the idea of a standardized wellness and chemical dependency curriculum for nurse anesthesia programs. Task force members included past AANA President Terry Wicks, the late Arthur Zwerling, Tony Chipas, Gary Clark, Sandy Tunajek, Adrienne Hartgerink, and then student representative Michael Lord. Although the task force originally had over 16 hours of material, a repeat survey of program directors by Hartgerink[4] in 2010 found that most programs felt 5–10 hours dedicated to this topic was adequate given other programmatic time constraints. The task force eventually developed six health and wellness modules including post-tests that became available in January 2013 (listed in **Table 3.9**).

Table 3.9 Health and Wellness Modules

Module 1	Health and Wellness: The Role and Responsibility of the Anesthesia Professional
Module 2	Stress: Understanding Causes and Consequences
Module 3	Stressors Encountered in the Healthcare System and How to Cope More Effectively
Module 4	Risk & Exposure: The Signs, Symptoms, Pathophysiology and Co-morbidities of Substance Abuse
Module 5	Management of Chemical Dependency & Addiction
Module 6	Understanding the Environment for Successful Building & Sustaining of a Personal Wellness Plan

Available at http://www.aana.com/resources2/health-wellness/Pages/Wellness-and-Chemical-Dependency-Curriculum.aspx

The availability of these modules coincided with the COA requirement that evidence- based wellness and substance use disorder information be taught in nurse anesthesia educational programs. The modules cover the five topic areas the COA states could be included in a wellness and substance use curriculum: importance of wellness to the health care professional; healthy lifestyles; coping mechanisms; identification and intervention of substance use disorder; and reentry into the workplace after treatment for substance use disorder.[36] The modules are available on www.aanalearn.com and are updated periodically to assure information is current. They are appropriate for both students and faculty. Students receive a discounted rate and can work through the modules individually or in class to facilitate discussion.

Faculty are encouraged to take time to investigate the myriad resources available on the website. There is a section entitled Ideas for Presenting the Wellness and Chemical Dependency Curriculum that faculty may find helpful. Additional health and wellness videos, articles, and modules are continually being added to the library of resources available to faculty and students.

Summary

Historically, the physical changes in response to stress were an essential adaptation for meeting natural threats. Likewise, in today's world the stress response can be an asset for raising levels of performance during critical events such as graduate school, job interviews, important meetings, or in situations of actual danger or crisis. However, if stress becomes persistent, all parts of the body's functional ability (brain, heart, lungs, vessels, and muscles) become chronically overworked or underworked. This may produce physical or psychological damage over time. Short-term acute distress can also be harmful if it leads to inappropriate behaviors.

Stress is not itself an illness but is a condition that can give rise to real illness. Various psychological and behavioral changes affecting work performance and interpersonal relationships may be noticed by colleagues, including inability to concentrate, overworking, irritability or aggression, becoming withdrawn or unsociable, or reluctance to accept constructive criticism and advice. The long-term consequences of stress include cynicism, apathy, depression, emotional exhaustion, hostility, alcohol and substance abuse, obsessive compulsive disorders, and other dissociative behavioral patterns.

The nurse anesthesia profession needs a proactive, supportive, structured process designed to assist student registered nurse anesthetists in dealing with the multiple stressors inherent to their education. Nurse anesthesia educational leaders should keep in mind that the goal is not to eliminate all stress, but to help students develop a variety of skills to cope with the negative aspects of stress related to education. The guiding principle of stress reduction is a preventive approach so that the negative aspects of stress can be avoided. Raising awareness and giving students' realistic warnings, recommendations, and reassurances supported by constructive feedback improves faculty-student relationships. Although the faculty cannot be responsible for the overall well-being of students, faculty members do have a responsibility to recognize signs of stress and to help students deal with a stressful issue in a constructive manner.

Faculty should provide active intervention, establish student support groups, and employ mechanisms to reduce stress. For example, faculty can avoid continual reference to the national certification examination, provide positive and frequent feedback in a constructive and honest manner, specify expectations, and assist students to understand that learning clinical skills and new technologies are progressive steps on the path to success.

As the role of graduate education in our society continues to evolve, the needs of graduate students are changing, too. Support for student registered nurse anesthetists can no longer be restricted to academic and financial issues. The program must also consider how it might help students deal with the pressures and stresses of graduate school.

The profession's move to doctoral education for entry into practice has the potential to further increase the workload and challenges for programs, students, and faculty. Faculty who are distressed will be less effective in what they do. Stress can obstruct teaching and empathetic listening. Tension and ill health can undermine job performance. Most of all, faculty should not only have a thorough understanding of stress but also demonstrate the ability to implement appropriate practices in their own lives, thus modeling positive stress management for their students. Healthy stress management is one of the most important lifelong learning skills that any individual may acquire.

Students should be proactive and advocate for their educational programs to address self-care issues because the management of stress is associated with less professional burnout, greater job satisfaction, enhanced academic performance, and better mental and physical health. It is also important for graduate students to take active steps to remain healthy and fit for duty.

As health care practitioners, the more we know and understand about stress, the more proactive we all can become in achieving balance and perspective in our professional careers. Stress prevention and coping strategies are important to understand if we are to have meaningful discussions regarding health and well-being with all those who participate in education be they students, teachers, administrators, or policy makers.

Occupational stress, burnout, and fatigue are risks to the anesthesia profession. The ability to develop effective coping strategies, and avoid the maladaptive, increases professional satisfaction and personal wellness. Ineffective coping and unrecognized risk can lead to depression, substance use disorder, or even suicide.

Although it is impossible to change the stress that comes with anesthesia education or the inherent personalities that individuals bring, it is possible to improve the knowledge that students and educators have on how to better arm themselves to cope with stress, to recognize the vulnerabilities, and to control the risk factors. Hopefully this knowledge will help anesthesia students and providers avoid the pitfalls of destructive behavior through recognizing the importance of wellness and stress management.

References

1. Chipas A, McKenna D. Stress and burnout in nurse anesthesia. *AANA J.* 2011;79(2):122–128.
2. Tunajek S. Moving forward by looking back. *AANA NewsBull.* July 2014:38–39.
3. Health & Wellness and Peer Assistance. American Association of Nurse Anesthetists. http://www.aana.com/resources2/health-wellness/Pages/default.aspx. Accessed January 15, 2016.
4. Hartgerink AG. Overcoming barriers to instituting a Wellness and Chemical Dependency Curriculum (WCD) in Nurse Anesthesia Educational Programs. [capstone project] 2011.
5. American Association of Nurse Anesthetists. Nurse Anesthesia Educational Programs—Survey of Wellness Curriculum. [survey] November 2015–January 2016. Park Ridge, IL.
6. Swanlund E. Personal communication. October 11, 2015.
7. Chipas A, Cordrey D, Floyd D, Grubbs L, Miller S, Tyre B. Stress: perceptions, manifestations, and coping mechanisms of student registered nurse anesthetists. *AANA J.* 2012;(80)4(Spec ed):S49–S55.
8. Beck DL, Hackett MB, Srivastava R, McKim E, Rockwell B. Perceived level and sources of stress in university professional schools. *J Nurs Educ.* 1997;36(4):180–186.
9. Benjamin L, Walz GR. Counseling Students and Faculty for Stress Management. Ann Arbor, MI: ERIC Clearinghouse on Counseling and Personnel Services; 1987. ERIC Document Reproduction Service ED279917.
10. Finkelstein C, Brownstein A, Scott C, Lan YL. Anxiety and stress reduction in medical education: an intervention. *Med Educ.* 2007;41(3):258–264.
11. Jones MC, Johnston DW. Reducing distress in first level and student nurses: a review of the applied stress management literature. *J Adv Nurs.* 2000;32(1):66–74.
12. Perez E, Carroll-Perez I. A national study: stress perception by nurse anesthesia students. *AANA J.* 1999;67(1):79–86.
13. Repak N. Emotional fatigue: coping with academic pressure. Grad Resources. http://www.gradresources.org/articles/emotional_fatigue.shtml. Accessed Sept 26, 2016.
14. Kless JR. Use of a support group to reduce student stress in a nurse anesthesia program. *AANA J.* 1989;57(1):75–77.
15. Wildgust BM. Stress in the anesthesia student. *AANA J.* 1986;54(3):272–278.
16. Misra R, McKean M, West S, Russo T. Academic stress of college students: comparison of student and faculty perceptions. *Coll Student J.* 2000;34:236–245.
17. Kieffer Phillips J. Exploring student nurse anesthetist stressors and coping using grounded theory methodology. *AANA J.* 2010;78(6):474–482.
18. Martin-Sheridan D. Factors that influenced six nurse anesthesia programs to close. *AANA J.* 1998;66(4):377–384.
19. Horton BJ. The importance of mentoring in recruiting and retaining junior faculty. *AANA J.* 2003;71(3):189–195.

20. Shirey M. Stress and burnout in nursing faculty. *Nurse Educ.* 2006;31(3):95–97.

21. McLean J. Forgotten faculty: stress and job satisfaction among distance educators. *Online J Distance Learning Adm.* 2006;9(2):1-8. http://www.westga.edu/~distance/ojdla/summer92/mclean92.htm. Accessed September 29, 2016.

22. Davies M, Spence Laschinger HK, Andrusyszyn M. Clinical educators' empowerment, job tension, and job satisfaction. *J Nurses Staff Dev.* 2006;22(2):78–86.

23. McCall WG, Alves SL, Brooks DY, Fallacaro MD, Gray GC, Ritter D. An analysis of factors influencing nurse anesthesia educational program director turnover: 1976–77. *AANA J.* 1997;65(6):537–542.

24. Owens B, Herrick C, Kelly J. A prearranged mentorship program: can it work long distance? *J Prof Nurs.* 1998;14(2):78–84.

25. Tunajek S. Student stress: a question of balance. *AANA NewsBull.* 2006;60(5):20–21.

26. Quinlan D. Peer assistance: part I and part II. In: Foster S, Faut-Callahan M, eds. *A Professional Study and Resource Guide for the CRNA.* Park Ridge, IL: American Association of Nurse Anesthetists; 2001:425–484.

27. Larsson J, Rosenqvist U, Holmstrom I. Being a young and inexperienced trainee anesthetist: A phenomenological study on tough working conditions. *Acta Anesthesiologica Scandinavica.* 2006;50(6):653-658. doi:10.1111/j.1399–6576.2006.01035.x.

28. Luck S, Hedrick J. The alarming trend of substance abuse in anesthesia providers. *J Perianesth Nur.* 2004;19(5):308–311.

29. Ross TK, Gries CA, Nanos J, O'Leary A, Teitler M. The reported incidents of substance abuse among student registered nurse anesthetists in the United States from 1991 through 1996 [abstract]. *AANA J.* 1997;65(5):503.

30. Lazarus R. *Psychological Stress and the Coping Process.* New York, NY: McGraw-Hill; 1966.

31. McKinzie C, Altamura V, Burgoon E, Bishop C. Exploring the effect of stress on mood, self-esteem, and daily habits with psychology graduate students. *Psychol Rep.* 2006;99(2):439–448.

32. Hodgson C, Simoni J. Graduate student academic and psychological functioning. *J Coll Student Dev.* 1995;36(3):244–253.

33. Baldisseri MR. Impaired healthcare professional. *Crit Care Med.* 2007;35(Suppl 2):S106–S116.

34. Neumann Y, Finaly-Neumann E, Reichel A. Determinants and consequences of students' burnout in universities. *J Higher Educ.* 1990;61(1):20–31.

35. Kendrick P. Comparing the effects of stress and relationship style on student and practicing nurse anesthetists. *AANA J.* 2000;68(2):115–122.

36. The Standards for Accreditation of Nurse Anesthesia Educational Programs. Council on Accreditation of Nurse Anesthesia Educational Programs. Park Ridge, IL: American Association of Nurse Anesthetists; 2004 (revised 2016).

37. Biddle C, Aker J. The national study of sleep-related behaviors of nurse anesthetists: personal and professional implications. *AANA J.* 2011;79(4):324–331.

38. Sinha A, Singh A, Tewari A. The fatigued anesthesiologist: a threat to patient safety? *J Anaesthesiol Clin Pharmacol.* 2013;29(2):151–159.

39. Patient Safety: Fatigue, Sleep, and Work Schedule Effects [position statement 2.17]. American Association of Nurse Anesthetists. http://www.aana.com/resources2/professionalpractice/Pages/Patient-Safety-Fatigue-Sleep-and-Work-Schedule-Effects.aspx. Accessed February 10, 2016.

40. Stevens MS. Normal sleep, sleep physiology, and sleep deprivation. Medscape. http://emedicine.medscape.com/article/1188226-overview. Accessed May 10, 2012.

41. Code of Ethics for the Certified Registered Nurse Anesthetist. American Association of Nurse Anesthetists, http://www.aana.com/resources2/professionalpractice/Pages/Code-of-Ethics.aspx. Accessed February 10, 2016.

42. Conner M. Self-efficacy stress, and social support in retention of student registered nurse anesthetists. *AANA J*.2015;83(2):133–138.

43. Sapolsky RM. *Why Zebras Don't Get Ulcers: The Acclaimed Guide to Stress, Stress-Related Diseases, and Coping*. 3rd ed. New York, NY: WH Freeman; 2004.

44. Bandura A. *Social Foundations of Thought and Action: A Social Cognitive Theory*. Englewood Cliffs, NJ: Prentice-Hall; 1986.

45. McDonough JP. Personality, addiction and anesthesia. *AANA J.* 1990;58(3):193–200.

46. Burges N, Savickas M. Personality and medical specialty choice: a literature review and integration. *J Career Assess.* 2002;10(3):362–380.

47. Sandi C, Pinelo-Nava M. Stress and memory: behavioral effects and neurobiological mechanisms. *Neural Plast.* 2007;16(6):1–20.

48. Lupien SJ, Fiocco A, Wan N, et al. Stress hormones and human memory function across the lifespan. *Psychoneuroendocrinology.* 2005;30(3):225–242.

49. McEwen BS, Sapolsky RM. Stress and cognitive function. *Curr Opin Neurobiol.* 1995;5(2):205–216.

50. Higgins Roche BT. *Substance Abuse Policies for Anesthesia.* Winston-Salem, NC: AANA; 2007.

51. Tunajek S. Why wellness? *AANA NewsBull.* September 2009. http://www.aana.com/resources2/health-wellness/Pages/Wellness-Milestones.aspx.

52. Benfield W. The power of balance in the aspiring anesthetist. *AANA NewsBull.* January 2016. http://www.aana.com/resources2/health-wellness/Pages/Wellness-Milestones.aspx.

53. Uranga T. Occupational stress and the resilience to overcome, *AANA NewsBull.* July 2015. http://www.aana.com/resources2/health-wellness/Pages/Wellness-Milestones.aspx.

54. Bozimowski G, Groh C, Rouen P, Dosch M. The prevalence and patterns of substance abuse among nurse anesthesia students. *AANA J.* 2014;82(4): 277–283.

55. Hartgerink A, Switzman J. Self-Care techniques for a balanced body and mind. *AANA NewsBull.* March 2016:32–33.

56. Polk LV. Toward a middle-range theory of resilience. *ANS Adv NursSci.* 1997;19(3):1–13.

57. Gillespie BM, Chaboyer W, Wallis M. Development of a theoretically derived model of resilience through concept analysis. *Contemp Nurse*. 2007;25(1–2):124–135.

58. Gillespie BM, Chaboyer W, Wallis M, Grimbeek P. Resilience in the operating room: developing and testing of a resilience model. *J Adv Nurs*. 2007;59(4):427–438. doi:10.1111/j.1365–2648.2007. 04340.x

59. Gates GS. Teaching-related stress: the emotional management of faculty. *Rev Higher Educ*. 2000;23(4):469–490.

60. Cragg CE, Andrusyszyn MA. Humbert, J. Experience with technology and preferences for distance learning delivery methods in a nurse practitioner program. *J Distance Learning*. 1999;14(1):1–13.

61. Bower, BL. Distance education: facing the faculty challenge. *Online J Distance Adm*. 2001. http://www.westga.edu/~distance/ojdla/summer42/bower42.html. Accessed September 6, 2016.

62. Larsson J, Sanner M. Doing a good job and getting something good out of it: on stress and well-being in anesthesia. *Br J Anaesth*. 2010;105(1):34-37. doi:10.1093/bja/aeq125.

63. Williams G. Counseling Consulting Professionals.www.garywilliams.net/Adaptive CopingSkills.pdf. [blog post] Accessed May 12, 2011.

64. Garcia-Ortero M, Teddlie C. The effect of knowledge of learning styles on anxiety and clinical performance of nurse anesthesiology students. *AANA J*. 1992;60(3):257–260.

65. Positive thinking: stop negative self-talk to decrease stress. Mayo Clinic. http://www.mayoclinic.org/healthy-lifestyle/stress-management/in-depth/positive-thinking/art-20043950?pg=1. Accessed July 5, 2016.

66. Lee R. *The SuperStress Solution*. New York, NY: Random House; 2010.

67. Neft M. 2016 Jan Stewart memorial lecture preview: an interview with George Ceremuga. *AANA NewsBull*. 2016;70(4):40–41.

68. Faber N. Mindfulness in anesthesia: a safety and satisfaction initiative. *Current Reviews for Nurse Anesthetists*. 2015.

69. Richards K, Campenni E, Muse-Burke J. Self-care and well-being in mental health professionals: the mediating effects of self-awareness and mindfulness. *J Ment Health Couns*. 2010;32(3):247–264.

70. Kabot-Zinn J. *Coming to Our Senses: Healing Ourselves and the World Through Mindfulness*. New York, NY: Hyperion; 2005.

71. Kabot-Zinn J. Mindfulness-based interventions in context: past, present, and future. *Clin Psychol Sci Pract*. 2003;10(2):144–156.

72. Weil A. Three Breathing Exercises. Weil Lifestyle. http://www.drweil.com/drw/u/ART00521/three-breathing-exercises.html. Accessed December 15, 2015.

73. Bennett MP, Zeller JM, Rosenberg L, McCann J. The effect of mirthful laughter on stress and natural killer cell activity. *Altern Ther Health Med*. 2003;9(2):38–44.

74. Betro R. The role of nature in coping with psycho-physiological stress: a literature review on restorativeness. *Behave Sci*. 2014;4(4):394–409.

75. Fry WF. Humor and the brain: a selective review. *Int J Humor Res*. 2002;15(3):305–333.

76. Robinson V. *Humor and the Health Professions: The Therapeutic Use of Humor in Health Care*. 2nd ed. Thorofare, NJ: Slack; 1990.

77. Wanzer MB, Frymier A, Wojtaszczyk A, Smith T. Appropriate and inappropriate uses of humor by teachers. *Commun Educ*. 2006;55(2):178–196.

78. Singh B. Peer support: taking advice from a friend. *MIT Faculty Newslett*. 2006;18(4):184–189.

79. Whittemore R, Rankin S, Callahan C, Leder M, Carroll D. The peer advisor experience providing social support. *Qual Health Res*. 2000;10(2):260–276.

80. Baumeister RF, Dale K, Sommer K. Freudian defense mechansisms and empirical findings in modern social psychology: reaction formation, projection, displacement, undoing, isolation, sublimation, and denial. *J Pers*. 1998;66(6):1081–1095.

81. AANALearn: Online Continuing Education. Wellness and Chemical Dependency Task Force. Stressors Encountered in the Healthcare System and How to Cope More Effectively [module]. 2012.

82. Valdes JA. The concept of reentry in the addicted anesthesia provider. *AANA J*. 2014; 82(2):95–100.

83. American Association of Nurse Anesthetists Peer Assistance Advisors. (2010). Program directors survey: Chemical dependency/wellness curriculum [survey]. AANA Wellness and Chemical Dependency Task Force.

84. Bell DM, McDonough JP, Ellison JS, Fitzhugh EC. Controlled drug misuse by Certified Registered Nurse Anesthetists. *AANA J*. 1999;67(2):133–140.

85. Cleck J, Blendy J, Making a bad thing worse: adverse effects of stress on drug addiction. *J Clin Invest*. 2008;118(2):454–61.

86. Sinha R. How does stress increase risk of drug abuse and relapse? *Psychopharmacology*. 2001;158(4):343–359.

87. Tunajek S. Peer support: validity and benefit. *AANA NewsBull*. 2007;61(5):29–31

88. Bell, D. *Review of current state of drug misuse by CRNAs* [survey]. 2007. Knoxville, TN: University of Tennessee.

89. American Association of Nurse Anesthetists. Re-entry Recommendations and Resources. www.AANA.com/Reentry. Accessed July 22, 2016.

90. Hamza H, Monroe T. Reentry and recidivism for Certified Registered Nurse Anesthetists. *AANA NewsBull*. June 2011:34–36.

91. Suicide Prevention. Substance Abuse and Mental Health Services Administration. www.SAMHSA.gov/suicide-prevention. Accessed September 17, 2016.

92. Institute of Medicine. Kohn LT, Corrigan JM, Donaldson MS, eds. To Err Is human: Building a Safer Health System. Washington, DC: National Academies Press; 2000.

93. Devencenzi T, O'Keefe J. To err is human: supporting the patient care provider in the aftermath of an unanticipated adverse clinical outcome. *Int J Emerg Ment Health*. Spring 2006;8(2):131–135.

94. American Association of Nurse Anesthetists. Adverse Medical Events/Critical Incidents-How to Cope. http://www.aana.com/resources2/health-wellness/Pages/Adverse-Medical-Event-How-to-Cope.aspx. Accessed November 12, 2015.

95. Gazoni FM, Durieux ME, Wells L. Life after death: the aftermath of perioperative catastrophes. *Anesth Analg* 2008;107(2): 591–600.

96. Gazoni FM, Amato PE, Malik ZM, Duriex ME. The impact of perioperative catastrophes on anesthesiologists: results of a national survey. *Anesth Analg.* 2012;114(3):596–603.

97. Everly GS, Jr., Flannery RB, Jr., Eyler VA. Critical incident stress management (CISM): a statistical review of the literature. *Psychiatr Q.* Fall 2002;73(3):171–182

98. Regel S. Post-trauma support in the workplace: the current status and practice of critical incident stress management (CISM) and psychological debriefing (PD) within organizations in the UK. *Occup Med* (Lond). 2007;57(6):411–416.

99. Conway J, Federico F, Stewart K, Campbell MJ. *Respectful Management of Serious Clinical Adverse Events (Second Edition).* IHI Innovation Series white paper. Cambridge, MA: Institute for Healthcare Improvement; 2011. www.IHI.org.

100. Medically Induced Trauma Support Services (MITSS). http://www.mitsstools.org. Accessed November 18, 2015.

101. Rice J, Uranga T. Reflections on health and wellness. *AANA NewsBulletin.* November 2015;24–25.

102. Clark GD. Substance abuse education for nurse anesthetists: differences in knowledge of substance abuse between student nurse anesthetists who have completed a substance abuse workshop and those who have not. *Subst Abus.* 1996;17(3):167–174.

103. Clark GD, Stone JS. Assessment of the substance abuse curriculum in schools of nurse anesthesia. *Journal of Addictions Nursing.* 1999;11(3):123–135.

104. Stokes DL, Hogan GT. The effect of education on perceptions of chemical dependency in anesthesia. *AANA Journal.* 2007;(5):A56.

105. Dunn D. Substance abuse among nurses: defining the issue. *AORN.* 2005;82(4): 573-582. doi:10.1016/S0001-2092(06)60028-8

106. Tetzlaff J, Collins GB, Brown DL, Leak BC, Pollock G, Popa D. A strategy to prevent substance abuse in an academic anesthesiology department. *J Clin Anesth.* 2010;22(2):143–150.

107. Pullen LM, Green LA. Identification, intervention and education: essential curriculum components for chemical dependency in nurses. *J Contin Educ Nurs.* 1997;28(5):211–216.

108. American Association of Nurse Anesthetists. Substance Use Disorder Workplace Resources. http://www.aana.com/resources2/health-wellness/Pages/SUD-Workplace-Resources.aspx. Accessed September 18, 2016.

109. American Association of Nurse Anesthetists. Peer Assistance. http://www.aana.com/resources2/peer-assistance/Pages/default.aspx. Accessed January15, 2016.

110. American Association of Nurse Anesthetists. Emotional and Mental Well-Being. http://www.aana.com/resources2/health-wellness/Pages/Emotional-and-Mental-Well-Being.aspx. Accessed September 20, 2016.

CHAPTER 4

Legal Issues for Educators

Mary Jeanette Mannino, JD, CRNA

Keywords: Contract law, education law, supervision of students, TEFRA, vicarious liability.

Key Concepts

- Applicable laws come from many different types of sources and should be well researched and updated often to ensure the best understanding and most accurate compliance.
- In-depth screening and frequent evaluation is an important part of maintaining a student program.
- A clear understanding of the student's capabilities, duties, and roles are important to a successful and safe learning environment.
- Students should be supervised by appropriate parties at all times to avoid legal issues.
- It is important to know who is "captain of the ship" and in what situations this applies. Legal liability can be perceived in many ways, so documentation and knowledge are key.
- CRNAs should have an education in the way law applies to them and their businesses. They should be aware of their responsibilities and roles. They should have an accurate understanding of contract law, common business practice, and negotiation technique.

Introduction

There are many components to understanding the legal aspects of nurse anesthesiology education, including the rights and responsibilities of the university, the faculty, the students, clinical rotations, and the profession. As in many other areas of nursing, there are myths and misunderstandings regarding the law and its application to practice.

Because nurse anesthesiology education and practice are based on the scientific method, it is frequently difficult for educators, practitioners, and students to understand the nuances inherent in legal study and conclusions. While science is generally very current and frequently tested, the law is often years behind clinical practice and is ever evolving. Legal precedents may be shattered, laws enacted with a political and economic genesis, and appeals lengthy and expensive.

While not comprehensive in its scope, this chapter will emphasize the important areas of concern regarding the law and anesthesia education. It is not intended to replace legal counsel from individual institutions or be considered legal advice. Rather, a look at some of the applicable laws and analysis of relevant legal cases will provide educators and students a frame of reference and resources to answer some of the major legal questions.

Sources of Law

There are four sources of American law: constitutional law, administrative law, statutory law, and common law. In addition to those sources, each state has a separate constitution and procedures for enacting and enforcing their own laws.

In nurse anesthesiology education, there may be some overlap in federal and state constitutional law. For example, civil rights and discrimination may be covered by both entities. Except for federal jurisdiction areas such as the military, the Native American system, and the District of Columbia, the United States government does not generally get involved in licensure and other administrative legal areas that are relegated to state jurisdiction; however, the federal government does have considerable legal influence over educational funding, grants, and health care reimbursement. In recent years, we have seen major changes in Medicare reimbursement for anesthesia services. In the late 1980s, a federal law was passed allowing Certified Registered Nurse Anesthetists (CRNAs) to receive direct reimbursement from Medicare for anesthesia services. Subsequently, rule changes regarding reimbursement for supervision of nurse anesthesiology students were enacted. The entire issue of reimbursement for nurse anesthetists by a medically directing physician anesthesiologist, referred to as Tax Equity and Fiscal Responsibility Act of 1982 (TEFRA), has generated considerable confusion over a reimbursement issue becoming a quasi standard of care determination. While reimbursement is beyond the scope of this chapter and is, in itself, a complicated issue, it is none the less important for educators to be familiar with current law and to assure that there is no fraudulent billing in the name of the students or the program.

Each state has the duty of protecting its citizens and, as such, has set up licensure boards to develop criteria for licensees, including setting educational standards and enforcing rules and regulations. Most state nurse practice acts identify nurse anesthesiology as legal and may identify the educational and certification requirements. A common misconception is that the boards of nursing exist to protect and promote nursing. In reality, the board's duty is to the public and to assure them that an individual licensed by the state has met minimum requirements.

Most anesthesia programs (the military and Veterans Affairs being the exception) require that students maintain their basic nursing license and be in good standing with the state in this regard. After graduation and certification, state nursing boards may require a separate designation as a nurse anesthetist. The American Association of Nurse Anesthetists (AANA) State Government Affairs Department maintains current files on the requirements of each individual state and is an excellent resource for this information. (http://www.aana.com/advocacy/stategovernmentaffairs/Pages/default.aspx)

Common Law

Historically, common law is a holdover from British rule. It has been called "judge made law" and is based on the law of precedent. There are also instances when the facts of a case are distinct from all previous cases and the court will form an opinion as a "matter of first impression." Many of the cases reviewed and analyzed in this chapter are based on common law.

Evidence

In all areas of law, evidence is used as proof of facts. In the medical realm, many documents provide that this proof of patient care or policies be upheld. The medical record is frequently the first item that is requested in a medical malpractice case, but a new area of law is emerging in relation to social media and electronic records. Electronic records will probably be held to the same standard as written records, although there is little law on this topic to date.

The issue of social media postings as evidence in cases is an emerging area of the law. Educators will acknowledge that the students of the current generation are competent electronic users, and while this is useful in literature review, research, and studying, there are legal and personal perils that they should understand.

In the process of discovery in legal cases, social media evidence may be obtained by opposition attorneys. Also, in other legal proceedings, such as contract issues, criminal charges, nursing board actions, and billing fraud cases, social media postings may also play a part in establishing fault or defense. A wise educator will include some of the following information in a student handbook and discuss this in an orientation class.

- There is no reasonable expectation of privacy in social media postings.
- Privacy settings should be encouraged.
- Direct access to a social media account should not be given without a proper court order.
- Use of profanity and libelous statements can be used against a student.
- Use of personal electronic equipment (mobile phones, tablets, computers) should be addressed as a program policy and facility policy.
- Phone data, including text messages can be used as legal evidence.[1]

As new technology emerges, it can be expected that new areas of law and regulations regarding their use in medical facilities will be forthcoming.

Case Law

State and federal courts publish many decisions based on issues relative to interpretation of statutes, rules, and regulations. Many of the antitrust cases argued by nurse anesthetists have been a result of the need to determine whether there was a violation of federal antitrust laws in denying privileges to CRNAs.

Postsecondary Education Law

Academic law has evolved also, as colleges and universities have moved from totally private institutions to those that are federally funded. Recent examples include faculties that have elected to be part of collective bargaining units and athletic regulations that have been expanded to include females.

Whether or not postsecondary law has been codified, institutions have set up their own governances, due process procedures, and rules. As universities become more research-oriented with federal and private funding support, additional legal and ethical standards apply.

Nurse anesthesiology educational programs additionally must comply with the standards established by the Council on Accreditation of Nurse Anesthesia Educational Programs (COA). This places an additional burden for educators to ensure that there is no conflict between the university and the COA.

Hospital/Facility Law

Nurse anesthesiology education includes a major clinical component requiring facilities where the students learn the technical skills necessary in the practice of anesthesiology. It is in the clinical area where many students and educators realize that technical skills are as important as academic foundation. Depending on the structure of the program, students may complete the academic portion in a front-loaded type of program prior to clinical, or in an integrated program where classes and clinical are held simultaneously.

It is incumbent upon the program directors and clinical coordinators to have a strong understanding of the hospital and anesthesia department standards, rules, and regulations. These include operating room policies, infection control, and use of equipment and supplies. Each facility will have its own method of documenting the course of an anesthetic and the students must be aware of this information and the importance of compliance.

While it would be best that students not get involved in anesthesia department politics and reimbursement issues, the faculty should attempt to protect the students from these issues. In rapidly changing health care economics, anesthesia departments are facing changes from local to national corporate takeovers, contract issues, and revenue issues.

Education Law Regarding Student Status

The university and its appropriate department will have admission standards for application to nurse anesthesiology programs. While these standards are required by the Council on Accreditation, many programs establish higher standards and admission requirements. These standards must be in writing and the applicants need to have a thorough understanding of the content. Institutional admission standards require assurance that certain legal criteria are met. These include (1) the selection process must not be arbitrary or capricious; (2) the institution is bound under a contract legal theory to adhere to its published admission policies; and (3) the institution may not discriminate on the basis of race, sex, age, sexual orientation, disability, or citizenship.[1]

While there is a paucity of case law specifically regarding nurse anesthesiology education, the following is a case regarding student status and dismissal from an anesthesia program.

"JJ" (the plaintiff) brought action against a nurse anesthesia program (program) alleging violations of Title II of the Americans with Disabilities Act as well as a state common law claim for negligent misrepresentation, breach of contract, and promissory estoppel.*

The facts show that the plaintiff was admitted to the program in 1999. The program was of two years duration with the graduates being awarded a master of science degree in biology from the university and a certificate of nurse anesthesia from the hospital. After completing the academic program, the plaintiff began the clinical portion and was scheduled to graduate in May 2001. At some point in March 2001, the plaintiff's performance level in the clinical area began to decline due to extreme anxiety. On March 8, 2001, the plaintiff met with the medical and program directors to discuss clinical performance. After that meeting, a memorandum was prepared stating that the student appeared to be suffering the effects of an acute stress response or some form of chronic anxiety disorder, and professional counseling and/or psychological evaluation were recommended. In the memorandum, it was questioned in writing whether or not the student was capable of successfully attaining his educational goals.

About three weeks later, the plaintiff once again met with the directors and was informed that his clinical work had been suspended. At that time, they provided him with three options: (1) continue his academic course of study in order to complete the requirements for a master of science degree from the university and take a leave of absence from the clinical phase until September 1, 2001, when he would be able to restart the nine-month clinical phase; (2) continue the academic course of study and completely resign from the program; or (3) completely resign from both further academic study and the program. The plaintiff chose the first option, took a leave of absence and returned to the program September 2001. On December 11, 2001, however, the plaintiff was dismissed from the program.

Alleging that at no time was he offered any type of professional counseling or a psychological evaluation, he filed a legal action for emotional distress and requested compensatory and punitive damages.

To argue his case, the plaintiff entered into evidence the student handbook that states that the faculty and administration of the program "will assist a student whenever possible...." The plaintiff contended that despite this clause in the handbook and despite the defendant's knowledge of his physical disability, the program failed to accommodate him during the three-month period between his return from his leave of absence until the time he was dismissed from the program.

* Promissory estoppel is a legal doctrine in contract law whereby there may be reliance made on the terms of the contract.

The court of appeals dismissed all of the plaintiff's allegations, but there are legal lessons here that are important to anesthesia educators.

Legal Lessons: The student handbook and clinical evaluations will be used as evidence in legal proceedings regarding student actions, such as probation and dismissal. If at all possible, students who have difficulty with the clinical portion of the program should be identified early and remedial action taken.

Case: Termination of a student who refused drug testing

In the following case that has broad implications for nurse anesthesia programs, the university where the programs are housed, the clinical facilities, and faculty members, a jury recently awarded a large sum to an anesthesia student. *AB v Bloomsburg University* (2015).

The facts of the case, as set down by a previous court ruling *AB v Bloomsburg University* (2012), are:

"AB" (the plaintiff) was a student enrolled in the nurse anesthesia program at Bloomsburg University in Bloomsburg, Pennsylvania. The clinical component of the program was partnered with Geisinger Medical Center in Danville, Pennsylvania. According to the plaintiff, she was summoned out of her clinical area September 24, 2012 by her program director. He informed her of his concern over a change in her demeanor and appearance and requested that she submit to a drug test. AB refused the test and asked to speak with her parents about it. After speaking to her parents and wanting to clear her record of drug use accusations, she decided to submit to the test. According to the subsequent lawsuit, her efforts to contact the director and others and her decision to have the test were met with silence and rebuff. Three days later, September 27, 2012, AB received a letter signed by the program director and the director of the nursing program at Bloomsburg University, informing her that she had been expelled from the program due to her alleged failure to take a drug test. AB filed suit, alleging that she was never given the opportunity by Bloomsburg University to appeal, and that her due process rights under the equal protection law of the United States Constitution were violated. She also alleged breach of contract. The defendants (University of Bloomsburg and Hospital) moved to dismiss the complaint, based on the Eleventh Amendment to the U.S. Constitution dealing with sovereign immunity. In granting that motion, the court held that because Bloomsburg University was a state-sanctioned university, it was immune from claims against the institution and those who functioned under official capacity.

The court did agree with the plaintiff that her due process rights may have been violated. It also agreed that her "liberty interest" claim should go forward. Liberty interest concerns the loss of reputation, good name, and integrity. Specifically, the court used the information that there was a public dissemination of false information that AB-had a substance abuse issue.

The allegation that there was a breach of contract between AB and Bloomsburg University was dismissed. In its ruling, the court said that the student handbook did not establish a contractual relationship. Further, they wrote that the drug policy of the hospital was not considered a contract.

With this ruling, AB was able to proceed in her legal action against the hospital. In the subsequent action, a jury found for AB and against the hospital and awarded damages based on their analysis of the facts.

The jury based damage awards on its belief that AB would have been dismissed from the program if she had been given the procedural due process rights. They ruled that AB did suffer injuries as a result of the denial of her due process rights. It awarded $415,000 in compensatory damages and $1.1 million in punitive damages. Those awards were against the hospital and not the directors, as individuals.

Analysis and Lessons for Educators

While this case applies Pennsylvania law to the facts, it is reasonable to expect that similar rulings may apply in other states. The reported facts only represent what is recorded in court documents and may not reflect the entire situation.

Clear in the court's ruling was the constitutional protection under the due process clause of the U.S. Constitution's 14th Amendment. Program administration from the university to clinical facilities will be held to affording students due process in allegations related to both an academic and clinical nature. Not only should the policies be clear as to the standards by which a student will be held, but the process for upholding those standards must be delineated and followed. It stands to reason that clear and careful documentation of all communication between the program and students be recorded and kept confidential.

Supervision of Students

Supervision of students in the clinical area is a legal concern for the supervising CRNAs, medical anesthesiologists, and the institution. It is frequently easier to administer the anesthetic oneself, than to supervise a student. Also, supervising anesthesia providers are concerned that a worthwhile learning experience for the students may not always be in the best interests of the patient.

This is another area where common sense should outweigh any legal concerns. No harm should be allowed to happen to a patient, under any circumstances; however, there are many situations where there may be different ways to administer an anesthetic to a patient for a certain procedure. It is reasonable to expect that the student will have researched these various options, have a clear understanding of the pros and cons, and is both academically and technically prepared to perform the procedure. If a student is not prepared to justify the technique and to appropriately plan for it, it may be prudent for the student to be relieved of direct administration of the anesthetic.

There have been some legal cases that directly address the issue of supervision of nurse anesthesiology students. Clinical faculty and program directors should be aware of the outcome of any such cases and ascertain if there may be lessons to learn for dealing with similar situations. From a legal perspective, there are various components of the supervision issue that may create problems and, from a risk management perspective, be dealt with in advance. These include: assignment of students appropriate to educational level and patient physical status; level of supervision needed; student preparation for cases; identification of high-risk patients and procedures;

medical record documentation; ability of the student to troubleshoot a problem; and evaluation of the student, post-procedure.

No chapter about the legality of supervision of nurse anesthesiology students would be complete without a discussion of the Worthy case—*Central Anesthesia Associates, PC v Worthy*, 333 S.E.2d 829, (1985). While it is an old decision, several key elements regarding who may legally supervise a student registered nurse anesthetist are addressed. It involves an institution in Georgia where anesthesia assistants practice, along with CRNAs and MD anesthesiologists, and where student registered nurse anesthetists receive clinical experience as well. Georgia law addressed the legality of nurse anesthesiology practice in a statute that stated:

> "Anesthesia may lawfully be administered by a Certified Registered Nurse Anesthetist, provided such anesthesia is administered under the direction and responsibility of a duly licensed physician with training and experience in anesthesia."

The facts show that a woman gave birth without anesthesia and without complication. The next day she underwent a tubal ligation, which was performed by her obstetrician/gynecologist assisted by an intern employed by the hospital. A professional corporation consisting of anesthesiologists administered the anesthesia through a registered nurse enrolled as a student registered nurse anesthetist in a school operated at the hospital by the anesthesiologists' corporation. At the time of induction, the student registered nurse anesthetist was under the supervision of a physician's assistant employed by the corporation. During the tubal ligation procedure, Mrs. Worthy suffered a cardiac arrest resulting in brain damage.

In the subsequent malpractice suit, the issue of whether or not a physician's assistant (AA) could legally supervise a CRNA student arose. The court essentially ruled that the statute did not permit anesthesia assistant supervision of student registered nurse anesthetists. The Standards and Guidelines of the COA are consistent in policy with this ruling.

Legal Lesson: From an educator's perspective, careful adherence to state law regarding supervision is critical.

Vicarious Liability

Students, faculty, surgeons, and administrators frequently discuss the issue of liability from the perspective of who is actually liable and has to pay in a medical malpractice suit. This particular topic is one that is based on myths and history, rather than current legal doctrine. There are several ways to look at this topic, including legal precedent, history, custom, and procedural strategy. Historically, this issue is related to the captain of the ship doctrine and has been expanded in recent years to include economic concerns and politics. A 1940s case defined captain of the ship doctrine. At that time, hospitals were immune from lawsuits because they were considered charitable institutions. Under the doctrine of charitable immunity, a hospital could not be sued for the acts of its employees. The court ruled that a private practice physician could be sued because immunity did not apply to him and that he was considered the captain of the ship. *McConnell v Williams,* 361 Pa. 355 (1949). Note: The doctrine of charitable immunity for hospitals has been reversed in recent years.

In the current medical malpractice arena, hospitals no longer have charitable immunity and can be sued for the acts of their employees under the laws of agency. Yet the issue of the surgeons' assumed liability for hospital employees and independent contractors continues to be discussed in the anesthesia community. Unfortunately, the misused term *supervision* has made this topic even more controversial. Because this topic has many facets, this chapter will address only a few of them and will not attempt to include reimbursement and political issues; however, there is a difference depending on whether the party named in a lawsuit is an anesthesia student or a CRNA. Furthermore, the assumed liability of others for the acts of a CRNA is related to the employment status and contractual language.

Case: Who is liable for the negligent acts of a student?

Another legal case involving anesthesia education is *North Broward Hospital District v Kalitan* (2015). In this case, the appeals court focused on noneconomic damages in a medical malpractice case and the issue of liability for a nurse anesthesia student.

The facts, as reported by the appeals court are as follows: This is a malpractice case brought by Susan Kalitan (plaintiff), against North Broward Hospital District (hospital), an anesthesiologist, the anesthesia group that contracted with the hospital, a CRNA who was clinical coordinator for the Barry University nurse anesthesia program, and a student registered nurse anesthetist.

The patient was scheduled for a carpal tunnel surgical procedure of the wrist under general anesthesia. During endotracheal intubation, the patient's esophagus was perforated. The hospital records do not indicate which anesthesiologist team member, CRNA, or SRNA actually intubated the patient, but the anesthesiologist testified that it was he who performed the procedure.

When the patient awoke in the recovery area, she complained of excruciating pain in her chest and back. The anesthesiologist was notified and, unaware of the perforated esophagus, ordered a drug for the chest pain and concluded that there was no cardiac issue. The patient was subsequently discharged from the hospital and taken home by a neighbor.

The following day, the plaintiff was found to be unresponsive when checked by the neighbor. She was taken to the emergency room of a nearby hospital and, after diagnosis of the problem, had surgery to repair the esophagus. Subsequently, the plaintiff was in a drug-induced coma in the intensive care unit for several weeks and required additional surgery and therapy to help with eating and to regain mobility. She testified to having continuing issues from pain, loss of independence, severe mental disorders, and physical limitations.

A jury awarded the plaintiff $4,718,011 in total damages, which included the noneconomic damages of $2 million for past pain and suffering and $2 million for future pain and suffering.

On a vicarious liability issue, the jury found that the CRNA was acting as the university's agent or employee when supervising the student.

This current case before the Florida Court of Appeals deals with both the issues of vicarious liability and a statutory cap on noneconomic damages.

This court ruled that the university was not vicariously liable for the acts of the nurse anesthetist. While there was some legal maneuvering on the part of both the plaintiff and defendant university, the facts show that the CRNA was an employee of the anesthesia group and was rendering anesthesia services to the hospital. This court agreed and held that the university was not liable for the acts of the CRNA.

Regarding the issue of noneconomic damages, the court reinstated the total damage award as found by the jury, and as limited by the doctrine of sovereign immunity.

Analysis and Lesson for Educators

Reading appellate court decisions can be difficult; finding a practical conclusion, even more so. There are several elements of this case that should interest educators.

- Clinical component. The court record of the actual clinical scenario is lacking in specifics. Since the anesthesiologist admitted under testimony to actually performing the endotracheal intubation, it is unclear why the CRNA and the student were named in this case. From a practical perspective, the anesthesia record did not indicate any problems or who actually performed the procedure. Clinical coordinators should be made aware of the importance of an accurate anesthesia record, including who actually performed the anesthesia-related procedures.
- Vicarious liability. The area of agency, or who is liable for the acts of others, is a common legal issue in the anesthesia profession. The plaintiff usually names everyone involved in an incident and frequently looks for the "deep pocket." In this case, they looked to the university to be liable for the acts of the CRNA, in his role as clinical coordinator. The court rejected that argument by stating that the CRNA was actually an employee of the anesthesia group and imputed liability on the group for his actions.
- It is highly recommended that all clinical coordinators have a letter of agreement or contract, establishing their relationship with the university. This is especially important if the clinical coordinators are not employees or members of the faculty of the university, but volunteers. It would also be prudent to have a well-defined organizational structure as part of the student handbook for nurse anesthesia educational programs.
- Noneconomic damages. This issue is the basis for tort reform legislation and is determined on a state-by-state basis. This immediate case did not answer the constitutionality of a cap on noneconomic damages, and it is likely that this issue will come up again to the Florida Supreme Court. When instructing anesthesia students on the law of negligence, they should understand the three types of damages that can be awarded in a malpractice case: actual, special or noneconomic, and punitive. In states where there has been a cap on noneconomic damages, it is argued that there will be fewer nuisance lawsuits.

Agency Law

Under the laws of agency, generally the employer is responsible for the acts of the employee that are performed within the scope of the employment. Because of the unusual nature of anesthesia practice, a CRNA has many employment options, including being employed by a facility (hospital/ambulatory surgery center), a medical group, a CRNA group, or self-employed. Because of the need for nurse anesthetists, many CRNAs practice in several different arrangements at the same time. This becomes an issue because of the need to assure there is malpractice insurance coverage. Because many of the employment opportunities for CRNAs are different than for nursing, students need to be educated on the job market and the pros and cons of the various relationships.

Whether one is a student or CRNA, knowledge of the current law on vicarious liability and the ability to successfully argue its application to practice is critical to the individual and the profession. This topic will provoke emotional arguments that make no legal or financial sense; however, a surgeon's ego may interfere with his or her understanding of the law, when it comes to the captain of the ship analogy. There have been a number of legal rulings on the issue with most of them stating that the surgeon is not automatically the captain of the ship.

For example, in *Lauro v Knowles*, 739 A.2d 1183, Rhode Island (1999), Lauro (plaintiff) sought to impose captain of the ship liability for an eye injury she received in the operating room.

Case: Dr. Knowles operated on the plaintiff to alleviate carpal tunnel syndrome in her right wrist. He performed the surgery at St. Joseph Hospital (hospital). There was an anesthesiologist and a student registered nurse anesthetist involved in providing anesthesia. When the plaintiff awoke from anesthesia, she had suffered a corneal abrasion of her right eye. The injury was allegedly sustained in connection with the administration of anesthesia.

Dr. Knowles testified at his deposition that he assumed the plaintiff was prepped and had already been given anesthesia when he walked into the operating room. He said that he had nothing to do with the administration of anesthesia or with the anesthesiology team stationed at the head of the operating table. Rather, he claimed, these functions were the responsibility of the anesthesiologist and the other members of that team who were present. The Rhode Island court agreed with other jurisdictions that it must be a finding of fact that the surgeon exercised control over the anesthesia process and in this case, there was no evidence of that control.

Other cases have affirmed the importance of the surgeon exerting control over anesthesia in order to be legally considered captain of the ship. *Parker v Vanderbilt University* 767 S.W. 2d 412, Court of Appeals of Tennessee (1988) and *Franklin v Gupta* 81 Md. App. 345, 567 A 2d 524 (1990). In Franklin, the Maryland court noted that the operating room environment is changing to a point where the surgeon can no longer have actual control over technical equipment and the persons who operate it.

In *Parker v Vanderbilt*, there was an allegation that a student registered nurse anesthetist intubated the esophagus of a patient leading to brain damage. The Appeals Court ruled that the surgeon was not vicariously liable for the acts of the student or CRNA. They referred to "control" when they wrote the following: "While we agree that a surgical nurse, under the direct supervision of the surgeon, who acts according to the surgeon's specific directions, is certainly the servant of the surgeon, we are not willing to place a nurse anesthetist in this category, particularly where there is no showing that the surgeon directed the procedures to be utilized by the nurse anesthetist or had a genuine opportunity to alter the course of events."

From a practical standpoint, it is wise for all parties to understand that the surgeon will not be liable for the acts of the nurse anesthetist unless he or she has participated in the anesthetic. This statement assumes the nurse anesthetist understands that he or she is responsible/liable for his or her own acts and must be certain that there is sufficient insurance coverage.

Contract Law

Contracts are part of daily commerce and may be found in all aspects of one's professional career. Knowledge of contract law is essential to program directors, faculty, and students. It is usually prudent for contracts to be written or reviewed by an attorney who is familiar with state law and the area of interest specific to the subject; however, it is prudent for everyone to know how to read a contract, have an understanding of the terms, and be aware of the legal remedies if there is a breach.

A contract is a legally enforceable agreement between two or more parties that creates an obligation to do or not to do certain things. In order for a contract to be legal, the parties must be legally competent to enter into a contract and there must be mutual agreement of the terms. While there are situations where verbal contracts are legal, for the purposes of this chapter, we will assume that the terms of the agreement have been put into writing.

Because a written contract can appear to be complicated, many people do not take the time to carefully read and understand their legal obligations. Most contracts contain certain standard clauses that are modified to suit the special needs of the circumstances. The following outline lists the clauses that may be seen in a contract of interest to the nurse anesthesiology profession.

I. Name and purpose of the contract

II. Parties

III. Recitals (statements of background, often containing "whereas" clauses)

IV. Starting date

V. Length of contract

VI. Terms of relationship

VII. Duties of each party

VIII. Termination clause

IX. Covenants

X. Applicable law

XI. Remedies for breech or nonperformance

XII. Signatures and dates signed

Specific Types of Contracts

While the standard clauses appear in most contracts, there will be certain articles that are specific to each type of contract. Each institution and individual has different contractual needs. **Tables 4.1–4.3** contain examples that may be relevant to educators and students.

Table 4.1 University and Clinical Site Contracts

I. Duties of university
• Preparation of students for clinical sites • Appointment of clinical coordinators • Salary of clinical coordinators • Malpractice insurance for students
II. Duties of clinical site
• Supervision of students • Participation in clinical conferences • Participation in clinical evaluation of students • Stipend (if any) • Provision of department policies and procedures • Student participation in clinical site activities

Table 4.2 Student Contract for Stipend Assistance

I. Obligations of student
• Graduate from accredited anesthesia program • Successfully pass certification examination • Work for facility or group for a specified period of time • If unable to fulfill work obligations, buy-out terms, specified
II. Obligations of facility/group
• Stipend at agreed amount at specified time • Provide guaranteed employment upon student graduation and certification • Employment salary and benefits may be specified or negotiated at the time of employment

Table 4.3 Employment Contract Between CRNA and Hospital

I. Obligations of CRNA
• Maintain license and certification
• Hospital privileges in good standing
• Provide anesthesia services to surgical and obstetrical patients at the hospital
• Provide peri-anesthesia services, including pre- and post-anesthesia assessment
• Provide postoperative pain management
• Maintain anesthesia equipment
• Order anesthesia supplies
• Provide hospital billing office with appropriate information to allow for billing
• Be available for anesthesia services Monday through Friday and every other weekend
II. Obligations of facility/group
• Provide state-of-the-art anesthesia equipment and monitors
• Provide anesthesia supplies and medications
• Provide operating room and PACU personnel to assist in anesthesia procedures
• Salary and Benefits
• Annual salary of $__________
• Benefits to include, _____ paid days off, _____ days and $_____ for professional activities, such as continuing education
• Full invested in pension program
• Health insurance for family
• Malpractice insurance
• Clinical privileges through medical staff with due process right

Case: In reviewing contract law cases involving nurse anesthesiology education, the following case is illustrative of a student requesting not to fulfill the terms of a post-education agreement.

A hospital entered into a contract with its then-employee registered nurse (AC), by which the hospital agreed to provide tuition assistance for anesthesia school. The terms of the contract included tuition assistance in the form of a monthly stipend and health and dental insurance while AC was in anesthesia school.

The contract provided that if AC works for the hospital for a period of five years after completion of her studies, her loan would be forgiven. The agreement also stated that if she failed to rejoin the hospital as an active employee after graduation, she would be responsible for paying the hospital for the advances, plus accrued interest.

When she graduated from her anesthesia program, she sought employment elsewhere because it appeared that there were no nurse anesthetist positions available at the hospital. The hospital brought a breach of contract action against the nurse anesthetist, seeking repayment for the money given. The nurse anesthetist responded, stating that the hospital breached the contract by failing to offer her a position as a nurse anesthetist.

A trial court ruled in favor of the hospital awarding them $29,879.84 plus interest for a total of $43,396.49. The nurse anesthetist appealed this ruling.

The Court of Appeals in affirming the trial court's decision in favor of the hospital discussed the fact that in order for a contract to be valid, both parties must agree to its terms. Part of the higher court's analysis was the fact that according to the writing of the contract, the nurse agreed to remain an employee of the hospital, but not necessarily as a nurse anesthetist. Since there was not an anesthesia position available at the time, the appellant had the option of working as a nurse under the terms of financial agreement. *Sweetwater Hospital Association v Carpenter*, TN Ct of Appeals. No. E2004-00207-COA-R3-CV (2005).

Legal Lessons: This case points out how the terms and the intent of the contract must be understood. The nurse anesthetist relied on a verbal assurance that the hospital would provide her a nurse anesthetist position; however, the final decision for hiring would be made by the physician anesthesiologist director of the department. Students should be counseled to understand the importance of any financial agreement for tuition assistance and the payback terms. This case is a good example of an unexpected outcome for the student, who fully expected to be employed as a nurse anesthetist and not an RN to fulfill the payback terms of her agreement.

A student must understand the professional and ethical considerations of breaching a contract or failing to fulfill the terms or essence of the agreement. As a professional, nurse anesthetists are held to high standards in business as well as clinical practice. While an act may, on its face, not be illegal or worthy of a lawsuit, poor judgment on the part of the anesthetist can have long-lasting effects on the individual's professional career.

Noncompete Clauses

Clearly the most misunderstood areas of contracts are noncompete clauses. While these covenants may be upheld by the law, they may depend on the jurisdictions and facts surrounding their inclusion. Also, it is imperative that as more CRNAs become business owners, having such a clause may be a good business decision in preventing employee or subcontractor anesthetists from underbidding or otherwise attempting to get the contract.

Noncompete clauses generally have two components: time and distance. A typical clause may read, "after conclusion of this contract, for whatever reason, the anesthetist will not provide anesthesia services in a 50 mile radius of the hospital for two years." As one can imagine, these clauses have the effect of restricting the anesthetist from providing anesthesia services that would essentially compete with the original group or hospital.

Whether or not to sign or modify a noncompete clause depends on the circumstances of the individual, the anesthesia market, and the negotiating skills of all parties.

Gene Blumenreich, past AANA General Counsel, presented a very balanced approach to this subject. His paper would be a good subject for classroom discussion. In his article, he discusses several approaches to negotiating these particular clauses.[2] Mr. Blumenreich recommends that nurse anesthetists understand the legal implications of these covenants and makes suggestions on how they may be used as a bargaining tool in employment contract negotiations.

Negotiations

It is imperative that anesthetists develop negotiation skills to assist with the various business and practice options and opportunities. These skills are useful when the anesthetist is obtaining a contract for employment or private practice, or membership in an HMO, PPO, or other managed care entity. This section will describe the negotiation process and assist the reader in developing the necessary skills to effectively negotiate a business contract.

Negotiation is a process through which parties determine whether an acceptable agreement can be reached. Information is exchanged, evaluated, and used as the basis for final decisions.

Effective negotiation involves the gathering and exchange of information to assess the parties and the potential for agreement. This information includes the (1) positions; (2) needs; (3) interests; and (4) goals of the parties.

Most negotiations in an anesthesia business will probably be performed by the anesthetist or spokesperson for a group; however, there may be circumstances when an attorney or consultant may be retained for that purpose. Learning how to be an effective negotiator may make the difference in a successful business venture and is probably one of the most critical elements as practice situations change.

Characteristics of an Effective Negotiator

There are many scholarly works that discuss the characteristics of an effective negotiator. Table 4.4 summarizes the key points.

Table 4.4 Characteristics of an Effective Negotiator

• Preparation and planning skills
• Knowledge of subject matter being negotiated
• Ability to think clearly and rapidly under pressure and uncertainty
• Ability to express thoughts verbally
• Listening skills
• Judgment and general intelligence
• Integrity
• Ability to persuade others
• Patience
• Decisiveness
• Ability to earn respect and confidence of opponent
• General problem solving and analytic skills
• Self-control, especially of emotions and their visibility
• Insight into other's feelings
• Persistence and determination
• Ability to perceive and exploit available power to achieve objective
• Insight into hidden needs and reaction of own and opponent's objective(s)
• Ability to lead and control members of own team or group

Planning

Experts often cite planning as one of the most critical aspects in successful negotiations. In the planning process careful attention must be given to the purpose of the contract, goals of both parties, national and local market trends, financial considerations, and underlying agendas. At this time, a strategy should be developed and parameters established.

Teaching Law to Nurse Anesthetist Students

Legal classes are taught as part of the curriculum in nurse anesthesiology programs. Law may be taught as a separate course or integrated in other classes. The author has been on the faculty of Gonzaga University since the early 1980s and teaches a separate two- credit law and business class every year. This class will be integrated into the new DNP curriculum at Gonzaga. Drawing on this lengthy experience, several recommendations are suggested. The class should be taught to senior students. Students who have not been in the clinical area have little basis for understanding standards of anesthesia practice. Because most schools do not teach much about the business of anesthesia, this is a good opportunity to include it in the curriculum. Since nurse anesthetist practice is unique in many respects, it is recommended that this course not be taught in conjunction with other advanced practice nurses.

The purpose of this course is not to teach law to the anesthesia students, but to teach how the law is applied to our profession and practice. It is especially important for the students to understand the legal basis for CRNA practice and how the law is constantly evolving.

It is also important to teach this class based upon CRNA practice instead of practice as a student, where rules of supervision are different. Students must be made aware of the fact that there are differences in state laws and institutional policies and procedures that may be different from their educational clinical sites. The AANA is the best resource for information and legal rulings relating to CRNA practice. Students and graduates should be very familiar with the legal column in the *AANA Journal* and information on www.aana.com in the member and public sections.(http://www.aana.com/newsandjournal/legalbriefs/Pages/default.aspx)

The syllabus from the law and business class required for the anesthesia students at Gonzaga University in Spokane, Washington follows. The content is updated every year so current cases and rulings will be applicable. Students are expected to participate in case presentations, contract preparation, and negotiations, as well as to analyze precedent setting rulings that affect CRNA practice.

Class Outline

American Legal System

A. How laws are made
B. Court system
C. Common Law
D. Constitutions
E. Adversary system

Legal History of Nurse Anesthetists

- Anesthesia as the practice of medicine or nursing
- Antitrust cases and the CRNA's right to compete with anesthesiologists
- Legislation obtaining Medicare direct reimbursement
- Military status of CRNAs
- Legal and legislative challenges to education, practice, reimbursement, opt-out status, and other cases

A. Anatomy of a Lawsuit
   1. Preliminary stage
   2. Trial
   3. Appeals
   4. Disposition (settlement)
   5. Arbitration

B. Statutory and Regulatory Law
   1. Nurse practice acts
   2. Other statutes
   3. Administrative law related to licensure
   4. Legal basis for nurse anesthesiology practice

C. Criminal Law and Anesthesia
   1. Practicing medicine without a license
   2. Criminal battery

D. Consent Law
   1. Consent as a defense to battery
   2. Informed consent
   3. Consent for research

E. Negligence
   1. Elements of negligence
   2. Anesthesia practice and negligence
   3. Litigation of anesthesia cases

4. Res ipsa loquitur
5. Prevention of anesthesia lawsuits
6. Defense of anesthesia lawsuits

F. Vicarious Liability
1. The law of agency
2. Captain of the ship doctrine
3. Supervision and implied liability
4. Practical aspects of vicarious liability

G. Business Principles
1. Setting up a private practice
2. Proposal preparation
3. Obtaining business
4. Business structures
5. Sole proprietorship
6. Partnership
7. Corporations

H. Projections
1. Income
2. Expenses
3. Roadblocks to private practice
4. Getting assistance
5. Accountant
6. Attorney
7. Business consultants

I. Employment Law
1. Practice options for nurse anesthetists
2. Employment rights

J. Other areas of law
1. Product liability
2. Antitrust law
3. Intentional torts

K. Contract Law
1. Purpose of contracts
2. Types of contract
3. Elements of an employment contract
4. Contract for anesthesia services
5. Negotiations
6. Review of other anesthesia-related contracts

L. Anesthesia Economics
    1. Economic principles
    2. Supply/demand
    3. Competition
    4. Self-interest
    5. Reimbursement for anesthesia services
    6. Third-party payment

M. Case presentations and final examination projects

Summary

Teaching law to nurse anesthesiology students is a challenge because of the changing political, legal, and economic environments. There are many individuals and institutions who will use legal excuses or threats to influence CRNA practice. If the students, graduates, and faculty understand the basic tenets of law and where to find resources, the entire profession will benefit.

Suggested Resources

- Kaplin WA, Lee BA. *The Law of Higher Education*. 3rd ed. Hoboken, NJ: Wiley; 1995. (This is a comprehensive resource and reference for all legal aspects of higher education. There is no specific area for anesthesia or related clinical education; however, it can be useful for general university legal issues.)
- www.aana.com (AANA is the professional organization for nurse anesthetists. This website has invaluable information regarding legal, education, practice, and reimbursement issues.)
- Blumenreich GA. Legal Briefs. http://www.aana.com/newsandjournal/Pages/aanajournalonline.aspx (These columns, written by the AANA General Counsel, are one of the best resources for current legal cases regarding nurse anesthetists and should be mandatory reading for both students and CRNAs.)
- University library. University libraries are some of the best resources for legal research and assistance to students and faculty. If there is a law library connected with the university, or a law library within a local public library, these are also excellent sources of information.
- Cohen H. *You Can Negotiate Anything*. Secaucus, NJ: Lyle Stuart; 1980. (This book is frequently quoted in other books on negotiations. It is considered to be one of the best books on negotiation techniques.)
- Ilich J, Jones BS. *Successful Negotiating Skills for Women*. Boston: MA; Addison-Wesley; 1981. (This is an excellent book directed primarily to women.)
- Jandt FE, *Win-Win Negotiating: Turning Conflict Into Agreement*. New York, NY: John Wiley & Sons; 1985.

- Leeds D. *Smart Questions: A new Strategy for Successful Managers*. New York, NY: McGraw Hill. (This book utilizes the power of questions in the negotiating process. It is very readable and contains valuable information for the non-professional negotiator.)
- Levin E. *Negotiating Tactics: Bargain Your Way to Winning*. New York, NY: Ballantine; 1980.
- Schoenfield M, Schoenfield R. *Legal Negotiations; Getting Maximum Results*. Colorado Springs, CO: Shepard's/McGraw-Hill; 1988 . (This book is primarily written for lawyers who do all types of negotiations on behalf of their clients. It is well-organized and presents a systematic approach to negotiating.)
- Mannino MJ. *The Business of Anesthesia: Practice Options for Nurse Anesthetists*. Park Ridge, IL; AANA Publishing; 1994. *(*out of print*)*

References

1. Kaplin WA, Lee BA. *The Law of Higher Education*. 3rd ed. Hoboken, NJ: Wiley; 1995.

2. Blumenreich G. Nurse anesthetists in the middle: Covenants not to compete. *J Am Assoc Nurse Anesth*. 1998;66(6):541–544.

3. DiBianca M. Discovery and preservation of social media evidence. *Bus L Today*. 2014;1:1–4.

CHAPTER 5

Educational Requirements for Nurse Anesthesia Programs

Francis Gerbasi, PhD, CRNA

Keywords: Accreditation, doctoral, education, fellowships, quality, standards.

Key Concepts

- The Council on Accreditation of Nurse Anesthesia Educational Programs (COA) establishes the standards and requirements that all accredited nurse anesthesia programs must meet.
- On January 1, 2022 and thereafter, all students matriculated into an accredited nurse anesthesia program must be enrolled in doctoral programs.
- Quality assessment by programs' continuous self-assessment and review is an essential requirement.
- Monitoring student achievement includes COA requirements that programs must meet for certification examination pass rates, attrition, and employment rates.
- Accreditation requirements include but are not limited to program administrators' qualifications and responsibilities, student admission requirements, and the curriculum (ie, didactic and clinical).

Introduction

In 1933 the National Association of Nurse Anesthetists (NANA) was established. A primary goal of NANA was to develop nurse anesthesia educational objectives.[1] During the next 65 years the education of nurse anesthetists transitioned from apprenticeships to the awarding of graduate degrees at accredited universities. In 1998, all nurse anesthesia educational programs were required to award master's degrees, and in 2009 the COA established the requirement that students accepted into an accredited program on January 1, 2022 and thereafter must graduate with doctoral degrees.[2,3] In addition, at its January 2014 meeting the COA adopted standards and procedures for the accreditation of postgraduate Certified Registered Nurse Anesthetist (CRNA) fellowships.[4] Please refer to the 2004 *Standards for Accreditation of Nurse Anesthesia Educational Programs* (2004 standards) and the *Standards for Accreditation of Nurse Anesthesia Programs: Practice Doctorate* (PDS) for additional information regarding the history of nurse anesthesia accreditation.[2,5] This chapter will provide the reader with a better understanding of the accreditation standards and requirements for programs awarding master's and doctoral degrees, and how programs demonstrate compliance with accreditation requirements.

Accreditation Standards, Policies, and Procedures

The accreditation requirements for nurse anesthesia programs have been governed by the COA for over 40 years. The COA is the only accrediting agency recognized by the U.S. Department of Education (USDE) and the Council for Higher Education Accreditation (CHEA) to accredit nurse anesthesia educational programs in the United States and Puerto Rico. The scope of the COA's accreditation includes nurse anesthesia programs that award post-master's certificates, master's degrees, and/or doctoral degrees, including programs offering distance education. The standards (ie, master's, doctoral, and fellowships) are measures used by the COA to assess the quality of nurse anesthesia education.[2,4,5] The standards were developed with input from the stakeholders that are affected by them, including CRNA practitioners and educators; student registered nurse anesthetists; program administrators and faculty; hospital administrators; state boards of nursing; members of the National Board of Certification and Recertification for Nurse Anesthetists (NBCRNA); and the AANA Board of Directors. In January 2014, the COA approved the PDS and the *Standards for the Accreditation of Post-Graduate Fellowships* (PGFS).[4,5] Revisions were also approved to the 2004 standards.[2]

To be accredited by the COA a nurse anesthesia program must demonstrate it is in full compliance with the standards. An example of how accredited programs awarding master's or doctoral degrees demonstrate compliance with the program effectiveness and evaluation standards is the development and implementation of a systematic evaluation process (refer to PDS, H. Evaluation Standards, pp. 25–26, and 2004 Standards, Standard IV: Program Effectiveness, pp. 10–11).[2,5] The evaluation progress must include formative and summative evaluations of students, and evaluation of the program by students, faculty, alumni, and employers. Programs are required to demonstrate how they use evaluation data to improve quality and effectiveness.

In addition to establishing standards for nurse anesthesia programs, the COA establishes policies and procedures used to implement the standards. The

Accreditation Policies and Procedures are used to foster educational quality and to facilitate implementation of the Standards.[6] The policies and procedures are also established to meet the requirements of external agencies such as USDE and CHEA and to safeguard the rights, responsibilities, and interests of students, faculty, administrators, the profession, the public, and other members of the community of interest. Substantive revisions of the *Accreditation Policies and Procedures* that could have a major effect on programs are subject to review, hearing, and comment by the Council's community of interest. Nurse anesthesia programs are expected to follow the *Accreditation Policies and Procedures* in carrying out their educational activities and submitting accreditation-related requests to the COA.

It is essential that program administrators and faculty have a good understanding of the accreditation standards, policies, and procedures. The standards for nurse anesthesia programs awarding master's and doctoral degrees and the *Accreditation Policies and Procedures* are posted on the COA's website (https://home.coa.us.com). In addition, the COA publishes Program Directors' Updates three times per year. The Program Directors' Updates provide program administrators and faculty with information regarding changes in accreditation and education requirements. In addition, programs are assigned an accreditation specialist. The accreditation specialists provide support for programs by clarifying requirements and processing programs' accreditation-related activities such as continued accreditation reviews and requests for new clinical sites.

Standards for Accreditation of Nurse Anesthesia Programs: Practice Doctorate (PDS)

The COA first published standards for practice-oriented and research-oriented doctoral degrees in 2004. In June 2007, the AANA Board of Directors unanimously adopted a position supporting doctoral education for entry into nurse anesthesia practice by 2025. This decision was based on more than two years of investigation thoroughly exploring the interests and concerns surrounding doctoral preparation of nurse anesthetists. The COA's Standard Revisions Task Force (SRTF) developed standards for the accreditation of programs awarding doctoral degrees and fellowships between 2011 and 2013.[7] The PDS were developed with input from the community of interest. In January 2014, the COA approved the PDS. On January 1, 2022 and thereafter, all students matriculating into an accredited program must be enrolled in a doctoral program. As of May 5, 2017, there are 53 programs approved to award doctoral degrees for entry into practice and 24 programs offering post-master's doctoral degrees for CRNAs.

Standards for the Accreditation of Post-Graduate Fellowships (PGFS)

In addition to developing new doctoral standards and revisions to the standards for programs awarding master's degrees, the SRTF also developed the PGFS.[4] A fellowship accredited by the COA contains advanced education and training in a focused area of specialty practice or concentration. The PGFS support fellowship offerings in areas of specialty practice such as pediatrics, obstetrics, and pain management or concentrations such as leadership. The fellowship is developed for CRNAs. Nonclinical fellowships may be applicable to other advanced practice registered nurses (APRN). Although each postgraduate fellowship may be unique, the standards are intended to promote quality and consistency for accreditation purposes. The PGFS apply to postgraduate fellowships conducted face-to-face and by distance education.

General Educational Requirements for Nurse Anesthesia Programs

Accreditation of nurse anesthesia programs provides quality assurance concerning the educational preparation of nurse anesthetists for entry into practice through continuous self-assessment and review. Accredited programs are required to perform ongoing evaluation and assessment to determine their integrity and educational effectiveness. Each program must continuously monitor and evaluate its didactic and clinical curriculum, including curriculum content, admissions policies, faculty, and clinical sites used for student educational experiences. Common methods that programs use to meet this requirement include student evaluations of the didactic and clinical instruction, exit student evaluations of the program, alumni evaluations, and employer evaluations of the graduates. These aspects of programs are evaluated periodically by the COA to determine their compliance with accreditation standards (ie, master's and doctoral) and their relevance to anesthesia practice.[2,5]

The processes for the accreditation of a nurse anesthesia program are focused on ensuring the program's compliance with the accreditation standards. The first step in the process for accreditation of a new nurse anesthesia program is for the sponsoring institution to file a letter of intent with the COA. The letter of intent must be from the chief executive officer of the sponsoring institution, and reflect the institution's legal authority to grant the degree and its commitment to providing the necessary resources to establish a program that meets accreditation requirements. For the continued accreditation of established nurse anesthesia programs, the CEO of the sponsoring institution must submit a letter indicating that it has the legal authority to grant the degree.

Following the COA's acceptance of the letter of intent, both new and established programs start an accreditation review process. The process includes the submission of evidence of eligibility, a self-study, and onsite review. The onsite review is conducted by experienced nurse anesthesia educators and practitioners approved by the COA to serve as onsite reviewers. Only after all of these activities have been completed will the program be reviewed by the COA. The COA Board reviews all of the documentation and makes an accreditation decision based on the program's ability to demonstrate compliance with the standards. For new programs the length of initial accreditation is normally five years. The length of accreditation for established programs can range from two to ten years. The COA's decisions regarding the length of accreditation awarded are based on programs' compliance with the standards as reflected in the "Decisions for Accreditation of Nurse Anesthesia Educational Programs" policy.[6]

It is important to note the accreditation decision process does not consider workforce issues (ie, assessment of supply and demand for CRNAs). This would be inconsistent with USDE and CHEA recognition requirements that the accreditation process and decision be focused on a program's ability to demonstrate compliance with accreditation standards. In addition, considering the supply and demand for CRNAs would have antitrust implications for the COA.

Ongoing monitoring of accredited programs is accomplished through programs' submissions of their annual reports, mid-point student and faculty evaluations, and progress reports to the COA. Annual reports provide data regarding the programs, including the names of university and program officials, degrees offered, and the academic units in which nurse anesthesia programs are housed. In addition, programs report student attrition and graduate employment rates. Programs' students and faculty provide anonymous evaluations of the programs and their clinical sites at the mid-point of the programs' accreditation cycle. The COA reviews the evaluations and requests progress reports on identified areas of concern. The COA can request a program provide a progress report for reasons in addition to student and faculty evaluations such as unresolved issues related to partial or noncompliance with the standards and criteria.

Program Resources and Student Capacity

At its May 2013 meeting, the COA approved a "Program Resources and Student Capacity" policy.[6] The policy supports the requirement that programs must verify there are adequate resources to support the size and scope of the program to appropriately prepare students for practice and to promote the quality of graduates. The process used to establish programs' class size is identified in the policy. Programs can submit requests to increase their assigned class size. Requests to increase class size must be approved prior to the enrollment of additional students.

Monitoring Student Achievement

The COA requires programs to document student achievement in multiple ways. Indicators of student achievement include identifying the number of students who complete the program, the number of graduates who pass the National Certification Examination for Nurse Anesthetists (NCE) in accordance with the COA's "Certification Examination" policy, and the number of graduates who secure employment as a CRNA within six months, post-graduation. Programs are also required to conduct graduate (alumni) and employer evaluations to assess programs' ability to prepare nurse anesthetists who are competent and capable of functioning in a variety of anesthesia settings.

The COA conducts periodic assessment of recent graduates' preparedness for entry into practice. The most recent published assessment was conducted from August 2011 to February 2012. The results indicate 98% of graduates and 97% of employers identified graduates were prepared for entry into practice. Ninety-six percent of the employers indicated they would hire the same graduates again.[8]

The COA believes an important measure of student achievement is the ability of graduates to pass the NCE. The COA established a policy and procedures for monitoring programs' NCE pass rates in 2003. The COA made major revisions to the policy in 2006, 2013, and 2016. The most recently revised policy identifies the mandatory pass rate of 80% of all of a program's first-time takers when considering the three most recent graduation cohorts.[9] Programs must meet or exceed the COA mandatory pass rate. Programs that fall below the mandatory pass rate will be placed on monitoring. If improvement is not demonstrated within the established timeframe the program's accreditation is subject to an adverse accreditation action.

In 2007, the COA implemented the monitoring of programs' attrition and employment rates.[10] Programs are required to report student attrition and employment rates on the COA annual report. High attrition rates are identified by the COA, and employment rates less than 80% based on a five-year average require programs to provide status reports to the COA. If improvement is not shown within a specified time, a program's accreditation is subject to an adverse accreditation action.

Programs must demonstrate they meet the COA's requirements for each of these three student achievement indicators (ie, NCE pass rate, attrition, and employment rates). This stringent evaluation process helps to ensure the effectiveness of nurse anesthesia education and the COA's compliance with USDE recognition requirements for accrediting agencies.

Program Administrators' and Clinical Coordinators' Requirements

The 2004 standards and the PDS have requirements for nurse anesthesia program administrators and assistant administrators. Both standards require that nurse anesthesia programs employ CRNAs in program administrator and assistant program administrator positions. Doctoral degrees are required for the CRNA program administrators (program administrator and assistant program administrator) in all doctoral programs by 2018. The CRNA program administrator must have the leadership authority and accountability for the administration of the program. Administration of a nurse anesthesia program includes the management of faculty and students, fiscal program management, maintenance of COA accreditation, and other higher education accreditation requirements of the university, faculty continuing education, and program evaluation, at a minimum. The CRNA program administrators' graduate degrees must be from an institution of higher education accredited by a nationally recognized accrediting agency.

The program must appoint a CRNA clinical coordinator for each clinical site. All clinical coordinators were required to have a master's degree by 2015. Program administrators must provide the COA with an official transcript demonstrating compliance with this requirement. Exceptions to the master's degree requirement can be requested. An exception, if granted, will be effective for five years from the date of COA approval.

Admission Requirements

The standards identify the minimum admission requirements applicants must meet for acceptance into a nurse anesthesia program. The standards require that applicants admitted to a nurse anesthesia program be graduates of an accredited school of nursing and possess a baccalaureate degree in nursing or an appropriate major, an unencumbered license as a registered professional nurse in the United States, its territories or protectorates, and a minimum of one year full-time work experience, or its part-time equivalent, as a RN in a critical care setting. Most applicants have acquired two or more years of clinical experience.

Requirements for the Didactic Curriculum

The didactic curriculum of nurse anesthesia programs must meet the standards and provide students the foundation upon which to build sound and safe clinical practice. Based on the COA's 2015 Annual Report data, most nurse anesthesia programs awarding master's degrees range from 64 to 96 credit hours, and programs awarding doctoral degrees range from 80 to 130 credit hours.[11] The master's and doctoral standards identify required courses and number of content hours in the basic nurse anesthesia academic curriculum[2,5] (Tables 5.1 and 5.2).

Table 5.1 Standards for Accreditation of Nurse Anesthesia Educational Programs: Practice Doctorate—Minimum Curriculum Course Contact Hour Requirements[5]

Required content	Minimum number of contact hours
Advanced physiology/pathophysiology	120
Advanced pharmacology	90
Basic and advanced principles in nurse anesthesia	120
Research	75
Advanced health assessment	45

Note: Required content areas are identified in the PDS.

Table 5.2 Standards for Accreditation of Nurse Anesthesia Educational Programs: 2004—Minimum Curriculum Course Contact Hour Requirements[2]

Required content	Minimum number of contact hours
Pharmacology of anesthetic agents and adjuvant drugs including concepts in chemistry and biochemistry	105
Anatomy, physiology, and pathophysiology	135
Professional aspects of nurse anesthesia practice	45
Basic and advanced principles of anesthesia practice, including physics, equipment, technology, and pain management	105
Research	30
Clinical correlation conferences	45

Note: Required content areas are identified in the 2004 standards.

In addition, required content areas are identified without a specific number of hours. Courses required to meet the academic requirements identified in the APRN Consensus Model include three separate comprehensive graduate-level courses in advanced physiology/pathophysiology, advanced health assessment, and advanced pharmacology (refer 2004 Standards, Standard III, Criteria C14–C15, and PDS, Curriculum Standards E.2.1–E,2.2).[2,5,12]

Courses in anesthesia practice provide content such as induction, maintenance, and emergence from anesthesia; airway management; anesthesia pharmacology; teaching of regional anesthesia techniques; and anesthesia for special populations such as obstetric, geriatric, and pediatric patients. Students are instructed in the use of anesthesia machines and other related biomedical monitoring equipment and are evaluated didactically using such traditional evaluation methods as examinations, presentations, care plans, and papers.

Nurse anesthesia programs must be able to show that they provide an extensive, educationally sound curriculum combining both academic theory and clinical practice. Evidence includes student, faculty, alumni, and employer evaluations. The curriculum must be provided in a logical manner. Classroom and clinical experiences must be sequential starting from basic and moving toward more advanced knowledge and skills as the student progresses in the program. The policies and procedures of each program must use outcome criteria to promote student learning while enhancing the program's quality and integrity.

The methods used to provide nurse anesthesia education are changing as new technologies such as distance education and simulation are being applied in higher education. Based on the COA's 2016 Annual Report, 75% of nurse anesthesia programs use some form of distance education in providing didactic instruction.[11] The distance education offerings vary from several core nursing courses to programs in which the majority of the didactic curriculum is provided using distance education. Programs must be approved by the COA prior to offering distance education. Program administrators must follow the established accreditation policies and procedures for submission of distance education applications.

The majority of programs report using some form of simulation.[11] Simulation offerings vary from use of mannequins to demonstrate regional anesthesia techniques to full-body simulators. At present, simple models and simulated experiences may be used to satisfy the minimum case requirements for placement of central venous pressure catheters and part of the requirement for endoscopic techniques.[13]

Requirements for the Clinical Curriculum

Nurse anesthesia students must develop the knowledge, skills, and abilities for entry into practice, and must participate in all phases of their clinical cases including preoperative, intraoperative and postoperative anesthesia care. The standards establish programs' minimum requirements for the clinical curricula and help ensure that graduates are prepared to administer all types of anesthesia, including general, regional, selected local, and moderate/deep sedation to patients of all ages for all types of surgeries. The clinical curriculum ensures students are taught to use all currently available anesthesia drugs, to manage fluid and blood replacement therapy, and to interpret data from sophisticated monitoring devices. In addition, students obtain experience in the insertion of invasive catheters, the recognition and correction of complications that occur during the course of an anesthetic, the provision of airway and ventilatory support during resuscitation, and pain management.

Supervised clinical experience provides student registered nurse anesthetists with the opportunity to incorporate didactic anesthesia education into the clinical setting. During their clinical anesthesia experience, students must be supervised by CRNAs or anesthesiologists who are immediately available. The clinical supervision ratio of students to instructors must be coordinated to ensure patient safety and should not exceed two students to one CRNA or anesthesiologist. Effective January 1, 2015, students enrolled in nurse anesthesia programs must meet increased clinical requirements to be eligible to sit for the NCE. A student must have performed a minimum of 600 anesthetics and 2000 clinical hours, which must include specialties such as pediatric, obstetric, cardiothoracic, and neurosurgical anesthesia.[2,5]

Programs must establish processes to accurately count, track, and evaluate students' clinical experiences and performance. In 2015, the COA established *Guidelines for Counting Clinical Experiences* to enhance consistency in how students quantify their clinical learning expereinces.[13] Clinical evaluations must include both formative and summative assessments. Clinical faculty must provide accurate and complete clinical assessments of students' performance.

Summary

The nurse anesthesia profession has flourished for more than a century by having a foundation built on its educational programs that meet stringent educational standards. Advancements in nurse anesthesia education have helped strengthen the profession. As programs transition from awarding master's to doctoral degrees for entry into nurse anesthesia practice, it is important that program administrators and faculty continue to ensure their programs meet accreditation requirements and graduates have the entry-into-practice competencies to provide safe, competent, and ethical anesthesia and anesthesia-related care to patients for diagnostic, therapeutic, and surgical procedures.

References

1. The National Association of Nurse Anesthetists. *Constitution and Bylaws*. Park Ridge, IL: AANA Archives. 1933.

2. Council on Accreditation of Nurse Anesthesia Educational Programs (COA). *Standards for Accreditation of Nurse Anesthesia Educational Programs, 2004*. Park Ridge, IL: Council on Accreditation of Nurse Anesthesia Educational Programs; 2016.

3. Gerbasi F. Program Directors' Update. Park Ridge, IL: Council on Accreditation of Nurse Anesthesia Educational Programs; 2009:53.

4. Council on Accreditation of Nurse Anesthesia Educational Programs (COA). *Standards for Accreditation of Post-Graduate CRNA Fellowships*. Park Ridge, IL: Council on Accreditation of Nurse Anesthesia Educational Programs; 2014.

5. Council on Accreditation of Nurse Anesthesia Educational Programs (COA). *Standards for Accreditation of Nurse Anesthesia Programs: Practice Doctorate*. Park Ridge, IL: Council on Accreditation of Nurse Anesthesia Educational Programs; 2016.

6. Council on Accreditation of Nurse Anesthesia Educational Programs (COA). *Accreditation Policies and Procedures*. Park Ridge, IL: Council on Accreditation of Nurse Anesthesia Educational Programs; 2017.

7. Gombokoto RL, Walker JR, Horton BJ, Martin-Sheridan D, Yablonky MJ, Gerbasi F. Council on Accreditation of Nurse Anesthesia Educational Programs adopts standards for the practice doctorate and post-graduate CRNA fellowships. *AANA J*. 2014;82(3):177–183.

8. Cook KA, Marienau MS, Wildgust B, Gerbasi F, Watkins J. Assessment of recent graduates preparedness for entry into practice. *AANA J*. 2013;81(5):341–345.

9. Gerbasi F. Program Directors' Update. Park Ridge, IL: Council on Accreditation of Nurse Anesthesia Educational Programs; 2016:75.

10. Implementation of Policies for the Monitoring of Nurse Anesthesia Programs' Attrition and Graduate Employment Rates. Council on Accreditation of Nurse Anesthesia Educational Programs; May 2007.

11. Council on Accreditation of Nurse Anesthesia Educational Programs (COA). Annual Report. Park Ridge, IL: Council on Accreditation of Nurse Anesthesia Educational Programs; 2016.

12. American Association of Colleges of Nursing (AACN). *APRN [Advanced Practice Registered Nurse] Consensus Model*. Washington, DC: American Association of Colleges of Nursing. 2008.

13. Council on Accreditation of Nurse Anesthesia Educational Programs (COA). *Guidelines for Counting Clinical Experiences*. Park Ridge, IL: Council on Accreditation of Nurse Anesthesia Educational Programs; 2015.

CHAPTER 6

Evidence-Based Nurse Anesthesia Practice: Learning, Practicing, and Teaching

John J. McFadden, PhD, CRNA

Keywords: Evidence-based, evidence-based models, levels of evidence, nurse anesthesia practice, patient outcome, pedagogy, quality care, teaching, translational research.

Key Concepts

- Evidence-based practice is critical to improving patient outcomes.
- Implementation of evidence-based practice requires a thorough assessment of best available evidence.
- Evidence exists in many forms; the strength and applicability of evidence requires practitioner judgment.
- In contrast to research utilization, evidence-based practice incorporates the experience and judgment of the health care practitioner and the patient's desires.
- Evidence-based practice requires several key skill sets in order to be successful.
- Nurse anesthesia educators must be deliberate in designing pedagogical strategies that assist students to acquire evidence-based practice skills.
- Adoption of evidence-based practice may pose challenges; however, the rewards for patients are significant.

Introduction

This chapter will give a historical background of evidence-based practice (EBP), define EBP, and discuss the reasons for and against use of EBP. It also will outline the steps of the EBP process, describe how to implement an evidence-based approach to clinical practice, and explain how to appraise the strength of evidence-based literature. Finally, considerations for teaching EBP are provided as a resource for nurse anesthesia educators.

Beginnings of Evidence-Based Practice

Certified Registered Nurse Anesthetists (CRNAs) have a long-standing history of delivering high-quality anesthesia services. Evidence-based practice facilitates a clinician's ability to provide high-quality care while integrating multiple aspects of the patient's preferences and the family's preferences.

The widely cited Institute of Medicine (IOM) report titled, *To Err is Human: Building a Safer Healthcare System*, which attributes as many as 98,000 US deaths annually to medical errors, served to awaken the American public to the risks associated with health care.[1] As a result, health care consumers and purchasers began to question the quality of care rendered, and therefore, the continued competence of its practitioners. In a follow-up IOM report titled, *The Health Professions Education: A Bridge to Quality,* the following recommendation was issued:

> Department of Health and Human Services (DHHS) and leading foundations should support an interdisciplinary effort focused on developing a common language, with the ultimate aim of achieving consensus across the health professions on a core set of competencies that includes patient-centered care, interdisciplinary teams, evidence-based practice, quality improvement, and informatics.[2]

With the issuance of the Health Professions Education report, multiple communities of interest began to embrace the IOM's call for EBP competence. This movement is further reinforced by the emphasis on translational research in the required curriculum for the nursing practice doctorate or Doctor of Nursing Practice degree[3,4] and more recently in the IOM report, *The Future of Nursing: Leading Change, Advancing Health.*[5] EBP has given rise to the creation of many clinical practice guidelines, which are based on the analysis and summary of quantitative reports and the implementation of hospital- and clinician-level performance measures based on available evidence.

The rapid proliferation of the evidence-based concept within the literature is demonstrated by Alper et al,[6] whose MEDLINE search in 2003 using the key words "evidence based" returned almost 54,000 citations. More than 42,000 of these were published since 1993. This rapid expansion of knowledge available to the clinician is daunting. In an evidence-based approach to care, where a clinician is expected to continually apply the best evidence to the care of patients, the activity of continually assessing the best available evidence becomes challenging. For example, Alper et al[6] estimated the amount of time it would take for a physician trained in medical epidemiology to evaluate all primary care-related literature to be over 620 hours per month. This is equivalent to over 15 full-time equivalents (FTEs) based on a 40-hour work week. More recently, MEDLINE describes how more than 806,000 new scientific articles were published in one year alone in 2015.[7] Erren, Cullen, and Erren rightly pose the question: How does one "effectively surf today's information tsunami"?[8]

Choudry, Fletcher and Soumerai[9] assessed the proposition that physicians with more clinical practice experience may be less likely to render high-quality patient care. Their results revealed that as experience increased, clinical performance decreased, bringing into question the accuracy of the belief that a more experienced practitioner will deliver the highest quality care. Heater, et al[10] reported a 28% improvement in patient outcomes when care is rendered based on the best and latest evidence. Two decades later, with a similar nod to the benefits of using evidence over experience, Lugtenberg, Burgers and Westert[11] were able to demonstrate that Dutch evidence-based clinical guidelines can be effective in improving the structure and process of care.

The half-life for the nursing profession is estimated to be between two and five years.[12] Professional half-life is defined as the point at which half of a practitioner's beginning knowledge becomes dated as a result of changes in the field or by simply being forgotten. Due to the rapidly changing health care arena, practitioners entering into practice today may be competent; however, that competence may not be long lasting.[13] Rapidly changing medical and technological advances have the ability to significantly impact a health care practitioner's explicit knowledge base in a short time. In this world of health care quality measurement, it is critical that CRNAs commit to lifelong learning and become well versed in the application of an EBP approach to care.

Understanding the Evidence-Based Practice Movement

Nurse anesthetists, like other health care providers, exercise decision-making as part of their daily practice. Each patient encounter generates clinical questions that require thoughtful answers. The uniqueness of every patient undergoing an anesthetic makes decision-making an ongoing, continuous process. How do nurse anesthetists gather and interpret data, draw conclusions, reference the most up-to-date scientific data, and ensure that the "right" action plan is constructed for each patient? How is the need for information to make the correct decisions met? Although it may appear to the untrained eye that the clinical nurse anesthetist is on autopilot after induction and before emergence, a commitment to vigilance requires nonstop observation, decision-making, and reaction during the provision of care.

Making a decision is a cognitive and emotional activity that involves selecting one pathway over others in an attempt to solve a problem and achieve a desired outcome. There are many factors that influence a decision: bias and preconceptions; previous experiences; logic and reasoning; values and ethics; available resources; emotions; and knowledge. Some theorize that personality or even genes may also influence how an individual makes decisions.[14,15] Clearly, decision-making is a dynamic, complex phenomenon that involves many attributes. In health care, the practitioner balances input from many of these variables. In addition, clinical decision makers may rely on input from other colleagues, published research articles, textbooks, product literature, or even gut instinct. The weight placed on any one of these variables will vary, depending on the decision at hand and its urgency.

When did the process for decision making in health care become an area of interest? Some trace the origins of the decision-making process to the start of the scientific revolution in the mid-1500s. This era marked a transition in the way science is conducted and how complex questions about life are answered. Simply relying on the views of authority figures (the "received view") or tradition was no longer acceptable. Other experts, however, prefer to consider the focus on using data for decision making as a more sophisticated, recent trend. Specifically in the medical profession, epidemiologist Archie Cochrane, who had roots in Scotland and Britain, is credited with beginning the evidence-based movement with the publication of his book, *Effectiveness and Efficiency: Reflections on Health Services.*[16] His ideas and support eventually led to the development of Cochrane,[17] previously known as the Cochrane Collaboration.

Cochrane[17] is a worldwide network of health care professionals, researchers, and people interested in health who serve as collaborating contributors of independent and trustworthy information about health. This forum was originally established as a means of organizing medical research in a way that would be helpful to health care professionals seeking the best available evidence for clinical decision-making. The mission of Cochrane is to "promote evidence-informed health decision-making by producing high-quality, relevant, accessible systematic reviews and other synthesized research evidence." The Cochrane Groups include: Cochrane Review Groups, with a focus on preparing and maintaining systematic reviews; the Cochrane Centres, which coordinate activities within a defined geographical or linguistic area; Cochrane Fields and Networks, which disseminate information and focus on other dimensions of health care; and Cochrane Methods Groups, which provide policy advice and methodology support for Cochrane Reviews. The Cochrane Library houses the collection of six databases that contain the evidence used by health care professionals for clinical decision-making. The six databases include: Cochrane Databases of Systematic Reviews (CDSR), Cochrane Central Register of Controlled Trials (CENTRAL), Cochrane Methodology Register (CMR), Database of Abstracts of Reviews of Effects (DARE), Health Technology Assessment Database (HTA), and the NHS Economic Evaluation Database (EED).

Several terms have been used to label the process of using data to support decision-making in health care. The term *evidence-based medicine*, which began appearing in the medical taxonomy in the early 1990s, has been attributed to the McMaster Medical School in Hamilton, Ontario. These methodologies were put into practice through the development of the Evidence-Based Medicine Working Group, led by David Sackett and Gordon Guyatt.[18] The group was renamed the Evidence-Based Clinical Practice Working Group.[18] Sackett became the founder of the Oxford Centre for Evidence Based Medicine. Throughout the 1990s, interdisciplinary teams were being established by the Agency for Health Care Policy and Research in an attempt to develop evidence-based clinical guidelines. This agency was later renamed the Agency for Healthcare Research and Quality. It continues to serve as a clearinghouse for clinical guidelines (https://www.guideline.gov). This development in medicine has influenced other professions, including nursing, to adopt the evidence-based model. Other terms currently associated with the process include *evidence-based practice, evidence-based nursing, evidence-based health care, evidence-based teaching*[19,20] and *evidence-based nurse anesthesia practice*. The basis for all of these terms is the same: using the best scientific evidence to support making clinical decisions, rather than basing clinical care on tradition and authoritative dictates.

A Common Definition for Evidence-Based Practice

Nurses have been called upon to use research to improve nursing care for decades.[21,22] Current professional practice and educational standards for nurses and advanced practice nurses, including for nurse anesthetists, memorialize the requirements for practitioners of nursing to engage in evidence-based practice.[3,4,23–29] One universal definition of evidence-based practice does not exist. Although sometimes used interchangeably, EBP does not equal research utilization. Research utilization is a part of EBP and involves applying research findings to practice. EBP is an overarching process that consists of multiple steps, including the application of research findings to practice. EBP also considers multiple forms of "evidence." Significant work has been previously completed by many authors to refine the concept of evidence-based medicine or practice over the years. Many scholars offer their own definition, each emphasizing different attributes.

Sackett and coauthors see evidence-based medicine as "the integration of best research evidence with clinical expertise and patient values."[30] Sackett et al offer additional definitions. Patient values are the "unique preferences, concerns and expectations each patient brings to a clinical encounter and which must be integrated into clinical decisions if they are to serve the patient."[30] Best research evidence is "clinically relevant research, often from the basic sciences of medicine, but especially from patient-centered clinical research into the accuracy and precision of diagnostic tests (including the clinical examination), the power of prognostic markers, and the efficacy and safety of therapeutic, rehabilitative and preventive regimens."[30] Clinical expertise is defined as "the ability to use our clinical skills and past experience to rapidly identify each patient's unique health state and diagnosis, their individual risks and benefits of potential interventions, and their personal values and expectations."[30]

Sigma Theta Tau International proposes that evidence-based nursing practice is "an integration of the best evidence available, nursing expertise, and the values and preferences of the individuals, families and communities who are served."[31] Pravikoff et al offer this definition: "Evidence-based practice is a systematic approach to problem solving for health care providers, including RNs, characterized by the use of the best evidence currently available for clinical decision making, in order to provide the most consistent and best possible care to patients."[32] The American Association of Nurse Anesthetists (AANA) defines *evidence-based nurse anesthesia practice* as the "integration and synthesis of the best research evidence with clinical expertise and patient values" in order to optimize the care of patients receiving anesthesia services.[33] Additionally, the AANA adopted an evidence-based policy and process for the development of practice-related documents.[34,35] As the definition of evidence-based practice evolves, the main constituents of the definition remain stable: a decision-making process for clinicians that considers research data, clinician expertise, and patient input.

The Changing View of Science

Like other scientists, nurses have a history of searching for cause and effect relationships to guide the decision-making process in providing care. Florence Nightingale exemplified this process by combining her understanding of mathematics, the classics, and her knowledge about hospital care to conduct studies about urban and hospital sanitary conditions. Statistical analysis was the basis for her correlations between mortality and lack of ventilation, lack of natural light, and overcrowded conditions as described in her work *Notes on Hospitals*.[36] These cause-and-effect studies led to Nightingale being considered the first biostatistician.[37]

Nightingale based her ideas about nursing on the scientific theories of her time and paralleled the ideas of the medical community. Positivism held the dominant position as the philosophy of science of the time. The ontology of positivism is that the world is real and knowable and exists independently of the observer. Positivists believe the world is governed by natural laws, resulting in cause-effect relationships, and believe it is predictable. The goal of this worldview is to uncover truths and facts as quantitatively derived relationships between variables. Like her contemporaries, Nightingale was convinced of the power of this approach to science coupled with the use of statistics.

As the profession evolved, nursing scholars questioned the congruence between the profession's holistic foundation and the positivist approach to science. How can the human health experience be reduced to measurable concepts independent of history, culture, and social and personal contexts? A reductionist approach can become so dissociated from the object it is attempting to explain that it no longer provides useful information. In addition to predicting and controlling the relationships between variables, there is a recognized need to explain and understand the meaning of the phenomena of human health through a postmodern approach. This can only be done within the context in which these phenomena occur. As a profession that involves intimate relationships between unique individuals with varying life experiences, nursing is well suited for the postmodern worldview. This is the paradigm that helps shape the dualism between the science and art of nursing.

So where does this leave today's nurse anesthetist attempting to use a rapid and consistent problem-solving approach to clinical practice problems, many of which involve life and death situations? There is no doubt that quantitative research using the scientific method and a positivist approach provide knowledge about many biophysical processes in which the profession is involved. This knowledge is invaluable to the nurse anesthetist. The limitation of these approaches is that they can never fully explain what an individual experiences when faced with the transition between health and illness and the various aspects involved in receiving modern health care. A context-dependent, postmodern approach may be used when trying to understand the interpersonal relationships involved in providing nurse anesthesia care. These methods add richness to capturing the experiences of people as they receive health care. A plurality of approaches will enrich the profession so that knowledge development is supported with a solid understanding of the lived human experience; therefore, the phrase embraced by the modern scholar applies— "the question drives the method."

As a result of the multiple approaches to generating knowledge and research data, it is a challenge for many health care providers to identify and apply the appropriate data or set of evidence needed to make a decision. Searching a knowledge base, weeding through the available science, reflecting on one's own clinical expertise, and contemplating the uniqueness and singularity of the patient and situation at hand require a formidable skill set.

Several scholars have identified barriers that exist for nurses to accomplish this task. These barriers include lack of time, limited resources, undeveloped skills in data searching and the research process, inexperience in applying the evidence, lack of authority to implement process changes, and patient noncompliance.[38–41] These challenges are not necessarily unique to nurses, but applicable to a wide range of health care providers, including nurse anesthetists.

Identifying the appropriate data and applying it to the situation at hand is one of the more demanding tasks involved in clinical decision-making. Some decisions made by nurse anesthetists allow for creativity; no singular approach emerges as best. Providing reassurance in the preoperative holding area or discussing a medical error that has occurred are examples of situations that demand judgment, concern about the individual patient's needs, and other considerations that are context-dependent. Other decisions, however, leave less room for the imaginative spirit. Choosing a dose of an intravenous agent or managing a rare coexisting disease during a general inhalation anesthetic may allow for some ingenuity, but these generally are situations that require data that have been tried and tested. It is a challenge finding the right blend of evidence to make decisions in nurse anesthesia practice. Thus, nurse anesthetists and most health care providers consider a variety of research approaches—quantitative analysis, qualitative analysis, and mixed method approaches—and integrate these findings with their own judgment and the desires of the patient to make decisions about how to provide care.

Wyszewianski and Green[42] describe four types of physician practitioners with regard to utilization of available evidence. These descriptions are of interest to the nurse anesthesia profession and may be applicable as well.

1. The seeker actively engages the professional literature and readily accesses electronic as well as print collections. This type of practitioner usually easily embraces the concept of an evidence-based approach to care, in that they easily translate information gleaned from the literature into practice. They actively engage in independent evidence appraisal.
2. The receptive practitioner in similar fashion will apply new information to the clinical setting; however, this information must originate from a respected and trusted source rather than being independently assessed.
3. The traditionalist will place greater weight on experience, skill, and authoritative advocates for change when making clinical decisions or considering an alteration to clinical practice.
4. The final type of practitioner described by Wyszewianski and Green[42] is the pragmatist. The pragmatist shares in the belief that clinical practice is grounded in a scientifically sound foundation; however, pragmatists are less likely to adopt practices if they view them as being disruptive to the flow of care or impact patient satisfaction.

Practicing nurse anesthetists and those registered nurses pursuing graduate studies in the field may derive benefits by comparing these approaches to their own personal approaches to reviewing the available evidence and incorporating it into practice.

Evidence-Based Practice: Why or Why Not?

There are several reasons that support the need to use research results or evidence when making a decision that impacts another person's health and well-being. The continued focus on error reduction inspired by the IOM[1] has promoted health care practices that are based on sound scientific knowledge. Accrediting and regulatory agencies, including Magnet Recognition by the American Nurses Credentialing Center (ANCC), also promote the use of evidence-based decisions in practice. This promotes scholarship in clinical practice. In many ways, the evidence-based practice movement attempts to minimize the distance between scholarship and practice, researcher and clinician; that is, knowledge generators and knowledge users must interface on a more consistent basis and share perspectives.[43]

The ethical principle of autonomy, or self-determination, requires that a patient provide informed consent before receiving health care. Informed consent involves frank, open discussion about risks, benefits, outcomes, and alternatives of care. These discussions between provider and patient cannot occur without some evidence supporting a care decision. Decisions regarding treatments and interventions should include the goal of being cost-justifiable since funding and resources for health care are not limitless. Utilization of health care resources needs to be supported by data that defend an intervention's benefit and cost-effectiveness. Last, patients and payers, as consumers of health care, have the right to be aware of the processes used by a provider and the outcomes achieved. In the broadest sense, these are aspects considered when evaluating quality of care.

Evidence-Based Practice: Implementation Considerations

Not everyone views evidence-based practice as a panacea for ending the health care industry's woes. Holmes and colleagues[44] cautioned against having a false sense of security in believing that quantitative, positivist research serves as the strongest evidence available for decision-making. In fact, Holmes et al[45] highlight hidden political concerns of evidence-based practice. They suggest that the creation of practice guidelines can discipline, govern, and regulate nursing work, however, suppress creativity and critical thinking. Finally, unless practitioners possess the skills to read, evaluate, weigh, and apply research, the process is not effective. This skill deficit sets up a disconnect between research and practice. This ultimately may inhibit a practitioner's resourcefulness and his or her ability to synthesize and integrate knowledge.[46]

The adoption of an evidence-based approach to clinical practice often faces numerous barriers. According to Pravikoff, et al,[32] there are two types of barriers health care practitioners may encounter when attempting to implement an evidence-based practice. A practitioner may experience personal barriers, which impede the implementation of evidence-based practice. These barriers may include such things as a diminished value or knowledge for research into practice, a lack of database search skills (including internal database structure or function understanding), lack of computer skills necessary to conduct searches, access-related issues (eg, computer, library, or database), difficulties understanding the literature, or an inability to evaluate and synthesize the literature.

In addition to personal barriers, there are also institutional barriers, which pose a challenge to the implementation of an evidence-based framework supporting clinical practice. The facility may not place a high import toward adopting an evidence-based practice; it may lack the necessary budget or support services in order to accomplish this approach; or it may not hold the philosophical belief in the positive ramifications of adopting an evidence-based approach to care. In a recent study of medical residents, Windish et al[47] discovered most residents lacked the necessary knowledge to interpret statistics published in the medical literature. Although the sample size was small, the study is telling in a health care era with widespread support for an evidence-based approach to patient care.

Just as there are barriers to the implementation of an evidence-based approach to care, there are also facilitators to the adoption of this care approach, both internally and at the organizational level. According to Fineout-Overholt et al[48] these facilitators may include fostering the relationships between academic and clinical settings, the commitment of facility administration, or the identification of an evidence-based mentor in order to foster the development of evidence-based skills in health care practitioners.

Given these inhibiting and facilitating factors, how will practitioners transition into an evidence-based practice? Diffusion describes the process by which an innovation or information is communicated over time among members of a group. Diffusion occurs in a fashion graphically similar to a sigmoid curve, such that early adopters of the innovation fall to the lower left portion of the curve and late adopters to the upper right. According to Dearing, the characteristic "S" shape of the curve results from modeling of the innovation in the field over time, as influenced by the group's leaders.[49]

Roger's Diffusion of Innovations theory has been used to study research transfer and dissemination of information.[50] Diffusion theory requires several key components which include: an innovation; adopters; a group or system with leaders and perceived pressure to adopt the innovation; personal adoption processes which include innovation awareness and implementation; and a diffusion system. Balas and Boren[51] report it takes some 17 years to translate research findings into widespread clinical practice. Rogers discusses five attributes of an innovation which may impact the rapidity with which it is adopted:[50]

1. The perceived advantages (eg, cost) of the innovation
2. The degree of compatibility with the adopter's values and needs
3. The complexity (or simplicity) of the innovation
4. The ability of the adopter to experiment with the innovation, or its "trialability"
5. The degree to which the innovation is observable or visible to others

Considering evidence-based practice as an innovation within this context may help explain why it has been slow in achieving widespread adoption.

The Nuts and Bolts of Evidence-Based Practice

Many models exist or are in development to describe the process for evidence-based practice. Melnyk and Fineout-Overholt describe five critical steps that form the foundation for the process of evidence-based practice (**Table 6.1**).[52]

Table 6.1 Evidence-based Process Steps

1. Form a PICO question
2. Identify and retrieve best available evidence
3. Appraise the evidence
4. Integrate clinical expertise and patient values and needs with research
5. Evaluate intervention's effectiveness

These five steps are explained in more detail below:

1. Converting the need for information into an answerable question. The question should address the population of interest, the intervention of interest, the condition of interest, the outcome of interest, and a timeframe. The authors suggest the acronym PICO (ie, patient population, intervention of interest, comparison intervention or status, and outcome for focusing the formation of the question).
2. Identify and collect the best evidence that addresses the question.
3. Critically evaluate or appraise the evidence. Consider the validity, reliability, rigor, relevance, and clinical applicability of what is known about the issue. Determine the gaps versus the consistencies in the evidence available.
4. Integrate the research with clinical expertise and the unique values and needs of the patient.
5. Evaluate the effectiveness and efficiency of the intervention and the process.

To be successful in applying an evidenced-based process to clinical practice, a clinician must follow a fairly structured process which begins with formation of a clinical question. In order to uncover all existing evidence which relates to a clinical question, it is imperative the clinician frame the question appropriately. If the question is too broad, a clinician may have difficulties working through the abundance of literature returned while conducting a database search.

As suggested by Melnyk and Fineout-Overholt,[52] the utilization of the PICO format may be helpful. In addition, practitioners may consider the addition of an appropriate timeframe when framing the questions (ie, PICOT). One PICO-style example is as follows: In the pediatric patient (patient population), how effective is dexamethasone (intervention) versus ondansetron (intervention comparison) in preventing nausea (outcome)?

The next step a practitioner must take is to locate the evidence. This step requires access to electronic databases such as PubMed, Excerpta Medica Database (Embase), or the Cumulative Index of Nursing and Allied Health Literature (CINAHL). A clinician must select the most appropriate database in order to maximize success in uncovering the existing evidence. A practitioner must become familiar with the types of studies and access each database will afford. For example, the CINAHL contains nursing, allied health, and biomedicine studies. In comparison, PsycINFO contains citations within the field of psychology or the psychological aspects of related disciplines. Secondary to selecting an appropriate database to mine the evidence which relates to the clinical question the practitioner is attempting to answer, is the ability to identify key search terms. Practitioners must be savvy at selecting the appropriate search key words which have the greatest potential in uncovering the existing literature. Several helpful evidence-based internet resources are listed below. (**Table 6.2**).

Table 6.2 Useful Resources

Resource	URL
Centre for Evidence-Based Medicine (CEBM)	www.cebm.net
Joanna Briggs Institute (JBI)	http://www.joannabriggs.org
Agency for Healthcare Research and Quality (AHRQ)	http://www.ahrq.gov/
The Cochrane Collaboration	http://www.cochrane.org/
PubMed database	http://www.ncbi.nlm.nih.gov/pubmed/
OVID	www.ovid.com

Once the practitioner has successfully conducted a literature search associated with the clinical question at hand, the practitioner must undergo a thorough assessment of that literature. Generally, considering evidence which is quantitative in nature, systematic reviews or meta-analyses on the associated topic are considered to be the strongest evidence, provided they are rigorously conducted. Randomized clinical trials are usually considered the next evidence tier, followed by cohort studies, case control studies, case series, case reports, ideas, editorials, or opinions, respectively. From a historical perspective, qualitative studies have played less of a role in the evidence-based practice movement; however, the health care arena has recently begun to embrace the value qualitative reports can add to an EBP approach.

Ranking the Evidence: Strong versus Weak

When examining the body of research around a given topic, it is necessary to sift through the data and information to separate stronger sources from weaker ones. The investigator must ascribe value to each piece of evidence and determine if it is appropriate for the question at hand. This step is wrought with implications not only for the researcher and the practitioner, but also for educators and policymakers. In essence, this step holds the power to continue a current practice or change a clinician's care decisions.

The strength of a research study or other source of data is not based on the conclusion reached, but rather on the extent to which appropriate methodology is used to conduct the study or generate the source. To minimize the influence of bias when accomplishing this goal, experts in evidence-based research recommend the use of a ranking system. Many examples of ranking systems are available from a variety of sources such as governmental agencies, academic centers, and health systems. The type of data examined drives the style of the ranking system. Once a body of research has been ranked, the ranking labels then can be used by practitioners to make decisions.

Most existing ranking systems, or taxonomies, are designed according to type of research design, ie, quantitative or qualitative studies. In general, the Agency for Healthcare Research and Quality recommends that assessing the strength of a body of evidence should include three domains:[53]

- *Quality*: the extent to which a study's design, conduct, and analysis have minimized selection, measurement, and confounding biases (internal validity).
- *Quantity*: the number of studies that have evaluated the question, overall sample size across studies, magnitude of the treatment effect, and strength from causality assessment, such as relative risk or odds ratio.
- *Consistency*: whether investigations with both similar and different study designs report similar findings (requires numerous studies).

In general, most evidence ranking and grading systems used in today's literature will use one of three coding systems. These coding systems may be letters (eg, A, b), numbers (eg, 1, II), or a combination of letters and numbers (eg, 1a, IIb). The difficulties posed by these coding systems is that they are often not universally reproducible and must be adapted based on the question at hand, and the types of literature which will answer the question at hand. An example of one type of evidence ranking methodology is provided in the Appendix at the end of this chapter.[54] **(See Appendix A).**

Critical appraisal of the quantitative literature requires addressing questions such as the following: Are the results of the study valid? Are the results reliable? Will the results apply to this patient population?

The postmodern paradigm associated with qualitative research has yielded many evaluative techniques and criteria. The evolution of these criteria is exemplified in the seminal writings of Guba and Lincoln,[55] among others.[56–61] Although no single method is "right," a trustworthy qualitative work includes, but is not limited to, assessment of such concepts as credibility (ie, accuracy of researcher actions), transferability (ie, are the results meaningful to other populations?), dependability (ie, under similar circumstances another researcher would reach the same conclusions), and confirmability (ie, conclusions are rooted in the data).

There are several tools which have been developed in order to assess various documents such as guidelines (ie, the Appraisal of Guidelines Research and Evaluation [AGREE] instrument), randomized controlled trial reports (ie, Consolidated Standards of Reporting Trials [CONSORT]), and meta-analyses of randomized controlled trials (ie, Quality of Reporting of Meta-analyses [QUORUM]). These tools have been developed to assist the practitioner in evaluating the quality of that particular piece of evidence (ie, guideline).

A Note About Rigor

The *rigor* of a research study refers to the extent that error or bias has been minimized. Quantitative and qualitative research will have different methods of assessing rigor because the two approaches have different philosophical underpinnings, methods of data collection, and techniques for analysis. To assess the rigor of all studies (quantitative, qualitative, or mixed-methods), using the same scale or ranking system will overlook the variation between these research methods, and it risks the erroneous evaluation of the studies as deficient. To that end, many experts propose multiple frameworks for evaluating research based on the nature of the research itself.

The Relationship Between Evidence-Based Practice and Ethics

Most nurses associate ethics with nursing practice. The ethical dilemmas of modern nursing practice include the use of genetic information, distribution of health care resources, application or refusal of advanced technology, and safeguarding confidential information. But ethics extends to research and evidence-based practice, as well. The principles of autonomy, beneficence, non-maleficence, justice, veracity, and fidelity frame the duties that nurses have to patients in implementing a decision-making process.

Every decision made in nursing involves risk. Some decisions that aim to be beneficial are instead actually harmful. Certainly, some decisions involve inconsequential risks; others, however, may impact quality of life. A thoughtless conversation, inconsiderate approach, or negative comment may invoke psychological or emotional hurt. A wrong decision that involves pharmacology, timing, or an invasive procedure may lead to suffering, pain, or even death. These all serve as examples that counter the principles of non-maleficence and beneficence. Patients also have a right to expect that their health care providers are competent, disclose the facts behind their care choices, and are efficient and cost-effective in their care. Not doing so contradicts the principles of fidelity, veracity, and autonomy.

Nurses who engage in decision making without adequate evidence are operating in a state of ignorance, basing interactions, treatments, and practices on no facts or false facts. Nurses have a moral imperative to use evidence to support their care decisions. If evidence is lacking, nurses have a duty to collect and share evidence. It is simply unethical for a nurse to base clinical decisions on false assumptions or inaccurate knowledge.

There are other ethical questions that are associated with the use of research and the implementation of an evidence-based practice approach. Are there adequate safeguards to protect individual patient information when sharing case reports and small sample studies? How will evidence be used and who will benefit? For example, a policymaking group could be enticed to use weak evidence to support a decision that decreases health care costs at the expense of improved patient outcomes for a small patient population. A pharmaceutical company could base a marketing strategy on a weak study that leads providers and patients to make choices based on false assumptions. These examples require consideration of the ethical principle of justice as the rights of an individual or group are balanced against the rights of another individual or group. Last, the temptation exists for practitioners to apply the steps of evidence-based practice as a formula for resolving ethical dilemmas. Use of recipes or algorithms alone cannot replace the thoughtful, situation-specific debate of ethical principles by bioethics committees and similar groups. To do so would violate the spirit of considering the individual patient's needs and the practitioner's expertise that is germane to quality health care decision-making.

Considerations for Educators

Nurse educators, including those who teach in nurse anesthesia programs, are expected to integrate evidence-based practice and information literacy into both undergraduate and graduate program curricula. Accreditation standards require graduates to be competent in the application of the evidence-based process as a clinical problem-solving approach.[3,4,23,24,28] The objectives of the educational program should reflect this competency. Courses, expected student learning outcomes, assignments, and assessments should all be aligned to reflect the program's objectives. Carefully constructed statements that describe the desired, measurable student learning outcomes will help guide faculty as they design their courses. No longer the "sage on the stage," faculty will need to be deliberate in the design of pedagogical strategies that assist students to acquire the cognitive, psychomotor, and affective skills necessary to engage in EBP. Assessments will benefit students most if they are authentic or meaningful, reflecting a real-world activity germane to the learner and not just a number score.

Students enrolled in a nurse anesthesia educational program, depending on when they completed their entry level professional nursing program, may be more skilled in the research process than evidence-based practice. Additionally, studies continue to identify barriers faced by US registered nurses in consistently using EBP.[62,63] An initial self-assessment exercise may help graduate nursing students determine which of their skills require further development and which do not. The challenge is the paucity of tools available to assess EBP competency. Melnyk[64] described three tools that have been developed for the medical profession: the Berlin questionnaire, the Fresno tool, and the Assessing Competency in Evidence-Based Medicine (ACE) tool, but concluded there remains a need to develop valid and reliable EBP competency assessment tools that are relevant to nurses and advanced practice nurses. Leung and colleagues[65] completed a systematic review of instruments for measuring knowledge, skills and/or attitudes for evidence-based practice. Although they conclude that there is no proven, reliable instrument currently available, the review provides educators with a plethora of resources and a basis for those interested in developing such a tool.

There are numerous strategies suggested for the faculty to consider when designing a foundational EBP course or integrating EBP assignments throughout the curriculum. If the faculty is committed to integrating EBP throughout the curriculum, it makes sense to allow students to self-assess their skills early and place foundational EBP content in the beginning of the curriculum. The EBP process can then be threaded throughout the program in course assignments and assessments, reinforcing skill development. Students may be introduced to the process of searching the literature by completing the PubMed online tutorials, quick tours, webcasts and videos, and handouts.[66] Likewise, online tutorials are available for the research database Cumulative Index of Nursing and Allied Health Literature or CINAHL.[67] Chang and Levin[68] suggest designing learning experiences that increase in complexity over time. They also propose activities that allow for indirect experiences or social modeling, whereby students observe others engaging in the EBP process. Other teaching strategies include case studies, simulation with validated checklists, game-based learning, and web-based learning modules such as podcasts, self-directed learning modules, and voice-over electronic slide show presentations.[69–73]

Not all faculty possess the confidence and skills to teach EBP. There is also divergence between what is taught in the classroom and what is observed in the clinical setting. Although EBP has gained momentum, practitioners may or may not consistently use an evidence-based approach in daily practice. Melnyk et al[74] surveyed nurse practitioner educators to assess their knowledge, beliefs, and teaching practices regarding EBP. The study also examined the relationships that exist among these variables and the inhibiting and facilitating factors related to teaching EBP. The authors determined an initial need to ensure faculty possess skills in EBP. Mentorship from colleagues, well-developed syllabi, and access to resources were identified as interventions for helping faculty develop EBP skills and confidence. The authors also urged faculty to consistently role-model EBP in both didactic and clinical courses and to evaluate a program's curricular content to ensure that it introduces and reinforces the EBP process and not just the research process. Additionally, Koffel and Reidt[75] describe the benefits of designing an interprofessional EBP workshop to improve faculty's skills in teaching EBP.

Summary

The discourse regarding the risks and benefits of employing an evidence-based practice process for decision-making in any health care specialty, including nurse anesthesia, is bound to continue as long as the process exists. Just as the scientific method has evolved since its early inception in the 16th century, the evidence-based practice model will evolve and continuously be refined. No professional should embrace the process because it is the popular trend in health care. Instead, the conscious decision to subscribe to the process should be because it is in the best interest of the patients for whom we care. Educating current and future nurse anesthetists to use the EBP process to daily practice requires nurse anesthesia educators to employ a variety of pedagogical strategies. Developing skill in the EBP process requires a combination of theoretical understanding and application in the clinical setting. The real challenge for nurse anesthetists who practice evidence-based nurse anesthesia will be in embracing multiple ways of knowing, synthesizing the best evidence with clinical judgment, and honoring the singularity of each patient entrusted to their care.

References

1. Kohn LT, Corrigan JM, Donaldson MS, eds. *To Err Is Human: Building a Safer Health System.* Washington, DC: National Academies Press; 2000. http://www.nap.edu/catalog/9728.html. Accessed June 20, 2016.

2. Greiner AC, Knebel E. Health Professions Education: A Bridge to Quality. Washington, DC: National Academies Press; 2003. http://www.nap.edu/books/0309087236/html/. Accessed June 20, 2015.

3. American Association of Colleges of Nursing. The Essentials of Doctoral Education for Advanced Nursing Practice. Washington, DC: American Association of Colleges of Nursing; 2006.

4. Council on Accreditation of Nurse Anesthesia Educational Programs. Standards for Accreditation of Nurse Anesthesia Educational Programs: Practice Doctorate. Park Ridge, IL: Council on Accreditation of Nurse Anesthesia Educational Programs; 2014.

5. Institute of Medicine. The future of nursing: leading change, advancing health. Washington, DC: National Academies Press; 2010. http://www.nap.edu/download/12956. Accessed January 20, 2016.

6. Alper BS, Hand JA, Elliott SG, Kinkade S, Hauan MJ, Onion DK, Sklar BM. How much effort is needed to keep up with the literature relevant for primary care? *J Med Libr Assoc.* 2004;92(4):429–437.

7. U.S. National Library of Medicine. Fact Sheet: MEDLINE. https://www.nlm.nih.gov/pubs/factsheets/medline.html. Updated June 23, 2016. Accessed July 1, 2016.

8. Erren TC, Cullen P, Erren M. How to surf today's information tsunami: on the craft of effective reading. *Med Hypotheses.* 2009;73(3):278–279.

9. Choudry NK, Fletcher RH, Soumerai SB. Systematic review: the relationship between clinical experience and quality of health care. *Ann Intern Med.* 2005;142(4):260–273.

10. Heater BS, Becker AM, Olson RK. Nursing interventions and patient outcomes: a meta-analysis of studies. *Nurs Res.* 1988;37(5):303–307.

11. Lugtenberg M, Burgers JS, Westert GP. Effects of evidence-based clinical practice guidelines on quality of care: a systematic review. *Qual Saf Health Care.* 2009;18(5):385–392.

12. Lysaght RM, Altschuld JW. Beyond initial certification: the assessment and maintenance of competency in professions. *Eval Program Plann.* 2000;23(1):95–104.

13. Lundgren BS, Houseman CA. Continuing competence in selected health care professions. *J Allied Health.* 2002;31(4):232–240.

14. Roiser JP, de Martino B, Tan GC, Kumaran D, Seymour B, Wood NW, Dolan RJ. A genetically mediated bias in decision making driven by failure of amygdala control. *J Neurosci.* 2009;29(18):5985–5991.

15. MacKillop J. Integrating behavioral economics and behavioral genetics: delayed reward discounting as an endophenotype for addictive disorders. *J Exp Anal Behav.* 2013;99(1):14–31.

16. Cochrane AL. Effectiveness and Efficiency: Random Reflections on Health Services. London, England: Nuffield Provincial Hospitals Trust; 1972.

17. Cochrane. About us. http://www.cochrane.org/about-us. Accessed June 18, 2016.

18. Sackett D, Richardson WS, Rosenberg W, Haynes, R.B. Evidence-Based Medicine: How to Practice and Teach EBM. New York: Churchill Livingstone; 1997.

19. Marzano R, Pickering DJ, Pollock, JE. Classroom Instruction That Works. Alexandria, VA: ASCD; 2001.

20. Cannon S, Boswell, C. Evidence-Based Teaching in Nursing: A Foundation for Educators. 2nd ed. Burlington, MA; Jones & Bartlett; 2016.

21. Abdellah FG. Overview of nursing research 1955–1968. *Nurs Res.* 1970;19(3):239–252.

22. Lindeman CA. Priorities in clinical nursing research. *Nurs Outlook.* 1975;23(11):693–698.

23. American Association of Colleges of Nursing. The Essentials of Baccalaureate Education for Professional Nursing Practice. Washington, DC: American Association of Colleges of Nursing; 2008.

24. American Association of Colleges of Nursing. The Essentials of Master's Education in Nursing. Washington, DC: American Association of Colleges of Nursing; 2011.

25. American Association of Nurse Anesthetists. Scope of Nurse Anesthesia Practice. http://www.aana.com/resources2/professionalpractice/Pages/Scope-of-Nurse-Anesthesia-Practice.aspx. Updated June 2013. Accessed June 28, 2016.

26. American Association of Nurse Anesthetists Code of Ethics for the Certified Registered Nurse Anesthetist. http://www.aana.com/resources2/professionalpractice/Pages/Code-of-Ethics.aspx. Updated 2005. Accessed June 28, 2016.

27. American Nurses Association. *Nursing: Scope and Standards of Practice.* 2nd ed. Silver Spring, MD: ANA; 2010.

28. Council on Accreditation of Nurse Anesthesia Educational Programs. Standards for Accreditation of Nurse Anesthesia Educational Programs. Park Ridge, IL: Council on Accreditation of Nurse Anesthesia Educational Programs; 2004.

29. Melnyk BM, Gallagher-Ford L, Long LE, Fineout-Overholt E. The establishment of evidence-based practice competencies for practicing registered nurses and advanced practice nurses in real-world clinical settings: Proficiencies to improve healthcare quality, reliability, patient outcomes, and costs. *Worldviews Evid Based Nurs.* 2014;11(1):5–15.

30. Sackett DL, Straus SE, Richardson WS, Rosenberg W, Haynes RB. *Evidence-based Medicine.* Edinburgh: Churchill Livingstone; 2000.

31. Sigma Theta Tau International Honor Society for Nursing website. Evidence Based Nursing Position Statement. http://www.nursingsociety.org/aboutus/PositionPapers/Pages/EBN_positionpaper.aspx. http://www.nursingsociety.org/connect-engage/about-stti/position-statements-and-resource-papers/evidence-based-nursing-position-statement. Updated July 6, 2005. Accessed July 8, 2008.

32. Pravikoff DS, Tanner AB, Pierce ST. Readiness of U.S. nurses for evidence-based practice. *Am J Nurs.* 2005;105(9):40–51.

33. American Association of Nurse Anesthetists. Evidence-based Practice. http://www.aana.com/resources2/professionalpractice/Pages/Evidence-Based-Practice.aspx.

34. American Association of Nurse Anesthetists. Policy on Evidence-based process for practice-related documents. http://www.aana.com/myaana/AANABusiness/governance/Pages/Policies-and-Guidelines.aspx. Updated 2014.

35. Thiemann LJ, McFadden JJ. Advancing evidence-based nurse anesthesia practice. *AANA J*. 2010;78(4):279–282.

36. Nightingale, F. *Notes on Hospitals*. John W. London, England: Parker and Son; 1859.

37. Cohen IB. Florence Nightingale. *Sci Am*. 1984;250(3):128–133.

38. Gerrish K, Ashworth P, Lacey A, Bailey J, Cooke, J, Kendall, S., McNeilly, E. Factors influencing the development of evidence-based practice: a research tool. *J Adv Nurs*. 2007;57(3):328–338.

39. Fink R, Thompson CJ, Bonnes, D. Overcoming barriers and promoting the use of research in practice. *J Nurs Adm*. 2005;35(3):121–129.

40. Olade, R. Evidence-based practice and research utilization activities among rural nurses. *J Nurs Scholarsh*. 2004;36(3):220–225.

41. McKenna HP, Ashton S, Keeney S. Barriers to evidence-based practice in primary care. *J Adv Nurs*. 2004;45(2):178–189.

42. Wyszewianski L, Green LA. Strategies for changing clinicians' practice patterns. A new perspective. *J Fam Prac*. 2000;49(5):461–464.

43. Reed PG, Lawrence, LA. A paradigm for the production of practice-based knowledge. *J Nurs Manag*. 2008;16(4):422–432.

44. Holmes D, Murray, SJ, Perron A, McCabe J. Nursing best practice guidelines: reflecting on the obscene rise of the void. *J Nurs Manag*. 2008;16(4):394–403.

45. Holmes D, Murray SJ, Perron A, Rail G. Deconstructing the evidence-based discourse in health sciences: truth, power and fascism. *Int J Evid Based Healthc*. 2006;4:180–186.

46. Hudson K, Dike G, Haas B, Varnell, G. Navigating the evidence-based practice maze. *J Nurs Manag*. 2008;16(4):409–416.

47. Windish DM, Huot SJ, Green ML. Medicine residents' understanding of the biostatistics and results in the medical literature. *JAMA*. 2007;298(9):1010–1022.

48. Fineout-Overholt E, Melnyk BM, Schultz A. Transforming health care from the inside out: advancing evidence-based practice in the 21st century. *J Prof Nurs*. 2005;21(6):335–344.

49. Dearing JW. Evolution of diffusion and dissemination theory. *J Public Health Manag Prac*. 2008;14(2):99–108.

50. Rogers EM. *Diffusion of Innovations*. 5th ed. New York, NY: Free Press; 2003.

51. Balas EA, Boren SA. *Managing Clinical Knowledge for Healthcare Improvement*. Stuttgart, Germany: Schattauer Publishing Company; 2000.

52. Melnyk BM, Fineout-Overholt E. *Evidence-based Practice In Nursing and Healthcare: A Guide to Best Ppractice.* Philadelphia, PA: Lippincott Williams & Wilkins; 2005.

53. West S, King V, Carey TS, et al. Systems to Rate the Strength of Scientific Evidence. [Evidence Report/Technology Assessment 47.] Rockville, MD: Agency for Healthcare Research and Quality; 2002.

54. Welcome to CEMB. Centre for Evidence-Based Medicine http://www.cebm.net/?0=1025%2F%3F0%3D1025. Maya 2001. Accessed July 7, 2016.

55. Guba EG, Lincoln YS. *Effective Evaluation: Improving the Usefulness of Evaluation Results Through Responsive and NaturalisticApproaches.* San Francisco, CA: Jossey-Boss; 1981.

56. Lincoln YS. Emerging criteria for quality in qualitative and interpretive research. *Qualitative Inquiry.* 1995;1(3):275–289.

57. Lincoln YS, Guba EG. Paradigmatic controversies, contradictions, and emerging confluences. In: Denzin NK, Lincoln, YS, eds. The *Landscape of Qualitative Research.* 2nd ed. Thousand Oaks, MI: Sage; 2003:253–291.

58. Rolfe G. Validity, trustworthiness and rigour: quality and the idea of qualitative research. *J Adv Nurs.* 2006;53(3):304–310.

59. Sandelowski, M. The problem of rigor in qualitative research. *Adv Nurs Sci.* 1986;8(3):27–37.

60. Sandelowski M. In response to: deWitt L. & Ploeg J. (2006) Critical appraisal of rigor in interpretive phenomenological nursing research. *J AdvNurs.* 2006;55(2):643–645.

61. Schwandt TA. Farewell to criteriology. *Qual Inq.* 1996;2(1):58–72.

62. Melnyk BM. Fineout-Overholt E, Gallagher-Ford L, Kaplan L, et al. The state of evidence-based practice in US nurses: critical implications for nurse leaders and educators. *J Nurs Adm.* 2012;42(9):410–417.

63. Yoder LH, Kirkley D, McFall DC, Kirksey KM, StalBaum AL, Sellers D. CE: Original Research: staff nurses' use of research to facilitate evidence-based practice. *Am J Nurs.* 2014;114(9):36–37.

64. Melnyk BM; Gallagher-Ford L. Implementing the new essential evidence-based practice competencies in real-world clinical and academic settings: moving from evidence to action in improving health care quality and patient outcomes. *Worldviews Evid Based Nurs.* 2015;12(2):67–69.

65. Leung K, Trevena, L, Waters, D. Systematic review of instruments for measuring nurses' knowledge, skills and attitudes for evidence-based practice. *J Adv Nurs.* 2014;70(10):2181–2195.

66. US National Library of Medicine. National Institutes of Health. PubMed Online Training. https://learn.nlm.nih.gov/rest/training-packets/T0042010P.html. Accessed July 6, 2016.

67. EBSCO Publishing, CINAHL/MEDLINE Databases.. http://support.epnet.com/cinahl/. Accessed July 6, 2016.

68. Chang A, Levin RF. Tactics for teaching evidence-based practice: improving self-efficacy in finding and appraising evidence in a master's evidence-based practice unit. *Worldviews Evid Based Nurs*. 2014;11(4):266–9. doi: 10.1111/wvn.12050.

69. Raurell-Torreda M, Romero-Collado A. Simulation-based learning as a tactic for teaching evidence-based practice. *Worldviews Evid Based Nurs.* 2015;12(6):392–394.

70. Davidson SJ, Candy, L. Teaching EBP using game-based learning: improving the student experience. *Worldviews Evid Based Nurs.* 2016;13(4):285–293. doi: 10.1111/wvn.12152.

71. Welch CE, Van Lunen BL, Hankemeier DA, Wyant AL, Mutchler JM, Pitney WA, Hays DG. Perceived outcomes of web-based modules designed to enhance athletic trainers' knowledge of evidence-based practice. *J Athl Train.* 2014;49(2):220–233. doi: 10.4085/1062-6050-49.2.14.

72. Kleinpell R, Ely EW, Williams G, Liolios A, Ward N, Tisherman SA. Web-based resources for critical care education. *Crit Care Med.* 2011;39(3):541–553. doi: 10.1097/CCM.0b013e318206b5b5).

73. Long JD, Gannaway P, Ford C, Doumit R, Zeeni N, Sukkarieh-Haraty O, Milane A, Byers B, Harrison L, Hatch D, Brown J, Proper S, White P, Song H. Effectiveness of a technology-based intervention to teach evidence-based practice: The EBR tool. *Worldviews Evid Based Nurs.* 2016;13(1):59–65. doi: 10.1111/wvn.12132. .

74. Melnyk BM, Fineout-Overholt E, Feinstein NF, Sadler LS, Green-Hernandez C. Nurse practitioner educators' perceived knowledge, beliefs, and teaching strategies regarding evidence-based practice: implications for accelerating the integration of evidence-based practice into graduate programs. *J Prof Nurs.* 2008;24(1):7–13. doi: 10.1016/j.profnurs.2007.06.023.

75. Koffel J, Reidt S. An interprofessional train-the-trainer evidence-based practice workshop: Design and evaluation. *J Interprof Care.* 2015;29(4):367–369. doi: 10.3109/13561820.2014.962127.

Appendix A: Oxford Centre for Evidence-based Medicine Levels of Evidence (March 2009)*

Level	Therapy/ Prevention, Aetiology/ Harm	Prognosis	Diagnosis	Differential diagnosis/ symptom prevalence study	Economic and decision analyses
1a	SR (with homogeneity*) of RCTs	SR (with homogeneity*) of inception cohort studies; CDR† validated in different populations	SR (with homogeneity*) of Level 1 diagnostic studies; CDR† with 1b studies from different clinical centres	SR (with homogeneity*) of prospective cohort studies	SR (with homogeneity*) of Level 1 economic studies
1b	Individual RCT (with narrow Confidence Interval‡)	Individual inception cohort study with >80% follow-up; CDR† validated in a single population	Validating** cohort study with good§§ reference standards; or CDR† tested within one clinical centre	Prospective cohort study with good follow-up****	Analysis based on clinically sensible costs or alternatives; systematic review(s) of the evidence; and including multi-way sensitivity analyses
1c	All or none§	All or none case-series	Absolute SpPins and SnNouts††	All or none case-series	Absolute better-value or worse-value analyses ††††
2a	SR (with homogeneity*) of cohort studies	SR (with homogeneity*) of either retrospective cohort studies or untreated control groups in RCTs	SR (with homogeneity*) of Level >2 diagnostic studies	SR (with homogeneity*) of 2b and better studies	SR (with homogeneity*) of Level >2 economic studies
2b	Individual cohort study (including low quality RCT; eg, <80% follow-up)	Retrospective cohort study or follow-up of untreated control patients in an RCT; Derivation of CDR† or validated on split-sample§§§ only	Exploratory** cohort study with good §§ reference standards; CDR† after derivation, or validated only on split-sample§§§ or databases	Retrospective cohort study, or poor follow-up	Analysis based on clinically sensible costs or alternatives; limited review(s) of the evidence, or single studies; and including multi-way sensitivity analyses
2c	"Outcomes" Research; Ecological studies	"Outcomes" Research		Ecological studies	Audit or outcomes research
3a	SR (with homogeneity*) of case-control studies		SR (with homogeneity*) of 3b and better studies	SR (with homogeneity*) of 3b and better studies	SR (with homogeneity*) of 3b and better studies
3b	Individual Case-Control Study		Non-consecutive study; or without consistently applied reference standards	Non-consecutive cohort study, or very limited population	Analysis based on limited alternatives or costs, poor quality estimates of data, but including sensitivity analyses incorporating clinically sensible variations.

Level	Therapy/ Prevention, Aetiology/ Harm	Prognosis	Diagnosis	Differential diagnosis/ symptom prevalence study	Economic and decision analyses
4	Case-series (and poor quality cohort and case-control studies§§)	Case-series (and poor quality prognostic cohort studies***)	Case-control study, poor or non-independent reference standard	Case-series or superseded reference standards	Analysis with no sensitivity analysis
5	Expert opinion without explicit critical appraisal, or based on physiology, bench research or "first principles"	Expert opinion without explicit critical appraisal, or based on physiology, bench research or "first principles"	Expert opinion without explicit critical appraisal, or based on physiology, bench research or "first principles"	Expert opinion without explicit critical appraisal, or based on physiology, bench research or "first principles"	Expert opinion without explicit critical appraisal, or based on economic theory or "first principles"

Produced by Bob Phillips, Chris Ball, Dave Sackett, Doug Badenoch, Sharon Straus, Brian Haynes, Martin Dawes since November 1998. Updated by Jeremy Howick March 2009.

*	By homogeneity we mean a systematic review that is free of worrisome variations (heterogeneity) in the directions and degrees of results between individual studies. Not all systematic reviews with statistically significant heterogeneity need be worrisome, and not all worrisome heterogeneity need be statistically significant. As noted above, studies displaying worrisome heterogeneity should be tagged with a "-" at the end of their designated level.
†	Clinical Decision Rule. (These are algorithms or scoring systems which lead to a prognostic estimation or a diagnostic category.)
‡	See note #2 for advice on how to understand, rate and use trials or other studies with wide confidence intervals.
§	Met when all patients died before the Rx became available, but some now survive on it; or when some patients died before the Rx became available, but none now die on it.
§§	By poor quality cohort study we mean one that failed to clearly define comparison groups and/or failed to measure exposures and outcomes in the same (preferably blinded), objective way in both exposed and non-exposed individuals and/or failed to identify or appropriately control known confounders and/ or failed to carry out a sufficiently long and complete follow-up of patients. By poor quality case-control study we mean one that failed to clearly define comparison groups and/or failed to measure exposures and outcomes in the same (preferably blinded), objective way in both cases and controls and/or failed to identify or appropriately control known confounders.
§§§	Split-sample validation is achieved by collecting all the information in a single tranche, then artificially dividing this into "derivation" and "validation" samples.
††	An "Absolute SpPin" is a diagnostic finding whose Specificity is so high that a Positive result rules-in the diagnosis. An "Absolute SnNout" is a diagnostic finding whose Sensitivity is so high that a Negative result rules-out the diagnosis.
‡‡	Good, better, bad and worse refer to the comparisons between treatments in terms of their clinical risks and benefits.
†††	Good reference standards are independent of the test, and applied blindly or objectively to applied to all patients. Poor reference standards are haphazardly applied, but still independent of the test. Use of a non-independent reference standard (where the 'test' is included in the 'reference,' or where the 'testing' affects the 'reference') implies a level 4 study.
††††	Better-value treatments are clearly as good but cheaper, or better at the same or reduced cost. Worse-value treatments are as good and more expensive, or worse and the equally or more expensive.
**	Validating studies test the quality of a specific diagnostic test, based on prior evidence. An exploratory study collects information and trawls the data (eg, using a regression analysis) to find which factors are 'significant.'
***	By poor quality prognostic cohort study we mean one in which sampling was biased in favour of patients who already had the target outcome, or the measurement of outcomes was accomplished in <80% of study patients, or outcomes were determined in an unblinded, non-objective way, or there was no correction for confounding factors.
****	Good follow-up in a differential diagnosis study is >80%, with adequate time for alternative diagnoses to emerge (eg, 1–6 months acute, 1–5 years chronic)

Grades of Recommendation*

A	consistent level 1 studies
B	consistent level 2 or 3 studies ***or*** extrapolations from level 1 studies
C	level 4 studies ***or*** extrapolations from level 2 or 3 studies
D	level 5 evidence ***or*** troublingly inconsistent or inconclusive studies of any level

Extrapolations are where data are used in a situation that has potentially clinically important differences than the original study situation.

*Appendix A reprinted with permission from the Centre for Evidence-based Medicine. Accessed July 2, 2008 and July 7, 2016 from www.cebm.net.

CHAPTER 7

Admissions Criteria for Nurse Anesthesia Programs

Shawn Collins, DNP, PhD, CRNA

Keywords: Admissions criteria, cognitive, critical thinking, CRNA, noncognitive, nurse anesthesia program, qualitative, quantitative, subjective.

Key Concepts

- It is a challenge to determine the best candidates for limited nurse anesthesia program positions in a market where applicants far exceed available quotas. To narrow the pool of applicants, nurse anesthesia (NA) program admission committees need to select individuals they believe will be successful not only in completing the programs, but also passing the National Certification Exam and practicing nurse anesthesia.
- Rather than relying on a few sources of evidence, nurse anesthesia program admission committees should consider a variety of information about applicants. The information considered should include both cognitive and noncognitive criteria until such time that research demonstrates otherwise.
- Good practice demands that admissions decisions be made on evidence rather than speculation. In choosing the admission criteria, admission committees should have a firm justification of the predictive validity of the chosen criteria in relation to the academic and programmatic performance outcomes.
- The relative value that each school places upon specific applicant characteristics, skills, and experience must be consistent with the supports and demands of the program of study offered by the school.
- Recruiting qualified applicants is just the beginning step in retaining students and seeing them through to program completion. After students are admitted they ought to be afforded resources that will foster their persistence in the nurse anesthesia program as well as promote their academic success.

Introduction

As nurse anesthesia educators, we all want the best for our students; at the same time, we also want to protect the public. Faculty understands that admission and retention of exceptional candidates strengthen our profession. It is challenging to determine the best candidates for limited nurse anesthesia program positions in a market where applicants far exceed available quotas, given the high emotional, financial, and personal impact on both the program and the participants. Sifting through the numerous and impressive applications to find those who are a good fit for the nurse anesthesia profession is not an exact science. But what methods are currently used to narrow the applicant pool, and what may be missing?

Meeting the criteria for acceptance into some graduate school programs with limited student quotas can be challenging for graduate school candidates. Perhaps just as challenging for graduate school admission committees is setting appropriate standards for acceptance into those programs. Applications to nurse anesthesia (NA) programs far exceed available positions. To narrow the pool of applicants, NA program admission committees need to select individuals they believe will be successful not only in completing the programs, but also passing the National Certification Exam and practicing nurse anesthesia. This screening process requires admission committees to devise methods and criteria for choosing candidates who will successfully complete the NA program. The primary cognitive criteria considered for admission to nurse anesthesia programs typically include Graduate Record Exam (GRE) scores, science grade point averages (SGPA), overall GPAs (OGPA), letters of recommendation, a personal interview, and completion of a predetermined number of years of acute care nursing experience.

Attrition rates in master's programs range from 10%-75% and rates for doctoral programs range from 40%-70%.[1] Because of the significant financial, emotional, and personal impacts of taking the intensive NA programming, and the negative effects high attrition rates have on both the program and the participants, determining the most successful candidates for a limited number of positions is very important. However, current admission criteria may not provide the substantive data necessary for predicting student progression through nurse anesthesia programs.

The need for the quantitative side of educating nurse anesthetists is obvious—they are mandated by bodies such as the Council on Accreditation of Nurse Anesthesia Educational Programs (COA) and monitored by the National Board of Certification and Recertification for Nurse Anesthetists (NBCRNA)—but what about the qualitative side? If the qualitative aspect of nurse anesthesia education is important, how do we as educators measure that? After all, how we interact with other professionals is just as important as how we educate didactically and clinically.

There is general agreement in the literature that the admission process should include both cognitive and noncognitive criteria.[2,3] Some researchers propose that admissions criteria need to include not only hard data such as grade-point averages, but also some way(s) to measure a candidate's level of "sensitivity to feelings and needs" of the people around him or her—additional triangulation instruments in the admission officer's toolbox.

This chapter focuses on the admissions process for nurse anesthesia educational programs. It will review commonly used admission criteria, as well as provide a review of research on newer admission variables. These variables cover both cognitive and noncognitive criteria. (See **Table 7.1.**)

Traditionally Used Nurse Anesthesia Admission Criteria

Quantitative GRE

One of the most researched admission criterion for academic performance in graduate nursing education is the GRE. The GRE has attempted to be the standard in predicting success in graduate programs; however, its accuracy in predicting success of student GPA and success in graduating from programs has been incomplete. Several studies have shown that the GRE is no better than other criteria, or worse, the least predictive of all admission criteria in predicting graduate school success.[4–9] Many graduate nursing programs are eliminating the GRE from admissions processes due to its questionable effectiveness in predictive value and its perceived barriers to application.

One study of graduate nursing students demonstrated the GRE only predicted 5% to 8% of the explained variance in program GPA, and thus, was not an effective indicator of graduate school academic ability or success.[4] This same study provided anecdotal evidence that the GRE was a significant barrier to graduate school application. A large study of master of science in nursing students that included student registered nurse anesthetists found that if applicants had an undergraduate GPA of 3.25 or higher in combination with a nursing GPA of 3.0 or higher, the GRE score added little predictive value.[5]

Table 7.1 Traditional Admission Variables and Their Value

Admission Variable	Recommendation
GRE	Old GRE scoring format has little to no predictive value. Research needed on new scoring format, so no recommendation as to its utility.
Years of Experience	Mandatory one year. Research demonstrates increasing years of experience does not necessarily predict better performance.
Overall GPA	Use a minimum overall GPA of >3.25
Science GPA	Use as a weighted criterion
Science Courses	No data to justify certain courses as they relate to success in a nurse anesthesia program
Personal Essay	Validity is questionable, but may be beneficial in in determining potential for doctoral level writing, especially if standard grading criteria is used. If GRE is used, the analytical writing score may be a better predictor.
Interview	Useful, but utilize a structured interview format and a rubric to enhance validity and reliability.
Critical Thinking Skills	Useful in anesthesia, but is mostly a subjective determination. May be better to use a valid and reliable tool to evaluate.
Letters of Recommendation	Validity is low, and there is little data to support their use. Bias is common. If used, have the applicant elaborate in a face-to-face format.

In terms of nurse anesthesia programs and the GRE, most studies have shown little to no predictive value for success in terms of academic progression, clinical performance, or performance on the national certification examination.[10–12] Additionally, standardized tests have demonstrated bias against women and minorities.[13] One study did find a weakly positive correlation between GRE quantitative score and national certification examination scores.[14] Another study found that as total GRE scores increased, so did the nurse anesthesia program GPAs of nurse anesthesia students.[12] This author went on, however, to recommend the removal of the GRE as an admission criterion as the correlation was weak. Newton and Moore found that students with undergraduate GPAs of at least 3.28 had significantly higher GRE verbal and GRE quantitative scores than students with an undergraduate GPA less than 3.28.[15]

It seems there is a deficit of validity testing among those using GRE scores, with statements of questionable validity by the participants, and statements that the GRE is seen as a barrier to applicants, all leading to create an ambiguous purpose for the GRE as an admission criterion. Despite the lack of evidence regarding the GRE's predictive value in nurse anesthesia, little research has been done on the new GRE format as it relates to student success in nurse anesthesia programs. This complicates the trend to remove the GRE as an admission criterion until further research is conducted on the new GRE format and its ability to predict success in nurse anesthesia programs.

Years of Acute Care Experience

Currently, students admitted to nurse anesthesia programs are required to have at least one full-time year of acute care experience. The thought behind this requirement is time to develop critical thinking experience and some level of maturity as a registered nurse. However, research on the amount of acute care experience and GPA in nurse anesthesia school has demonstrated that as the years of experience increase, there is a decrease in nurse anesthesia GPA. In fact, increasing years of acute care experience represented a negative correlation with academic progression.[12] The conclusion from this study was that years of acute care experience demonstrate little value from an academic standpoint, but no studies have been performed to demonstrate how these students perform in the clinical component of training.

The finding that more experienced students have more difficulty with academics is supported by other studies.[16,17] Older and more experienced students may face many more adjustment demands in returning to school than younger students who have recently completed an undergraduate degree. These older students may face more adjustment-related stresses such as loss of income and employment status, as well as attempting to balance family responsibilities and full-time student status.

A 1999 paper[18] stated "research studies have not yet identified a uniform set of skills and knowledge inherent in the traditional 1 year of critical care experience" required for admission to a nurse anesthesia program. This is still the case today, although the COA recently created a more narrowly defined acute-care experience requirement.

Nurse anesthesia program admission committees have started to require more than the minimum required one year of acute care experience. This is often done on the premise that the applicant pool is so strong and numerous that increasing years of experience helps narrow down the applicant pool; however, this approach can potentially limit an excellent candidate from entering a given program. Sometimes a "diamond in the rough" with the minimum one year of acute care experience is worth molding into a brilliant Certified Registered Nurse Anesthetist that will represent your program well.

Overall Grade Point Average (GPA)

The second most researched admission criterion for academic performance in graduate nursing programs is the GPA. Cumulative GPA is the most extensively used measure of graduate school academic performance. In general, GPAs are a more reliable predictor of graduate nursing program success than GRE scores.[19] Evidence points to preadmission academic grades as being predictive in subsequent academic performance in all professional disciplines, including nursing.[2] An association between undergraduate GPA and dismissal from graduate nursing programs has also been demonstrated.[5] One study in particular demonstrated undergraduate GPA is more predictive of success (operationalized as first-year graduate GPA, graduate GPA at graduation, and graduation) in graduate nursing programs than GRE scores.[20]

However, numerous studies on the predictability of overall undergraduate GPA as it relates to academic performance in nurse anesthesia programs have been performed with various results. In the majority of studies, evidence strongly supports preadmission overall GPA as a predictor of subsequent academic performance in nurse anesthesia,[2,3,11–15,21] although the explained variance in nurse anesthesia studies has not been as strong as in other nursing studies. One study in particular indicated a statistically significant relationship between the admission GPA and the current GPA for student registered nurse anesthetists.[22] Some programs, however, define preadmission overall GPA differently. Some programs look at all coursework completed prior to application to the nurse anesthesia program, while others only look at the last 60 hours of completed work. This leads to confusion depending on the definition of preadmission overall GPA.

The relationship between preadmission academic performance and clinical performance has not been studied extensively, and is less clear than its correlation with graduate academic program performance.[2] Some studies have demonstrated a positive link between preadmission GPA and clinical performance,[23–28] while others show little to no correlation.[26,29,30] An example of preadmission overall GPA and its value in predicting clinical performance in nurse anesthesia students is found in a 2013 article by Collins et al.[11]

An important applicable finding in this study is the value of preadmission overall GPA in predicting clinical factors that in turn predict NCE performance: the ability to transfer didactic knowledge to the clinical setting ($P<.001$), efficiency ($P<.004$), the ability to troubleshoot equipment ($P<.020$), and the technical skills factor ($P<.002$). The regression models for overall GPA predicting all four of these clinical variables were also statistically significant.

The statistically significant predictive value of overall GPA of these clinical variables and the models (the ability to transfer didactic knowledge to the clinical setting ($P = .017$), efficiency ($P = .033$), the ability to troubleshoot equipment ($P = .013$), and the technical skills factor ($P = .008$) suggests that overall GPA is an important preadmission criterion for NA programs. Anesthesia simulation may be beneficial in increasing proficiency in these areas.

One real issue with undergraduate overall GPA is the restrictions in defining academic performance when accounting for variations in grading standards across courses, faculty, and programs.[19] How does one compare for a degree, or more specifically, a GPA obtained at X university as compared to Y university? If overall GPA is used in admissions decisions, it is advisable to use the last 60 hours of work versus the GPA for all work.[13,31] Experienced educators understand that the transition from high school to university can be challenging for some with a new environment, newfound freedoms, and more choices. As a result, academic performance—and its indication of academic potential—can suffer in the first two years of university experience.

Despite its limitations, of all the cognitive criteria used in nurse anesthesia program admissions, preadmission overall GPA seems the most promising. There seems to be a consistency across multiple studies that preadmission overall GPA, and possibly science GPA for some professional disciplines, provides a valid measure of cognitive abilities in the admissions process for health professional programs.[2]

Science GPA

Undergraduate science GPA has demonstrated mixed results when comparing it to academic success in graduate programs. Numerous studies have found science GPA, examined separately from overall GPA, is a good predictor of academic performance in medical students, nursing students, and physiotherapy students.

While the analytical ability in the hard sciences is undoubtedly important, it is questionable that strong performance in these courses yields students who work well with frail or vulnerable patient populations.[30,32] In fact, the practice of using the science GPA is questionable. A study by Moruzi and Norman[29] demonstrated it was far more important to look at how well students performed in their undergraduate language and humanities courses in predicting overall success later in their medical school program.

As they relate to nurse anesthesia, studies have varied in their findings with science GPA and performance in nurse anesthesia programs. Zaglaniczny[17] found that the science GPA students attained during their nurse anesthesia program accounted for 24% of the variance in the overall score of the national certification examination, but the NCE has changed since this study was conducted. In terms of preadmission science GPA, one study indicated that as the preadmission science GPA increases, the current GPA in the nurse anesthesia program also increased.[12] This result is consistent with the findings of Haritos et al[21] and Reese.[3]

As with overall GPA, however, there needs to be consistency with the definition of courses being used for the science GPA calculation. It is difficult to account for variations in grading standards across courses, faculty, and programs. Although there are inconsistent results with using science GPA as an admission criterion, of the currently used cognitive criteria it has been demonstrated to be one of the more significant predictors of student success.

Requiring Particular Courses

Nurse anesthesia programs tend to be foundationally heavy in physical sciences. In order to allow applicants a broader foundation prior to nurse anesthesia school matriculation, some programs require applicants to have taken particular courses such as organic chemistry or statistics. These requirements may be germane to a particular university's requirements, but there is no data to justify certain courses as they relate to success in a nurse anesthesia program.

Subjective Letters of Recommendation

Letters of recommendation provide another method to more deeply evaluate an applicant than a rating scale alone, help to validate information in an application, or obtain new information about past performance. The evaluation of past performance is particularly important in effectively predicting job performance in professional practice programs.

In most nurse anesthesia programs, letters of recommendation are still used in the student selection process; however, there is little evidence to support their use. One author goes as far as to say "there is a clear and gross imbalance between the importance placed on letters and the research that has actually documented their efficacy."[33] One of the main issues with letters of recommendation is their poor reliability.[34] Studies have also reported poor predictive validity.[35,36] One study did note a difference in research ability and work habits of those admitted compared with those not admitted to a doctoral education program. Rejected applicants' references were lower in ratings on research ability and work habits.[37] Although standardization of the form helps, this admission criterion seems to be biased toward superficially positive comments, possibly as a result of the threat of litigation, but more likely as a result of applicants choosing their own references, with a bent toward avoiding possibly negative references. Furthermore, evaluators tend to favor letters written by people they know,[38] despite any evidence that this leads to superior findings regarding the applicant.

Two meta-analyses[39,40] found the validity of letters of recommendation to be low when compared with other selection methods. Research also demonstrates that characteristics of the individual writing the letter have an effect on its evaluations. Such letter qualities (eg, length, vividness, examples used) result in more positive evaluations of the letters of recommendation.[41] Research also shows that letters of recommendation can be written differently for men and women,[42] with the average letter written for male applicants being longer than for female applicants.[43] Race bias also occurs with letters of recommendation.[41]

Ambiguity of letters of recommendation, defined as the lack of relevant, precise, or detailed information, can lead to bias based on characteristics such as race and gender. In order to decrease bias, one must reduce ambiguity through the creation of a structured letter of recommendation. In other words, the letter of recommendation should be standardized.[41] As part of the standardized letter of recommendation, provide an area for the evaluator to present information about the applicant that is inconsistent with stereotypes. Much like structured interviews, if letters are structured to elicit information about specific criteria related to improved student performance, their validity may improve.[33] Specific criteria should focus on assessments of motivation, drive, and persistence, as cognitive characteristics are already evaluated by other measures such as GRE, overall GPA, and science GPA.

Another way to decrease bias might be to require readers to elaborate on their evaluations. Elaboration forces the evaluator to slow down their thought processes and evaluate the candidate in a more deliberate manner.[41] This, of course, would take more time and resources, both on the part of the evaluator and the admissions committee. Another method to decrease bias and increase interrater reliability would be to use the median score from several evaluators, which would accomplish the same goal of reducing bias. Finally, letters that use rating scales versus purely descriptive letters may fare better in predictive power.[33]

Personal Essay

Many schools require some form of a personal essay or statement that might allow students to demonstrate their writing ability. The validity of such written personal statements, however, is questionable. Powers and Fowles studied 302 graduate student applicants from a variety of disciplines, all of whom were required to submit a personal statement as part of their application. Of the applicants studied, 59% admitted they received help of some kind in editing or revising. Only 38% denied getting help of any kind.[44] There is a plethora of self-help advice available to applicants now as well. In both the literature and on the Internet, students can find information on how to craft personal statements—including examples—so as to gain favor with admissions committees.

Despite the pitfalls of personal statements, there are redeeming qualities, although there is little formal research on personal statement validity.[44] One study reported a modest correlation between creative thinking skills and originality and literacy achievement.[45] This study also found that students whose personal statements were well written subsequently had first-year GPAs that were higher than predicted.

Additionally, inter-rater reliability can be an issue when evaluating the written statements. If the personal essays/statements are to be scored as a part of the admissions process, it is advisable that there are multiple readers, taking the median score so as to minimize bias. Also, providing clear scoring guidelines for the reader, possibly in the form of a rubric, will help decrease inter-rater reliability issues.

While the personal essay may be indicative of the final grade in writing intensive courses such as theory,[15] the GRE writing score may be a better indicator of writing ability. A trained reader grades GRE analytical writing scores, based on two essays. A computer program also grades the computer version. If human and computer agree, the human score is used. If there is a disagreement between human and computer scores, then a second human rater is added, and the human ratings are averaged. With the paper GRE version, an average of two human ratings is calculated, with a third added for discrepancies.

Interview

The interview is used primarily to assess noncognitive characteristics and critical thinking skills. At the same time, the interview can be used to proactively recruit applicants who are perceived as strong candidates or a good fit for the culture of the given program. This might then be considered a part of the rational or judgmental model of admissions decisions, where judgments of people with expertise or knowledge about the requirements for success in a given position or role is central. Other rationale for using the interview include determination of applicant

- experience and knowledge of the profession;
- source of motivation;
- interpersonal behavior;
- responsibility and commitment; and
- educational, economic, and social background.[46]

According to Truell and Woosley,[47] the literature reveals the personal interview to be the most effective screening tool for business school admission. Although many programs use the same rationale for using interviews, the format and structure of interviews vary widely. Some programs utilize an open nonstructured format while others use a more standardized approach with predetermined questions for all applicants. Some programs choose to conduct one-on-one interviews while others conduct small-group interviews or a panel of interviews with rotations. In contrast, at least one study determined medical applicant interviews do not predict clinical performance.[48] All of these points indicate a lack of internal reliability for the interview.

As a noncognitive tool, the interview is a commonly used tool in nurse anesthesia admissions; however, it needs to be used in the right way. Edwards[49] reported that 98% of medical school admissions committees used the interview as an admissions tool, but only 20% of those were evaluating its effectiveness in determining success. To be useful, the interview should include some sort of rubric scoring system so its validity and reliability can be determined.

Reliability concerns stem from interviewer variability. Some authors attribute this variability to interviewer experience. Interviewing variables such as social or personality traits of interviewers or their own demographic or educational backgrounds can influence their decisions. For example, one study found female interviewers assigned lower ratings than males, and also that the student interviewers were more lenient than others.[50] Furthermore, access to academic information prior to the interview tends to lend bias.[51,52]

There is mixed evidence as to the predictability of personal interviews. Some authors report positive correlations between preadmission interview scores and subsequent academic and clinical performance,[53–56] while others have concluded there is no predictive value of success.[54,57–61]

Despite its face validity as a measure of noncognitive ability, there is much controversy regarding the personal interview's reliability and predictive validity. In order to overcome bias and use best practice, interviewer training and utilizing interviewers with prior experience are important considerations to improve reliability. Also, the use of a structured interview format improves reliability.[51,52]

Interviewers typically rate applicants using a Likert scale. While this provides quantitative data for comparison, it tends to be unreliable. Raters tend to agree more about the lowest and highest quality applicant interviews. Therefore, low and high ratings are more reliable, and weighting low and high responses improves validity. Ignoring the moderate interview rankings entirely during the admissions process is preferable to using them when computing larger weighted sum scores.[62]

Critical Thinking Skills

Every day, nurse anesthesia providers encounter situations that require them to make important decisions. These situations necessitate the need to practice critical thinking (CT)—a higher order skill that transcends simple problem solving—using reasoned judgment and evaluation in order to deal with serious medical situations.[63,64] Thinking critically means being well-informed, inquisitive, open-minded, and orderly in order to tackle the complexities of clinical practices and, therefore, be able to make appropriate judgments for their patients.[65,66] Moreover, medical professionals should provide evidence and logical arguments to support their judgments, assertions, and decisions.[67]

CT is a reflective process that leads to reasoned decisions. CT is especially important in situations where the problem is unclear and/or there are multiple solutions to the problem. Good CT requires an understanding of concepts that constitute the problem, an understanding of why a particular process or decision is made.

Although dozens of specific skills and dispositions are involved in critical thinking,[68,69] there are eight general activities that critical thinkers should be able to perform. These activities for students include:

- asking questions and being willing to wonder
- defining problems clearly
- examining evidence
- analyzing assumptions and biases
- avoiding emotional reasoning
- avoiding oversimplification
- considering alternative interpretations
- tolerating uncertainty[70]

CT is important in nurse anesthesia so sound judgments are made, with evaluation of the outcomes. CT also helps to differentiate relevant from irrelevant data, identify clues in the data, identify what data may be missing, provide for the comparison of possible outcomes, and recognize emerging clinical patterns while arriving at decisions that provide the best approach for a given situation. Nurse anesthesia requires all of these components in a sometimes fast-paced decision-making environment.

What does an applicant with good CT skills look like? (**Figure 7.1**) Unfortunately, there are not many specific tools available for evaluating CT. Evaluation of CT is mostly a descriptive/qualitative process. The applicant should ask good questions, and be willing to search for the answers, especially in a Socratic learning environment. Using alternative ways to view information while considering different perspectives to the problem and/or solution are important and should be encouraged; questioning current practice, expressing their own ideas or perspectives, and keeping an open mind while extending their thinking beyond their experiences is important. Many of these applicant attributes could potentially be evaluated in an interview situation with a clinical scenario.

Figure 7.1 Activities of Critical Thinkers

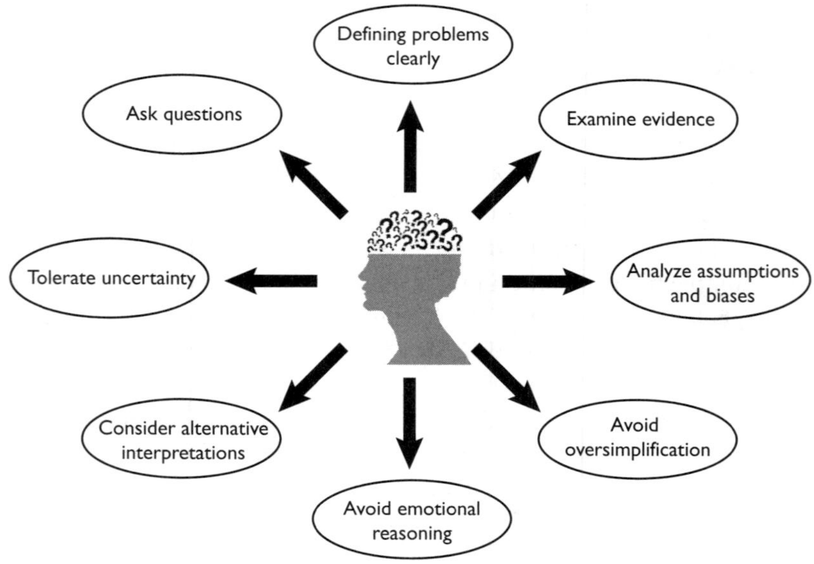

Of the few available CT assessment tools, one interesting tool is the Critical Thinking Disposition Assessment (CTDA) scale. The scale comprises 19 statements rated on a 7-point Likert scale, with three factors: systematicity and analyticity; inquisitiveness and conversance; and maturity and skepticism. The CTDA was found to be a valid and reliable instrument to measure the critical thinking disposition of medical care professionals and students.[71]

Nontraditional Admission Criteria

The Institute of medicine (IOM) published a landmark study recommending that health care professional licensing bodies work with certifying credentialing organizations to develop more effective methods of identifying unsafe providers and to take corrective action.[72] The IOM also recommended that the identification of unsafe health care providers should actually take place during the university admission process or in the early stages of clinical training. By doing so, health care professionals who are identified as unsafe can be restricted from university admission, or corrective action can be taken immediately upon the identification of unsafe behavior.[72]

Many of the current admission criteria used today tend to focus more on academic ability rather than clinical and interpersonal ability. With varied results using cognitive criteria in determining which applicants are successful in nurse anesthesia programs, it is not surprising that nurse anesthesia faculty have started to look elsewhere for criteria that may be more predictive in determining the successful transition of nurse anesthesia students through the intense nurse anesthesia curriculum. This part of the chapter reviews some nontraditional cognitive and noncognitive items that some programs are using or considering using in admissions decisions (**Table 7.2**, p. 151).

Multiple authors[3,12,22,73,74] have researched the value of cognitive-related factors in predicting the success of nurse anesthesia students; however, noncognitive factors, such as personal interviews and recommendations, have also been included in these studies. This inclusion of noncognitive factors matches Cadman and Brewer's[75] assertion that because of the increasingly complex and pluralistic nature of nursing, nurses need a balance of cognitive and noncognitive thinking. In light of Cadman and Brewer's assertion, it is understandable why some are raising concerns about including more focus on noncognitive criteria in admissions as well as in program progression and graduation.

Current selection criteria for nurse anesthetist student candidates include critical hard data, but neglect important affective information accessible through well-researched noncognitive tests.

As Burns[22], Lebeck[73], and Reese[3] have pointed out, the traditional criteria for selecting students to be admitted to a nurse anesthesia study program have been shown to be inadequate in determining which nurse anesthesia students will successfully complete and graduate from a degree program. As nurse anesthesia programs transition from the master's degree to the doctor of nursing practice (DNP) degree, nurse anesthesia educators have an opportunity to incorporate an examination of current admission criteria as part of the strategic planning.[22]

Clinical Math/Science Test

Some may consider the use of a math test on admission as repetitive, especially if the program uses the quantitative GRE score as an admission criterion. The ability to quickly perform math, with or without a calculator, is an everyday function of nurse anesthesia practice. Therefore, the argument has been made to evaluate the baseline of knowledge in terms of clinical math ability. No research has been performed on the use of a clinical math test as it relates to program success or successful completion of the national certification examination.

Simulation Scenario

One method for determining the personal characteristics and critical thinking skills of an applicant is through the use of simulation scenarios. Personal characteristics may include leadership ability, communication skills, and interpersonal and teamwork skills. The anesthesia profession requires a blend of cognitive and noncognitive skills, as we face clinical problems requiring cognitive knowledge, while also working in a stress-filled team environment. Simulation scenarios work to elicit both cognitive and noncognitive skills,[76] and thus can be considered a blended method of applicant evaluation. High-fidelity simulation attempts to replicate real-life clinical scenarios using fidelity human simulators managed by computer-adaptive software.[77]

High-fidelity simulation has been shown to promote skill attainment and mastery, as well as promote patient safety and teamwork. More anesthesia programs are choosing to include simulation scenarios as part of the admissions process, and although there are numerous studies on its use in other health care interviews, there is one study on its use as part of the nurse anesthesia program interview.

One medical school admissions study that looked at the use of high-fidelity simulation in the selection process demonstrated that simulation may be a better tool for determining noncognitive skills than the face-to-face interview.[78] In a pilot study on simulation use in nurse anesthesia program interviews, cognitive (describing possible physiologic causes, developing and verbalizing a treatment plan, and successfully implementing the treatment plan) and noncognitive skills (ability to ask for help or request resources as needed, receptive to assertions and ideas from team members, effective use of communication skills, and ability to function as a team leader) were evaluated.[79]

The nurse anesthesia simulation study demonstrated a correlation between face-to-face interview scores and simulation scores, but no correlation between face-to-face interview scores and other noncognitive categories such as writing samples and professional involvement. As previously noted, the simulation environment provides more data than just cognitive ability. The study did not address any connections between the use of high fidelity simulation in the interview process and successfully completing a nursing anesthesia program or national certification examination scores. Further research is needed in the area of high fidelity simulation in the nurse anesthesia admissions process as it relates to success in the nurse anesthesia program.

CCRN

In this era of increasingly complex and challenging health care, certification attests to a nurse's knowledge and ability, showing patients, their families, and employers that a nurse is qualified, experienced, and competent and has met the rigorous requirements to achieve this distinguished credential.[80] Attaining licensure as a registered nurse, much like passing the national certification examination, assures minimum competency in the given field. The AACN states that nurses, however, must acquire additional specialized knowledge, skills, and experience to care competently for critically ill patients. It is through CCRN certification that specialized knowledge, skills, and experience are validated.[81]

CCRN certification is a credential granted by the AACN Certification Corporation. More than 80,000 acute and critical care nurses are presently certified worldwide in adult, pediatric, or neonatal nursing. The 3-hour CCRN exam contains 150 items; 125 items are scored and 25 are used to gather statistical data on item performance for future exams. The items are based on the AACN Synergy Model for Patient Care, with 80% focusing on clinical judgment and 20% focusing on professional caring and ethical practice.[82]

Although it is important to have the COA-mandated one year of acute care experience, that year, or years, of experience does not always mean the same amount of knowledge or quality of experience. The CCRN can play a role in leveling the evaluation of critical care experience. Another possible benefit of recommending that applicants have CCRN certification is that they have demonstrated they can pass a standardized test specific to nursing practice.

Empowerment has been a topic of interest in recent years. Research demonstrates that those who have taken the CCRN exam and passed are more likely to feel empowered and are less likely to leave their position or nursing profession.[83] This could be a link in demonstrating satisfaction with acute care settings and job satisfaction, with a subsequent dedication to completing an advanced practice program such as nurse anesthesia. This potential connection needs further research.

The major disadvantage to using CCRN certification in admissions decisions is the lack of research on how CCRN certification affects outcomes, such as successful transition through and graduation from a nurse anesthesia program and performance on the national certification examination. Research needs to be performed to determine the CCRN value in concrete terms as it relates to nurse anesthesia programs. As part of this research, it would be beneficial to have official scores from the applicant's CCRN certifying examination.

Table 7.2 Operationalization of the EI Variables

	Area Scores	Branch Scores	Task Scores
	Experiential	Perceiving	Faces
			Pictures
		Facilitating	Sensations
			Facilitation
Overall EI	Strategic	Understanding	Blends
			Changes
		Managing	Emotion Management
			Emotional Relations

Used by permission. From Collins S. Emotional intelligence as a noncognitive factor in student registered nurse anesthetists. *AANA J.* 2013;81:465-72.

Personality Testing

Historically, organizations have based hiring and training on test scores that measure cognitive intelligence. Traditionally defined as an IQ, cognitive intelligence tests represent attempts to indicate one's capacity to learn, understand, recall, and solve problems. Starting in the latter part of the 20th century, an understanding of what constitutes an intelligence evolved, so that researchers today consider certain aspects of intelligence that go beyond the cognitive components.[84]

One of the noncognitive tests with well-documented content and construct validity is the Meyers-Briggs Type Indicator (MBTI). As individuals, we relate to and interpret the world around us in different ways, and this is commonly referred to as our personality. The differences in our personalities can be identified with the Myers-Briggs type indicator. MBTI is the most widely used professional personality test. More important for the purposes of this discussion, research suggests that noncognitive characteristics such as personality traits may influence academic performance.

The MBTI uses Carl Jung's theory of psychological type to assess and define personality. The Meyers-Briggs test identifies an individual's preference in four planes: Introversion versus Extroversion; Intuitive perception versus Sensing perception; Thinking versus Feeling; and Perceiving versus Judging.

Jung developed psychological type based on four functions: Feeling (F), Thinking (T), Intuition (I), and Sensing (S). It also includes four attitudes: Extroversion (E), Introversion (I), Judging (J), and Perceiving (P). Extroverts are oriented primarily toward the outer world and enjoy meeting new people, thinking aloud, and being active. Introverts are oriented toward the inner world and tend to focus on concepts, ideas, and internal experiences. Judging and perceiving concerns lifestyle choices with judging types preferring more order and set deadlines, while perceiving types prefer more flexibility and surprises. Sensing and Intuitive types concern information gathering with sensing types and prefer hard facts; intuitive types prefer more abstract concepts. Thinking and feeling are considered the rational processes that determine how certain conclusions and judgments are made regarding the information collected. Thinking types prefer to make decisions based on in personal objective positions. Feeling types tend to respond well to people's values in our deck at assessing the human impact of decisions.[85,86] Studies on nursing and dental students demonstrated the highest type in both professions was Introversion-Sensing-Thinking-Judging (ISTJ),[87,88] with Judging types scoring higher in academic performance than Perceiving types, and Extrovert types being more satisfied from a student perspective than Introvert types.[89]

On a cautionary note, using tests such as the MBTI for admissions risks the validity of the instrument, as it was not created for admissions. Although the MBTI is one of the most heavily used personality instruments available (used by 89% of Fortune 500 companies) and has been applied in hundreds of different ways over the past few decades, it may not be well-suited to selecting nurse anesthesia students.

Proper use of the MBTI for making selection decisions requires expert interpretation and judgment. It is also hard to link MBTI results directly to key job-related behaviors. The inability to clearly link early personality measures to job performance criteria was identified as a serious shortcoming and effectively killed the use of these tools as selection measures for several decades. The past few decades have seen the evolution of a new breed of work-related personality tools that have been developed with the major components that describe performance at most modern jobs in mind. Unfortunately, the MBTI is not one of these, and this is the biggest reason why it should not be used in most admission selection situations.

The MBTI can also screen out great candidates. The idea is to figure out if someone's personality "fits" a specific job position or not, but although this may work for some professions, it won't work for most of them. For example, if someone is applying to a nurse anesthesia program, the school wants to know if that person has the potential to remain calm during an emergency. But what personality type makes a good nurse anesthetist? Additionally, the tests will likely give those with "mainstream" personality types a more positive reading, while creative, think-outside-the-box candidates "who may potentially become leaders and do extraordinary things for an employer may be weeded out."[90]

MBTI results may be flawed. In these types of tests, there's always a chance that potential students may simply respond how they think the school wants. Therefore, the test results won't be a true representation of their personalities. Many of the most popular personality tests weren't created to be used in the hiring process. For example, the Myers-Briggs test was developed for training and development, not hiring; therefore, its application to screen candidates is questionable.

There are privacy risks and the potential for discrimination with the MBTI. Since these questions are usually asked in a way where the significance of the answers is unclear, candidates may reveal "private thoughts, beliefs and emotions, through his or her responses to questions." Experts also fear that these tests may discriminate against certain groups, because candidates will answer questions depending on how comfortable they feel in the situation.[90] Although the law does not make it illegal to administer personality tests during the admission process, schools should seriously consider the number of issues, from validity and reliability of these tests to concerns about invasion of privacy and possible discrimination against minorities.

Another area closely related to personality testing is found in a study performed by Clayton et al that looked at nurse anesthesia program academic faculty perceptions of characteristics needed for critical success in military nurse anesthesia programs. The study indicated that military nursing anesthesia program faculty believe that clinical awareness and personality characteristics were the most important qualities for critical success.[91]

Finally, the California Personality Inventory (CPI) instrument has been using multiple studies comparing personality to clinical performance in anesthesia programs. A study by Reich et al[92] examined anesthesiology residents, clinical performance, and results of the CPI. The CPI contains 434 true-false questions that can be used to determine non-pathological or normal aspects of a person's personality. A study by Gogh et al[93] found Dominance, Social Presence, and Achievement via independence were the highest CPI scales in anesthesia residents. Another study examined the same data and determined that the alpha personality type—those who are typically independent, reliable, and self-disciplined—predicts high-performance anesthesiology residents.[94] This study also found high-performance residents scored better than low-performance residents in the categories of Dominance, Independence, Empathy, Responsibility, Socialization, Achievement Motivation, and Well-Being.

In a construct, similar to personality testing, a study using four focus groups of faculty from four different universities—including CRNA faculty—examined necessary characteristics for success in graduate nursing programs. The focus groups determined that personal characteristics were considered most important, professional characteristics and clinical skills moderately important, and kinds of clinical experience of lesser importance. The most important characteristic under personal was "ethical"; under professional, "clinically confident"; under clinical, "interpersonal communication"; and under clinical experience, "to work in a setting with physician nurse interaction." It is interesting to note that personal characteristics, while viewed as the most important in determining success in graduate nursing programs, are also the most difficult to measure objectively. The greatest difference between seasoned nurses and new graduates tends to be learned skills such as communication, judgment of one's abilities, self-confidence, and collaboration.[95] The bottom line for nurse anesthesia educators is that there seems to be no predictive value for using personality testing as an admission criterion.

Emotional Intelligence

Current admission criteria for nurse anesthesia programs reflect traditional variables thought to be useful in determining the best candidate for acceptance. In the past 15 years, a wealth of studies showed there is little predictive value for nurse anesthesia student success in terms of OGPA, GRE scores, and other factors related to intelligence quotients (IQ).[3,96,97] However, researchers have given very little study of the noncognitive skills that influence the success and capacity for successful interactions, especially the role of emotional intelligence in understanding the success of NA students.

Moss[98] stated that people have known intuitively for some time that success is not directly attributable solely to the kind of intelligence measured by IQ tests. Universities could fill undergraduate programs three times over if based solely on GPA and standardized test scores, which indicates that exceptional grades and test scores no longer discriminate between applicants.[32] This leads to a desire to find other types of intelligence that impact success; emotional intelligence has been suggested as a candidate for this role. This will require determining the relationship of emotional intelligence profiles between applicants and successful nurse anesthesia students.

Emotional intelligence as defined by Salovey and Mayer, leading experts in the field, is "the subset of social intelligence that involves the ability to monitor one's own and others' feelings and emotions, to discriminate among them and to use this information to guide one's thinking and actions."[99] Increasingly, students are required to be active participants in directing their own educational success, and this is especially true when professional clinical issues are in play. Mayer and Kilpatrick[100] suggested that emotionally intelligent people were better equipped to deal with the challenges of clinical nursing practice and independent study. Cadman and Brewer[75] noted that individuals in professional nursing need to be able to blend and integrate both theory and practice. They believed students recruited into nurse anesthesia programs needed to be effective in both areas, and emotional intelligence may be a linking aspect in making that connection.

Emotional intelligence rather than IQ is believed to be the determinant of who advances most quickly within an organization.[101] (**Figure 7.2**) Attributes such as self-awareness, perseverance, and emotional stability are more accurate predictors of success than other variables, such as IQ and academic achievement.[32] Neuwirth[102] said that although cognitive intelligence as measured by IQ is important in success, no matter how intelligent one may be, if a person cannot interact in a meaningful way with others, the results are less than optimal. This is especially important in a discipline that works in a team-based environment such as nurse anesthesia.

Figure 7.2 Emotional Intelligence Skills

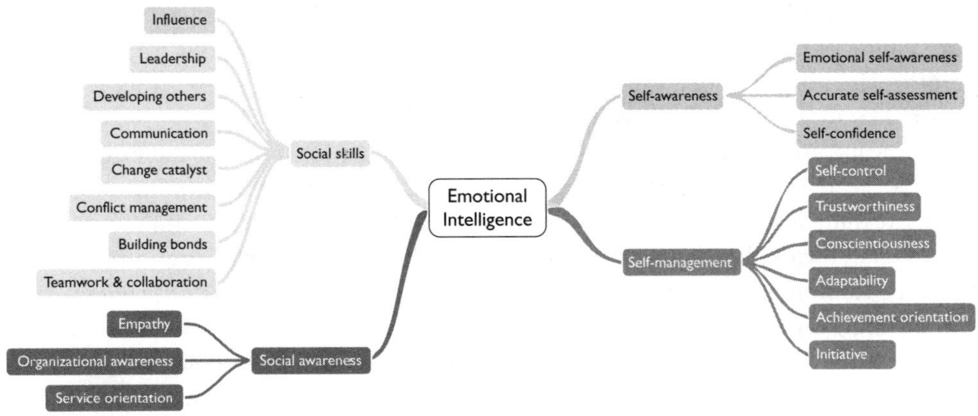

There may also be a connection between critical thinking skills and emotional intelligence. There is speculation that emotion might be a powerful motivator for quality decision-making; emotion may propel decision-makers to expand and reconsider their reasoning, and therefore to think critically.[103,104] Zimmerman and Phillips[105] presented evidence that affective learning can actually encourage the ability to think critically. Management of emotion involves not only recognizing and understanding emotion, but also using it to solve problems.[106]

Faculty across the country report increasing levels of disrespect and confrontation regarding acceptable performance, as the student struggles to compete in an academic structure that emphasizes high GPA as a measure of success.[107] Society today values individualism, personal accomplishment, and materialism that lead to an air of perfectionism. These characteristics are in opposition to the team-oriented worker who values working toward the good of the organization as a whole.

Emotional intelligence studies in higher education demonstrate EI is related to academic success.[104,108–111] Certain branches of emotional intelligence are more predictive than others. Those branches include facilitating emotions and managing emotions, and the studies show moderate effect sizes.[1,74,112,113] Students higher in facilitating and managing emotions may be better equipped to manage the emotions that accompany their lives, thus enabling them to concentrate, learn, and excel at school.

Emotional intelligence has also been shown to be a predictor of success in the workplace. Diana Durek, a consultant with a company that provides emotional intelligence consultation for the United States Air Force, stated: "IQ by itself is not a strong predictor of workplace performance. While many professions require a certain degree of cognitive ability, once one is in a given role, EI becomes the better predictor of success."[84] This is corroborated by Nooryan, Gasparyan, Sharif, and Zoladl,[114] who concluded that the ability to effectively deal with emotions in the workplace assists in coping with stress and education, and emotional intelligence decreased anxiety in physicians and nurses, a finding corroborated by Montes-Berges and Augusto.[115] Another study by Weng et al[116] found that higher EI was significantly associated with less burnout ($P<.001$) and higher job satisfaction ($P<.001$) among doctors. This finding was duplicated in nurses as well.[115]

The path to emotional intelligence competency is not merely to add a few courses on communication or interpersonal skills to an already intense program like nurse anesthesia training. Studies have shown that learning emotional intelligence skills takes time and a lot of effort.[75,117] Cadman and Brewer stated that "emotional intelligence cannot be developed quickly enough through interpersonal skills training and therefore, it is essential that nurse educators create assessment strategies that will identify emotional intelligence at recruitment."[75(p321)]

Interestingly, many students who are required to submit to emotional intelligence testing report feeling satisfied with the experience.[32] There are numerous emotional intelligence screening instruments that can be used for applicant admission testing. Two of the more commonly used EI tools are the MSCEIT and the EQ-i. Experts caution that tools should be carefully selected to fit the needs of the particular institution or program.[107]

The homogeneity of the nurse anesthesia applicant pool and the lack of solid data that suggests predictive value of cognitive factors emphasize the potential importance of noncognitive data[10] such as EI. Current research demonstrates a tangible link between a student's emotional intelligence scores and that student's likelihood of succeeding in both college and professional environments. A wide body of research in the general population shows that through EI screening and/or coaching, student success can be improved, and attrition rates curtailed. However, emotional intelligence studies in nurse anesthesia are limited, and further research is needed prior to definitively recommending its use in the admissions process.

Grit

The nebulous term "fire in the belly" has been used in nurse anesthesia educator circles as a term describing the often difficult to elicit ability of a student to persevere no matter what happens. What if perseverance were used as a predictor rather than an outcome, and how do we measure it? Often, as nurse anesthesia educators, we rely on the personal interview in an attempt to determine perseverance. This can be difficult in the short timeframe nurse anesthesia educators spend with each applicant. There may be another way.

Duckworth, Peterson, Matthews, and Kelly[119] introduced the construct of grit, defined as trait-level perseverance and passion for long-term goals, and showed that grit predicted achievement in challenging domains over and beyond measures of talent. For instance, at the U.S. Military Academy, West Point, cadets higher in grit were less likely to drop out than their peers with less perseverance, or grit, even when controlling for SAT scores, high school rank, and a measure of Big Five conscientiousness. In four separate samples, grit was found to be either perpendicular to or slightly inversely correlated with intelligence.

Duckworth et al[119] proposed that grit is distinct from traditionally measured facets of Big Five conscientiousness in its emphasis on stamina. In particular, grit entails the capacity to sustain both effort and interest in projects that take months or even longer to complete. This is especially intriguing as it relates to nurse anesthesia training and its move toward a mandatory 36-month training regimen.

Grit is related to but distinct from the need for achievement.[120] Individuals high in grit do not swerve from their goals, even in the absence of positive feedback. In narrowing applicants to those who will succeed, it has been demonstrated that when you consider individuals of equal talent, the grittier ones do better. Grit is not just having resilience in the face of failure, but also having deep commitments, a passion for long-term goals.[121]

Research demonstrates that grit does not relate positively to IQ but is highly correlated with the Big Five personality trait of conscientiousness. Grit does, however, demonstrate incremental predictive validity of success measures above and beyond IQ and conscientiousness. Duckworth et al state, "Collectively, these findings suggest that the achievement of difficult goals entails not only talent but also the sustained and focused application of talent over time."[119(p. 1087)] Furthermore, six different studies demonstrated that "individual differences in grit accounted for significant incremental variance in success outcomes over and beyond that explained by IQ, to which it was not positively related."[119]

There are two different Grit instruments. The 8-item Grit–S is both shorter and psychometrically stronger than the 12-item Grit–O. In confirmatory factor analyses, the Grit–S fit the data better than the Grit–O. Moreover, the reduction of items from the Grit–O to the Grit–S does not come at the expense of predictive validity. Given its superior psychometric properties, comparable predictive validity, and fewer items relative to the Grit–O, the authors recommend the Grit–S as an economical measure of perseverance and passion for long-term goals.[122]

With the intense programming required of nurse anesthesia students, grit may show promise as a predictor for perseverance, or "fire in the belly." Longitudinal research is currently being conducted on grit in anesthesia students and its predictive value in determining progression through anesthesia programs.

One study closely related to grit is by Hulse, et al,[10] which noted that students with higher trait anxiety scores are half as likely to be successful as compared with students with lower trait anxiety scores. Another finding from this study demonstrated that students with greater internal locus of control versus external locus of control were twice as likely to succeed. In other words, students who felt some control of their situation, as compared with others controlling their situation, were more successful (Table 7.3).

Table 7.3 Nontraditional Admission Variables and Their Value

Admission Variable	Recommendation
Clinical Math/ Science Test	Not enough research to recommend its use.
Simulation Scenario	Time and resource intensive. If resources are available, research demonstrates positive links with non-cognitive skills and healthcare program success.
CCRN	Shows promise in comparing registered nurses with different ICU experiences, but research is needed comparing CCRN scores with successful transition through a program and NCE scores.
Personality Testing	Multiple issues with using personality tests, the least of which is validity in admissions. Not recommended.
Emotional Intelligence	One study has demonstrated its usefulness in NA students, but more research is needed before a definitive recommendation can be made.
Grit	In theory, Grit is intriguing. Too early to recommend its use in NA admissions. Research is currently being conducted as it relates to NA programs.

Weighting Admission Criteria

Rubrics have been discussed to some extent, as they are important in supporting validity and reliability, both from a rational/judgmental model of decision-making and a statistical/mechanical model. The use of rubrics helps to avoid inherent subjectivity that can engender perceptions of unfairness on the part of student applicants when final decisions are made.[123] There is an abundance of research, some of which is presented here, that statistically supports the predictive power of several criterions if used in conjunction with each other.

It may be that a nurse anesthesia program needs to determine which factors are most important in successfully transitioning through its given program. From that point, create a rubric that emphasizes the chosen criterion, and weight it accordingly. Defending a quantitative number is—in theory—much easier than defending a subjective number.

Summary

There continues to be a lack of consensus on the admission criteria that predict successful transition—academically and clinically— through a nurse anesthesia educational program and successful passing of the national certification examination. However, good practice demands that decisions be made on evidence rather than speculation. In choosing the admission criteria, admission committees should have a firm justification of the predictive validity of the chosen criteria in relation to the academic and programmatic performance outcomes. Rather than relying on a few sources of evidence, nurse anesthesia program admission committees should consider a variety of information about applicants. The information considered should include both cognitive and noncognitive criteria until such time that research demonstrates otherwise.

Traditional admission criteria certainly have their place in determining admission to nurse anesthesia programs, but there are other variables that warrant further research and consideration. In particular, noncognitive data such as emotional intelligence, psychological empowerment, resilience, and overall well-being should be examined for their potential to determine the best candidates with the highest probability of successfully transitioning through a nurse anesthesia program.

Recruiting qualified applicants is just the beginning step in retaining students and seeing them through to program completion. After students are admitted they ought to be afforded resources that will foster their persistence in the nurse anesthesia program as well as promote their academic success.

In short, the relative value that each school places upon specific applicant characteristics, skills, and experience must be consistent with the supports and demands of the program of study offered by the school. The educational institution and the nurse anesthesia discipline definition of academic and clinical performance, including those performance outcomes that extend beyond the formal academic setting, may need to be explored. What attributes does the discipline want to see in future leaders, researchers, clinicians, and academicians?

References

1. Beauvais AM, Stewart JG, DeNisco S, Beauvais JE. Factors related to academic success among nursing students: a descriptive correlational research study. *Nurse Educ Today.* 2014;34(6):918–923.

2. Salvatori P. Reliability and validity of admissions tools used to select students for the health professions. *Adv Health Sci Educ Theory Prac.* 2001;6(2):159–175.

3. Reese CA. An Examination of the Perceived Importance of Applicant's Preadmission Characteristics as Predictive of Success in nurse Anesthesia Graduate Education Programs [dissertation]. Richmond, VA: Virginia Commonwealth University; 2002.

4. Katz JR, Chow C, Motzer SA, Woods SL. The graduate record examination: help or hindrance in nursing graduate school admissions? *J Prof Nurs.* 2009;25:369–372.

5. Suhayda R, Hicks F, Fogg L. A decision algorithm for admitting students to advanced practice programs in nursing. *J Prof Nurs.* 2008;24:281–284.

6. Holmes CB, Beishline MJ. Correct classification, false positives, and false negatives in predicting completion of the PhD from GRE scores. *Psychol Rep.* 1996;79:939–945.

7. Morrison T, Morrison M. A meta-analytic assessment of the predictive validity of the quantitative and verbal components of the Graduate Record Examination with graduate grade point average representing the criterion of graduate success. *Educ Psychol Meas.* 1995;55(2):309–16.

8. Smaby MH, Maddux CD, Richmond AS, Lepkowski WJ, Packman J. Academic admission requirements as predictors of counseling knowledge, personal development, and counseling skills. *Counselor Education and Supervision.* 2005;45:43–57.

9. Ji CC. Predictive validity of the Graduate Record Examination in education. *Psychol Rep.* 1998;82:899–904.

10. Hulse JA, Chenowith T, Lebedovych L, Dickinson P, Cavanaugh B, Garrett N. Predictors of student success in the U.S. Army graduate program in anesthesia nursing. *AANA J.* 2007;75(5):339–46.

11. Collins S, Faut-Callahan M. A call for change: clinical evaluation of student registered nurse anesthetists. *AANA J.* 2014;82:65–72.

12. Burns SM. Predicting academic progression for student registered nurse anesthetists. *AANA J.* 2011;79:193–201.

13. Creech CJ, Aplin-Kalisz C. Developing a selection method for graduate nursing students. *J Am Acad Nurse Pract.* 2011;23:404–9.

14. Fuller KM. Identification of pre-admission criteria predictive of success in graduate nurse anesthesiology program [Dissertation]. Available from ProQuest Nursing & Allied Health Source: Publication No. AAT 9532128; 1995.

15. Newton SE, Moore G. Undergraduate grade point average and graduate record examination scores: the experience of one graduate nursing program. *Nurs Educ Perspect.* 2007;28:327–331.

16. Pelech W, Stalker CA, Regehr C, Jacobs M. Making the grade: the quest for validity in admissions decisions. *J Soc Work Educ.* 1999;35:215–226.

17. Zaglaniczny KL. Factors which predict performance on the National Certification Examination for Nurse Anesthetists. *AANA J.* 1992;60:533–540.

18. Elnitsky C, Cato J, Nichols BS. Essential skills and knowledge of applicants. *AANA J.* 1999;67:273–278.

19. Megginson L. Exploration of nursing doctoral admissions and performance outcomes. *J Nurs Educ.* 2011;50:502–512.

20. Rhodes ML, Boullough B, Fulton J. The graduate record examination as an admission requirement for the graduate nursing program. *J ProfNurs.* 1994;10:289–296.

21. Haritos G, Shumway SH, Austin PN, Ellis WE. Nurse anesthesia admission qualifications. *AANA J.* 1995;63:244–248.

22. Burns SM. Predicting academic progression for student registered nurse anesthetists. *AANA J.* 2011;79(3):193–201.

23. Balogun JA. Predictors of academic and clinical performance in a baccalaureate physical therapy program. *Phys Ther.* 1988;68:238–42.

24. Hansen MJ, Pozehl BJ. The effectiveness of admission criteria in predicting achievement in a master's degree program in nursing. *J Nurs Educ.* 1995;34:433–437.

25. Higgs ZR. Predicting success in nursing: from prototype to pragmatics. *West J Nurs Res.* 1984;6:77–95.

26. Katz GM, Mosey AC. Fieldwork performance, academic grades, and preselection criteria of occupational therapy students. *Am J Occup Ther.* 1980;34:794–800.

27. Mitchell KJ. Traditional predictors of performance in medical school. *Acad Med.* 1990;65:149–158.

28. Peat M, Woodbury MG, Donner A. Admission average as a predictor of undergraduate academic and clinical performance. *Physiother Can.* 1982;34:211–214.

29. Woodward CA, McAuley RG. Can the academic background of medical graduates be detected during internship? *Can Med Assoc J.* 1983;129:567–569.

30. Kulatunga-Moruzi C, Norman GR. Validity of admissions measures in predicting performance outcomes: the contribution of cognitive and noncognitive dimensions. *Teach Learn Med.* 2002;14:34–42.

31. Wilson T. A student selection method and predictors of success in a graduate nursing program. *J Nurs Educ.* 1999;38:183–7.

32. DeProspero Rogers, P. Beyond grades and scores: expanding the role of emotional intelligence. *Journal of College Admission.* 2014;224:6–10.

33. Kuncel NR, Kochevar RJ, Ones DS. A meta-analysis of letters of recommendation in college and graduate admissions: reasons for hope. *International Journal of Selection & Assessment.* 2014;22:101–107.

34. Ross CA, Leichner P. Criteria for selecting residents: a reassessment. *CanJ Psychiatry.* 1984;29:681–686.

35. Kirchner GL, Holm MB. Prediction of academic and clinical performance of occupational therapy students in an entry-level master's program. *Am J Occup Ther.* 1997;51:775–9.

36. Standridge J, Boggs KJ, Mugan KA. Evaluation of the health occupations aptitude examination. *Respiratory Care.* 1997;42:868–872.

37. Young IP. Predictive validity of applicants' reference information for admission to a doctoral program in educational leadership. *Education Research Quarterly.* 2005;29:16–25.

38. Nicklin JM, Roch SG. Letters of recommendation: controversy and consensus from expert perspectives. *International Journal of Selection and Assessment.* 2009;17:76–91.

39. Hunter JE, Hunter RF. Validity and utility of alternative predictors of job performance. *Psychol Bull.* 1984;96(1):72–98.

40. Reilly RR, Chao GT. Validity and fairness of some alternate employee selection procedures. *Pers Psychol.* 1982;35:1–62.

41. Morgan WB, Elder KB, King EB. The emergence and reduction of bias in letters of recommendation. *J Appl Soc Psychol.* 2013;43:2297–2306.

42. Madera JM, Hebl MR, Martin RC. Gender and letters of recommendation for academia: agentic and communal differences. *J Appl Psychol.* 2009;94:1591–1599.

43. Trix F, Psenka C. Exploring the color of glass: letters of recommendation for female and male medical faculty. *Discourse & Society.* 2003;14:191–220.

44. Powers DE, Fowles ME. The personal statement as an indicator of writing skill: a cautionary note. *Educational Assessment.* 1997;4:75–87.

45. Willingham WW, Breland HM. *Personal Qualities and College Admissions.* New York, NY: College Board;1982.

46. Elam CL, Johnson MM, Wiese HJ, Studts JL, Rosenbaum M. Admission interview reports: a content analysis of interviewer comments. *Acad Med.* 1994;69:S63–S5.

47. Truell AD, Woosley S. Admission criteria and other variables as predictors of business student graduation. *Coll Stud J.* 2008;42:411–418.

48. Basco WT, Gilbert GE, Chessman AW, Blue AV. The ability of a medical school admission process to predict clinical performance and patients' satisfaction. *Acad Med.* 2000;75:743–747.

49. Edwards JC, Johnson EK, Molidar JB. The interview in the admission process. *Acad Med.* 1990;65:176–177.

50. Elam CL, Johnson MMS. An analysis of admission committee voting patterns. *Acad Med.* 1997;72:S72–S75.

51. Elam CL, Andrykowski MA. Admission interview ratings: relationship to applicant academic and demographic variables and interviewer characteristics. *Acad Med.* 1991;66:S13–S15.

52. Shaw DL, Martz DM, Lancaster CJ, Sade RM. Influence of medical school applicants' demographic and cognitive characteristic on interviewers' ratings of noncognitive traits. *Acad Med.* 1995;6:532–536.

53. Heale JA, Blumberg P, Wakefield J, McAuley R. The relationship between admission selection scores and performance of family medicine residents. Hamilton, Ontario, Canada: McMaster University; 1989.

54. Levine SB, Knecht HG, Eisen RG. Selection of physical therapy students: interview methods and academic predictors. *J Allied Health.* 1986;15:143–151.

55. Powis DA, Waring TC, Bristow T, O'Connell DL. The structured interview as a tool for predicting premature withdrawal from medical school. *Aust N Z J Med.* 1992;22:692–698.

56. Tompkins LS, Harkins CJ. Predicting academic success in a nontraditional program. *J Allied Health.* 1990;19:15–24.

57. Agho AO, Mosley BW, Smith-Paul B. Use of interview in selecting students for occupational therapy programs. *Am J Occup Ther.* 1998;52:592–594.

58. Gabard DL, Porzio R, Oxford T, Braun R. Admission interviews: questions of utility and cost in masters of physical therapy programs in the United States. *Physiother Res Internat.* 1997;2:135–149.

59. Kulatunga-Moruzi C. Toward valid selection criteria for academic and professional excellence in medicine [unpublished master's thesis]. Hamilton, Ontario, Canada: McMaster University; 1998.

60. Posthuma BW, Noh S. Interview scores and academic grades as selection criteria for admission to an occupational therapy program. *Can J Occup Ther.* 1990;57:285–292.

61. Rolfe IE, Pearson S, Powis DA, Smith AJ. Time for a review of admission to medical school? *Lancet.* 1995;346:1329–1333.

62. Stansfield RB, Kreiter CD. Conditional reliability of admissions interview ratings: extreme ratings are the most informative. *Med Educ.* 2007;41:32–38.

63. Alfaro-LeFevre R. *Critical Thinking in Nursing: A Practical Approach.* 2nd ed. Philadelphia, PA: Saunders; 1999.

64. Beyer B. *Critical Thinking.* Bloomington, IN: Phi Delta Kappa Educational Foundation; 1995.

65. Fero L, O'Donnell J, Zullo T, et al. Critical thinking skills in nursing students: comparison of simulation-based performance with metrics. *J Adv Nurs.* 2010;66:2182–93.

66. Wangensteen S, Johansson IS, Björkström ME, Nordström G. Critical thinking dispositions among newly graduated nurses. *J Adv Nurs.* 2010;66:2170–2181.

67. Fischer SC, Spiker VA, Riedel SL. *Critical thinking training for Army officersvolume two: a model of critical thinking*; 2009. Arlington, VA: U.S. Army Research Institute for the Behavioral and Social Sciences Research Report No. 1882.

68. Halpern DF. *Thought and Knowledge: An Introduction to Critical Thinking.* Hillsdale, NJ: Lawrence Erlbaum Associates, Inc.; 1989.

69. Ennis RH. A taxonomy of critical thinking dispositions and abilities. In: Baron B, Sternberg, R., eds. *Teaching Thinking Skills.* New York, NY: Freeman; 1986.

70. Wade C. Using writing to develop and assess critical thinking. *Teachf Psychol.* 1995;22:24–8.

71. Shao-Ping Y, Hung-Chang L,Ya-huei W, Ming-Jen C. Development of a scale to measure the critical thinking disposition of medical career professionals. *Soc Behav Pers.* 2014;42:303–312.

72. Kohn LT, Corrigan JM, Donaldson MS. To err is human: building a safer health system. Washington, DC: National Academies Press; 2000.

73. Lebeck LL. Correlation of student factors with performance on the National Certification Examination for nurse anesthetists. ProQuest UMI No. 30951222003.

74. Collins S. Emotional intelligence as a noncognitive factor in student registered nurse anesthetists. *AANA J.* 2013;81:465–472.

75. Cadman C, Brewer J. Emotional intelligence: a vital prerequisite for recruitment in nursing. *J Nurs Manag.* 2001;9:321–324.

76. DeCarlo D, Collingridge DS, Grant C, Ventre KM. Factors influencing nurses' attitudes toward simulation-based education. *Simul Heal.* 2008;3:90–96.

77. Hoffmann R, O'Donnell JM, Kim Y. The effects of human patient simulators on basic knowledge in critical care nursing with undergraduate senior baccalaureate nursing students. *Simul Healthc.* 2007;2:110–114.

78. Ziv A, Rubin O, Moshinsky A, et al. MOR: a simulation-based assessment centre for evaluating the personal and interpersonal qualities of medical school candidates. *Med Educ.* 2008;42:991–998.

79. Penprase B, Mileto L, Bittinger A, et al. The use of high-fidelity simulation in the admissions process: one nurse anesthesia program's experience. *AANA J.* 2012;80:43–48.

80. Moneke N, Parsons W, Moran M, Davidek A. Promoting CCRN certification at New York Presbyterian Hospital-Weill Cornell Medical Center. *Criti Care Nurse.* 2014;34:77–9.

81. Safeguarding the patient and the profession: the value of critical care nurse certification. *Am J Crit Care.* 2003;12:154–164.

82. CCRN Introduction. AACN Certification Corporation, 2015. http://www.aacn.org/wd/certifications/content/ccrnintro.pcms?menu=certification. Accessed August 20, 2015.

83. Fitzpatrick JJ, Campo TM, Graham G, Lavandero R. Certification, empowerment, and intent to leave current position and the profession among critical care nurses. *Am J Crit Care.* 2010;19:218–226.

84. Gordon W. Climbing high for EI: MHS creates customized emotional skill job profiles to help the U.S. Air Force and American Express lower training costs and increase retention. *Talent Development*. 2010;64:72–73.

85. Boyd R, Brown T. Pilot study of Myers-Briggs type indicator personality profiling in emergency department senior medical staff. *Emerg Med Australas.* 2005;17:200–203.

86. Rushton S, Morgan J, Richard M. Teacher's Myers-Briggs personality profiles: identifying effective teacher personality traits. *Teach Teach Educ.* 2007;23:432–441.

87. Lee JY, Lee YM, Kim DK. The relationship between personality types and the academic achievement levels of dental students. *Korean Journal Human Development.* 2009;16:179.

88. Lim JY, Yoo IY, Oh SN. Relationship between personality type, SAT score and GPA of student nurses. *J Korean Acad Nurs.* 2001;31:835–845.

89. Kim MR, Han SJ. Relationships between the Myers-Briggs type indicator personality profiling, academic performance and student satisfaction in nursing students. *International Journal of Bio-Science and Bio-Technology.* 2014;6:1–12.

90. Stabile SJ. The use of personality tests as a hiring tool: is the benefit worth the cost? *University of Pennsylvania Journal of Labor and Employment Law.* 2002;4:279–313.

91. Clayton BL, Lypek DJ, Connelly LM. Faculty perceptions of characteristics needed for clinical success at military nurse anesthesia programs. *AANA J.* 2000;68:515–523.

92. Reich DL, Uysal S, Bodian CA, et al. The relationship of cognitive, personality, and academic measures to anesthesiology resident clinical performance. *Anesth Analg.* 1999;88:1092–1100.

93. Gough HG, Bradley P, McDonald JS. Performance of residents in anesthesiology as related to measures of personality and interests. *Psychol Rep.* 1991;68:979–994.

94. McDonald JS, Lingam RP, Gupta B, Jacoby J, Gough HG, Bradley P. Psychologic testing as an aid to selection of residents in anesthesiology. *Anesth Analg.* 1994;78:542–547.

95. Crosby FE, Dunn JD, Fallacaro MD, Jozwiak-Shields C, MacIsaac AM. Preadmission characteristics of advanced practice nursing students. *J Am Acad Nurse Pract.* 2003;15:424–431.

96. Gunn I. The history of nurse anesthesia education: highlights and influences. *AANA J.* 1991;59:53–61.

97. Horton B. Upgrading nurse anesthesia educational requirements (1993–2006). *AANA J.* 2007;75:247–251.

98. Moss MT. *The Emotionally Intelligent Nurse Leader.* San Francisco, CA: Jossey-Bass; 2005.

99. Salovey P, Mayer JD. Emotional intelligence. *Imagination, Cognition, and Personality.* 1990;9:185–211.

100. Mayer J, Kilpatrick M. Hot information processing becomes more accurate with open emotional experience. Durham: University of New Hampshire; 1994.

101. Weisinger H. *Emotional Intelligence at Work.* San Francisco, CA: Jossey-Bass; 1998.

102. Neuwirth ZE. The silent anguish of the healers: patients suffer when physicians fall prey to stress. *Newsweek.* 1999:79.

103. Akerjordet K, Severinsson E. Emotional intelligence: a review of the literature with specific focus on empirical and epistemological perspectives. *J Clin Nurs.* 2007;16:1405–1416.

104. Chabeli MM. Higher order thinking skills competencies required by outcomes-based education from learners. *Curationis.* 2006;29:78–86.

105. Zimmerman BJ, Phillips CY. Affective learning: stimulus to critical thinking and caring practice. *J Nurs Educ*. 2000;39:422–5.

106. Vitello-Cicciu JM. Exploring emotional intelligence: implications for nursing leaders. *J Nurs Adm*. 2002;32:203–210.

107. DeSouza ER. Frequency rates and correlates of contrapower harassment in higher education. *J Interpers Violence*. 2011;26:158–88.

108. Walker M. Emotional Intelligence and Academic Success in College [dissertation]. ProQuest UMI No. 326848 12006.

109. Cohen J, ed. Educating Minds and Hearts: Social Emotional Learning and the Passage Into Adolescence. New York, NY: Teachers College Press; 1999.

110. Vandervoort DJ. The importance of emotional intelligence in higher education. *Curr Psychol*. 2006;25:4–7.

111. Edgar L, Herbert R, Lambert S, MacDonald J, Dubois S, Latimer M. The joint venture model of knowledge utilization: a guide for change in nursing. *Nurs Leaders (Tor Ont)*. 2006;19:41–55.

112. Beauvais AM, Brady N, O'Shea ER, Griffin MT. Emotional intelligence and nursing performance among nursing students. *Nurse Educ Today*. 2011;31:396–401.

113. Codier E, Odell E. Measured emotional intelligence ability and grade point average in nursing students. *Nurse Educ Today*. 2014;34:608–612.

114. Nooryan K, Gasparyan K, Sharif F, Zoladl M. The effect of teaching emotional intelligence (EI) items on job related stress in physicians and nurses working in ICU wards in hospitals. *International Journal of Collaborative Research on Internal Medicine and Public Health*. 2011;3:704–13.

115. Montes-Berges B, Augusto JM. Exploring the relationship between perceived emotional intelligence, coping, social support and mental health in nursing students. *J Psychiatr Ment Health Nurs*. 2007;14:163–171.

116. Weng HC, Hung CM, Liu YT, Cheng YJ, Yen CY, Chang CC, Huang CK. Associations between emotional intelligence and doctor burnout, job satisfaction, and patient satisfaction. *Med Educ*. 2011;45:835–842.

117. Goleman D. *Working with Emotional Intelligence*. 2nd ed. New York, NY: Bantam Books; 1998.

118. Collins S. Emotional intelligence as a noncognitive factor in student registered nurse anesthetists. *AANA J*. 2013;81:465–472.

119. Duckworth AL, Peterson C, Matthews MD, Kelly DR. Grit: perseverance and passion for long-term goals. *J Pers Soc Psychol*. 2007;92:1087–1101.

120. McClelland DC. *The Achieving Society*. Oxford, England: Van Nostrand; 1961.

121. Perkins-Gough D. The Significance of Grit: A Conversation with Angela Lee Duckworth. *Educ Leadersh*. 2013;71:14–20.

122. Duckworth AL, Quinn PD. Development and Validation of the Short Grit Scale (Grit-S). *J Pers Assess.* 2009;91:166–174.

123. Cunningham CJ, Manier A, Anderson A, Sarnosky K. Rational versus empirical prediction of nursing student success. *J Prof Nurs.* 2014;30:486–92.

CHAPTER 8

Generational Dynamics in Nurse Anesthesia Education

Lisa Mileto, DNP, CRNA

Keywords: Andragogy, baby boomers, Generation X, Generation Y, Generation Z, heutagogy, traditionalists.

Key Concepts

- A generation is a cohort of people born during a specified range of years and who are deeply influenced by shared experiences.
- The United States (U.S.) has a five-generation workforce including the traditionalist generation, the baby boomer generation, Generation X, Generation Y, and Generation Z, each with a unique set of characteristics and values.
- Cross-generational conflict in the academic environment can hinder both student achievement and faculty job satisfaction.
- Commonalities exist between Generation Y and Generation Z learning styles, allowing for andragogical and heutagogical instructional models that work for both groups.
- Anesthesia educators must shift from being lecturers to designers of learning methods, a paradigm shift from focusing on teaching to emphasizing self-managed, flexible learning.

Introduction

The children now love luxury; they have bad manners, contempt for authority; they show disrespect for elders and love chatter in place of exercise. Children are now tyrants, not the servants of their households. They contradict their parents...and tyrannize their teachers.

—Socrates

Disapproval of young people's behavior is a recurring societal theme.[1] In today's environment, educators are confronted with meeting the learning needs of a generationally diverse group of learners. Assisting educators to navigate generational diversity, with its challenge and promise, is the focus of this chapter. Generational differences affect anesthesia education and have an impact on both clinical and classroom andragogy. The first steps in harmonizing diverse student and instructor populations are to understand what motivates members of different generations and to institute instructional methods that focus on self-directed learning in place of lecturing.

A generational transformation is occurring in health care across America. For the first time in history, the workforce consists of five generations working together. A national dialogue continues among generation experts, academicians, researchers, and leaders, suggesting that generational needs should be taken into account to improve the quality of education. Exploring Certified Registered Nurse Anesthetist (CRNA) doctoral education from a generational perspective can provide added value, allowing educators to capitalize on unique, generation-specific opportunities to recruit and retain highly qualified anesthesia students and create favorable outcomes for the profession of nurse anesthesia. Understanding generational differences may diffuse intergenerational conflicts that can emerge when values are not aligned. The shift to doctoral education coincides with the necessary move from hierarchical instruction to self-determined learning.

Each generation has innate core values influenced by the era in which they were born and experiences throughout their formative years. Strauss and Howe's Generational Theory[1] examines the factors that drive people's behavior. A generation is a cohort group that shares birth years and is deeply influenced by and bound together by shared experiences.[2] The events people experience throughout their formative years partly determine who they are, how they see the world, and what they value. Events that capture the attention and emotions of millions of people throughout their youth contribute to the development of a generational personality.[1] War, natural disaster, pop culture, economics, public heroes, music, and technology are examples of defining events. These events shape a generation and have a profound effect on a person's value system.[1]

There is little change in a generation's values throughout the lives of its members. Generational characteristics are frequently attributed to a group's age. Statements such as, "These young people today..." illustrate how age is incorrectly attributed to a generational cohort's behavior. It is often the group's core values guiding the behavior.[2]

Overview of Five Generations

For the first time in history, the U.S. has transitioned from a two-generation workforce to a five-generation workforce, which includes the traditionalist generation, the baby boomer generation, Generation X, Generation Y and Generation Z.[3] This multigenerational workforce is due, in part, to increased longevity.[1] In the early 1900s, the average life expectancy was under 50 years. Life expectancy in 2016 is nearly 80 years.[4] **Table 8.1** provides a depiction of generational groups delineated by birth years.

Table 8.1 Comparison of 5 Generations

Generation	Birth years	Current age (2016)	Population (million)
Traditionalists	1920–1945	71–99	75
Baby Boomers	1946–1964	52–70	80
Generation X	1965–1980	36–51	46
Generation Y	1981–1995	21–34	76
Generation Z	1996–TBD*	20 and under	TBD

*TBD = To Be Determined

Traditionalists

Maturity: Be able to stick with a job until it is finished. Be able to bear an injustice without having to get even. Be able to carry money without spending it. Do your duty without being supervised.

—Ann Landers

The traditionalists were born between 1920 and 1945.[5] Defining events that occurred in their formative years included the Roaring Twenties, the Great Depression, World War II, and Prohibition.[5] Families gathered to listen to the radio, children read Superman comics, and baseball brought a new hero, Babe Ruth.

The Great Depression left a permanent impression on the minds of traditionalists. In 1933, President Franklin Delano Roosevelt promised the depression-weary people of the United States a New Deal.[5] Roosevelt implemented banking reform laws, emergency relief, work relief, and agricultural programs. The Social Security Act provided for long-term financial protection and the Servicemen's Readjustment Act of 1944, commonly known as the G.I. Bill, provided college or vocational education for returning World War II veterans.[5]

Influenced by the events of their time, the traditionalists developed characteristics such as a strong commitment to civic duty, patience, and respect for authority.[1] Traditionalists are quiet, private, hardworking, and patriotic. They have a no-nonsense, practical approach to life that contributes to their conservative, formal behavior and dress. Traditionalists are a staunch political force and active in the American Association of Retired Persons (AARP).[2] Traditionalists are motivated to save their money, pay cash, and buy products made in the U.S.. The core beliefs of the traditionalists are outlined in **Table 8.2**, next page.

Table 8.2 Core Beliefs of Traditionalists

Core Beliefs of Traditionalists
Sacrifice
Hard work
Conformity
Law and order
Respect for authority
Patience
Duty before pleasure
Compliance with rules

Baby Boomers

They will redefine old and cool and success before they are done with the world they have sworn to make over in their own Sharper Image.

—**David Stillman**

The baby boomer generation (boomers) was born between 1946 and 1964.[6] After nearly 200 years of a declining population, the post-World War II boom produced 1 baby every 17 minutes for 19 years.[2] Raising children was no longer a necessity for survival. Growing up in a time of economic expansion and prosperity, major social movements, and national optimism, boomers were cherished by their parents and represented the hope for the future that their parents fought to preserve.[6]

Defining events that occurred during the boomers' formative years included the Cold War, the war in Vietnam, the Cuban Missile Crisis, and air raid drills.[6] Boomers were raised in an era of great change. They witnessed the civil rights movement and they were empowered by campaigns and protests. Rosa Parks, the assassinations of Martin Luther King Jr. and John F. Kennedy, the McCarthy hearings, and Woodstock all left an indelible mark.[6]

During this era, woman's rights took center stage.[7] President Kennedy established the President's Commission on the Status of Women and appointed Eleanor Roosevelt as the chair. The commission reported substantial discrimination against women in the workplace and made recommendations for improvement in hiring practices, paid maternity leave, and affordable childcare. Soon after, new laws such as the Equal Pay Act of 1963 and Title VII of the Civil Rights Act of 1964 cleared the path for women to enter the workforce in record numbers. Women made difficult choices between the differing roles of stay at home mother and paid employee.[8]

The 1960s also was a time of great technological advancement. Inventions during this time included the handheld calculator, bar coding, and random access memory (RAM). Outer space captured the imaginations of the public and scientists. Some of the most dramatic advances were in the area of manned space flight.[7] In contrast to their traditionalist parents, boomers embraced radical social change.[9] They challenged traditional family attitudes and embraced different lifestyles. The boomers witnessed a cultural shift from poodle skirts and hula hoops to peace signs, rock and roll, anti-war campaigns, and love-ins.[7] The emerging drug culture and sexual freedom coincided with introspection and spiritual evaluation.

Privileged by wealth and prosperity, today's boomers cherish anything trendy—multifunctional smartphones, luxury cars, vintage wines, designer merchandise—and they are willing to work for it. They take a 60-hour workweek in stride.[9] Boomers focus their energy on expanding their longevity and enhancing their retirement. This is a reflection of their drive for personal gratification and wellness. Boomers are concerned about their workplace environment. They value participation, fairness, and equality. Boomers are team players who believe in inclusion and collaboration. Conversely, they are fiercely competitive and will go to great lengths to get what they want.[2] **Table 8.3** lists the core values of boomers.[9]

Table 8.3 Core Beliefs of Baby Boomers

Optimism
Teamwork
Personal gratification
Health and wellness
Personal development
Work
Spirituality

Generation X

A person should not believe in an "-ism," he should believe in himself. I quote John Lennon, "I don't believe in the Beatles, I just believe in me."

—**Ferris Bueller,** ***Ferris Bueller's Day Off***

Born between 1965 and 1980 and comprising an estimated 46 million people, Generation X (Gen X) is often referred to as the sandwich generation.[9] During their formative years, Gen X witnessed corporate layoffs and corruption, inflation, the energy crisis, and nuclear proliferation.[2] Rapidly rising divorce rates and women entering the workforce changed family dynamics.[10] Cynicism rose from political gridlock and corruption, turmoil in religious sectors, and fear of a dissolving Social Security and Medicare system. These defining events contributed to Generation X's prevailing skepticism. Institutions that were previously stable began to fail, leading to distrust, disappointment, and a survivor mentality. Watergate, the fall of the Berlin Wall, the Challenger disaster, and Operation Desert Storm were all sentinel events that influenced Gen X.[9]

Today, Gen X values balance in their lives, particularly between their work and personal lives; they do not define themselves by their work.[10] They are frugal and are not influenced by trendy brand names or hype. Having little regard for corporate life, they often challenge or work around authority and the status quo.[9] Gen X are independent problem solvers who excel at multitasking and leveraging new technology. The hipster counterculture subgroup stereotypically has tattoos, beards, large horn-rimmed glasses, and casual dress. Valuing intellect, creativity, and independent thinking, hipsters consider mainstream consumers culturally ignorant.[11]

Generation X is often labeled as disloyal, uncommitted, and cynical. On the contrary, they are voracious learners, creative, and resourceful.[10] Gen X members are no less motivated to succeed than previous generations; they simply choose to define success in their own terms. The core beliefs of Gen X are outlined in **Table 8.4**, next page.

Table 8.4 Core Beliefs of Generation X

Balance
Techno-literacy
Fun
Casualness
Self-reliance
Pragmatism

Generation Y

They want to study, travel, make friends, make more friends, read everything (super-fast), take in all the movies, listen to every hot band, and keep up with everyone they have ever known.

—Mark Edmundson

Generation Y, born 1981–1995, comprise nearly one-third of the current population.[10] Defining events in the formative years for Generation Y (Gen Y) included threats and acts of terrorism (particularly September 11, 2001), the arrival of a new century, and school shootings.[10] This cohort was raised in a child-focused environment. Parents were involved in their children's lives in a style of parenting coined "helicopter parenting," creating an environment of protection and guidance. Gen Y have received extensive accolades for their achievements and have been the recipients of a cultural shift toward the promotion of positive self-esteem.[10]

Gen Y is often referred to as the narcissistic generation. Several studies by Twenge et al[12] conducted between 1982 and 2009, including a nationwide meta-analysis (N=49,818) and an examination of data from one college campus (N=4,152), demonstrated significant increases in American college students' narcissistic traits over the generations.[12] The Narcissistic Personality Inventory results indicated that, by 2006, two-thirds of the students had above-average scores on this inventory, ranking 30% higher than students in 1982. The results support generational differences reflecting changes in culture.[12] Social media such as Facebook and YouTube and SnapChat encourage self-promotion. Generation Y's sense of entitlement is fed by their baby boomer parents, who spend billions of dollars each year on their children.[10]

In contrast to baby boomers, Generation Y values changing employment frequently to seek the work environment that meets their desired lifestyle.[8] In addition to having a sense of civic responsibility and social engagement, they are tech-savvy as well as tech-dependent. According to a 2014 Deloitte/Bentley University survey,[13] 6 out of 10 Gen Y cited their company's sense of purpose as part of the reason they chose their job. In the same study, just 12% identified "my own personal gain" as a primary leadership priority, and 66% indicated they would like to start their own business.[13]

David Infante is a journalist for Mashable and a Gen Y member.[11] He describes Gen Y as "Yuccies: Young Urban Creatives." Yuccies are the cultural offspring of "yuppies" and "hipsters":

"Generation Y, borne of suburban comfort, indoctrinated with the transcendent power of education, and infected by the conviction that not only do we deserve to pursue our dreams; we should profit from them. Getting rich quick would be great. But getting rich quick and preserving creative autonomy? That's the yuccie dream. [They] are intent on being successful like yuppies and creative like hipsters."[11]

Generation Y is culturally diverse, with 36% nonwhite or Hispanic.[14] Valuing diversity and embracing collaboration, they tolerate differences of opinion. They are compliant and respectful of authority, yet they do not hesitate to challenge authority.[14] Members of Gen Y are exceptionally altruistic and collectively hopeful. The core beliefs of Gen Y are outlined in **Table 8.5**.

Table 8.5 Core Beliefs of Generation Y

Core Beliefs
Optimism
Confidence
Achievement
Sociability
Diversity
Civic duty

Generation Z

You deserve to make a living being yourself. Your ideas are valuable. Follow your dreams.

—David Infante

Generation Z (born after 1996) comprise the current 20 and under group.[15] According to The National Education Association, 25% of the U.S. population is considered members of Generation Z (Gen Z).[12] Whereas Gen Y is optimistic, Gen Z is realistic. Having grown up post-9/11, in the middle of the Great Recession and surrounded by school violence, they are aware of troubling times. Global terrorism, sustainability concerns, cybercrime, and the energy and education crisis are defining events for Gen Z. These events contribute to Gen Z being cautious and security-minded, yet striving to improve the world.[12] Their role models are everyday characters like The Hunger Games' Katniss Everdeen, who face what seem like inescapable scenarios, but rise above them to create a better world.[13] Growing up with major innovation, hyper-connectivity, and social change, Gen Z are inquisitive, creative, and globally aware.[13]

Gen Z are closer to their parents than the previous generation, yet they have less need for direction because they have instant access to questions they have about most everything. They experience "velcro parenting,"[14] where the amount of time parents spend with their children has reached new heights. Creative work models, home schooling, and unemployment have increased parent/child time.[14]

Significant parental unemployment has impacted Gen Z, unlike the previous two generations. Their perspective on personal finance (conservative), career choices (realistic), and lifestyle (moderate) have been influenced by the Great Recession.[15] Cybercrimes like identity theft are a dangerous reality that are not well policed or regulated. Gen Z has Internet street smarts and they plan to tackle such issues globally.[15] Nearly half of Gen Z feel that school violence will have the biggest impact on their generation, more than social networking and the election of the first black president.[13]

Generation Z has never known a world without smart devices and the Internet.[16] Their social network is web-based (Twitter, Snap Chat, Instagram, Vine), allowing Gen Z to become global citizens and contributing to their expectation to work and have social communication anytime and anyplace.[16] Selfies and emojis as forms of communication are shared daily, even hourly. Generation Z receives most of their media on mobile devices and prefer media that they can interact with as opposed to passive TV or print texts.[16] Binge-watching entertainment without commercials is commonplace. Consumerism has changed tremendously for Gen Z; Uber and Airbnb are trusted companies that are simply service applications (apps). Due to access to a constant influx of global news, Gen Z are more socially aware than the generations before them.[16]

Generation Z is self-directed, stating they want to design their own college study plans, study entrepreneurship, and work for themselves.[15] Sixty-five percent of grade school students will work in jobs that don't exist today.[16] Nearly one-third report finding a job as their top concern.[15] The recession will have Gen Z competing for jobs with boomers, Gen X, and Gen Y. Gen Z will back their boss, and seek jobs where bosses "have their backs." Flexibility is important; employers worry that Gen Z is so flexible, retention might be challenging.[17] Gen Z will not be as loyal to employers as generations before them. Eighty-three percent of today's students believe that three years or less is the appropriate amount of time at their first job.[17]

Higher education costs are becoming prohibitive and student debt is high, therefore Gen Z looks for alternative ways to enter the professional working world. Nearly one-fourth are most concerned about the cost of education and the long-term financial impact it can have on their future.[17] The education crisis arrives as Gen Z starts college, and as the profession of nurse anesthesia transitions to the entry level doctoral degree. More than half of Gen Z report that student loan debt is a major consideration in their education and career decisions.[17] Nearly 40% are focused on the opportunity for growth (not salary) when asked about their first job.[17]

College student Ashton Carrick describes behaviors and characteristics of Gen Z in a *New York Times* opinion article:[18] "I think it's the stress. It permeates everything we do as college students. Many small, elite colleges are insanely competitive to get into in the first place and they remain competitive as students try to outdo one another with grades, scholarships, extracurricular activities and internships. Having been one of those hypercompetitive students, I can tell you that it never feels like enough. The person sitting next to you in class is always doing more and doing it better. I became obsessed with stacking my resume, even more so than I was in high school. I saw it as a reflection of whether I would succeed in life. And I'm not alone. The obsession seems largely driven by fear—fear of a crumbling job market, of not meeting parents' expectations, of crippling loan debt."

Such an intense preoccupation with success—or at least what we've been told success looks like—is not without its consequences. Rates of mental illness in young adults have spiked in the last couple of years. According to a 2013 survey by the American College of Health Association, 57% of female and 40% of male college students reported feeling overwhelmingly anxious, while 33% of females and 27% of males reported feeling seriously depressed. The association also found that suicide rates in young adults had tripled since the 1950s, with the National Alliance on Mental Illness estimating that a quarter of college students have had suicidal thoughts.[18]

Trends toward seeking highly successful careers that do not require a decade of expensive education, academic credentials, and debt may be preferred by Gen Z. Such career paths are possible due to the simplicity of obtaining free knowledge. Free or low-cost online classes are increasing at an exponential rate.[19] These Massive Open Online Courses (MOOCs) are changing the nature of education. They can be viewed as a disruptive innovation that might disaggregate teaching from assessment and accreditation.[19] These online courses are shaking up traditional power dynamics of education, as venture capitalists seek to exploit this business model.[19]

The impact of institutional failure that Gen Z has been surrounded by remains to be seen. The education bubble, declining economy, political gridlock, and corporate corruption will undoubtedly have a lasting impression. Generation Z is already a formidable force at age 20, and they have an agenda. Anesthesia programs have the opportunity to plan for the arrival of Gen Z and design the educational platform accordingly. The core beliefs of Gen Z are outlined in **Table 8.6.** Who is the next group? Generation Alpha.

Table 8.6 Core Beliefs of Generation Z

Realism
Resilience
Fiscal responsibility
Flexibility
Collaboration
Global awareness

Generational Conflict

Cross-generational conflict in the academic environment can hinder both student achievement and faculty job satisfaction. Bridging the gap creates a collaborative environment that stimulates learning and creates harmony. **Table 8.7** depicts the viewpoints of five generations.

Table 8.7 Viewpoints of Five Generations

	Traditionalists	Boomers	Gen X	Gen Y	Gen Z
Future Outlook	Practical	Optimistic	Skeptical	Hopeful	Realistic
Turnoffs	Profanity	Political incorrectness	Cliché, hype	Techno-illiteracy, intolerance	Corruption
Work ethic	Dedicated	Driven	Balanced	Determined	Self-employment
Relationships	Personal sacrifice	Gratification	Reluctant to commit	Crave community	Cautious
View of authority	Respectful	Love/hate	Unimpressed	Team-oriented	Cautious

It is not uncommon for baby boomers and traditionalists to have a perception that members of Gen X and Gen Y lack commitment.[2,7] Clinical educators and faculty complain that students do not want to stay to finish cases and have a casual attitude. Occasionally labeled as disrespectful in the classroom, Gen X, Gen Y, and Gen Z students are often bored by traditional lecture styles and lengthy class times. Instructors can be offended by students' frequent use of mobile devices and their impersonal communication style.[20,21]

The root of generational conflict is the mix between past, present, and future. The boomers have grown to see themselves as the be-all generation, "the older sibling who has been dethroned by a new arrival."[20,21] Boomers feel displaced by Gen X, whom they believe are disrupting the world the boomers improved. In contrast, Bristow[21] states that "Boomer blaming" by Gen X has a negative impact on "consequences for the construction of knowledge, the focus of social policy, and the experience of generational contact." Gen X is highly skeptical of the boomers. They prefer self-reliance above the boomer's attachment to teams, and they have refused to bow to the boomer-driven work ethic. Boomers judge Gen X as cynical and less committed.[21] Generation X is committed to preserving their life outside of work and the classroom, and believe that they bring more promise and energy through this life balance.[9,10]

Both boomers and Gen X believe that members of Gen Y lack direction and are overly reliant on frequent positive feedback. They feel that Gen Y members are needy and have an air of entitlement. Hira[22] states, "This is the most high-maintenance workforce in the history of the world. The good news is they're also going to be the most high-performing." Viewed by boomers and Gen X as ambitious and demanding, Gen Y and Z members question everything. On the other hand, they exhibit values such as honesty, caring, moral courage, patriotism, and democracy.[2,15] Gen Y and Gen Z members believe they will do a better job of upholding these values, and that the older generations have talked the talk, but that they will walk the walk.[15]

Such struggles that occur between generations are being played out in hospitals across America. A philosophical shift is occurring in health care. Generational influences are creating marked changes in physician work schedules and resident and medical student education. A 2008 *Wall Street Journal* article by Goldstein[23] states, "U.S. medicine is in the middle of a cultural revolution, as young physicians, intent on balancing work and family, challenge the assumption that a doctor should be available to treat patients around the clock." Physicians are searching for and finding jobs that have a predictable schedule. For example, medical residents pushed for and received limited weekly hours and time off post call in 2002.[22] Even with the limited hours, a survey of medical residents in 2006 found that lack of free time was the biggest concern for 63% of respondents.[23] Anesthesia students also have concerns about the hours required for anesthesia education. The Council on Accreditation of Nurse Anesthesia Educational Programs currently requires student clinical and classroom time commitment not exceed 64 hours per week.[24]

Educational Strategies for Generational Differences

Anesthesia educators should be knowledgeable about generational differences when designing doctoral anesthesia programs and curricula for Gen X, Gen Y, and Gen Z students. A cohort of post-master's doctoral students will likely have generational diversity. Meeting doctoral students' educational needs requires an understanding of their values and learning styles. Nurse anesthesia program administrators and faculty are increasingly grappling with generational differences in the classroom, online, and during clinical education of nurse anesthesia students. Conflict can arise when values are not understood. Friction may be aggravated by new technology and work patterns that mix workers of different generations in frequently changing teams.[25] There are several strategies for implementing classroom instruction that are generationally adept. Less hierarchal instruction and more self-direction, as well as collaborative learning, can be beneficial.

Over the past decade, anesthesia educators may have had a more reactionary response to the educational needs of Gen Y, but they now have the opportunity to proactively design programs that fit the learning styles of Gen Z. The exponential advancements in technology have likely had the greatest impact on the learning styles of the most recent generations.[16] Today's students are products of thousands of hours of exposure to continuously updated information via the Internet.[16,25] The use of the latest technology is second nature to most; therefore, they expect technological sophistication in their anesthesia program. Instructors must shift from being primarily lecturers to being designers of learning methods, a paradigm shift from focusing on teaching to emphasizing learning.[25,26] Andragogy is the theory and practice of adult learning. Heutagogy is the theory of self-determined learning.[27] Problem-centered learning instead of content-centered learning, respectively, is an important distinction between the theories. The lines between teacher and student are more fluid and the focus is on shared learning, exploration, and discussion.[27]

Ryan and Tilbury's[28] report to the Higher Education Academy provides an overview of new pedagogies that promote learner empowerment by using flexible learning platforms such as future-facing education, decolonizing education, social learning, transformative capabilities, and crossing boundaries. Learner empowerment and co-creation allow for the flexibility doctoral students need to be producers of, as well as consumers of knowledge.[27] Flipped learning, for example, reverses the typical "reading assignment followed by lecture followed by testing."[29] Flipped learning is scaffolded learning that includes video lectures, podcasts, or narrated presentations and infographics that are viewed by students prior to class-based activities. The classroom element is repurposed into concept clarification and applied learning. The classroom becomes more of a workshop-style approach with interactive activities. Flipped learning is helpful for complex concepts, creating more effective use of class time.[29]

Accommodating different learning styles can be a challenge. Although baby boomer instructors favor more traditional and static training methods like PowerPoint presentations, handouts, and outlines, Gen Y and Gen Z students prefer interactive, technology-based forms of learning.[25] Micro-learning, problem-based learning, flipped classrooms, and mobile learning promote retention for Gen Y and Z.[27–29] Discussion groups using scholarly blogs and information tools such as wikis can meet their need for participation and engagement with classmates online. Exam software with analytics allows for rapid test feedback for both students and faculty.

The education paradigm is moving from education 1.0 to 3.0 rapidly.[30] Traditional educators are accustomed to a top-down approach with knowledge moving from teacher to students. The real and virtual classrooms of education 3.0 are less hierarchal. Teaching is not merely teacher-to-student, but also student-to-student, student-to-teacher, and people-technology-student.[30] The meaning of education is not dictated, as in education 1.0, but socially constructed and contextually reinvented in education 3.0.[30] Technology and the school are not in the physical classroom or simply online (brick and click), but everywhere (infused into society and part of the digital universe).[30]

Teaching Generation X Students

A dominant force in college classrooms for the past 20 years, Gen X has been studied extensively in terms of learning style and values. Generation X students are creative, self-sufficient, easily adaptable and technoliterate.[2] They show a preference for self-paced, independent learning, which is characteristic of doctoral education. Online learning modules with diagrams and video, study questions, and case scenarios are effective teaching tools for Gen X. They often prefer online courses.[21] In the classroom, Gen X students identify with an instructor who effectively utilizes technology and who provides a creative, engaging presentation. They value immediacy, efficiency, and quality in educational design.[21]

In contrast, Gen X students are turned off by instructors who micromanage or use pressure tactics to teach in clinical or the classroom. This group is not motivated by fear or long-term reward strategies.[9] For example, although appreciative of examination content clues, they do not learn from threats about passing grades or instructors who create test anxiety. Pragmatic and down-to-earth, Gen X prefers educational strategies that focus on outcomes that reflect real-world skills necessary for success.[21]

Teaching Generation Y Students

Generation Y is a cohort of students that began entering colleges in 2000. There is considerable research attempting to determine the values, learning styles, and marketing potential of this generation.[14,16] Although similarities exist in the teaching methods favored by Gen X, Gen Y, and Gen Z, Gen Y has unique educational needs. Growing up in a world of instant gratification, Gen Y members perceive that their issues or needs are not valued if there is a delay in response longer than what they consider appropriate.[32,33] Their expectations for rapid results for test grades, written evaluations, or course handouts can be a source of frustration for instructors. twenty-four-hour access to university, hospital, faculty, and educational resources is a common expectation.

Gen Y generally does not work well under rigid educational or management structures.[28] They prefer flexibility and open collaboration that allow peers to share information.[29,30] It is not surprising that four-hour classroom lectures with slides, handouts, and minimal student interaction do not enhance Gen Y learning.[27] Methods to facilitate Gen Y's learning are group assignments with Socratic questioning and class presentations that allow Gen Y to work in teams.[27,28] Guided independent study in advance of complex case discussions allows for flexible, independent study combined with group learning, tapping into their preference for teamwork.[28] In addition to this problem-based learning style, instructors can use flipped classroom instruction, resource guides in the form of podcasts and vodcasts, and the use of scholarly blogs and wikis. The effective use of mobile learning provides opportunities for critical thinking, discussion, and case examples.[31] Online courses permit the flexibility that Gen X and Gen Y need by allowing them to work on their own time, reducing the traditional classroom instruction time.

Members of Gen Y and Gen Z are, by nature, holistic learners, exploring with their minds and responding by doing.[16] Both generations learn well in a participative, positive learning environment in which they can think and investigate possibilities.[21,27,28] With the availability of high-fidelity human-patient simulation and interactive e-learning, instructors have numerous tools that meet the needs of today's students. Dramatic innovations in technology, increasingly potent pharmacologic agents, complex medical cases, and advances in surgery and anesthesia make human-patient simulation an important educational tool. Students can safely practice high-acuity, low-frequency skills in a carefully monitored environment. Simulation allows for team training and the development of highly effective communication across disciplines and generations.

Generation Y students are well-prepared, confident, and willing to do what it takes to succeed. They are accustomed to devoting their time and energy toward accomplishing their goals and being rewarded for doing so. Gen Y students want more direction than their Gen X predecessors.[26] They need encouragement to seek greater autonomy and self-reliance.[33] This group may find the transition to doctoral education difficult. As high-achieving undergraduate students who found academic success with little effort, they may have unrealistic expectations about what it takes to handle the rigors of nurse anesthesia education. Generation Y students may benefit from information on study techniques and time-management skills, the development of study groups, and other forms of collaborative learning. **Table 8.8** shows the learning characteristics of Gen Y.

Table 8.8 Learning Characteristics of Generation Y

Generation Y
Holistic learners
Based in real-world tasks
Spontaneous
Kinesthetic
Graphic and visual

Generation Y students tend to be overachievers, but they have been overly managed.[14,16,23] Often rewarded for participation instead of achievement in elementary education, they will challenge a grade or an evaluation. Gen Y expect grade inflation and instant success in the clinical setting. This group struggles with setting goals and identifying their individual strengths and weaknesses.[26] They request more supervision and structure than Gen X. Gen Y students aim to please, and following the rules replaces the rebellion of Gen X. They require more mentoring initially but have shown an ability to make dramatic and constructive changes in a short time.[26] Praise is high on the list of expectations from Gen Y.[26]

The Generation Z Learner

Gen Zs are the most home-schooled generation in the last century.[16] They dislike lecture-test classroom styles for learning and often prefer hands-on or mobile learning.[27,28,30] Their digital world can be customized, so they want their education customized.[16] Gen Zs expect to be able to learn and study whenever and wherever they choose. Because they are hyperconnected, they are wired for the rapid delivery of content and data from the Internet.[16,31] Their frequent multitasking has unfortunately led to short attention spans. This creates instructional challenges, as they are easily bored and ready to move on to the next topic.[16] Flipping the classroom, microlearning, and using problem-based learning can help Gen Z students focus their attention on a subject that has depth and complexity.[28,29,30]

Engage Gen Z students by having a learner-centered curriculum, not a teacher centered curriculum.[30] Extended lessons can be hard to manage for instructors and students, so educators are tailoring information into microlearning sessions. Instructors are creating shorter class days with fewer hours of lecture content in one day, and many universities are moving most coursework online.[28,30] Similar to Gen Y, Gen Z engage with scholarly blogging, vodcasting and podcasting, and digital media that allow students to connect with each other and with other students around the world.[27] Conversely, being from the digital generation does not mean Gen Z knows how to properly find or manage information online. Teaching Gen Z how to discover, manage and curate information, and find reputable sources is vital. **Table 8.9** has the learning characteristics of Gen Z.

Table 8.9 Learning Characteristics of Generation Z

Generation Z
Inquisitive Less hierarchal Hyperconnected Shared learning

Strategies for Teaching Gen X, Gen Y, and Gen Z

Students today need to be given high and clear expectations.[32,33] Frequent student-faculty contact to assess student critical thinking and frequent student reflective self-assessment are important educational tools. Recurrent and timely feedback about academic and clinical performance are essential. Gen X, Gen Y, and Gen Z prefer both independent learning and an interactive, energetic classroom style.[28] Neither group is intimidated by authority. This can occasionally lead to classroom antics that boomer instructors perceive as disinterest and even disrespect. Allowing time for fun and active student participation is essential for maintaining an attentive, engaged group.[31]

Today's students become engaged by lectures that include live or video demonstrations, pictures, and images. Current textbooks mirror web pages with key points, charts, highlights, and graphs. The visual image, not the printed word, is the preferred means of communication. The old approach relied on textual directions to walk students through steps in their assignments. A more modern, effective approach uses infographics to illustrate steps and give directions instead of a step-by-step list.[27,29]

Other easy-to-implement tools include establishing a regular presence on numerous social networking sites for the program that provides a forum for sharing ideas and concerns. Because Gen Y and Gen Z prefer frequent and detailed evaluation of their performance on both exams and clinical practice, a rigorous evaluation platform across the program is beneficial. Additionally, adhering to due dates for evaluations and providing access to and submission of evaluations online can help meet this generational learning style.

Summary

In summary, a generational transformation is occurring in classrooms across America. Generational differences impact anesthesia education and have an impact on both clinical and classroom pedagogy. Baby boomer faculty are teaching record numbers of Gen X and Gen Y students. Generation Z is ushering in a new era with new values. This great generational transition has significant implications for anesthesia educators and the transition to doctoral education. Instructors need to use current best-teaching strategies and develop innovative, flexible teaching methods that foster autonomous and self-regulated learners. To harmonize a diverse student population, educators should understand what motivates members of different generations and institute teaching techniques that meet their needs.

Each generation has innate core values based on the events and experiences of the era in which members spent their formative years. These core values affect learning styles, work ethic, perceptions of others, and how people communicate. Gen X, Gen Y and Gen Z offer core values that can bring positive changes to doctoral nurse anesthesia programs and the health care workforce. Anesthesia educators who anticipate generational differences will be equipped to meet their students' educational needs and diffuse intergenerational conflicts that can emerge when values are not aligned. Embracing generational differences, using innovative instructional methods to refine the way we educate, and implementing educational strategies described will help deliver success. Anesthesia educators are in for a challenge and a tremendous opportunity.

References

1. Strauss W, Howe N. *Generations: The History of America's Future, 1584 to 2069.* New York, NY: William Morrow; 1991:27–42.

2. Zemke R, Raines C, Filipczak B. *Generations at Work: Managing the Clash of Veterans, Boomers, Xers, and Nexters in Your Workplace.* New York, NY: AMACOM; 2000:1–150.

3. Brown P. *Generation X, Y and ZEKE: Zealously Enthused Kinda Educated.* WestBow Press; 2014.

4. Centers for Disease Control and Prevention. National Center for Health Statistics. http://www.cdc.gov/nchs/index. Accessed September 21, 2016.

5. Brokaw T. *The Greatest Generation.* New York, NY: Random House; 1998:1–18.

6. Brokaw T. *BOOM! Voices of the Sixties.* New York, NY: Random House; 2007:1–282.

7. Lancaster LC, Stillman D. *When Generations Collide.* New York, NY: HarperCollins; 2002:3–48.

8. Bonvalet C, Clement C, Ogg J. *Renewing the Family: A History of the Baby Boomers.* New York, NY: Springer; 2015.

9. Martin CA, Tulgan B. *Managing the Generation Mix: From Collision to Collaboration.* 2nd ed. Amherst, MA: HRD Press; 2006:1–160.

10. Walker J, Lewis L. *Dealing with X, Y, Zs. How to Manage the New Generations in the Workplace.* Upper Saddle River, NJ: FT Press; 2010.

11. Infante D. *The hipster is dead, and you might not like who comes next.* Mashable. http://www.mashable.com/2015/06/09/post-hipster-yuccie. June 9, 2015. Accessed August 14, 2016.

12. Twenge JM. Foster, JD. Birth cohort increases in narcissistic personality traits among American college students, 1982–2009. *Soc Psychol Personal Sci.* 2010;1(1):99–106.

13. Anatole E. Generation Z: Rebels With a Cause. Forbes http://www.forbes.com/sites/onmarketing/2013/05/28/generation-z-rebels-with-a-cause. May 28, 2013. Accessed March 27, 2016.

14. Potter C. The annals of anxiety: constructing velcro parents as a "problem" for higher education. *Chron High Educ.* http://www.chronicle.com/blognetwork/tenuredradical/2010/08/our-friend-over-at-historiann-asks-. August 23, 2010. Accessed March 23, 2016.

15. Hawkins BD. Here Comes Generation Z. What Makes Them Tick? The National Education Association. http://neatoday.org/2015/07/13/here-comes-generation-z-what-makes-them-tick. July 13th, 2015. Accessed April 2, 2016.

16. Koulopoulos T. Keldsen, D. *The Gen Z Effect: The Six Forces Shaping the Future of Business.* Brookline, MA: Bibliomotion, Inc; 2014.

17. Crouch B. How will Generation Z disrupt the workplace? *Fortune Magazine.* http://fortune.com/2015/05/22/generation-z-in-the-workplace/. Accessed May 22, 2015.

18. Carrick AK. Drinking to blackout. *The New York Times*. http://www.nytimes.com/2016/09/19/opinion/drinking-to-blackout.html. September 19, 2016. Accessed September 19, 2016.

19. Yuan L, Powell S. MOOCs and open education: implications for higher education. *Publications from the Centre For Educational Technology, Interoperability and Standards*. http://publications.cetis.org.uk/2013/667. March 2013. Accessed September 15, 2016.

20. Cogan B, Gencarelli T. *Baby Boomers and Popular Culture: An Inquiry Into America's Most Powerful Generation*. Santa Barbara, CA: Praeger; 2015.

21. Bristow J. *Baby Boomers and Generational Conflict*. London, UK: Palgrave Macmillan; 2015.

22. Hira NA. You raised them, now manage them. *Fortune*. 2007;155(10):38–46.

23. Goldstein J. *As doctors get a life, strains show: quest for free time reshapes medicine; a 'team' approach*. The Wall Street Journal. May 8, 2008:W1,W6.

24. Standards For Accreditation of Nurse Anesthesia Educational Programs. http://home.coa.us.com/accreditation/Pages/Accreditation-Policies,-Procedures-and-Standards.aspx. Revised May 2015. Accessed Dec. 21, 2015.

25. Elliot R, Norwood A, Mangum C, Haynie L. Generational (age) differences in nursing students' preferences for teaching methods. *J Nurs Educ*. 2006;45(9):371–374.

26. Tulgan B. *Meet Generation Z: The Second Generation Within the Giant "Millenial" cohort*. Rainmaker Thinking. http://rainmakerthinking.com/assets/uploads/2013/10/Gen-Z-Whitepaper.pdf. 2013.

27. Heick T. *The Difference Between Pedagogy, Andragogy, and Heuragogy. teachthought*. http://www.teachthought.com/pedagogy/a-primer-in-heutagogy-and-self-directed-learning. October 10, 2015. Accessed September 21, 2016.

28. Ryan A, Tilbury D. Flexible pedagogies: new pedagogical ideas. *The Higher Education Academy*. November 2013.

29. Hughes, H. *Flipping the classroom: participatory learning, technology and design*. In: Kyei-Blankson, L and Ntuli, E, eds. *Practical Applications and Experiences in K–20 Blended Learning Environments*. Hershey, PA: IGI Global; 2014:137–152.

30. Moravec, J. Moving Beyond Education 2.0. Education Futures. https://educationfutures.com/blog/2008/02/moving-beyond-education-20/. February 15, 2008. Accessed Sept 21, 2016.

31. Murphy M. Gen Z and the future of education. Bentley University, PreparedU. http://www.bentley.edu/prepared/how-online-learning-will-change-world. February 25, 2015. Accessed August 30, 2016.

32. Twenge JM. *Generation Me*. New York, NY: Simon & Schuster; 2014:15–56.

33. Marano HE. *A Nation of Wimps: The High Cost of Invasive Parenting*. New York, NY: Broadway Books; 2008:142–241.

CHAPTER 9

The Importance of Effective Communication

Michael D. Fallacaro, DNS, CRNA, FAAN
Betty J. Horton, PhD, CRNA, FAAN

Keywords: Accreditation, communication, education, evaluation, listening, patient safety, social media.

Key Concepts

- The importance of effective communication skills has been brought to national attention by a variety of groups, such as professional membership organizations, regional and specialized accrediting agencies, private foundations, and branches of the federal government.
- The acquisition of effective communication skills can improve the work performance of program administrators, didactic faculty, and clinical faculty in the office, classroom, and clinical areas. Skill development requires knowledge of effective communication methods and opportunities to practice the same. Fortunately, there are many opportunities in nurse anesthesia programs to practice these skills.
- Graduate student registered nurse anesthetists must develop advanced skills in communicating with their patients and with all health care professionals involved in patient care. Instructors must mentor graduate students to expand their skills and to recognize the importance of clear and accurate communication in preventing errors and increasing patient safety.
- Evaluation of both instructors and graduate students on communication skills is advisable. Feedback from evaluations can help learners succeed in attaining effective communication skills.

Introduction

It is all about relationships. Success and respect are not achieved by titles or the number of ribbons worn upon one's chest, but rather garnered through the texture of one's speech, and the sincerity in motive and personal actions one takes in closing the communication loop to reach effective mutual respect and understanding. Communication skills are an essential element of professionalism and a reflection of an individual's intellect, preparedness, and character. This makes advanced communication skills a desirable outcome of nurse anesthesia education. Effective communication skills are also important within professional organizations, which must relay information to, and solicit feedback from, their members and the public on various issues.

National Perspectives

The American Association of Nurse Anesthetists

The American Association of Nurse Anesthetists (AANA) is a professional membership organization. Communication with the AANA typically begins when graduate students first become Associate Members through their educational programs, and continues across their careers. It is a professional responsibility and expectation that all professionals be engaged in their professional membership organization. The AANA shares information about its many services for nurse anesthetists and communicates other important messages to members. AANA serves to protect and promote the welfare of its membership. Additionally, the AANA derives much of its authority from the public and, thus, has a responsibility to meet societal needs. Because of these two complementary but different missions, a potential conflict of interest exists in that a professional association such as AANA could hypothetically put the needs of its members ahead of the needs of the public. Thus, in 1975 three autonomous councils were formed: the Council on Accreditation of Nurse Anesthesia Educational Programs (COA), the Council on Practice (later named the Council on Certification of Nurse Anesthetists [CCNA]), and the Council on Recertification of Nurse Anesthetists (COR). In 2007, the CCNA and COR incorporated, forming the National Board of Certification and Recertification for Nurse Anesthetists (NBCRNA).[1]

Effective communication between these three separate but related entities is essential to assure that public needs are being met through well-educated, competent Certified Registered Nurse Anesthetists (CRNAs). To assure a common understanding, effective communication first begins by accurately informing CRNAs, graduate students, and the public of the autonomous but related nature of the AANA, COA, and NBCRNA. Many people mistakenly attribute all matters dealing with CRNA certification, education, and accreditation to the AANA. The AANA is a professional membership organization for CRNAs. Members volunteer their services to the AANA and share their opinions with organizational and elected leaders. CRNAs have found that belonging to their professional organization provides them with a common voice on matters that affect both education and practice. The COA and NBCRNA have autonomous functions related to CRNA education/accreditation and certification and recertification. Mutual respect and coordination between these entities and the AANA are essential for both the public and the specialty.

In an effort to foster a safety culture of open communication among patient team members, the AANA developed Patient Centered Perianesthesia Communication Practice Considerations. These considerations include patient safety initiatives such as checklists, pre-procedure communications (preoperative huddles), time outs, and transfer of care protocols.[2] These practice considerations promulgate a culture of open communication among all health care team members to foster safe surgical and anesthesia care.

The Council on Accreditation of Nurse Anesthesia Educational Programs

The Council on Accreditation of Nurse Anesthesia Educational Programs believes that the development of communication skills is important in the education of the nurse anesthetist as documented in their Standards for Accreditation of Nurse Anesthesia Educational Programs. Accredited programs must demonstrate that graduates effectively communicate with individuals influencing patient care and that they utilize appropriate verbal, nonverbal, and written communication in the delivery of perianesthetic care.[3] Graduates who have attained these skills are competent communicators in patient care situations. Instructors must help graduate students acquire good communication skills during classroom and clinical experiences.

The COA also has expectations for the way programs should communicate with the COA on matters of accreditation. There are several accreditation policies in place that outline this expectation, such as progress reports and deadlines for compliance with the standards and criteria of the COA.[4] The cardinal rule is that it is essential for CRNA educators to know the COA's standards and policies and to communicate with the COA in a timely manner.

The Commission on Collegiate Nursing Education

Some nurse anesthesia programs reside in schools of nursing that are accredited by the Commission on Collegiate Nursing Education (CCNE) and honor its requirements as a program within the larger institution. In 2013, CCNE enacted Standards for Accreditation of Baccalaureate and Graduate Nursing Programs.[5] Item I1-E in the standards requires that there be processes by which preceptor performance expectations are clearly communicated to preceptors and reviewed periodically. In addition, CCNE will continue to require documented use of certain professional nursing standards and guidelines. Among the standards are those delineated in The Essentials of Doctoral Education for Advanced Nursing Practice, as applicable to the type of degrees offered. There are multiple examples related to communication in these essentials. An example in the doctoral essentials states: "The Doctor of Nursing Practice program prepares the graduate to use advanced communication skills/processes to lead quality improvement and patient safety initiatives in health care systems."[6]

Accreditation Commission for Education in Nursing

Some nurse anesthesia programs are located in schools of nursing accredited by the Accreditation Commission for Education in Nursing (ACEN); therefore, they are affected by this accreditor's requirements. The accreditation standards promulgated by ACEN for master's degree programs, NLNAC Standards and Criteria: Master's Degree/Post-Master's Certificate Programs in Nursing indicate that the interchange of information between the accreditor and others is important.[7] Standard 1.3 requires its communities of interest to have input into the program processes and decision-making; standard 3.3 requires that changes in policies, procedures, and program information be clearly and consistently communicated to students in a timely manner; and standard 6.3 requires that evaluation findings be shared with its communities. The NLNAC Standards and Criteria: Clinical Doctorate Degree Programs in Nursing identify the same requirements in Standards 1.3, 3.3, and 6.3.[8]

The National League for Nursing Commission for Nursing Education Accreditation

In response to member requests for additional options in nursing program accreditation agencies, the National League for Nursing Commission for Nursing Education Accreditation (CNEA) was formally established in September 2013. The CNEA provides accrediting services for all types of nursing programs, including practical (vocational), diploma, associate, bachelor, master, and doctor of nursing practice programs. CNEA standards require students to have experiences with intraprofessional and interprofessional collaborative practice; each requires effective communication. Some nurse anesthesia programs may soon be located in schools of nursing accredited by the newest nursing accrediting agency, CNEA.[9]

The Institute of Medicine

Poor communication among health care professionals has been identified as a potential problem by the Institute of Medicine. It increases the risk of errors, patient complaints, and malpractice claims.[10] Analyses of adverse events in surgery revealed that underlying causes are often communication failures rather than technical problems.[11] These findings indicate that students need to become competent in both communication and technical skills to maximize patient safety. In fact, the relationship between communication and patient safety is so important that the Institute of Medicine strongly recommends striving for effective communication among health care professionals. The Institute of Medicine encourages educators to ensure that students become working professionals who are proficient in using information technology and working as part of an interdisciplinary team.[12,13,14]

The Institute for Safe Medication Practices

The Institute for Safe Medication Practices has analyzed medication errors made by student nurses for safe practice. A report indicated that having two people, student and instructor, involved in administering medications to a patient made communication breakdowns in patient care more likely. This finding should be seriously considered by all clinical instructors who need to carefully monitor communication between themselves and students to safeguard against errors in medication administration.[15]

The Anesthesia Patient Safety Foundation

As far back as 2007, the Anesthesia Patient Safety Foundation's *APSF Newsletter* noted that team training is helpful to improve communication. Importantly, effective communication was seen as a vital link to the delivery of safe, effective health care. According to the article, the goal for improving communication through training was to reduce medical errors.[16]

Others

Many accreditors, in addition to those previously described, have established learning outcomes that are not specific to the technical aspects of a specific profession alone. Students preparing to become engineers for example are required to have the ability to communicate effectively; students studying to become pharmacists must learn to think critically and communicate effectively; and physician residents must be able to demonstrate effective interpersonal and communication skills. Accreditors that evaluate universities also recognize the importance of teaching students to communicate. For example, Middle States Association of Colleges and Schools has a goal that graduates will be skilled in oral and written communication.[17] It would be difficult to find an accrediting agency that did not expect students to be more proficient in communication by graduation.

The Importance of Communication in Educational Programs

During an ordinary day, a typical nurse anesthetist spends time speaking with people in a variety of situations. A CRNA talks with patients, physicians, or coworkers; a clinical instructor talks with graduate students; or a program administrator meets and talks with didactic and clinical instructors. The CRNA also frequently communicates intentions in writing and, knowingly or unknowingly, with nonverbal body language. Thus, effective communication abilities contribute to a CRNA's success in the office, classroom, and clinical arena.

Program Administration

A program administrator who is a good communicator can develop a persuasive proposal that stands out from the competition to secure a budgetary increase or to win grant funding. According to Harvard Business School, the more readable your proposal, the better your chances of success.[18]

Program administrators who demonstrate an ability to listen to counsel as well as to give counsel can become effective communicators. In contentious matters, one needs to allow others to communicate concerns, fears and/or feelings of anger before one can gain an understanding of the issue(s) at hand. Once these matters are "on the table" a good communicator can attempt to find a win-win solution where focus is directed first at areas of agreement and away from areas of disagreement. Areas of disagreement are best addressed after trust is built and after areas of agreement are first established. Contentious issues often require compromise and a willingness to accept some degree of change. Mutual respect and understanding are paramount if one hopes to establish or sustain a relationship. Confidentiality in communications is also key; trust entails some personal risk when people open up and share their concerns. Once trust is violated some relationships may never be repaired.

Classroom

Written and verbal communications involve intellectual and practical skills that graduate students are expected to develop at the undergraduate level.[17] Many universities offer courses in interpersonal communication skills and public speaking. The goals of these courses are to prepare learners to organize and express ideas clearly and appropriately; master standard use of written and oral communication; and listen, observe, interpret, and understand others. Graduate students must continue learning to write and speak clearly and effectively. It is a responsibility of nurse anesthesia faculty to cultivate these skills through effective educational opportunities for graduate students to write and publicly present matters of relevance to their faculty and peers alike.

The educational relationship is a communicative relationship between human beings that requires mutual respect, trust, and concern. Nurse anesthesia instructors may not have terminal degrees in adult education, so they must learn as much as they can about good instructional practices themselves. One technique is to inform graduate students early in the educational experience that you have high expectations for student learning, including the acquisition of knowledge about effective communications.

To help graduate students polish their communication skills, faculty can plan practical activities such as role-playing in interviewing patients, developing written anesthesia care plans, and completing medical records accurately. Faculty will need to assess learner interviewing and writing techniques and developing opportunities for graduate students to refine these skills before assignment to the clinical arena. They can also provide other writing and speaking opportunities in the classroom, including class presentations, journal clubs, topical papers, and capstone projects involving written work.[17]

A characteristic of a quality curriculum is a culminating experience in which the graduate students integrate learning to produce an intellectual work such as a research or capstone project, a policy paper, or a scholarly dissertation. External examiners can verbally quiz learners, allowing them to demonstrate knowledge of their subject matter and thus evaluate their communication skills. This activity should represent an integration of learning throughout an educational program and represent a graduate student's most advanced work. Prior to evaluating these verbal communication skills, faculty can choose to design practical mentoring sessions where presentations can be delivered to faculty or other groups in a learning process for reflection and improvement. All too often faculty need to be reminded that *learning ceases when evaluation begins*. If faculty choose to only evaluate, when do graduate students have the opportunity to learn? Therefore opportunities to make mistakes and opportunities to "fail" should be provided in safe and non-evaluative environments well before competency is ever assessed.

Clinical Instruction

Effectively imparting knowledge to learners in the clinical environment often presents unique challenges to educators and graduate students alike. Evaluating performance is a necessary responsibility for CRNAs who are involved in clinical instruction. The goal is to provide feedback that helps graduate students grow and mature in practice. To do this, one should avoid making character judgments and communicate practice criticism in a positive, private and constructive way during the evaluation.[18] Novice graduate student anesthetists will make mistakes. This is expected and faculty need to create an environment that, without patient harm, allows learners to disappoint. Good judgment comes from experience and experience comes from the poor judgments people have made before. To avoid having learners become defensive in discussions, faculty need to first listen and allow trainees to self-evaluate their performance before any critique is offered. Graduate students will only feel safe talking with faculty when past conversations have demonstrated that the CRNA faculty member has their best interests in mind. Speaking thoughtfully and respectfully creates a learning environment in which graduate students feel safe to express agreement or respectful disagreement with faculty.[19]

Like with all effective communications, confidentiality and trust are a must. Faculty discussing graduate student performance with other CRNAs or other learners in open areas will erode trust and destroy relationships. These matters can violate graduate student confidentiality rights and lead to legal and ethical challenges.

Another responsibility of a CRNA is to be a role model. If faculty messages to members of the surgical team are delivered in a clear and concise manner, this will minimize misunderstandings. Faculty who model effective interprofessional communication and collaboration demonstrate how to enhance patient safety by preventing errors and the fragmentation of care. Graduate students will learn these effective communication techniques from example. To accomplish this, faculty need to be direct and honest in communicating with others.[20]

Effective clinical instructors use several communication strategies when interacting with graduate students. They review care plans and offer suggestions; ask pertinent, thought-provoking questions about the case; discuss how clinical events correlate with course work; explain clinical issues clearly; and discuss evaluations by offering positive feedback or constructive criticism about performance. Self-confident CRNA educators are not afraid to admit when they are wrong or at a loss to answer questions. Jointly seeking knowledge with the learner toward better patient care sends a strong and positive message to graduate students that patient safety is the priority.

Questions are few when expectations are known. Both didactic and clinical instructors should become familiar with the contents of their respective graduate student handbooks. Only by knowing the written policies can one apply them and communicate them fairly to all.

Review of the Basics

Verbal Communication

Effective verbal communication means speaking clearly and concisely, conveying information, or articulating an opinion.[21] Educators engage in verbal communication most commonly in face-to-face meetings or during telephone conversations. Regardless of the setting, a good communicator is comfortable speaking to others in a manner that helps listeners understand and willingly receive the message. Learning the skills necessary for good verbal communication takes time.

It takes practice to speak with a graduate student about a problem in a way that allows the person to readily accept criticism, reflect upon it, and make changes accordingly. Some instructors advise that faculty first write down the main points they want to make before speaking with the graduate student. This will keep the message focused, and the graduate student will find what is being said easier to understand if it follows a logical sequence. When delivering the message, one should consider starting by asking a question to engage the graduate student in conversation, so that he or she will be more receptive to what is being said. Starting with a judgmental sentence such as "That was a stupid thing to do!" is not helpful. To label a person or action as "stupid" shows that faculty have made no effort to understand a learner's position and eliminates any thoughtful exploration of how to correct the problem. It is appropriate and often necessary to offer constructive criticism to graduate students regarding academic or clinical performance. It is not appropriate to criticize a graduate student's personal integrity through name-calling. If a learner has done a poor job on a clinical case, it is appropriate to say, "You did a poor job in managing this case." It is not appropriate to say, "You did a poor job in managing this case because you are stupid or lazy." The latter is a personal attack and will serve to destroy communication and seriously damage relationships. Instead, educators can choose to inquire about the graduate student's performance by asking questions such as "Why did you decide to take that approach or action?" or "What do you think about how you managed that case?" This approach is nonthreatening and engages the learner in a reflective and constructive conversation where problems can be identified and performance improved while respecting the individual's personal integrity and self-worth.

It also goes without saying that it is always better to critique performance in private and to praise performance in public. Such public acknowledgement of positive actions instills confidence in learners and often results in better communication and stronger relationships with mentors.

Nonverbal Communication

Facial expressions, body postures, gestures, and eye contact are all examples of nonverbal communication known as body language. Researchers have found that the meaning of gestures depends on personal style and settings, what has gone before, and expectations for the future. Some researchers have found that facial expression and tone of voice are 90% of communication between people.[22]

Authors have also found that the meaning of body language depends on cultural norms, and there is evidence that patterns of nonverbal communication are highly variable among cultures and among different groups. Everyone does not follow the same rules. For example, in some cultures it is polite for a speaker to look directly at the listener, while the listener is expected to watch the speaker without looking away. This behavior may be unacceptable in a culture in which direct eye contact is avoided.[22]

Body language also conveys messages that support or contradict what a person says. As an example, arms crossed across the chest may mean that the person is not receptive to further information on the issue being discussed; however, body language can be easily misinterpreted. Distress signals may originate from events at home or other places rather than from work. This means that, although body language is useful, it cannot be precisely interpreted. Body language should be viewed in the context of the situation and seen as an indication of a potential problem, rather than as concrete evidence.[22] Do not ignore body language; just pay attention to all nonverbal forms of communication to see if they add meaning to the spoken words.

Listening

The effectiveness of verbal communication depends on how well people listen and what they hear rather than what is actually said. According to one report, the average person remembers only half of the content delivered immediately after hearing it, no matter how carefully he or she listened. About one-half to one-third of the content is forgotten within eight hours, and only 25% of what was said is remembered two months later.[22] In another study, respondents expressed more approval of those who listened more than they spoke. People who talked more than they listened during a conversation met with disapproval. Those who always insisted on quiet while they were talking or dominated a conversation met with strong disapproval.[23]

A good listener is physically active and this skill can be taught. Universities and colleges now provide courses in listening, and proprietary organizations sometimes offer workshops to teach listening as part of communication training. Listening skills include an attitude of curiosity and patience that promotes the acquisition of ideas rather than facts. Listening attentively is important to understanding. Effective listeners: [19]

- Express interest in the other person's views.
- Acknowledge the emotions that the other person appears to be feeling.
- Restate what they have heard to show that they understand.
- Express agreement when they agree.
- Build on what the other person appears to have left out.
- Compare their views with the other person's views and, if there are differences, do not suggest that the other person is wrong.

These activities are possible because people think much faster than they talk. The proper use of thinking time helps one concentrate on what is being said. Improper use of thinking time lets one's mind wander away from the speaker's message.

Listening ability is affected by emotions. People tend to ignore what they do not wish to hear, and accept what they hope to be true. One can help avoid this problem by withholding any judgment until after the speaker has finished. Listen instead of judging what is said, think about each point a speaker makes, and search for evidence of common beliefs. One will likely find that an early emotional judgment was right or wrong by listening objectively to what a speaker has said.[22]

A graduate student's listening ability is also affected by emotions when he or she receives a negative evaluation or must be disciplined. Because of this fact, it is good practice to have two faculty members present during a conference and create a written record of the session to verify the interaction if questions arise later.

Written Communication

Instructors and their graduate students use the written word in many ways. Being able to convey a message in writing using proper spelling and grammar is important in memos, letters, emails, reports, meeting minutes, care plans, evaluations, resumes, publications, grant proposals, and curriculum vitae. [21] The tone of writing should be appropriate to the occasion. It may need to be formal or informal, detailed, or a summary of ideas. For example, minutes contained in summaries of topics discussed at a meeting.[18]

Whether a program administrator or a didactic or clinical instructor, one should know how to write an accurate and detailed report and this takes practice. Before beginning to write, it is necessary to have a clear goal in mind. Describe the goal in one or two succinct sentences that explain the idea and its benefits for the reader. All ideas presented in the remainder of the report should relate to the main goal.[18]

The writing process includes four stages:[18]

1. The *madman* brainstorms and jots down ideas in no particular order with no judgment about their value or grammatical structure.
2. The *architect* organizes relevant ideas into an outline. The notes that were generated during brainstorming are placed into groups of related ideas. At this stage, some ideas will be discarded and others will be structured into a linear outline that makes sense.
3. The *carpenter* adds structure in the form of sentences. Once an outline and the main ideas have been developed, the carpenter begins writing to present the ideas logically, without worrying about grammar or style.
4. The *judge* rules on grammar and style. The manuscript is corrected and polished to communicate clearly what the writer wants to say.

A writer's language needs to convey ideas clearly and directly. Any arguments should proceed logically and should be persuasive. If one uses jargon, it must be understandable to the audience. Key points that are too long, too technical, difficult to read, or full of verbiage should be edited. Do not waste the reader's time with irrelevant information.

Write a first draft and as many others as necessary to increase clarity and cut unnecessary language. Simplify ideas by breaking long sentences with many clauses into several sentences. Read the report aloud when proofreading to help spot repetition, ambiguity, awkward phrasing, and other flaws. Credibility killers include misspellings, grammar and punctuation errors, use of the wrong name, and inconsistent formatting.[18]

Some written reports benefit from an executive summary whose purpose is to communicate key points from the larger report. It is not a preface or introduction and does not introduce new material. The length of an executive summary ranges from one or two paragraphs to one or two pages. The executive summary can be 10% to 15% of the length of the full report.[18]

Memos

Memos are short versions of correspondence that communicate a condensed message with a central idea. They should describe the situation, the issue or problem, the question, and the answer. A description of the situation should be concise but complete and factual. The issue or problem the memo addresses should be explained clearly. Next, ask what can be done about the issue, followed by possible solutions to the question.[18]

As with any written communication, readers will find memos compelling if the information and ideas are logically ordered. The message should be the focus of the memo. Trying to impress the reader or establish authority by expressing complex thoughts in a long narrative can make the memo hard to comprehend. "Please" and "thank you" should be included without question. Proper etiquette employing politeness will always improve communication. A "I hope this note finds you well" at the beginning of a memo and a "Best Regards" at the end will personalize and engage the reader in a positive way if, indeed, it is sincere.

Email

Email is a popular method of communication that is widely used in nurse anesthesia programs for the exchange of information among faculty, students, and clinical sites. Remember to keep an up-to-date address book and know how to use it.

Although the value of communicating by email is well recognized, the speed with which it can be sent and its often informal composition pose real and substantial risks. It is advised to use caution in electronically communicating anything one would not want to be read in the headlines of the local newspaper. Legally, email belongs to the organization that provides the system and the linkup. Writers do not have privacy, and courts can obtain email records from organizations. One may choose to keep printed copies of emails sent or received regarding important issues if there is a possibility of problems, appeals, or litigation.[22] Additionally, electronic messages may be damaged or deleted if hardware fails or systems are damaged through viral attacks.

Never send an email when tired or angry. Administrators should never reprimand, reward, or terminate someone by sending an email. There is no substitute for a face-to-face meeting to communicate to an instructor or a graduate student that a change in performance is necessary. Face-to-face meetings are particularly important with disciplinary proceedings that must be confirmed in writing.

Avoid common mistakes in email writing. For example, do not use dense blocks of uninterrupted text, and do not forget to include a descriptive subject line. Using white space and paragraphs makes it easier for the reader to identify key points and gain a more complete understanding of what you are communicating. A subject line that describes the main idea of your message gives the reader a good idea of what is to follow. Subject lines also are helpful to the reader in identifying your message among a long list of others at a later date.

Do not fail to proofread. Set the completed, spell-checked document aside for a few minutes, and then read through it again. Spell-checkers do not catch the wrong word spelled correctly. If the email must be error-free, proofread it slowly forward and backward. Proofreading on a computer screen is not easy. You may even want to avoid sending an email that must be error-free. Even deleted emails can be resurrected and widely read by people who you never intended to see them. It is wise to develop a habit of last checking the "To:" line before sending an email to avoid the potentially damaging or embarrassing act of sending content to a wrong person(s).

Social Media

Social media forums provide opportunities for faculty and graduate students to share information about their lives with a broad audience. Extreme caution should be exercised with sharing any patient care information that would violate federal protections and compromise privacy. This is not only illegal, but also unethical. Graduate students should be advised that sharing information on social media platforms is, in essence, sharing information with future patients and potential employers. Often, employers search social media backgrounds of applicants to get a better idea of a candidate's habits, character, and background.

Opportunities for Instructors to Increase Learning About Communication

Faculty involved in the education of nurse anesthesia graduate students have many opportunities to increase communication skills, such as formal courses, online classes, and books on the topic. Workshops or conferences often offer topics to attendees that are related to effective communication. There are plenty of opportunities to practice communication skills, such as written and verbal delivery of graduate student evaluations, oral communication during meetings, and programmatic self-study evaluations.

Learner Evaluations

Anonymous surveys of surgical residents and attending surgeons revealed that both residents and faculty valued communication skills as important to patient care. The surveys suggested that an evaluation instrument that measured communication skills may strengthen the feedback process.[24] These findings are also applicable to the evaluations of faculty and graduate students in nurse anesthesia programs.

Nurse anesthesia faculty play a dual role in the development of communication competencies. First, instructors should continually strive to strengthen their own ability to communicate effectively. Second, instructors should assist their graduate students in expanding their basic communication skills by providing ample practice opportunities. Performance indicators can be employed to measure the success of both instructors and learners in this area.

Evaluations of an instructor can include rating his or her communication skills in items to include:

- Demonstrates the ability to communicate ideas in a clear, concise manner.
- Views the educational process as an interactive exchange between student and teacher.
- Facilitates discussion, inquiry, and scholarship among students and faculty.

- Demonstrates excellent interpersonal communication skills with regard to students, faculty, and clinical staffs.

Evaluations of a graduate student's communication skills can include items such as:

- Conducts thorough preanesthetic interviews.
- Consults with instructor regarding findings and observations.
- Seeks assistance by asking appropriate questions; counsels patients in preparation for anesthesia.
- Communicates effectively with patients, discusses plans of care, and puts the patient at ease.
- Demonstrates interpersonal skill and effectiveness in communicating with the health care team.

Verbal Communication in Meetings

Meetings can be classified by size, and this can determine how much chance one will have to speak at a gathering. An assembly consists of at least 100 people who listen to speakers. A council consists of 40 to 50 people who listen to speakers, but can ask questions or make other contributions. A committee, ideally four to seven people, provides a setting where members can communicate freely under the guidance of a chairperson. Regardless of the size of the meeting, an agenda is most important in effectively conducting the proceedings. If responsible for writing the agenda, one should provide sufficient information to assist members in forming ideas before the meeting so that participants can be prepared to communicate their ideas.[22]

Both nurse anesthesia program administrators and clinical instructors participate in many types of meetings. The basic purpose of a meeting is for people to gather in a group to exchange knowledge and experiences. At times, a group uses a meeting to formulate ideas for problem-solving. Educators can spend an inordinate amount of time in meetings; however, in every human culture, people gather frequently in small groups and occasionally in larger groups physically and/or virtually, to best impart information to others. Meetings are valuable because people who attend and get involved in discussions become committed to the decisions and goals of the group. The frequency of meetings can define the degree of group unity.[22]

A group of people can often produce better ideas, better decisions, and solve problems more efficiently than an individual; the group can also produce worse outcomes or produce nothing at all if the meeting is ineffective. Good leadership and communication skills are necessary for participants to best use the time spent in meetings. When participants listen carefully, the discussion can remain centered on the topic or problem. This is facilitated when the group leader opens the meeting by calling attention to the importance of listening.[22]

During a meeting, the leader's role is to assist the group toward the best conclusion as efficiently as possible, to interpret and clarify, to move the discussion forward, and to bring it to a resolution that everyone understands. If an item is complex, the discussion leader should clearly articulate the main topics so that everyone can see the desired direction for the discussion to take. Differing viewpoints, presented politely, should be encouraged, and difficult conversations should not be avoided. Leaders who are skilled at communicating during meetings do not necessarily agree with every idea; they simply make it equitable for everyone to express their ideas. When people feel comfortable communicating, more information is gained and better decisions can be made. If people don't get involved in conversations, they will probably not be committed to the final decision.[19]

It is not uncommon for meetings to be held to discuss a draft document. Avoid allowing the group to redraft the document during the meeting. The group should agree on the document's faults and assign someone to produce a new draft later.[22] Follow-up plans are important at the end of every meeting to avoid inaction and failure to meet expectations. The leader must follow up on commitments and hold people accountable.

At the end of each agenda item, the leader or committee chairperson should give a brief summary of the decisions reached. These summaries can become part of the minutes. The person who records the minutes should include the time, date, location, attendees, and any absences. The date and place of the next committee meeting should be communicated at the end of the meeting and recorded in the minutes.[22]

Writing Self-Study Evaluations

Writing a self-study evaluation is an important part of maintaining accreditation of a nurse anesthesia program. A completed self-study evaluation communicates to the accrediting agency that the program is in compliance or has plans to come into compliance with requisite educational standards. A committee ideally completes self-study evaluations so that input is obtained from key institutional and program personnel as well as graduate students. Participating in writing a self-study evaluation provides opportunities for individuals to develop and refine their communication skills.

New program administrators should seek assistance from an experienced person, leader or colleague while also looking at examples of previous self-study evaluations. To avoid repeating the mistakes of the past, one should not blindly mimic what is found in a past study or in a computer database.[18]

To meet the accrediting agency's expectations and avoid unnecessary work, good communicators need to think about the accrediting agency as the audience and follow the instructions precisely. Failure to follow instructions when writing a self-study evaluation could result in material being rejected or returned. Failure to follow instructions also raises the question in the minds of reviewers of whether one will abide by future requirements.

Leaders are encouraged to create a realistic plan to write the self-study evaluation by establishing a timeline, responsibilities, and a budget. Time for writing multiple drafts, creating graphics, reviewing by the committee, obtaining approvals from superiors, and completing production activities such as copying, binding, or submitting information electronically need to be considered.

Case Study

John had accepted his position as administrator of the nurse anesthesia program a short time before the Council on Accreditation (COA) mandated that all nurse anesthesia programs move to the clinical (practice) doctorate as entry to practice by 2025. His goal as a leader was to move his program to doctoral entry as soon as possible. In this spirit, he proposed an entry to practice degree option that was approved by his school and university. The COA also approved his program and the stage was set for this innovative degree option to commence.

The Problem

In all of his planning, John had neglected to engage Grace, the chair of the department of anesthesiology at his largest clinical site, one essential to his program; rumors were circulating that she was not in favor of this proposal.

At first John thought about sending Grace an email about the proposal, since he felt a face-to-face meeting might be contentious. After taking time to think about this, John thought it better to schedule a face-to-face meeting with Grace. John met with Grace and began the conversation with a thank you. He acknowledged Grace's support of the nurse anesthesia program and he remarked how her leadership was making a difference in the lives of so many. John then briefly presented the new curriculum proposal and the COA directives in this regard. He then asked Grace if she had any suggestions, questions or concerns about the proposal. He then attentively listened to her, without interrupting, for 30 minutes.

Grace had no suggestions; however, she had several concerns. The first concern was related to nurses potentially confusing patients by calling themselves "doctor." The second concern was about CRNAs demanding higher salaries because of this new degree. Finally the third concern was that CRNAs would demand an expanded practice role with this new degree.

John listened and jotted a few notes documenting these three major concerns. He began addressing Grace by first assessing that he had heard her correctly and that the three concerns he had written down were indeed correct. To this Grace agreed.

One by one John addressed Grace's concerns. To the first he stated that he, too, was very concerned about confusing patients and that he would not support anyone misrepresenting themselves as physicians to patients. John stated that it is imperative that patients know who their anesthesia provider is. If it is a CRNA, that person has a professional and ethical responsibility to identify himself or herself as a CRNA verbally and also with a visible nametag. John cited the AANA's Code of Ethics and COA's standards as they relate to this matter. If a patient calls a CRNA "doctor," John explained that it is the CRNA's responsibility to clarify that he or she is not a medical doctor, since it may logically be assumed that patients may be confused about roles in a clinical setting.

To the second concern, John had done his homework and was aware that seniority, not type of degree, was the determining factor in CRNA salaries at the hospital in question. In fact, John pointed out that it was a certificate-educated CRNA who was the highest paid CRNA on staff due to the fact that the CRNA had worked in the hospital for nearly 30 years.

Finally, John explained that the proposed practice degree had absolutely nothing in it that would change CRNA scope of practice. Further, he explained that the Board of Nursing and Board of Medicine in his state set CRNA scope of practice.

Grace was appreciative of John for his answers, yet her nonverbal communication told John that she was still uncomfortable. He asked Grace about this and she replied that there was a national politic that would prevent her from supporting his proposal.

To this John replied that he understood completely and really just wanted her to know that he respected her position and thanked her again for her support of the program and for her honest and upfront sharing of concerns.

As Grace left John's office she thanked John and remarked, "You know I can't support your proposal right?" John said, "I understand and it's ok." To which Grace replied with a smile "Well, I don't have to oppose it either" and she walked away.

Problem Solving

John's experience with Grace proved to be pivotal in getting his doctoral proposal approved at his university. True to her word, Grace did not support John's proposal. Rather, she remained silent on it completely. In this way, Grace saved face with her colleagues by not supporting the move while at the same time demonstrated her respect for John and his efforts. A win-win by all accounts.

Lesson #1: People need to feel free to talk to others and know they will be met with empathy and understanding. Too many administrators fail to listen, although they announce that their doors are always open. The listener should not show displeasure through verbal responses or body language. Being a good listener can help you to avoid friction between individuals and build successful relationships.[21]

Lesson #2: A key to keeping communication open is to create an environment that allows people to lay their concerns, fears, and frustrations on the table for consideration. Once a person does this, then a meaningful dialogue can ensue to reach a common understanding. This creates a "together we can work this out" approach.

Lesson #3: In times of uncertainty, people fill communication voids with rumors. Rumors attribute the worst possible motives to those in control. Communicating the truth will lower people's anxiety, whether the news is good or bad. To dispel rumors, the most effective way to communicate is informally, one-on-one. Honest communication will help counteract rumors.[22]

Lesson #4: Often email is not the right medium for communication, especially in a contentious situation. It is better to talk face-to-face so you can fully understand the individual's perceptions. Consider confining email to concrete requests, queries, and responses that are not controversial. For chatting or networking, use the telephone. For potentially unpleasant conversations, meeting face-to-face allows your tone of voice, gestures, and facial expressions to convey a more complete message. A face-to-face meeting also helps you to understand the other person's position more fully through observation of his or her nonverbal signals.[18, 25]

Lesson #5: Efforts to change behavior and communication go hand-in-hand. First, the desired behavior should be clearly stated. Second, to make it a lasting change, there should be ongoing communication with the person or people who can tell you what is and is not working.[20] Finally, beginning and ending a communication with a thank you sends a strong message of appreciation and respect, something that matters most to all people as they interact with others.

Summary

Effective communication is an asset to nurse anesthesia program administrators, didactic instructors, clinical instructors, and their graduate students. It is a skill that can produce a better understanding of people while at work or at home, or while engaged in outside activities. It also enables one to create a supportive learning environment in which students can acquire the relevant knowledge, skills, and competencies to be excellent nurse anesthetists. Good communicators always look for opportunities to practice and improve the way they communicate and the way to teach their graduate students to communicate. There is a great deal of truth in the saying that "Communication works for those who work at it."[26]

References

1. Horowitz J, McAuliffe MS, Rupp R. *Ira P. Gunn, Nurse Anesthetist: Writings and Wisdom from a Legendary Nursing Leader.* Park Ridge, IL: American Association of Nurse Anesthetists; 2015.

2. Patient-Centered Perianesthesia Communication. Practice Considerations. Park Ridge, IL: American Association of Nurse Anesthetists; 2014.

3. Standards for Accreditation of Nurse Anesthesia Educational Programs. Park Ridge, IL: Council on Accreditation of Nurse Anesthesia Educational Programs; 2015. Standards for Accreditation of Nurse Anesthesia Educational Programs: Practice Doctorate. Park Ridge, IL: Council on Accreditation of Nurse Anesthesia Educational Programs; 2015.

4. Accreditation Policies and Procedures. Park Ridge, IL: Council on Accreditation of Nurse Anesthesia Educational Programs; 2015.

5. Standards for Accreditation of Baccalaureate and Graduate Nursing Programs. Washington, DC: Commission on Collegiate Nursing Education; 2013.

6. The Essentials of Doctoral Education for Advanced Nursing Practice. Washington, DC: American Association of Colleges of Nursing; 2006:14.

7. ACEN 2013 Standards and Criteria: Master's and Post-Master's Certificate. Accreditation Commission for Education in Nursing; Atlanta, GA; 2013.

8. ACEN 2013 Standards and Criteria: Clinical Doctorate. Accreditation Commission for Education in Nursing; Atlanta, GA; 2013.

9. National League for Nursing Commission for Nursing Education Accreditation. http://www.nln.org/accreditation-services/the-nln-commission-for-nursing-education-accreditation-(cnea). Accessed October 12, 2015.

10. Tamblyn R, Abrahamowicz M, Dauphinee D, et al. Physician scores on a national clinical skills examination as predictors of complaints to medical regulatory authorities. *JAMA.* 2007;298(9):993–1001.

11. Flin R, Yule S, Paterson-Brown S, Maran N, Rowley D, Youngson G. Teaching surgeons about non-technical skills. *Surgeon.* 2007;5(2):86–89.

12. To err is human: building a safer health system. In: Kohn LT, Corrigan JM, Donaldson MS, eds. *Institute of Medicine.* Washington, DC: National Academies Press; 1999.

13. Crossing the quality chasm: A new health system for the 21st century. *Institute of Medicine.* Washington, DC: National Academies Press; 2001.

14. Grenier AC, Knebel E, eds. *Health Professions Education: A Bridge to Quality.* Washington, DC: National Academies Press; 2003.

15. Institute for Safe Medication Practices. Error-prone conditions can lead to student nurse-related medication mistakes. *AANA NewsBulletin.* 2007;61(12):10–11.

16. McQuillan RJ, King H, Salas E, Gaba D, Gait K. Teamwork and team training in the operating room: can it make a difference in patient safety? *APSF Newsletter.* 2007;22(3):53.

17. Liberal Education Outcomes: A Preliminary Report on Student Achievement in College. Association of American Colleges and Universities. 2005; http://www.aacu.org/sites/default/files/files/LEAP/LEAP_Report_2005.pdf. Accessed March 9, 2009.

18. Harvard Business Publishing. *Written Communications That Inform and Influence: The Results-Driven Manager Series.* Boston, MA: Harvard Business School Press; 2006.

19. Patterson K, Grenny J, McMillan R, Switzler A. *Crucial Conversations: Tools for Talking When Stakes Are High.* New York, NY: McGraw-Hill. 2002.

20. Lancaster G, Kolakowsky-Hayner S, Kovacich J, Greer-Williams N. Interdisciplinary communication and collaboration among physicians, nurses, and unlicensed assistive personnel. *J Nurs Scholarsh.* 2015;47(3):275–284.

21. Dowling T. Career article 132: basic communication skills everyone needs. Seeking Success website, http://www.seekingsuccess.com/articles/artl32.php3. Accessed January 19, 2008.

22. Harvard Business Publishing. *Harvard Business Review on Effective Communication.* Boston, MA: Harvard Business School Press; 1999.

23. Glynn CJ, Huge ME. Opinions as norms: applying a return potential model to the study of communication behaviors. *Commun Res.* 2007;34(5):548–568.

24. Hutul OA, Carpenter RO, Tarpley JL, Lomis KD. Missed opportunities: a descriptive assessment of teaching and attitudes regarding communication skills in a surgical residency. *Curr Surg.* 2006;63(6):401–409.

25. You've got conflict: e-mail and conflict management. American Council on Education Department Leadership Project. http://www.acenet.edu/_resources/chairs/docs/holton_e-mail.pdf. Accessed March 9, 2008.

26. Speech communication portfolio: why is communication important? Department of Speech Communication at Southern Illinois University, Edwardsville. http://www.siue.edu/SPC/SPC/_Portfolio/why.html. Accessed January 23, 2008.

CHAPTER 10

Theory and Principles of Adult Education for Clinical Instructors

William Hartland Jr., PhD, CRNA

Keywords: Adult learning principles, characteristics of the effective clinical instructor, clinical instructor, clinical teaching continuum, domains of learning, learning environment, nurse anesthesia student, theory of adult learning.

Key Concepts

- The clinical instructor is not only accountable for the clinical education of his or her students, but for all other aspects inherent to anesthesia clinical practice.
- The clinical instructor can enhance student learning by creating a physical and psychological environment that promotes learning.
- Nurse anesthesia students are adults coming from a variety of ethnic and social backgrounds with a wealth of professional and nonprofessional life experiences.
- The clinical instructor must continually determine where on the clinical teaching continuum instruction should take place based on the student's knowledge base and level of performance.
- Adult learning principles can give the clinical instructor a framework from which to build and develop clinical teaching excellence.
- Twenty-two characteristics of an effective clinical instructor serve as guidelines that clinical instructors can use on their journey toward clinical teaching excellence.

Introduction

Health care professionals are cognizant of the crucial role that clinical experience plays in the education of their students. In nurse anesthesia education, these clinical experiences are often referred to as clinical practicums. It is during clinical practicums that the nurse anesthesia student is given the opportunity to apply classroom knowledge to actual practice. This application is conducted under the careful guidance and tutelage of a clinical instructor (CI).

Most nurse anesthetists can still remember their own experiences, as students, with the CIs to whom they were assigned. Some of these memories are pleasant while others are not. Many CIs gave their students a sense of excitement, satisfaction, and accomplishment in the clinical arena. These CIs helped their students reach new heights in their journey toward clinical proficiency. These were the instructors that students eagerly awaited to be assigned to. Unfortunately, there were also CIs whom many anesthetists felt contributed little, if anything, to their educational experience. Some of these CIs appeared apathetic and uncaring; others appeared to teach by intimidation, humiliation, and fear. These were the instructors that students dreaded to see on their daily clinical assignment sheets.

In 1999, Glemon stated that teaching competency was an extremely important issue for nurse anesthesia instructors. Glemon suggested that no instructor wants to be labeled as an incompetent teacher and no student wants to be subjected to the same. The problem arises when nurse anesthetists are placed in a teaching role that they are ill-prepared for.[1]

Unfortunately, few clinical instructors have been afforded formal educational opportunities concerning effective teaching in the clinical arena. Many CIs have presumed teaching effectiveness by virtue of their professional preparation and clinical expertise. They assume that expertise in one specialty area automatically makes him or her an expert in another. This reasoning is not restricted to the profession of nurse anesthesia. It is also prevalent in numerous professional occupations both in and out of the health care domain. In the profession of nurse anesthesia, CIs should be mindful that clinical competency does not automatically imply the ability to effectively teach in the clinical area.

Some instructors presume teaching effectiveness by virtue of emulating CIs they had in school. They often rationalize this modeling by stating, "This is the way I was taught; and if it was good enough for me, it is good enough for you." Such experiences can definitely be an asset if the CIs being used as role models were also effective clinical teachers. On the other hand, emulating an ineffective CI will most likely perpetuate more of the same.

Other CIs may claim that they learned how to teach in the clinical arena by trial and error. Their clinical teaching strategies were developed from their own successful and unsuccessful teaching experiences. Even though experience is a coach that CIs will learn from throughout their careers, there are more efficient learning methods available. Evidence-based documentation is available in the literature to help the CI build a firm foundation in effective clinical instruction without exclusively relying on the process of trial and error.

As stated earlier, clinical instruction is an essential component of the nurse anesthesia student's overall educational experience. As a result, it is essential that clinical instructors be well-versed in effective clinical teaching methodology. But, what is this methodology? How does one become an effective CI? Before examining these and other issues, we will begin by examining this individual known as "the clinical instructor."

The Clinical Instructor

The responsibilities that are shouldered by the CI are significant. CIs are not only accountable for the clinical education of their students, but for all other aspects inherent to anesthesia clinical practice.

Professional Roles of the Clinical Instructor

As an anesthesia professional, the CI fulfills many roles. These roles include those of an anesthesia provider, employee, and clinical teacher.

As an anesthesia provider, the CI's primary responsibility is the safe anesthetic care and management of his or her patients. This includes working effectively and efficiently with co-workers and team members, delivering anesthesia management that is specific to each individual patient, and being a strong patient advocate. It also necessitates that the CI remain current in the latest developments and innovations in the specialty of anesthesia practice.

As an employee, the CI has a responsibility to his or her employer. This responsibility encompasses adherence to the protocols, policies, and directives of the employer. Such adherence is expected as a requirement for employment. Deviation from these established standards may result in disciplinary action or termination of employment.

As an educator, the CI plays a pivotal role in the clinical education of nurse anesthesia students. The CI functions as a teacher and mentor by helping students integrate didactic knowledge into practice. The CI serves as a role model that students can use during their professional development. The CI is also a student advocate who promotes and enhances the student's clinical learning experiences.

Domains of Learning and the Clinical Instructor

Webster's New World Dictionary defines learning as the acquiring of knowledge or skill.[2] This acquisition involves change in behavior or performance. For our purposes, this knowledge or skill acquisition encompasses three domains of learning: cognitive, psychomotor, and affective. The cognitive domain of learning is primarily concerned with new knowledge, understanding, and ways of thinking. The psychomotor domain focuses on new skills and behavior patterns such as new ways of acting or performing a task. The affective domain centers on attitudes, values, and ways of feeling.[3]

All of these domains can be further subdivided into a hierarchy of categories moving from the simple to complex. (**Table 10.1**, next page) The cognitive domain begins with simple knowledge outcomes such as recall, and proceeds through increasingly complex levels of comprehension such as applying certain information to new situations and evaluating its appropriateness. The psychomotor domain begins with readiness for action and progresses to doing the skill, doing it proficiently, and finally being able to create new movements that fit a particular situation. The affective domain commences with the learner's willingness to pay attention, progressing to active participation, simple acceptance, and finally the incorporation of a specific value into the learner's lifestyle.[3]

Table 10.1 Taxonomy of Educational Objectives*

Cognitive Domain		
There are six cognitive levels (1: lowest – 6: highest)		
1	Knowledge	Ability to recall or recognize content the way it was initially presented.
2	Comprehension	Ability to understand the meaning of material.
3	Application	Ability to use material in new situations.
4	Analysis	Ability to break down material into its component parts so that its organizational structure may be understood.
5	Synthesis	Ability to arrange and combine content in such a way as to produce a new structure or idea.
6	Evaluation	Ability to judge the value of material for a given purpose.
Psychomotor Domain		
There are seven Psychomotor levels (1: lowest – 7: highest)		
1	Perception	Use of senses to obtain cues that guide a motor activity.
2	Set	Readiness to take a particular action.
3	Guided Response	Early stages (imitation/trial by error) in learning a complex skill.
4	Mechanism	Performing with some confidence and proficiency.
5	Proficiency	Skillful performance of motor acts that involve intricate movement patterns.
6	Adaption	Ability to modify movement patterns to fit special situations.
7	Origination	Ability to create new movement patterns to fit special situations.
Affective Domain		
There are five Affective levels (1: lowest – 5: highest)		
1	Receptivity	Willingness to pay attention to a particular educational activity.
2	Responding	Responding or reacting to a stimulus. Showing an interest in something.
3	Valuing	The worth an individual puts on a particular object, occurrence, or behavior.
4	Organization	Bringing together different values to build an internally consistent system.
5	Value or Value Complex	The value system is integrated into the learner's lifestyle.

*Adapted from *Taxonomy of Educational Objectives*[14]

All three domains of learning are pertinent to anesthesia clinical education. The CI teaches and reinforces new knowledge (cognitive domain), specific anesthesia skills and techniques (psychomotor domain), and professional values/attitudes (affective domain). To effectively teach in each of the three domains of learning, the CI must determine which domain subcategory best applies to the student he or she is assigned. In order to make this determination, the CI should determine the student's knowledge base and experience level. Various student classifications, such as junior and senior, only give the CI an estimate of where the individual student's educational level should be. Two students with equal time in a program may be functioning at very different knowledge or skill levels. This may be the result of the individual student's comprehension abilities, personal motivation, and previous critical care and clinical anesthesia experiences. Whatever the reason, the CI should make every effort to determine the student's present performance level. This can be accomplished by reviewing available program documentation concerning the student's performance, discussions with program faculty, talking with other instructors, or direct discussions with the student. Time constraints in the clinical arena often rule out documentation and discussions with program faculty as practical options. The CI can, however, gain valuable insight from discussions with other CIs or by simply asking students to evaluate themselves in terms of their present strengths and weaknesses.

CIs must remember that no matter how proactive they are in attempting to determine a student's performance level, they should always maintain a high level of vigilance during the actual anesthetic case management. Direct observation will give the CI valuable insight concerning the student's actual performance level.

Although it is not necessary to memorize all the subcategories in each domain, it is important to understand that the subcategories progress from the simple to the complex depending on the students' needs and levels of experience. Infants first learn to crawl before they walk and they walk before they run. The same principle applies to nurse anesthesia students. For example, let's assume the CI is assigned a patient presenting for a coronary bypass. The CI will be working with an advanced student who is experienced in the anesthetic management of the coronary bypass patient. In this scenario, the role of the CI will primarily be to help the student function at a higher level in each of the three domains of learning. In other words, the CI may challenge the student to consider the reasoning behind certain techniques, to identify acceptable alternative techniques, and even new ways to accomplish the same results. If the CI is assigned a student who has little experience with this type of patient, the CI's role will be significantly different. With an inexperienced student, the CI should begin at the lower levels of the three domains. The CI will assume a more active teaching role beginning with the most basic knowledge and skills necessary for the anesthetic manage of the coronary bypass patient.

The Learning Environment

Although the CI cannot force a student to learn, he or she can optimize the student's learning environment in order to enhance learning. This involves creating an environment that promotes learning. Ideally, the learning environment should include a supportive atmosphere and a climate of mutual respect. In other words, a learning environment should be physically and psychologically comfortable.

Physical Learning Environment

The physical learning environment encompasses many tangible factors such as classroom size, design, layout, décor, temperature, lighting, acoustics, and equipment. The more comfortable the physical environment, the more the learner can concentrate on the learning task at hand. It is extremely difficult for students to concentrate on material being taught when they are shivering because of low room temperatures or sweating from high temperatures. It is also difficult to concentrate when external or internal classroom noise is so loud it is difficult to hear the instructor.

The CI's classroom is the operating room or other specialty area requiring anesthesia service. These clinical classroom areas are less than ideal physical learning environments. Specific surgical procedures, patient needs and surgeon's requests may require extremes in temperature and lighting. Extremes in noise may be the result of loud conversations, music, or equipment such as orthopedic saws and drills. On the other hand, the surgeon may demand absolute silence in the room during critical portions of the operation. The size and design of the room has been predetermined by the institution. Specific surgical or diagnostic procedures govern the amount of equipment crowded into the OR suite. It is evident that the CI has little control over the physical environment. As a result, CIs are left to teach in an area that many educators consider a hostile learning environment.

Psychological Learning Environment

The psychological learning environment of the operating room also encompasses many factors. These factors include the cohesiveness, emotional status, and experience of the operating room team. They include the physical condition of the patient and the complexity of the surgical procedure and anesthetic requirements. Operating room team members are sometimes perceived as being overbearing, ill-tempered, and difficult. Due to a variety of causes, a patient's physical condition during surgery can change very rapidly.

Nurse anesthesia students quickly realize that they are no longer sitting safely in a classroom or in a laboratory practicing on a mannequin. The student is now working in the real world with real patients. All of these factors can have a significant effect on the student's stress level and learning comprehension.

A certain level of stress can be healthy by helping a student remain alert and motivated. Too much stress, however, can be harmful and actually hinder and block learning. Howard McClusky addresses the issue of stress and learning in his load, power, margin theory.[4] McClusky states that the key factors of adult life are the loads the adult carries and the power which is available to help the adult carry the load. Margin is the ratio between load and power. The greater the power in relationship to the load, the more margin will be available for the student to cope with the stress.[4,5]

Load factors for nurse anesthesia students can be external or internal. External load factors include personal family problems, financial hardships, and a hostile operating room learning environment. Internal load factors include lack of self-confidence or self-worth. Power factors for the nurse anesthesia student may include previous health care experiences, a good self image, financial stability, and support groups. Margin, or the amount of control the student has to successfully manage stress, can be increased by either increasing the power factors or by decreasing the load factors.

By increasing margin and thus decreasing stress, the student's ability to concentrate on learning also increases.

As with the physical environment, the CI also has limited control over factors of the psychological environment. These factors include the complexity of the procedure, the patient's presenting physical status, and the cohesiveness of specific team members. There is, however, one aspect of the psychological environment the CI does control. CIs have control over themselves and how they interact with their students and other team members. This provides the CI with a significant influence on the student's level of margin. The CI can increase a student's margin by increasing the student's power or by decreasing the student's load. For example, the CI can increase a student's power by answering questions, explaining/reviewing techniques and procedures, demonstrating empathy and respect, and giving constructive feedback. The CI can decrease student load by being a mediator between the student and a hostile operating room environment, reassuring the student, and helping the student seek assistance if personal problems appear to be affecting clinical performance.

The clinical learning environment is probably the most complex learning environment in which a student and instructor must function. It is dynamic, demanding, stressful, and sometimes unforgiving. CIs are very limited in the control they have over specific factors in both the physical and psychological learning environment. They do, however, play a pivotal role in enhancing student learning in both of these environments. Even in the most hostile clinical environment, it is the CI who sets the final tone for student learning.

The Nurse Anesthesia Student

Who are these students the CI deals with on a daily basis? Nurse anesthesia students come from a variety of ethnic and social backgrounds. They all have a wealth of professional and non-professional life experiences. Although their ages may vary, they are all members of a group known as adult learners.

Theory of Adult Learning

Adult learning theory has its roots back in the days of Plato and Aristotle. Since then many theories of learning have evolved. For the purpose of organization, these theories will be classified, in whole or part, into one of four categories. These categories are: Behaviorist, Cognitivist, Social Learning Theorist, and Humanist.[6,7]

According to the Behaviorist, learning consists of a change in behavior. What one learns is determined by elements in the environment and not by the learner. As a result, the focus is on external behavior and observable behavior. It is the role of the teacher to arrange contingencies of reinforcement in the learning environment so that desired behavior will occur. Edward Thorndike's stimulus-response theory fits this category, where the teacher provides the correct stimulus and the student is expected to respond accordingly. Another behaviorist theory is B.F. Skinner's operant conditioning theory where desirable behaviors are reinforced and rewarded while undesirable behaviors are punished or ignored.[7]

Contrary to the Behaviorist, the Cognitivist does not focus on the environment. The Cognitivist focuses on internal mental processes such as how information is processed, stored, and retrieved in the learner's mind. To the Cognitivist, the human mind is not simply a passive exchange terminal where stimuli arrive and appropriate responses leave. Instead, the thinking person interprets sensations and gives meaning to the events that impinge upon his or her consciousness. Cognitivists will put information together in their minds one way and then another way until a problem is solved.[7]

The Social Learning theorist's focus is on the social setting in which learning occurs. Theories in this category suggest that people learn from observing other people. In other words, learning is a function of the interaction of persons, the environment, and the behavior. Theories of modeling and mentoring often fall into this category.[7]

It is this author's contention that aspects of each of the major learning theory categories can be applied to clinical anesthesia education. It is the humanistic approach, however, that appears to more closely fit our nurse anesthesia learners. From the Humanist perspective, learning involves more than just cognitive processes and overt behavior. It is a function of motivation and involves choice and responsibility. The Humanist's focus is on human nature, human potential, human emotions, and affect. Included in this category is the theory of human motivation based on a hierarchy of needs by Abraham Maslow and Malcolm Knowles' theory of andragogy.[6]

Historically, the term pedagogy has been used as a synonym for the general category of teaching. Under the pedagogical model, the teacher assumes responsibility for all decisions concerning what will be learned, when it will be learned, and how it will be learned.

The concepts of andragogy are grounded in humanistic assumptions. Knowles states that pedagogy literally means the art and science of educating children. On the other hand, androgogy is a word derived from the Greek word 'aner' (with the stem andr-), which means "man." Thus androgogy is literally translated as the art and science of helping adults (man) learn. Andragogy focuses more on the process and less on the content being taught. In other words, andragogy is learner-focused instead of being teacher-focused. This comprehensive adult learning theory contends that adults require certain conditions to learn.[8]

With respect to anesthesia education, clinical teaching can be examined in terms of a teaching continuum (**Figure 10.1**). The pure pedagogical model can be positioned at the left end of the continuum and the pure andragogical model at the right. Between these two extremes lie various combinations of these two models as defined by Knowles. At the pedagogical end of the continuum, instruction would be totally CI directed. In this situation, it would be appropriate for the CI to assume a totally active teaching role while the student assumes the passive role of listening and observing. This approach to teaching may be appropriate in circumstances where the student is new to the clinical environment or unfamiliar with particular procedures or techniques. For example, if a patient presents for a subarachnoid block, it would be inappropriate for a student with no previous training or instruction to perform the block. In this situation, the CI would most likely have the student observe while the CI explains and executes the procedure.

Figure 10.1 Clinical Teaching Continuum

At the right end of the continuum we find the andragogy model. In its purest sense, andragogy actually entails self-directed learning.[8] For the purpose of anesthesia clinical education, we will define the extreme andragogical end of the teaching continuum as total supervision and monitoring by the CI. At this end of the continuum, the student is totally immersed in the anesthetic management of the patient, while the CI's role is one of vigilant monitoring and observation of the student's performance.

For the majority of clinical experiences, it is unlikely that the CI functions totally at either of these extremes of the clinical teaching continuum. Most clinical instruction occurs somewhere between these extremes; thus, the term continuum. The CI determines where on the continuum to teach based on his or her knowledge of the student's performance, progression, and growth in the program. The CI should also be cognizant of the fact that the clinical teaching continuum is dynamic. Various situations, such as changes in the patient's condition, may necessitate right or left movement along the continuum. For example, suppose the CI is assigned to an experienced anesthesia student. The patient is basically healthy and the surgical intervention is fairly routine. The CI elects to let the student manage the case with minimal assistance. In this situation the CI would be operating at the far right of the clinical teaching continuum. During the anesthesia induction, the student experiences problems with the laryngoscopy. The CI steps forward and assists the student by applying some cricoid pressure and verbalizing suggestions. The CI is now shifting left on the clinical teaching continuum. As difficulty with the laryngoscopy escalates, the CI now recommends an advanced difficult airway technique that the student is unfamiliar with. The CI performs the laryngoscopy successfully as the student observes the new airway technique. The CI has now shifted even further left on the continuum. Although it is the CI's goal to educate students to be independent practitioners, this is obviously not an overnight event. The process of nurturing this independence involves continuous movements and shifts along the clinical teaching continuum.

Principles of Adult Learning

Most educators agree that there is a difference between teaching adults and children. There is also a great deal of agreement that the andragogical model for teaching adults is closely linked to various assumptions and principles.[6,8,9] These adult learning principles can give the CI a framework from which to build and develop clinical teaching excellence.

Principle 1: Adults Want to Learn

One thing we know about adults is that they want to learn regardless of their age. The old wives tale that "you can't teach an old dog new tricks" may apply to canines but not to people. Although the capacity to learn does not diminish with age, the rate and speed of learning may vary depending on various physiological changes such as declines in visual and audio acuity. Various pathological conditions may also have an adverse effect on learning capacity. Overall, adults can and want to learn. Nurse anesthesia students are no different. They are enrolled in nurse anesthesia programs for one reason: to become a nurse anesthetist. It is rare that a student is being forced to attend anesthesia school against his or her own free will.

Principle 2: Readiness to Learn

Adults are ready to learn those things that they need to know in order to cope effectively with real-life situations. The road to becoming a Certified Registered Nurse Anesthetist (CRNA) is long and demanding. The magnitude of information that must be learned often appears overwhelming. Despite this apparent barrier, the student is aware that mastery of this information is necessary to accomplish the goal of becoming a CRNA. Therefore, most are willing, ready, and eager to proceed with the learning process.

Principle 3: Adult Learning Is an Active Process

Adults appear to be better motivated when they are actively involved in the learning process. Adults have a desire to have some control over their lives. Many hold perceptions of themselves as independent and self-reliant individuals. They enjoy making decisions and freely offer their opinions. This especially holds true for nurse anesthesia students who come from critical care units where their decision-making was valued and encouraged. In addition, many nurse anesthesia students have had various levels of supervisory experiences. Therefore, CIs must remember that one of their goals, in anesthesia clinical education, is to foster this independent decision-making capability in their students.

Principle 4: Adult Learning Is Goal-Directed

Adults appear to learn best when they have clear obtainable goals. In other words, prior to learning, adults not only need to know what they are going to learn, but also why they need to know it. Therefore, one of the first tasks of the CI is to help the learners become aware of their need to know.

Children usually do not question why they are learning something in school. If they do inquire, the teachers usually respond that they are learning it because someday they will need it or that is what they are supposed to learn in this grade in school. Although accepted by most children, adults are usually not satisfied with such responses. Most adults strive to accomplish a specific goal, such as becoming a CRNA. They want to stay focused on those matters that will directly help them reach that goal. They do not want to be sidetracked by what they perceive as unnecessary information. Obviously, the CI is a much better judge of what must be learned to become a CRNA than the student. Learning for the adult student may be hindered, however, if the student does not understand the reasoning behind why something is being taught.

It is also important that the adult learner understands exactly what the CI expects the learner to accomplish or learn during any given clinical session. This gives the learner specific expectations and goals that they can focus on. In the clinical arena, this can be accomplished by the use of formal objectives or merely verbally informing the student what the clinical expectations are for the day or specific anesthesia experience.

Principle 5: Adults Prefer Immediate Application of Learning

Learning that is applied immediately is retained longer and is more subject to immediate use than learning that is not. In other words, learned material appears to be retained longer if it is applied soon after it has been taught. In anesthesia education, one of the primary purposes of the clinical practicum is to provide the student an opportunity to apply this material or theory into practice. Whenever possible, the CI should always strive to let the student apply what he or she has been taught in a timely manner. Obviously, this is dependent on the CI's judgment concerning the appropriateness of the task to the particular clinical situation.

Principle 6: Subject Matter Should Be Presented in a Logical Sequence

Learning is facilitated when there is logic to the subject matter and the logic makes sense in relation to the adult learner's repertoire of experiences. Whether teaching in the classroom or clinical arena, the CI must always strive to present new material in a logical progressive sequence. For example, when first teaching an individual how to drive an automobile, the instructor would not tell the student to get in the car and drive around the block. There are obviously a number of issues that must be first dealt with, such as knowing state laws concerning operating a motor vehicle and understanding the basic operation of the vehicle including controls, instrumentation, safely devices, etc. Once these issues have been covered, the student can then proceed to behind-the-wheel training.

The same scenario is applicable to clinical instruction. Whenever a CI is planning to teach a new skill, he or she should first break the skill into its individual essential components. Once these components are identified, they should be organized into a logical sequence of events so that each builds on the other, ultimately resulting in the accomplishment of the desired skill. For example, obviously nurse anesthesia students must learn how to intubate a patient. The technique of intubation can be broken into many components. These components include but are not limited to equipment, preparation of equipment, patient positioning, insertion of the laryngoscope, airway exposure, insertion of the endotracheal tube, etc. The CI should present these components as a logical sequence of events that will facilitate the student's learning of that skill. If the CI is not sure about an appropriate logical sequence of material he or she should not hesitate to seek guidance from a colleague. If your proposed sequence of events makes sense to your colleague, it will most likely make sense to your student as well.

Principle 7: Adults Need to Be Aware of Their Progress

Learning is facilitated and reinforced when the learner is made aware of his or her progress. The CI cannot expect a student to change or improve performance if the student is not aware of what is right or wrong. Student learning can be facilitated and reinforced by the use of constructive and obtainable feedback.

Constructive feedback should not be belittling or degrading. When giving feedback to a student, the CI should always focus on the desired performance, behavior, or outcome. The CI should never focus on or attack the individual as a person. For example, if you observe that your student is not holding the laryngoscope properly while performing a laryngoscopy, the student obviously must be corrected. Such corrections are best accomplished by first noting those things the student is doing correctly and then addressing the areas needing improvement. As stated earlier, when the corrections are being made the CI should focus on the incorrect technique and behavior and not on the individual. In the above example, the CI could explain to the student that success with laryngoscopy will dramatically increase if he or she changes the grip on the laryngoscope. In this way the CI is addressing the incorrect behavior. Calling the student a "stupid clumsy idiot" may give the CI some type of satisfaction, but will do little to promote learning.

Feedback should also be specific and obtainable. Early in my teaching career I remember a student telling me that his CI had commented that he was "performing OK, for a large male student." He stated that he was not sure what to do about the "large" and "male" comment. We both laughed, but the question still remained as to the purpose and value of the feedback he was given. Feedback that is vague or unattainable serves little value in helping a student improve his or her performance.

Principle 8: Adult Learners Often Reach Learning Plateaus

The existence of periodic plateaus in the rate of learning necessitates frequent changes in the nature of the learning task to ensure continuous progress. It is a well-known fact that some students appear to grasp concepts faster than others. It is also known that adult learners periodically encounter temporary learning plateaus or obstacles that inhibit learning progression. In other words, they appear to have difficulties understanding a concept or procedure that is necessary for further learning to progress. Learning plateaus are very common and should be expected. Hopefully these plateaus are short-lived and are conquered as soon as the particular difficulty is overcome. The CI can be very instrumental in assisting a student in working through these learning plateaus.

How does the CI know when these learning plateaus surface? When such plateaus occur, the student will often admit to having trouble understanding a concept or procedure. Some students, however, may feel that such an admission could be perceived as a sign of weakness.

Whether a student actively seeks help or not, the CI should constantly be scanning for these plateaus. The CI can accomplish this by becoming a "reflective clinical instructor."

Reflective Clinical Instructor

Donald Schön, Professor of Urban Studies and Education at Massachusetts Institute of Technology, proposed that the most effective teachers live a life of reflection about their teaching practice. Schön labeled this premise as being a "reflective practitioner."[10,11] The nurse anesthesia clinical instructor should also be a reflective practitioner. CIs should continually evaluate and re-evaluate their teaching strategies.

They are constantly pulling in information from their environment to determine the effectiveness of their teaching. This information may be gleaned from the type of questions their students ask. It may come from observing students' affect and behavior. For example, do the students look or act confused? Are they giving you a blank stare? Have they become suddenly quiet? These signs and others may alert the CI of a present or imminent learning problem. Reflective clinical instructors should continually evaluate their clinical teaching strategies, techniques, and student outcomes. This reflection is a dynamic process occurring before, during, and after each clinical experience.

Once the CI has identified that a student is having difficulty in learning or is experiencing a plateau in learning, strategies to assist the student can be formulated. If a student is having trouble understanding certain material, often all that is required is a further explanation. The CI should be aware, however, that if the student did not understand the first explanation, the student most likely will not understand a verbatim repetition of the explanation. The CI should rephrase the explanation or use additional examples for clarification. It is also possible that a new teaching strategy would facilitate the student's learning. For example, instead of trying to reiterate how to perform a particular technique, it may be helpful to demonstrate how it is done. Once the barrier to the student's learning progression has been identified, the CI can proceed with an appropriate plan of action.

Principle 9: Adults Possess a Large Amount of Prior Knowledge and Experience

Learning new material is facilitated when it is related to what is already known. Adults accumulate a vast amount of knowledge and experiences throughout their lifetime. Adult learning appears to be facilitated when the instructor can present new information by building on past information the learner has already mastered. For example, let's say a patient will require an arterial line. The student tells the CI that he or she has never started an arterial line before. The CI learns that the student has had an assortment of experiences starting intravenous lines in the critical care area. The student also claims vast experience in managing arterial lines already in vitro. Learning how to start an arterial line will be facilitated if the CI builds on the student's past intravenous and arterial line management experiences as opposed to starting completely new. In this situation, the CI might first have the student recall his or her experiences with managing arterial lines to include the purpose of the line, care, and so on. Next, the CI may have the student review the basic procedure for starting an intravenous line. At this point, the CI might point out the differences in technique in starting an intravenous line as compared to an arterial line.

The CI must be aware that past experiences can also be a detriment to learning. This is especially true when these experiences were weak or flawed. In this situation, life experiences may form patterns of behavior that may require unlearning before new learning can proceed. In the above arterial line example, it is possible that the student developed some undesirable shortcuts or techniques while starting intravenous lines. The CI must first correct these undesirable behaviors before proceeding to arterial cannulation. Before using a student's past experiences, the CI must be sure such experiences are sound and form a good foundation from which to build.

Principle 10: Self Esteem

Adults want to be treated as adults. Adults have a strong sense of self-esteem. Self-esteem can be defined as pride in oneself, the quality of being worthy of respect, or the belief and confidence in one's own ability and value.[2] A student's self-esteem and ego are on the line whenever he or she is asked to risk trying a new behavior in front of peers or cohorts.

When an adult's self-esteem, self-image, or psychological well-being are attacked, the adult often moves into a survival mode. Whenever adult students are belittled, humiliated, embarrassed, or criticized in front of others, their primary focus switches from learning to self-preservation and survival. As a student advisor, I have had many students come to me with a common theme. During a particular clinical experience these students felt that their CI had belittled or humiliated them in front of the operating room staff or others. During the course of these discussions it was obvious that following the incident, student learning had been impaired and in some instances destroyed for the remainder of the experience.

This does not mean that students should not be corrected. As stated earlier, feedback should be constructive and not destructive. The CI should focus on the problem and never attack the individual. The CI should also make every effort to correct or counsel the student quietly and in private. Corrections should never be broadcast throughout the operating room. Once we attack a student's self esteem, we seriously damage the learning environment.

Characteristics of an Effective Clinical Instructor

In 1982, Katz identified 22 "best" and "worst" CI characteristics as perceived by a national sampling of program directors, clinical instructors, and students.[12] In 1993, Hartland and Londoner conducted a follow-up study that identified and ranked the importance of these characteristics as perceived by 354 anesthesia program directors, CIs, and students nationwide (**Table 10.2**). The respondents in this second study perceived all 22 characteristics of effective clinical instructors to be important. Mean scores indicated that all 22 characteristics were perceived to be either very important or highly important. When the researchers rank-ordered the mean scores of the characteristics for all respondents, some characteristics had moderately higher mean scores than others.

Table 10.2 Characteristics Perceived as Indicative of Effective Clinical Instructors and Their Operational Definition

Rank	Characteristic	Operational Definition
1	Clinical Competence/ Judgment	The clinical instructor is technically skilled, demonstrating sound application of theory and knowledge to practice.
2	Calm	The clinical instructor is poised and composed in the clinical area and reacts to stress in a very professional and skillful manner.
3	Ego Strength/ Self-Assurance	The clinical instructor demonstrates confidence in his/her own abilities and recognizes his/her own limitations.
4	Flexibility	The clinical instructor encourages his/her students to become familiar with various anesthesia techniques appropriate to the patient's needs.
5	Appropriately Encourages Independence	The clinical instructor assigns students responsibilities and encourages them to act and think for themselves according to their level of education and competence.
6	Engenders Confidence	The clinical instructor helps students develop self-confidence in their own ability to perform appropriately.
7	Motivates Students	The clinical instructor expects students to assume an active role in the discussion and problem-solving process while encouraging them to perform and communicate at their level of knowledge.
8	Empathy/Respect	The clinical instructor demonstrates sensitivity toward students, understands their needs, supports their self-esteem, and relates to them in a non-threatening manner.
9	Evaluation/ Counseling	The clinical instructor evaluates and counsels students systematically and objectively with appropriate, constructive, and timely feedback.
10	Enjoys Teaching	The clinical instructor conveys interest, motivation, and satisfaction in clinical teaching.
11	Stimulates Student Involvement	The clinical instructor encourages his/her students to participate actively in all aspects of anesthesia care.
12	Positive Role Model	The clinical instructor serves as an appropriate model of the type of anesthetist students want to emulate.
13	Open-Minded	The clinical instructor discusses different views relating to anesthesia care and encourages students to develop their own sound viewpoints.
14	Sensitivity	The clinical instructor demonstrates understanding of others' feelings and supports the students' self-esteem.
15	Scholarly Teaching/ Knowledge	The clinical instructor demonstrates a broad reading and knowledge base, referring and applying pertinent articles and research to patient care, and explains the basis for his/ her clinical actions.
16	Accessibility	The clinical instructor is available and devotes appropriate time to his/her students.

Rank	Characteristic	Operational Definition
17	Communication Skills	The clinical instructor demonstrates a variety of effective verbal and nonverbal communication patterns.
18	Individualizes Teaching	The clinical instructor sets objectives and adjusts teaching methods specific to the level and learning needs of each individual student.
19	Timely Feedback	The clinical instructor evaluates students' performance as close to the performance as appropriate.
20	Actively Teaches	The clinical instructor interacts with the students throughout the clinical period.
21	Stimulates Effective Discussions	The clinical instructor skillfully encourages and facilitates discussions.
22	Use of Student Care Plan	The clinical instructor analyzes, evaluates and allows students to implement the student's care plan whenever possible.

*Adapted with permission from *AANA Journal*[13]

When the mean scores of the characteristics for each group (directors, instructors, students) were arranged in descending order by the researcher, no significant difference was found between respondent groups. The researchers concluded that it appeared that all four professional groups valued the 22 characteristics and perceived them as critically important to clinical instruction. The results of these studies give the CI insight into what colleagues and students perceive to be the desirable characteristics of an effective clinical instructor. They serve as guidelines that nurse anesthesia clinical instructors can use on their journey toward clinical teaching excellence.[13]

Summary

Progressing toward the goal of becoming an effective clinical instructor requires effort, patience, and dedication. As clinical instructors we must remember that our students are adult learners and that various principles of adult learning apply. We should utilize the perceived characteristics of effective clinical instructors to help us identify those areas in our own clinical teaching that need improvement. We must also remember the importance of maintaining the learning environment and the power we possess to accomplish that end.

Becoming an effective CI is a journey that some believe never really ends. The CI should consistently strive for clinical teaching excellence, cognizant that the future of the nurse anesthesia profession will be in the hands of the students that are taught today.

References

1. Gelmon SB, Promoting teaching competency and effectiveness for the 21st century. *AANA J*. 1999;67:409–416.

2. *Webster's New World College Dictionary*. 4th ed. John Wiley & Sons; 2004.

3. Ramsbreg GC. Objectives to outcomes: Your contract with the learner. Professional Convention Management Association. Birmingham, Alabama; 1993;21–37.

4. Lorge J, McClusky HY, Jenson GE, Hallenbeck NC. *Psychology of adults: Adult education theory and method.* Washington, DC: Adult Education Association of USA; 1993.

5. McClusky HY. An approach to a differential psychology of the adult potential. In: Knowles M. *The Adult Learner: A Neglected Species*. 4th ed. Houston, TX: Gulf Publishing Co; 1990:146–162.

6. Merriam SB, Caffarella RS. *Learning in Adulthood*. San Francisco, CA: Jossey-Bass; 1991.

7. Robinson RD. *Helping Adults Learn and cchange.* (3rd Ed.). West Bend, WI: Omnibook; 1996.

8. Knowles MS, Holton EF, Swanson RA. *The adult learner: The Definitive Classic in Adult Education and Human Resource Development*. 6th ed. Burlington, Massachusetts: Elsevier Inc.; 2005.

9. Brookfield SD. *Understanding and Facilitating Adult Learning: A Comprehensive Analysis of Principles and Effective Practice.* San Francisco, CA: Jossey-Bass; 1986.

10. Schön DA. *Educating the Reflective Practitioner: Toward a New Design for Teaching and Learning in the Professions*. San Francisco: Jossey-Bass; 1987.

11. Brookfield S. *Becoming a Critically Reflective Teacher*. San Francisco, CA: Jossey-Bass; 1995.

12. Katz LE. Characteristics of clinical teachers in nurse anesthesia. *AANA J*. 1984;52:192–197.

13. Hartland W, Londoner C. Perceived importance of clinical teaching characteristics for nurse anesthesia clinical faculty. *AANA J*. 1997;65(6):547–551.

14. Bloom BS, Masia BB, Krathwohl DR. *Taxonomy of Educational Objectives: The Classification of Educational Goals, Handbook I Cognitive Domain, and Handbook II: Affective Domain.* Philadelphia, PA: David McKay Company; 1964.

CHAPTER 11

Learning Styles and Their Effect on Clinical Instruction

John P. McDonough, EdD, CRNA, ARNP
Lilia Loriz, PhD, ARNP, BC
Meghan Niemczyk, MPH
Kiran Macha, MBBS, MPH

Keywords: Clinical instruction, learning styles.

Key Concepts

- A learning style is a particular strategy a student adopts that arises from myriad psychological, behavioral, cognitive and affective factors.
- In an attempt to classify the divergent learning styles of individuals, tests and assessment tools have been devised.
- Learners can be classified as one of the following: diverger, assimilator, converger, or accommodator.
- Each style is associated with a preference for certain types of learning activities.
- Learners may seek areas of study that are influenced by their preferred learning styles and their personality traits.
- Learning style also may be affected by the situations to which the student is subjected to and the experiences that bring him or her success.
- No particular learning style is more associated with academic success than another.
- Health care education is much more formal and rank-driven than other disciplines.
- Teaching methods that include personalization are superior for students with a variety of learning styles.

Introduction

In 2016, there were 116 Certified Registered Nurse Anesthetist (CRNA) programs in this country.[1] With the growth in the number of accredited programs has come an increase in nurse anesthesia students. This growth has brought about a demand for more clinical sites to educate these students. In the last decade, there has been an expansion in the number of approved clinical educational sites to accommodate these students. Clinical sites have increased by more than a factor of four from fewer than 400 to a current total exceeding 2,121.[2] This increase in nurse anesthesia clinical educational sites has brought about a role change for many CRNAs. Those CRNAs who had previously been tasked with the provision of anesthesia care now find themselves in the role of clinical preceptor for nurse anesthesia students.[3] The knowledge, skills, and abilities required to administer anesthesia to patients are different from those required to teach others how to administer anesthesia. Clinicians who have found themselves in this position have expressed concerns regarding their lack of preparation in the theoretic concepts of the teaching process.[4]

Learning Styles

As practitioners have become more involved in the clinical teaching process, they have noted that not all students learn in the same way. These differences may be caused by differences in learning styles. Thelen was the first to use the term *learning style* in the literature.[5] Learning style is a particular strategy that has been adopted by a student that arises from myriad psychological, behavioral, cognitive, and affective factors.[6] These factors combine to create a "distinct and habitual manner of acquiring knowledge, skills, or attitudes through study or experience."[7] Although one might surmise that since the activities of thinking and learning are so similar, and any given individual will carry out the process in similar ways, this is not the case. By acknowledging learning styles, the preceptor is able to design experiences and methodologies that are more in accord with the method in which a particular student actually acquires knowledge. There are diagnostic tools that have been created to assess cognitive styles, and they frequently differ from the learning style in the same individual.[8,9] Therefore, the terms "cognitive style" and "learning style" are not interchangeable.[10,11]

In an attempt to classify the divergent learning styles of individuals, many tests and assessment tools have been devised. Through the use of a frequently used assessment tool, the Learning Style Inventory, learners can be classified as using one of the following identified styles: diverger, assimilator, converger, or accommodator.[12] When Kolb described the basis of his concept of learning styles, it can be said to be an outgrowth of the personality theories of Carl Jung. Kolb's work was also influenced by the writings of John Dewey, who recognized the need for learning to be grounded in experience, and by Karl Lewin who claimed that for learning to be effective, people must be actively involved.[13] Some people dealing primarily with post-secondary education tend to see learning style within the view expressed by Gordon Pask. Pask described the three conceptual styles as holistic, serialist, and versatile, and his description of learning as either being deep, surface, or strategic.[14] Kolb and

Pask are not the only contributors to the debate in the field of learning styles. Honey and Mumford created an instrument called the Learning Style Questionnaire.[15] The instruments developed by both Kolb and Honey are still used today. Some believe that the Kolb's Learning Style Inventory has a firmer grounding in psychometrics than the available alternatives.[15,16] Others have expressed doubts concerning the model upon which Honey and Mumford's instrument is based.[17] That said, while it remains in common use today, the Learning Style Inventory (LSI) devised by Kolb is not accepted by all as being valid.[18] However, the Kolb LSI currently remains one of the most commonly used instruments; the concepts utilized by the LSI will be explored here. The LSI uses a series of 12 sentences. Those taking the LSI are presented with these sentences and are asked to rank order a set of potential endings offered for each sentence.[12] The response chosen to complete each sentence is associated with one of the four types of learning styles below **(Table 11.1)**.

Table 11.1 Learning Approaches Associated With Specific Learning Orientations

Learning Orientation	Characterized By
Concrete experience	An experience-based, involved approach to learning
Abstract Conceptualization	A conceptually based, analytical approach to learning
Active experimentation	An action-based, active approach to learning
Reflective observation	An observation-based, impartial approach to learning

The four learning orientations described by Kolb can be seen as the X and Y axis of a graph. On the vertical axis, "concrete" and "abstract" are at the opposite ends. On the horizontal axis, "active" and "reflective" are the opposing poles. If these two lines are crossed at their midpoint, four quadrants are created as shown **(Figure 11.1)**.

Figure 11.1 Classification of Learning Styles

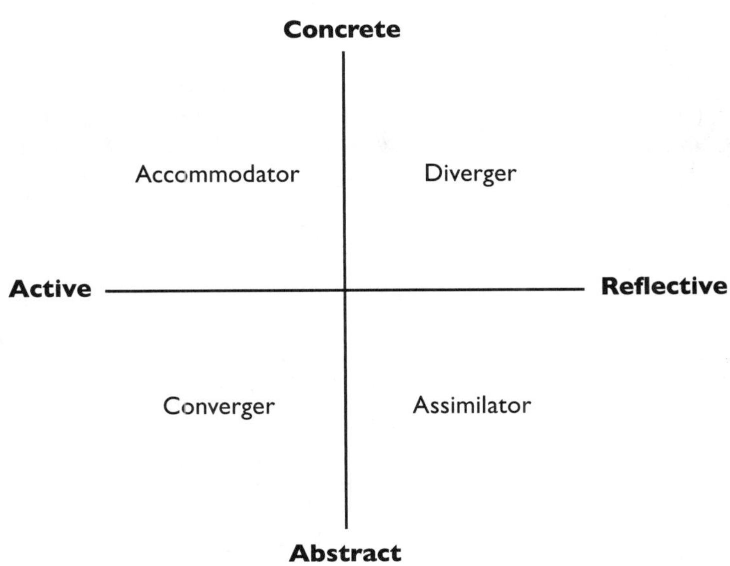

The score achieved on the LSI places a learner somewhere on each axis. This score will also place the learner somewhere in one of these four quadrants. Each quadrant is identified by a word that describes the style of learning that can be associated with someone achieving similar results. Each style is associated with a preference for certain types of learning activities.

Types of Learning Styles

Convergers are described as being pragmatic and prefer to learn through activities that involve abstract conceptualization and active experimentation. Convergers tend to seek the one single best answer to a question or a single solution to a problem. Convergers have been found to be less emotional, and they would rather have to deal with things than people.[14] Divergers are said to be reflective and favor observation and concrete experiences. Divergers tend to have learning strengths opposite those classified as convergers. Divergers are interested in people and have been described as emotional and imaginative.[12] Assimilators tend to be more theoretical and often favor abstract conceptualization and reflective observation. They do very well at inductive reasoning and tend to pose integrated explanations for observations that others may not appreciate.[12] Accommodators have been found to be activists who have a preference for learning activities that involve concrete experience and experimentation. They prefer to actually do things. These learners tend to take risks more than the other styles. When presented with a situation that does not fall clearly within the parameters of a particular theoretical concept or predetermined plan, these learners usually resort more to a process of trial and error. These learners are very much at ease with people, but can sometimes be viewed as being impatient.[12] As previously stated, individuals with different learning styles tend to value different types of learning activities. Specific activities are described detailing how various learning styles might best benefit from an exercise designed to teach endotracheal intubation (**Table 11.2**).

Table 11.2 Preferred Learning Activities Associated With Specific Learning Styles

Learning Style	Activity Preferred
Converger	Receiving practical tips from an expert laryngoscopist
	Using the "help" feature on software used to teach intubation
Diverger	Observing how other people intubate
	Thinking about the intubation just performed by the student
	Recording thoughts about experiences with intubations attempted
Assimilator	Understanding the theory and being clear on the concept of intubation
	Reading a text to get a clearer grasp of what was performed
	Reading to discover the pros and cons of different intubation techniques
Accommodator	Picking up a laryngoscope and attempting the procedure
	Practicing intubation procedure repeatedly
	Using people skills to induce experts to help develop a personal style

Differences In Learning Styles

When discussing learning styles, it is important to understand they may be fluid. Learners may, at any given time, employ a variety of learning styles, but they are not usually all present to the same degree.[16,19] There are data to support the proposition that learners vary their preferred style depending upon what stage of learning they are engaged in at any given time.[20] There are also indications that learners may seek certain areas of study that are influenced by their preferred learning styles, as well as certain personality traits.[21,22] Research has shown that learners educated for different professions demonstrate different learning styles when examined as groups.[23] For example, differences can be seen when comparing the learning styles of radiographers and nurses. In one study, 66 percent of radiographers were divided between the Kolb classifications of converger and assimilators, whereas the nurses were shown to be primarily composed of divergers and accommodators.[24,25] A group that contains a majority of divergers and accommodators more closely mimics the distribution of learning styles commonly seen in physicians.[24,25] For those classified as convergers, there is a preference to receive information as a symbolic representation of experience. They are more comfortable dealing with concepts and ideas than dealing with people and tend to be oriented toward technology.[24,25]

A student's preferred learning style may change based on the teaching methods used during the educational process.[26] Learning style may also be affected by the learning environment as well as the degree of success the student experiences. By examining the learning styles of nurse anesthesia students, the effect of experience and exposure to a set of educational strategies can be measured. When the Kolb LSI was given to a group of nurse anesthesia students who completed fewer than 12 months in their program, there was no dominant learning style preference noted for the group. However, when the LSI was administered to a group of nurse anesthesia students who had fully completed more than 12 months of their program, 80 percent of that group was divided between convergers and assimilators.[30] Also important to note, there is no particular learning style that is more associated with academic success than another. Accordingly, it is important for students to know that a particular style will not guarantee success. It might be helpful to encourage students to develop their least preferred style in an effort to maximize their chances of success in varying learning situations.[23]

Although it may seem counterintuitive, there is no general consensus regarding the need to align student learning styles with the teaching methods used in any particular educational setting. There are some data showing that when teaching styles do not match the learning style of the student, less than optimal results are achieved.[11,27] There are also studies that demonstrate a decreased failure rate when there is alignment of teaching and learning styles.[28] These findings are not universally agreed upon; other studies have documented that the matching of teaching and learning styles did not have a demonstrable effect upon academic performance.[29] As the results are inconsistent and inconclusive, there is no universal acceptance of a benefit derived from matching teaching and learning styles.[30] Rather than matching styles as a goal, it may well be more important to consider the needs of the instructor and the learner in the process. When curricula are designed in a way to facilitate these needs, there is an increase of self-reflective learning behavior reported in students.[31]

Since nurse anesthesia students are all adult learners, the question of matching teaching and learning styles may well be less important than for other university-level students. When compared with younger students, adult learners tend to have more flexibility with regard to learning styles. They may well be more able to adapt and succeed when teaching styles do not match their own learning style.[32] Since there is no correlation between age and gender as to specific learning styles, it is not possible to predict the preferred learning style of any beginning anesthesia student.[33]

Educational Differences

It should be noted that while an understanding of learning styles may be helpful for preceptors to understand how students learn, it is also important to understand that teaching at nurse anesthesia clinical educational sites is fundamentally different from teaching chemistry or biology in a classroom. Clinical learning experiences are essential to preparing nurse anesthetists who are ready to graduate and move into the clinical job setting after observing and interacting with preceptors.[34] The clinical site is the place where the skills demonstrated and mastered are based upon concepts that were introduced in the classroom. This clinical setting involves essential learning regarding the care of actual patients under the guidance of a credentialed practitioner who remains responsible for that care. This is a setting in which decisions involving life and death are made.[3]

Clinical education takes place in the real world, and patients do not come to hospitals for the purpose of meeting the educational and training needs of the profession. The patients are there to have anesthesia care provided in conjunction with a surgical or other diagnostic therapeutic procedure. Students are in attendance to assist and administer anesthesia to these patients. Sometimes the anesthesia provider works independently. Often, preceptors are the only ones present who are actually licensed by the government and credentialed by the facility to provide anesthesia care; they must direct nurse anesthesia students but are also personally responsible for the quality and outcome of that care.[35] While learning in the clinical area is by its very nature experiential, patient safety must always remain the highest priority. In such circumstances, because the stakes are so high, if there is any mismatch between learners' preferences and teaching styles, the students must adjust their expectations and amend their goals.

Health care education can be seen as being much more formal and competitive than other disciplines. In academic medicine there are frequently deans, department chairs, service chiefs, attending physicians, fellows, residents (characterized by postgraduate year cohort), and undergraduate medical students. In nursing, there are additional deans, chairs, program directors, faculty, doctoral students, master's students and undergraduate nursing students. In the clinical departments, respect must be shown to these diverse members of the health care team, particularly students.[36] In some departments, clinical preceptors may not always see learners as being deserving of respect and in need of mentorship. Although there is conflicting evidence as to the effect of matching learning and teaching styles to improve the chances of successful learning, studies show that a high level of personalization is a superior method for students with all varieties of learning styles. Engaging in the personalization of instructions may well be associated with a higher degree of success than an attempt to match teaching and learning styles.[37]

Multiple Learning Styles

The core of experiential learning allows students to be active in the educational and clinical process.[36] The level of involvement in these processes is not merely a function of teacher-student interaction. Much learning can come from student-student interaction as well.[38] Positive levels of teacher-student and student-student interactions are more likely to occur within the clinical department that see these interactions as valuable. In the past, CRNA educational programs as well as programs preparing registered nurses were diploma-granting programs and were based in hospitals. It was not uncommon at that time for nursing students and nurse anesthesia students to receive all their clinical instruction within the walls of the particular hospital that conducted its educational program. As both general nursing and nurse anesthesia evolved, the disciplines moved away from the hospital-based educational model to a university-based academic system, and the practice of having all student clinical educational experiences at a single institution became much less common. Students are now educated in programs that are based within institutions of higher learning that contract, through affiliation agreements, with multiple clinical facilities to provide educational experiences for their students.[39] There are now 116 accredited nurse anesthesia educational programs, and the Council on Accreditation of Nurse Anesthesia Educational Programs has accredited over 2,100 clinical sites. In such an arrangement, it is obvious that students from a single program will be exposed to clinical experiences in many sites that may well have different philosophies, staffing patterns, personnel expectations, and organizational structures. In order to be effective as sites for clinical instruction, these potentially diverse departments need to establish a climate where various forms of educational interaction, such as student-teacher, student-student, and teacher-teacher, are seen as valuable and supported.[40]

Nurse Anesthesia Education

Unlike students of many other disciplines obtaining clinical educational experiences in hospitals, nurse anesthesia students come as fully licensed professionals with years of experience. Depending upon their previous level of professional experience and educational background, it is quite conceivable that in some particular areas, the student may possess both theoretical and clinical expertise exceeding that of the clinical preceptor to whom they are assigned that day. However, in such situations, it is important for both the teacher and the learner to recall that the CRNA who is serving as the clinical preceptor is the individual most knowledgeable in the overall anesthesia management of the patient, and he or she bears the responsibility. Conversely, since the time that many clinical preceptors were students, significant and dramatic changes have occurred in the process of nurse anesthesia education.[39] As opposed to looking back with a combination of both dread and nostalgia at the way things used to be, it is much more productive for current clinical preceptors to seek the most effective and safety-driven methods to support the transition of current nurse anesthesia students into CRNA colleagues. Our students both need and deserve effective coaching and mentoring in the clinical area. That certainly does not mean that effective anesthesia professionals are created through a process of spoon-feeding information and not holding students responsible for their own learning success. Preceptors should ask questions that require critical thinking skills while encouraging students to present an evidence-based rationale for the decisions that they make. By combining the experiences of both preceptors and students, greater knowledge can be gained for the benefit of all.

Some students have a low level of expectations for themselves in terms of their clinical performance and are willing to see themselves as successful if they meet their expectations. There is much more required to be successful in nurse anesthesia than merely showing up in the clinical area. Unlike the experiences that some current students have had earlier in their lives, this profession is not in the habit of awarding trophies for mere participation. Asking difficult questions, expecting thoughtful and accurate responses, while helping students to become critical questioners themselves within an atmosphere of mutual respect has been shown to produce the best results.[41] Good clinical preceptors will set their sights on excellence as a goal and will encourage students to reach that goal. All students progress at different rates. There is no hard and fast timeline in which all students are expected to be simultaneously located. Accordingly, the same mold will not fit for all particpants.[42] By adapting the educational process to the needs of the specific situation, clinical preceptors can be a crucially important component in the metamorphosis of students into the expert anesthesia providers of the future.

Summary

Several distinct learning styles have been identified. Although there certainly may be some advantages for instructors in becoming familiar with these styles and their effect upon learner preferences, it is not a requirement for effective clinical instruction. It is more appropriate to expect the student in the clinical area to adapt his or her learning style to the teaching style of the clinical instructor than vice versa. As the individual tasked with responsibility for patient care, the preceptor must be comfortable in coordinating the process of teaching with the process of patient care. If the clinical instructor can incorporate specific teaching techniques that match the learning preferences of the students, all the better; however, data indicates that learners are capable of adjusting their preferences to match the teaching styles of the instructors.

References

1. Council on Accreditation of Nurse Anesthesia Educational Programs. CRNA School Search. http://home.coa.us.com/accredited-programs/Pages/CRNA-School-Search.aspx. Accessed September 6, 2016.

2. Council on Accreditation of Nurse Anesthesia Educational Programs. *Program Director's Update.* 2015;71:3.

3. Smith C, Swain A, Penprase B. Congruence of perceived effective clinical teaching characteristics between students and preceptors of nurse anesthesia programs. *AANA J.* 2011;79(4):62–68.

4. Starnes-Ott K, Kremer MJ. Recruitment and retention of nurse anesthesia faculty: issues and strategies. *AANA J.* 2007;75(1):13–16.

5. Fatt J, Poon T. Understanding the learning styles of students: implications for educators. *Int J Sociol Soc Policy*. 2000;20(11):31–35.

6. Fatt J, Poon T. Innovative teaching: teaching at its best. *Education*. 1998;118:616–625.

7. Sadler-Smith E. Learning styles: a holistic approach. *J Eur Ind Training*. 1996;20:29–36.

8. Peacock M. Match or mismatch? Learning styles and teaching styles in EFL. *Int J Appl Linguist*. 2001;11:1–20.

9. Suliman WA. Critical thinking and learning styles of students in conventional and accelerated programmes. *Internat Nurs Rev*. 2006;53(1):73–79.

10. Cook DA, Smith AJ. Validity of index of learning styles scores: multitrait-multimethod comparision with three cognitive/learning style instruments. *Med Educ*. 2006;40:900–7.

11. Sadler-Smith E. The relationship between learning style and cognitive style. *PersInd Dif*. 2001;30(4):609–616.

12. Kolb D, Smith D. User's Guide for the Learning Style Inventory. Boston, MA: McBer & Company; 1986.

13. Hoelker J. Classroom Ideas: writing stories for one another. *Modern English Teacher*. 2002;11:33–36.

14. Pask G. *Conversation Theory: Applications in Education and Epistemology*. New York, NY: Elsevier; 1976.

15. Duff A, Duffy T. Psychometric properties of Honey & Mumford's Learning Styles Questionnaire (LSQ). *Hum Res*. 2003;33:147–163.

16. Hauer P, Straub C, Wolf S. Learning styles of allied health students using Kolb's LSI-IIa. *J Allied Health*. 2005;34:177–182.

17. De Ciantis S, Kirton, M. A psychometric reexamination of Kolb's experiential learning cycle construct: a separation of level, style, and process. *Educ Psychol Meas*. 1996;56:809–820.

18. Koob J, Funk J. Kolb's learning style inventory: issues of reliability and validity. *Res Soc Work Pract*. 2002;12:293–308.

19. Grasha A, Yangarber-Hicks N. Integrating teaching styles and learning styles with instructional technology. *College Teaching*. 2000;48(1):2–10.

20. Mumford A. Putting learning styles to work: an integrated approach. *Ind Commercial Training*. 1995:27(8):28–35.

21. McDonough J. Personality, addiction and anesthesia. *AANA J*. 1990;58(3):193–200.

22. Heinström J. The impact of personality and approaches to learning on information behavior. *Information Research*. 2000;5(3).

23. Linares A. Learning styles of students and faculty in selected health care professions. *J Nurs Educ*. 1999;38(9):407–414.

24. Fowler P. Learning styles of radiographers. *Radiography*. 2002;8:3–11.

25. DiBartola LM. The Learning Style inventory challenge: teaching about teaching by learning about learning. *J Allied Health*. 2006;35(4):238–45.

26. Kolb AY, Kolb DA. "Learning styles and learning spaces: Enhancing experiential learning in higher education." *Academy of Management Learning & Education*. 2005;4(2):193–212.

27. Rassool GH, Rawaf S. Learning style preferences of undergraduate nursing students. *Nurs Stand*. 2007;21(32):35–41.

28. Ford N, Chen S. Matching/mismatching revisited: an empirical study of learning and teaching styles. *Br J Educ Technol*. 2001;2(1):5–22.

29. Joyce-Nagata B. Students' academic performance in nursing as a function of student and faculty learning style congruency. *J Nurs Educ*. 1996;35(2):69–73.

30. Thompson C, Crutchlow E. Learning style research: a critical review of the literature and implications for nursing education. *J Prof Nurs*. 1993;9(1):34–40.

31. Wagner F, Osterbrink J. Integrierte Unterrichtseinheiten: Ein Modell für die Ausbildung in der Pflege. Bern, Switzerland: Huber; 2001:213–217.

32. Spoon J, Schell J. Aligning student learning styles with instructor teaching styles. *J Ind Teacher Educ*. 1998;35(2):41–56.

33. Heffler B. Individual learning style and the Learning Style Inventory. *Educ Stud*. 2001;27:309–316.

34. Papp I, Markkanen M, von Bonsdorff M. Clinical environment as a learning environment: student nurses' perceptions concerning clinical learning experiences. *Nurse Educ Today*. 2003;23:262–268.

35. Abenstein JP, Warner MA. Anesthesia providers, patient outcomes, and costs. *Anesth Analg*. 1996;82:1273–1283.

36. Kalb KA, O'Conner-Von S. Ethics education in advanced practice nursing: respect for human dignity. *Nurs Educ Perspect*. 2007;28:196–202.

37. Horton C, Oakland T. Temperament-based learning styles as moderators of academic achievement. *Adolescence*. 1997;32:131–143.

38. Görres S, Keuchel R, Roes M. Auf dem Weg zueinerneuen Lernkultur: Wissenstransfer in der Pflege. Bern, Switzerland: Huber; 2002:179–182.

39. Horton BJ. Upgrading nurse anesthesia educational requirements (1933–2006)—Part 1: setting standards. *AANA J*. 2007;75(3):167–170.

40. Gillespie M. Student-teacher connection: a place of possibility. *J Adv Nurs*. 2005;52:11–219.

41. Myrick F, Tamlyn D. Teaching can never be innocent: fostering an enlightening educational experience. *J Nurs Educ*. 2007;46:299–303.

42. Raschick M, Maypole D, Day P. Field education: improving field education through Kolb Learning Theory. *J Soc Work Educ*. 1998;34(1):31–43.

CHAPTER 12

Ethics of Clinical Instruction

Kathy Wren, PhD, CRNA
Timothy Wren, DNP, RN

Keywords: Code of ethics, ethical dilemma, ethics.

Key Concepts

- Ethics, a discipline concerned with determining what is right and wrong, looks at moral duties and obligations.
- Professional organizations influence what is ethical through accepted standards of conduct expected of their members.[1–3]
- The Council on Accreditation of Nurse Anesthesia Education Programs (COA) requires nurse anesthesia programs to be governed by ethical standards.[4,5]
- The Coalition of National Health Education Organizations publishes a Code of Ethics, which includes (in Article I): "[a] promoting justice, [b] doing good, and [c] avoidance of harm."[6]
- The Coalition of National Health Education Organizations' Code of Ethics also states that clinical faculty have responsibilities in professional preparation of students (Article VI) to encourage and act as a role model for ethical conduct among those aspiring to enter the profession.[6]
- It is important to remember that, in addition to the professional role as a caregiver, clinical faculty also have obligations to inform patients as well as to correct any misunderstanding about who is responsible for their care and to be specific about what activities students will be performing in their care.[7]
- Clinical faculty are responsible for providing adequate student supervision based upon the student level, clinical situation, and patient health care demands.[7]

Introduction

Clinical instruction of nurse anesthesia students is rewarding and, at times, overwhelming. Training students to critically think and problem solve in the fast-paced and fluid environment of the operating room is challenging. In some circumstances, the Certified Registered Nurse Anesthetist (CRNA) clinical faculty will find there is not enough time to teach but only to act. During these times, the CRNA faculty will most likely need to suspend teaching duties in order to meet the demands of the clinical situation and then return to student instruction when the situation allows. Also, clinical experiences are not structured activities. Instruction in a classroom setting can be standardized and packaged so that students receive similar information. This is not the case with clinical experiences. Clinical experiences may vary widely between students based upon clinical sites, patient population, operating room schedules, clinical faculty, and a host of other uncontrollable factors. This means that clinical teaching will also vary widely. Due to the variability in clinical practice and clinical teaching, CRNA faculty will face many ethical dilemmas during clinical instruction of students. However, due to the variability in practice, it is extremely difficult to determine the right thing to do in individual circumstances. CRNA clinical faculty need to understand issues surrounding ethical decision-making in education so that they may be better prepared to deal with ethical problems that are sure to arise during clinical instruction of students.

Ethics

Ethics, a discipline concerned with determining what is right and wrong, looks at moral duties and obligations. Determining what is right and wrong involves cultural, societal, and social norms. For example, autonomy is highly valued in North American culture, but not in middle Asian society. Likewise, professional organizations influence what is ethical through accepted standards of conduct expected of their members. Most professional codes of ethics deal with issues such as competence, conflict of interest, confidentiality, responsibility to the profession, diversity, scholarship and research, and safety for clients.[1] For instance, the American Association of Nurse Anesthetists' (AANA) Code of Ethics for the Certified Registered Nurse Anesthetist[1] and Standards for Nurse Anesthesia Practice[2] outline ethical responsibilities of its professional members (**Table 12.1**).

Table 12.1 Sample of Ethical Guidelines for the Certified Registered Nurse Anesthetist (CRNA)[1,2]

- Protect the patient from harm
- Be a patient advocate
- Maintain patient confidentiality
- Refuse to engage in deception
- Participate in lifelong, professional educational activities
- Practice in accordance with professional practice standards
- Be responsible for one's actions
- Contribute to the body of knowledge
- Maintain the dignity and integrity of the profession
- Evaluate research findings and incorporate them into practice
- Maintain ethical business practices

Ethical codes are designed to help individuals determine how to best fulfill their ethical obligations in a particular situation or problem. Yet, a recent study found that many faculty (76%) believe ethical codes are not helpful in discouraging unethical practices.[8]

Given the fact that many students do not participate in a formal ethics course, most of what students learn about ethical behavior comes from what they observe of their faculty's actions in clinical practice. Often there is silent absorption of unethical behaviors and bad habits from those encountered in the clinical setting. Unless faculty model ethical actions, it is unlikely that students will learn ethical behaviors. Thus, faculty have vital roles in helping students learn clinical and professional ethics.

Ethics in Clinical Education

Due to the complex nature of clinical training, the number of individuals (patients, students, colleagues, health care professionals) and public interests involved (societal, professional, community, family), and the need for learner assessment and evaluation, clinical faculty frequently encounter ethical dilemmas in the clinical area. Thus, faculty must be aware of ethical guidelines established to assist in the resolution of ethical dilemmas.

Standards for Accreditation of Nurse Anesthesia Educational Programs

The Council on Accreditation of Nurse Anesthesia Education Programs (COA) is recognized by the U.S. Department of Education as the accreditation body for nursing anesthesia programs. In order to achieve and maintain accreditation, nurse anesthesia programs must demonstrate compliance with five master's level or eight practice doctorate level educational standards, and associated 54 criteria for master's or 119 criteria for practice doctorate. An entire educational standard dedicated to accountability and integrity requires nurse anesthesia programs to behave ethically toward its communities of interest.[4,5] Specific criteria impacting nurse anesthesia students are summarized in **Table 12.2**, next page.

Table 12.2 Ethical Responsibilities of Nurse Anesthesia Programs of Significance to Students[4,5]

- Students demonstrate professionalism, including a commitment to academic and personal integrity.
- Professional responsibility is demonstrated by the graduate's ability to: interact on a professional level with integrity, adhere to the Code of Ethics for the Certified Registered Nurse Anesthetist, apply ethically sound decision-making processes, function within legal and regulatory requirements, and accept responsibility and accountability for his or her practice.
- The program identifies, publishes, and distributes the rights and responsibilities of patients, applicants, faculty, students, conducting and affiliating institutions, and the accrediting agency.
- Maintain a reasonable student time commitment to studies and clinical responsibilities so as to ensure patient safety and promote effective student learning.
- Forbid students to obtain employment as nurse anesthetists.
- Prevent educational entities from falsifying their accreditation status.
- Develop and implement fair grievance and appellate policies.
- Develop and implement appropriate mechanisms for dealing with complaints against the program.
- Provide information to students concerning ethical responsibilities in loan repayments.
- Develop and implement nondiscriminatory policies.
- Policies and procedures regarding academic integrity are defined and used in all educational activities.

In fulfilling the requirements of the COA, clinical faculty should take an active role in monitoring students' clinical workload to ensure that learning is achieved and patient safety is maintained. This may involve monitoring and providing adequately spaced breaks and mealtimes on the clinical unit as well as end of shift relief. While service is an integral part of their training, students should not be used as a "cheap" or "captive" source of anesthesia coverage. Likewise, students should never be allowed to present themselves as nurse anesthetists to the patient or other health care personnel. Clinical faculty should also become actively involved in application, acceptance, and grievance processes of the anesthesia program. This will aid programs to develop and implement ethical policies and monitor compliance with its ethical responsibilities to its communities of interest.

National Task Force on Ethics in Health Education

In order to assist members of the health care education profession, the Council of National Health Education Organizations issued a code of ethics based on the core principles underlying ethical health care services. These principles include "[a] respect for autonomy, [b] promotion of social justice, [c] active promotion of good, and [d] avoidance of harm."[6] Within the code, the council delineates responsibilities to the public, profession, and employers as well as responsibilities in the delivery of health education, research and evaluation, and professional preparation. It is under the professional preparation section that the council lists ethical principles to guide education of health care professionals. Principles impacting teaching-learning relationships are summarized in **Table 12.3**.

Table 12.3 Ethical Principles for Teaching-Learning Relationships[4–6]

Clinical faculty should:

- Treat learners with respect;
- Treat all learners the same;
- Provide a quality education as defined by the profession and the community;
- Select students based on "academic performance, abilities, and potential contribution to the profession"[4];
- Create a safe educational environment;
- Create an educational environment that helps students to learn;
- Adequately prepare for the training of students;
- Use accurate and timely information;
- Give appropriate rationales for decisions;
- Conduct evaluations that are fair, consistent, and equitable;
- Provide objective and honest student counseling; and
- Provide adequate supervision based upon the learner's performance level.

Guidelines for Ethics in Clinical Teaching

The Department of Medicine at the University of Toronto further defines the role of clinical faculty and ethics in clinical training. In the excellent *Standards for Professional Behavior for Medical Clinical Faculty*, there is a list of specific behaviors and considerations related to professional responsibilities to the patient, student, and profession (Table 12.4).[10] Although written by medical education faculty in Canada, these guidelines are also applicable to health care training institutions and faculty in the United States.

Table 12.4 Professional Responsibilities of Clinical Faculty[10]

Clinical faculty should:

Model high standards of professionalism, such as

- Strive for excellence in practice
- Exhibit honesty, humility, and compassion
- Act with courtesy and respect
- Maintain privacy and confidentiality
- Embrace diversity
- Participate in self-reflection and improvement

Refuse to engage in unethical behaviors, such as

- Intimidation, threatening, bullying
- Interfering with reporting of improper conduct
- Sexual harassment
- Overstepping professional boundaries
- Making inappropriate statements
- Using unprofessional language
- Failing to report breaches of ethical and professional behavior

It is important to remember that, in addition to the professional role as a caregiver, clinical faculty also have obligations to inform patients about who is responsible for their care (the faculty as the licensed personnel) and to be specific about which activities students will be performing in their care.[7] Additionally, faculty must allow patients to refuse student involvement in their health care and inform patients that their health care information will be shared with the student learner when students are involved in the care of the patient.

Clinical faculty are also responsible for providing adequate student supervision based upon the student level, clinical situation, and patient health care demands.[7] This dictates that faculty must be an active participant in the design and implementation of the anesthesia plan so that patient and learner outcomes are optimized. Faculty must also provide accurate and timely feedback concerning student performance, critical thinking abilities, and anesthesia planning.

Clinical faculty should be honest and ethical in their own dealings with patients and students. They should expect and demand the same high level of ethical behavior from the learner. Clinical faculty should create an atmosphere of mutual trust and acceptance so that students will be able to discuss and report ethical concerns. This also implies that faculty are available to consult on ethical issues and concerns and help report and resolve ethical problems and violations.

Furthermore, ethical behavior is learned. It is incumbent upon didactic and clinical faculty to model and mentor ethical behavior in all their professional encounters and actions. Faculty help establish trusting relationships with students by treating them with respect and dignity. Not infrequently, however, positive faculty-student relationships are damaged when faculty communicate with other faculty about students' performance levels.[7] Among its many regulations, the Family Educational Rights and Privacy Act (FERPA) prohibits the sharing of academic information without prior written authorization from the student.[11] Yet, patient safety considerations would indicate the need for information sharing among faculty related to student performance. Also, an important adult education principle embraces the individualization of learning experiences/activities tailored toward the learner's need. In order to avoid a conflict between these two important viewpoints, faculty should:

- ensure that all specific student academic and evaluation information is shared only with those who truly have a need to know;
- communicate instead with other clinical faculty the student's need for additional learning experiences in critical thinking, medication dosing, airway management, and so forth; and
- avoid making statements such as, "This student is way behind the other students," "This student is not up to the level expected," " I don't think this student is ever going to make it," or other judgment/conclusion-type statements (**Table 12.5**).[7]

Table 12.5 Examples of Turning Evaluative Statements into Learning Objectives

Conclusion/Evaluative Statements	Learning Experiences/Activities
This student is below the expected level of performance.	The student requires additional experience(s) with a) endotracheal intubation; b) airway management with a mask; c) spinal block insertion; and d) recognizing and providing patient specific/appropriate treatment(s) for hypotension (for example).
The student doesn't understand anesthesia drugs.	The student needs additional review of pharmacological principles pertaining to drugs encountered during anesthesia, such as individualized dosing, side effects, contraindications. Also, this information must be included on the written patient care.
The student lacks critical thinking skills.	The student must verbally iterate the rationale for all choices in anesthesia care before implementing intervention(s) on the patient.

Theories of Ethical Decision-Making

Ethical dilemmas occur when there is a discrepancy between stakeholders of values, morals, opinions, and responsibilities. Stakeholders are individuals or entities that hold a vested interest in the situation. Stakeholders in an anesthesia clinical arena include didactic faculty, student, clinical faculty, patient, patient's family, hospital, nurse anesthesia program, community, and nurse anesthesia profession.

Most ethical decision-making models advocate following a process comparable to the traditional four-step model of nursing process (**Figure 12.1**) in resolution of ethical dilemmas.[12] The first step in dealing with an ethical dilemma is to fully identify and define the problem. Many times, what is first identified as the issue is not really the problem at all. If the real problem is not set down, energies will be wasted in dealing with side issues while the actual problem is not dealt with and left unresolved.

Figure 12.1 Ethical Decision-Making Model

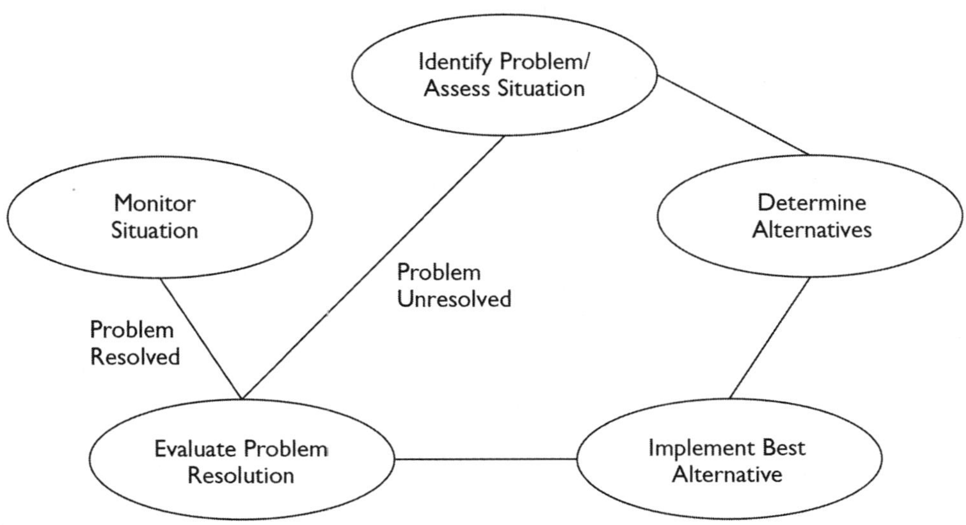

The second step in resolving an ethical dilemma is to list and assess available interventions aimed at resolution. Available interventions may be evaluated through looking at the underlying purpose of the dilemma, rules, and principles impacting the dilemma, and the probability of successful resolution related to each intervention.[12] In looking at the underlying purpose of the ethical dilemma, the clinical faculty will explore the big picture view of the problem. The faculty will explore the issues surrounding the problem and try to get to the heart of the problem. The faculty should ask, "What is the real problem here?"

In the third step, when viewing available options from the rules and principles perspective, the clinical faculty should look to available policies, procedures, rules, and regulations related to the problem. The code of ethics for the CRNA,[1] Standards for Nurse Anesthesia Practice,[2] and Scope of Nurse Anesthesia Practice[3] guidelines, as well as COA accreditation standards,[4,5] provide guidance for ethical dilemmas involving students and faculty in nurse anesthesia educational programs. The clinical faculty should ask, "What principles are pertinent to this problem?"

When reviewing options in the fourth and final step, the clinical faculty determines which interventions are available and then assesses each intervention according to the possibility of success.[12] Issues of practicality and feasibility of each option also aid in determining the likelihood of success. The clinical faculty should ask, "What is the likelihood that this intervention will bring about resolution of the problem?" and "What is most appealing and most detrimental about this intervention?"

Once options are delineated, the best intervention is selected and implemented. After full implementation of the intervention, the clinical faculty should evaluate the success or failure of the intervention in resolving the dilemma. If the dilemma has been successfully resolved, all that may be needed is further monitoring to ensure continued resolution of the matter. If the intervention is unsuccessful, then the clinical faculty should return to the first step of ethical decision-making and consider redefining the problem. Further data collection and collegial assistance may aid in redefining the problem more completely and exploring other potential interventions, which should increase the likelihood of successful intervention and resolution of the problem. At times, one may have to accept the fact that complete resolution of the problem may not be possible, as evidenced by ongoing debates concerning abortion or physician-assisted suicide. In very difficult situations or unresolved ethical dilemmas, the clinical faculty may wish to seek out the assistance of the university's ethics/bioethics department.

Ethical Dilemmas in Clinical Performance Evaluation of Nurse Anesthesia Students

Using clinical faculty to provide clinical instruction for health care professional students is not new. The training of medical students has, for many decades, relied on clinical faculty to assist with student education. Typically, medical students undergo two years of didactic training from college/university faculty, and then finish the remaining two years of training with monthly preceptorships, rotating between different hospital units and physician faculty.

Students in health care professions must not only master scientific and profession-specific content, but must be able to synthesize this knowledge and apply it in the health care setting. Students must acquire and practice clinical skills in the clinical setting. In turn, student performance must be evaluated in the clinical setting. Often it is the clinical faculty who must provide feedback for the performance evaluation.

In anesthesia training, programs often have full-time faculty who are responsible for didactic content, but with dozens of students and limited didactic faculty, it would be impossible for these few didactic faculty to provide all the needed clinical supervision and performance evaluations. Hence, clinical faculty have an important role in student nurse anesthesia education.

Historically the use of clinical faculty in nursing to provide feedback on student performance in the clinical arena is well documented.[13] Issues in the evaluation of student clinical performance arise from a number of areas. Some of these issues include:

- little or no training of clinical faculty in the process of student clinical performance evaluation;
- relative inexperience of clinical faculty in professional clinical practice and clinical preceptorship;
- student intimidation strategies targeted to influence faculty evaluation and feedback;
- cumbersome, inadequate, poorly designed student performance evaluation processes and tools; or
- faculty's fear of litigious actions related to student education, evaluation, and grading.

Many times it is difficult for clinical faculty to understand their responsibilities to patients and the profession when discussing clinical performance with students who are emotionally and monetarily invested in their education, as well unrealistic in understanding the limits of their abilities. As a consequence, clinical faculty often do not address performance inadequacies with students or document their concerns and observations on the student evaluation tool. In these types of situations, an ethical dilemma arises from the incongruence between students' needs and the needs of patients, the profession, and society.

The first step in dealing with an ethical dilemma is to fully identify and define the problem. In the performance of student clinical evaluations, clinical faculty have an ethical responsibility to create an educational environment that will help students learn as well as conduct evaluations that are fair, consistent, and equitable.[6,10] When a clinical faculty is reluctant to discuss and document inadequacies in a student's performance, an ethical dilemma arises. In this situation, the problem is reluctance to evaluate and document inadequate student clinical performance and may be due to little or no training of clinical faculty in the process of student clinical performance evaluation.

Once the problem has been identified and defined, possible interventions can be listed and assessed for successful resolution. In our example of inadequate student clinical performance evaluation and documentation due to lack of clinical faculty training, possible interventions may include:

- orientation to and explanation of the clinical evaluation tool;
- role-playing exercises;
- sample video vignettes of students' clinical performance followed by a discussion period of constructive evaluative comments;
- lecture series on student clinical performance documentation; or
- one-on-one faculty instruction in a clinical area on student clinical performance documentation.

Next, each intervention should be assessed as to its pros and cons. For example, reviewing the clinical evaluation tool will ensure that everyone in attendance has mastered the same content; however, faculty should be able to accomplish this basic task before meeting as a group, and free meeting time for higher level learning such as using the evaluation tool in sample clinical situations. An evaluation of possible interventions is summarized in **Table 12.6**.

Table 12.6 Intervention Evaluation

Intervention	Pros	Cons
Review of Clinical Evaluation Tool	All faculty start from same information Student able to receive faculty feedback on tool	Very basic level information Activity lacks engagement for those who have already reviewed tool
Role-playing exercises	Engages learning activity Brings emotional component to context	Needs audience volunteers willing to role-play Limited to face-to-face classes
Sample video vignette(s)	Useful in face-to-face and distance learning situations Video(s) may be used several times Video(s) may be stopped at key discussion points	Costly Requires use of production equipment/crew
Lecture series	Cost-effective Learners familiar and comfortable with this learning format	Not very learner-engaging Limited to scheduled time periods, limiting attendance
Faculty instruction	Individualized instruction Face-to-face interaction	Costly Time-consuming Limited to clinical situations as they present

After each possible intervention is assessed, the best intervention should be selected based upon available likelihood of success in relationship to available resources, such as associated costs, timeliness, support personnel, and space requirements. Once the intervention is implemented, the adequacy of its problem resolution should be evaluated. If the problem has not adequately been resolved, the process should be re-initiated.

One of the most common reasons for failing to achieve resolution is due to an incomplete delineation of the problem. For example, inadequate student clinical performance evaluations may result from faculty's fears of litigious actions related to student education, evaluation, and grading, instead of a lack of faculty training. As such, indicated interventions in this situation would be different than those identified above for lack of faculty training. In this scenario, interventions may possibly include a

- review of the legal basis for student clinical evaluations;
- lecture series on writing nonjudgmental/performance-based student clinical evaluations;
- lecture series on the purpose of student clinical evaluations; or
- journal club series on writing student clinical evaluations.

Thus, when resolution to an ethical dilemma fails to occur despite appropriate intervention, the first consideration should be to determine the adequacy of the problem definition.

Summary

Ethics, a discipline which looks at right and wrong, is useful to many people in many professions. In the health care industry, hospitals have ethics committees that review, discuss, and evaluate the morality of health care decisions and interventions. However, an ethics committee for clinical faculty does not exist to assist in the day-to-day decisions that are required in student learning environments. Schools have clinical guidelines and accrediting bodies, such as the Council on Accreditation (COA), have recommendations for dealing with students in the clinical environment but clinical faculty must rely on their own ethical meters when determining what is appropriate for each student, patient, and clinical experience.

In this chapter, an ethical dilemma from the clinical perspective was discussed to demonstrate the process of ethical decision-making. A model was presented, providing a visual representation of the ethical decision-making process. Interventions aimed at resolving the ethical dilemma were presented and evaluated to promote an improved understanding of the process.

The famous British author D. H. Lawrence said this about ethics, "Ethics and equity and the principles of justice do not change with the calendar." What is ethical, what is right, does not change with the passage of time. Clinical faculty have ethical responsibilities and moral duties to patients under their care as well as to students they are mentoring. These responsibilities remain despite the context or concerns related to relationship variables, grades, or threats of legal action.

References

1. Code of Ethics for the Certified Registered Nurse Anesthetist. Park Ridge, IL: American Association of Nurse Anesthetists; 2013.

2. Standards for Nurse Anesthesia Practice. Park Ridge, IL: American Association of Nurse Anesthetists; 2013.

3. Scope of Nurse Anesthesia Practice. Park Ridge, IL: American Association of Nurse Anesthetists; 2013.

4. Standards for Accreditation of Nurse Anesthesia Educational Programs. Park Ridge, IL: Council on Accreditation of Nurse Anesthesia Education Programs; 2015.

5. Standards for Accreditation of Nurse Anesthesia Programs: Practice Doctorate. Park Ridge, IL: Council on Accreditation of Nurse Anesthesia Education Programs; 2015.

6. Code of Ethics for the Health Education Profession. Council of National Health Education Organizations. http://cnheo.org/files/coe_full_2011.pdf. Accessed September 28, 2015.

7. Gaberson KB, Oermann MH, Shellenbarger T. Ethical and legal issues in clinical teaching. In: Gaberson KB, Oermann MH, Shellenbarger T, eds. *Clinical Teaching Strategies in Nursing*. 4th ed. New York, NY: Spring Publishing Company, LLC.

8. Nickols SY, Belliston LM. Professional Ethics: Caught and Taught. ERIC Clearinghouse on Information and Technology; 2001. ERIC Document Reproduction Service EJ625894.

9. Stirrat G. Reflections on learning and teaching medical ethics in UK medical schools. *Jour Med Ethics.* 2015;41:8–11.

10. Department of Medicine. Professional Behavior Standards. University of Toronto. Accessed September 28, 2015.

11. Family Educational Rights and Privacy Act Regulations. U.S. Department of Education. http://www2.ed.gov/policy/gen/guid/fpco/pdf/2012-final-regs.pdf. Accessed September 28, 2015.

12. Bosek M. Ethical decision making in anesthesia. In: Foster SD, Faut-Callahan M, eds. *A Professional Study and Resource Guide for the CRNA*. Park Ridge, IL: AANA Publishing; 2001:501–520.

13. Woolley AS. The long and tortured history of clinical evaluation. *Nurs Outlook.* 1977;25(5):308–315.

CHAPTER 13

Faculty Development

Judy Thompson, DNAP, APRN, CRNA

Keywords: Clinical faculty, education, faculty development, learning, teaching.

Key Concepts

- Faculty development is recognized as a vital part of nurse anesthesia education.
- Faculty are presently needed in our nurse anesthesia programs. Teaching us to teach serves our future as we prepare for doctoral education.
- Educational offerings are available and supported through our American Association of Nurse Anesthetists (AANA), councils, and educational institutions.
- The new doctoral standards mandate offerings in education for nurse anesthetists teaching in our programs.
- Many new educational resources and programs are available to assist educators and those seeking higher education.

Introduction

Much has changed since I wrote this chapter on faculty development back in 2006; so much so that the first edition's chapter seems to contain mostly information of historical significance now. I am actually very glad for the significant changes and incredible recognition that faculty development across the country has received in the last decade.

In the World of Education

What is faculty development? This was the simple question I asked in my first chapter 10 years ago. So much has changed. I do not need to ask this question any more of those in our field. Faculty development has taken on a new life across the country not only in our nurse anesthesia programs, but also in our association, the American Association of Nurse Anesthetists (AANA). Many of our programs have moved to academic institutions in a sole ownership capacity, or a hospital or health care system has partnered with an academic center to collaborate in a shared ownership, while sole ownership hospital-based programs with clinical affiliations at universities have decreased in numbers. Being affiliated with academic institutions has added much to the promotion of faculty development for both the clinician and the educator. Faculty development holds a very important place in these institutions. Educational institutions have been developing their faculty for years. The websites of many major universities and medical schools now have much information on faculty development programs. There are even organizations that will supply us with faculty and programs that teach us to teach, specifically, the Stanford Faculty Development Center for Medical Teachers.[1] They do a very good job of teaching us some of the essentials of teaching. Many institutions can be found with just a Google search.

The objectives of faculty development must still answer the same question as it did in the past: How will student improvement and/or achievement occur? This is, after all, the reason we develop faculty in the first place. The benefit of faculty teaching development programs is measured through surveys and student evaluations. Programs increase faculty members' value of teaching, rekindle their motivation and enthusiasm, and improve their knowledge, behaviors, and dissemination of skills.[2] Faculty development has been effective in improving faculty perceptions of the value of teaching.[3] Several models exist that can be implemented to support faculty teaching development. Institutions need to make informed decisions about which plan could be most successfully implemented in their college or school.

Faculty Focus is a website that offers much on faculty development and help with teaching in a number of areas, such as distance education, instructional design, educational assessment, teaching with technology, and flipping the classroom.[4] If you're interested in what works, and what doesn't, when it comes to teaching, learning, and leading—both in the traditional classroom and online — this might be a good place to start. Another good webite for developing faculty programs is California Northstate University College of Medicine.[5] This website provides many good ideas for supporting the creation of programs pertinent to faculty in health sciences and medicine and for our clinical faculty, in particular. There are, of course, many others that have become available in recent years.

Traditionally, faculty development for educators has been organized to include aspects that fit into the following categories: learning new clinical techniques, new contextual material (ie, new information, updates, recent discoveries) and new technological skills (ie, PowerPoint, multimedia, and presentations/simulations that could be used in teaching); educational techniques (ie, How do your students learn most effectively and how can you alter your teaching or examination style to maximize learning?); and personal management skills (ie, conflict resolution, communication, stress management). To create effective faculty development programs, it is important to get the faculty members' perspectives on what is actually needed. Without this input and the opportunity for faculty to collaborate and engage in growth and dialogue around common topics of interest, the essence of faculty development is lost.[6]

What do your clinical educators want to know? What is critically important for them to know in order to design your faculty development programs accordingly?

Evolution of Faculty Development: A Historical Perspective

The Council on Accreditation's standards relating to faculty development have undergone a number of substantive changes throughout the years. In the late 1960s, the standard required that all faculty of nurse anesthesia programs have preparations in evaluation and instruction. An intensive workshop lasting several days was organized by the AANA and held in Chicago. Classes were taught by an expert in the field of education. Following the course, attendees were required to spend several weeks in an anesthesia program other than the one they were affiliated with. They returned to Chicago after their internship, participated in more didactics, and took a written exam. A teacher's certificate was awarded following successful completion of this course. This course was an optional offering, but helped pave the way for other ideas on how to reach more faculty involved in teaching.

The I CARE workshops were also one of the early attempts to reach more faculty. Instituted in the 1970s, they were scheduled widely to include as many faculty in programs as possible. Schools were required to either send their faculty to these workshops or to have them participate within their own programs. The content included instruction, curriculum, testing, and measurement. Non-CRNA educators were contracted to put together and administer the I CARE program. College credit could be obtained if participants chose to seek approval with a university accepting the coursework.

In the early 1990s, revised standards broadened the language regarding faculty development. Coursework specific to evaluation and instruction was no longer mandated. The standards, in an attempt to be less prescriptive, had left it up to the schools to develop their faculty in ways of their own choosing. Faculty development could include a wider variety of clinical, technological, and scientific topics. Methodology of education was eliminated as a requirement.

With the mandate in the late 1990s that regional anesthesia administration be included in all curriculums, a new offering by the AANA was promoted called Teaching the Teachers. The program, which was held at an army base, was designed to teach nurse anesthesia educators how to teach regional anesthesia in their programs. A manual was written to accompany the course. Unfortunately, attendance was not as expected and the program was not repeated.

In the World of the CRNA Educator

Since the last edition of this book, we have been rapidly approaching full doctoral education by 2025 for all of the nurse anesthetists coming out of our programs. This means that all programs must offer the doctoral degree by 2022. Position statement: The AANA supports doctoral education for entry into nurse anesthesia practice by 2025.[7]

The new doctoral standards are different than those that we taught in the past when all of our programs were master's degree programs. The Council on Accreditation of Nurse Anesthesia Educational Programs (COA) has placed a much greater emphasis on faculty recognition and development and has added much-needed requirements for those who educate our students. Those requirements state: Core CRNA faculty (program administrator, assistant program administrator and course directors) involved in education must have formal instruction in curriculum, evaluation, and instruction.

Formal instruction in curriculum, evaluation, and instruction includes completed educational content evidenced on a transcript from an accredited institution of higher education, an AANA-approved continuing education (CE) program, or a CE program approved by another nationally recognized professional approval organization.[8]

The National Board of Certification and Recertification of Nurse Anesthetists (NBCRNA) and the new Continued Professional Certification (CPC) program give recognition to educators, preceptors, and those seeking higher education to meet the needs now and in the future for faculty in nurse anesthesia programs. Credits are now given for the following:

- Any role that involves direct clinical supervision or teaching behaviors for learners of any level or type. This includes, but is not limited to, student nurse anesthetists, medical students, or registered nurses gaining airway management experience.[9]
- Content development for educational purposes (eg, didactic/clinical faculty; journal clubs; seminars; M&M conferences; CE activities).[9]
- Academic credits must be delivered by an institution that is accredited by an agency recognized by the US Department of Education. Participants must receive a minimum grade of "C" or a "pass" on a pass/fail scale. Class B value is calculated based on the number of academic credit hours earned.[9]

Faculty development at both the Assembly of School Faculty (ASF) and the AANA's annual congress is widely promoted. Many programs have been in place now for a number of years that "teach the teacher"—from the Educator's Institute (a program sponsored by the ASF education committee which had faculty development topics and awarded a certificate for attendance many years ago) to topics on mentoring, developing care plans, leading inquiry and research, remediation for struggling students, flipping the classroom, grant writing, and numerous other topics on teaching and using simulation. The ASF has always been geared to teaching us to teach and providing much-needed information on what we need to know as educators. While attendance at this meeting has grown significantly, many of our clinical preceptors are not able to attend, or perceive that this meeting is for educators running our nurse anesthesia programs only. There is much to gain for the clinician teaching in our programs today.

Our first edition of *A Resource for Nurse Anesthesia Educators* was a big success for AANA Publishing, showing the desire that those teaching in our programs have for more information on the variety of educational topics contained in the text.

The New England Assembly of School faculty still runs the faculty development workshop annually, which is now approaching its 20th year. This workshop has gained in popularity for its diverse offerings of an educational and non-clinical nature. Topics have included:

- Evaluation
- Legal issues for educators
- Trigger films in education
- Stress management
- Conflict resolution
- Public speaking
- Using simulation in our teaching
- Teaching to generational differences
- Novice to Expert: How we learn
- The importance of communication
- Emotional intelligence

There exists a wide variety of offerings to expand on and teach the academic educators to be better teachers, but what about the clinical practitioner/educator? Many are placed into the position of teacher when they are assigned to precept a student from one of the ever-expanding nurse anesthesia programs. As more programs adopt clinical sites of all types to broaden the opportunities for their students, more nurse anesthetists and anesthesiologists are being put into a different role from that of the clinician they have been trained to be, to that of the educator that they are now expected to become. In academia, another very urgent concern as our programs rapidly move into the doctoral framework and into academic centers is the shortage of qualified faculty. Nursing realized that their push toward doctoral education for advanced practice nurses could not be realized by the initial deadline of 2015. The need for qualified faculty to teach in these doctoral programs was not going to be a reality within this tight timeline and, thus, the goal needed to be realigned. In 2014, the American Association of Colleges of Nursing (AACN) found that 13,444 qualified applicants were turned away from master's programs, and 1,844 qualified applicants were turned away from doctoral programs. The primary reason for not accepting all qualified students was a shortage of faculty.[10] At present, only nurse anesthesia continues to move toward the goal of doctoral education with a projected date.

Clinical educators are returning to completion programs in large numbers to obtain the needed degree to teach at the university level. While they have the skills to safely administer an anesthetic, they are novices in the role of faculty. Faculty development for all of these transitioning educators is critical. In a recent study published in the *International Journal of Nursing Education Scholarship*, it was reported that there are three core teaching needs of novice clinical teachers; the authors identified support strategies and recommendations to address these identified needs. The evidence suggests these three basic needs are: socialization, professional development, and the need for reflection and confidence building.[11] Socialization refers to the need to be supported and is defined as the need to acclimatize, to belong, and to connect with students. Professional development needs to include orientation, guidance from experienced peers, and feedback on their teaching practice. Mentor support of novice clinical faculty was found to be helpful as was evaluation by the institution. Finally, self-reflection allows novice teachers to recognize which skills and strengths they bring to teaching and what further developing of their teaching practice should include to build on their confidence.[11] Faculty development should be ongoing to continue to build confidence and increase self-awareness and promote teaching methods and evaluation.[11]

Medical schools across the country as well have developed offerings to work with didactic faculty and those in clinical roles to better serve those students assigned to their facilities. Articles are now abundant on educating the clinician to teach. AANA Learn[12] includes teaching modules for credits and helps those providers affiliated with academic institutions learn and improve on their teaching methods as well as meet the new COA requirements. There are modules available on didactic and clinical instruction, evaluation, and goals of writing and developing curriculum. These modules are available and award credit which meets the requirements of curriculum, evaluation, and instruction for educators now required by the COA.

To many of us, clinical teaching and all that goes along with it, is a new experience. How many of us were ever prepared to communicate our knowledge as practitioners, deal with learning styles, or challenge, motivate, reinforce, and evaluate one another? Many of us not only become clinical instructors within nurse anesthesia programs, but also take on roles of clinical coordinators, didactic instructors, and members of academic committees dealing with curriculum, evaluation, advertisement, due process, and admissions. With ever-expanding and challenging roles for nurse anesthetists, where do we learn to be this educator? And when given this role, where do we learn to do it well?

Sometimes just an introduction to clinical teaching, a Clinical Teaching 101, can be offered at the various clinical sites where our students learn the art and science of administering anesthesia. Program directors from the school can visit the sites and offer a presentation at one of the morning meetings or educational seminars as a way to take this introduction on the road. It is a good and simple way to start with those who work with our students on a daily basis. The presentation(s) can be interactive, as all of the clinical nurse anesthetists and physicians have been taught by others in their clinical learning, both good and bad. Discuss what made the preceptor that they learned from a good educator. What did he or she like best about those who had a positive effect? What made others ineffective or just plain bad? This always generates a lively discussion and can be a good lead-in to development of the clinical faculty. Something like this may change the direction of some who teach the way they were taught, which may not be something you want to perpetuate. Virginia Commonwealth University (VCU) has a series of educational trigger films[13] that have been very successful. They depict real clinical situations that many have encountered while working with new learners in the clinical area. Very few seasoned preceptors have not encountered some, if not all, of these situations and have had a chance to ponder and discuss with others. This has served as a valuable teaching moment for faculty.

Clinical faculty often need instruction on evaluation, so this, too, can be a form of faculty development offered by the conducting institution. Fair and constructive evaluation is critical to a program and to the safety of our patients; thus, this is a piece of faculty development that must not be ignored. Preceptors are on the front lines and need to know how to deal with fair and constructive evaluation; their know-how is vital. Sometimes this simple form of faculty development will inspire in those educators a desire to learn more and participate in some of the vast offerings available at meetings, on-line, or through webinars, articles, and scheduled workshops.

Some institutions have been introducing a teaching program for nurse anesthesia educators and new students into their curriculums. A perfect place to include this might be in the professional aspects portion of the curriculum. Most CRNAs in their lifetime careers will have some exposure to teaching, whether with students in an affiliated nurse anesthesia program or perhaps a medical student/resident doing an observation day or rotation through the anesthesia department. As CRNAs, most of us have never been exposed to any information on adult education or even on the topic of how adults learn. There is evidence to suggest that educational programs that target the needs of clinical educators can have a positive effect on teachers and improve the learning environment for students.[14]

As part of my role as a program director, I instituted a senior project at my institution. I was able to do this at the time because we were a hospital-based program and had students at several levels in one institution. This could be achieved in any clinical site that has students from your program that are at different levels in the clinical area. In the beginning of the project, I met with all of the students to discuss the roles of the senior (as teacher) and the first and second year students. We discussed in an open forum what they (all the students) felt helped them learn in the clinical area and what the preceptors did or did not do that encouraged and supported this learning. We created a set of objectives and discussed the process of evaluation and debriefing. The purpose of this preparation was to introduce the students to a teaching role. Support from the CRNA clinical preceptors was mixed, so we had to select those who supported the project. Their role would be to support the "student teacher," but to make sure that patient safety and care were first and foremost safeguarded in the process along with compliance of our nurse anesthesia standards. The clinical preceptors who were supportive of this effort were also briefed and encouraged to give feedback to both the student and the director. Senior students were assigned to a room with a first or second year student. Their role was as the preceptor and educator. They met before the case to discuss and review the student care plan and to offer suggestions. They worked hand-in-hand in the case with their student. CRNA preceptors met with the senior to review the plan as well. At the end of the day, the senior sat down with the student and reviewed/debriefed the case(s). What did they learn? Both learned an enormous amount and the project, which lasted about two months, was a real eye-opener to both groups of students. The first- and second-year students loved working with the upperclassmen; they felt they were less threatening and understood the complexities of the role of a student learner better than the CRNAs since they were in this role at the present time. The senior students felt that the role of preceptor was terribly underappreciated and very difficult. They got to see firsthand what CRNAs face daily, stepping back a bit to let someone else learn while being there to safeguard patient care and to be supportive. We practiced the art of evaluating constructively and communicating appropriately. This was a trial offering to give our students a chance to be an educator and to discuss the role and learn from it. I had this in place for three years and for each year that we implemented it, the evaluations were excellent. I considered it an innovation in education. It was difficult to support even in our environment. We needed supportive clinical preceptors who were willing to step back and allow for student teaching, supportive anesthesiologists (as we were in an anesthesia care team environment and this buy-in was even more difficult), the right kind of case, the agreement of the surgeon, and much support from the program as to the time commitment. My idea, while new to me, was not a new one according to the literature. Between 1978–2012, Michigan State University's (MSU) Primary Care Faculty Development program was a successful national on-campus/at home, part-time faculty development fellowship program. The overall goal of the program was to prepare primary care physicians for full time careers in academic medicine. The fellowship curriculum addressed the basic roles of instruction, research, and leadership and also other domains such as the use of computer technology and adjustment to working in the academic community.[15] The program was four weeks in length, and students learned and practiced teaching research and leadership skills via workshops, seminars, and small group activities. They were also given ample time to demonstrate their new skills. In the ideal world, this sounds like a wonderful opportunity, but we are nurse anesthetists first and foremost and the time this would take in our busy curriculums might be difficult at best.

Our Standards

Our standards and guidelines address faculty development. Standard III, Criteria VI states: "The educational environment provides opportunities for faculty development."[16] Faculty development is part of all programs now, mandated by our own standards as well as the requirements of most academic institutions. Our standards now address the content areas which include curriculum, evaluation, and instruction but what specifically should this cover within these broad areas? It is an area that is widely interpreted and leaves variation open for our programs.

In 1999, the Education Committee of the AANA surveyed the directors of nurse anesthesia programs and compiled a list of what the various programs did for faculty development. The Education Committee also surveyed what the directors would like to see made available for their faculties. The list was broad and varied. Some items under activities currently available to faculties included:

- Annual report preparation/self-study preparation
- Management/leadership/time management/computer competency workshops
- State meetings with various faculty topics
- Research grants
- Student research presentations

- Statistics workshops
- Simulator, computer, and crisis resource management training
- In-services on the evaluation tools
- Journal clubs
- New employee orientation
- Various programs within the universities on faculty development issues
- Use of technology to teach

The list compiled within the same survey that addressed which activities directors and faculty would like to see made available included support of the programs that were out there, but asked specifically for very different things. This list repeatedly included some of the following:

- Successful innovative teaching strategies
- Stronger Internet-based forums for communication among faculty
- Workshops to help develop assistant directors advance to directors, and faculty to advance to administrative positions
- Workshops on teaching the adult learner
- Testing programs and item writing
- Beginning research programs for students
- Teaching regional anesthesia
- Management skills and public speaking
- Objective evaluation
- Creation of a faculty pertinent video on educational/teaching how-to's
- Instructional techniques
- Counseling students
- Dealing with learning styles and the difficult student
- Legal and ethical issues in the clinical evaluation process.

While this list is older, faculty are still often in need of and request just these things that were listed almost 20 years ago. Many of the items on the past list have become a reality and have been in place now for some time. New directors and assistant directors are invited each year to a workshop held by the COA to prepare them for the roles that they will hold in the education of our students and accreditation of our programs. There are also workshops to help programs and faculty transition to doctoral education. Webinars are frequently available for many topics such as item writing given by NBCRNA, and grant writing and management given by the AANA Foundation. Mentorship of students at the Assembly of School Faculty is a regular event that encourages students to learn from experienced educators and to get involved in CRNA education. AANA Learn has been added to our offerings and contains not only clinical information, but information on education and teaching. Our first addition has expanded and grown to include more topics that our members have requested. We have expanded on simulation and provided our colleagues with innovations in teaching such as online learning and flipping the classroom. Teaching to different generations and the use of technology are some of the topics often requested by educators.

Teaching Us to Be Teachers Today

We still need the tools to teach us to be educators, and to be the best and most effective teachers that we can be. Our clinical faculty are the ones we model: the ones who give us the skills we will take with us as clinicians; the ones who give us the "pearls" of administrating a safe anesthetic; the ones who will allow us to make decisions, try techniques, correlate our didactic knowledge in the clinical arena, and gain autonomy through their mentorship; and, to one day teach our colleagues.

Clinical faculty often have dual roles within their anesthesia programs. Many prepare and deliver individual didactic presentations or teach entire courses within the curriculum of an anesthesia program. These faculty often seek information on communication, preparation, and evaluation among other offerings related to faculty development. Administrators of programs, clinical coordinators, and clinical faculty who serve on the schools' various committees may seek expanded types of faculty development. These might include curriculum design, examination preparation, item and objective writing, interviewing, public speaking, utilization of technology in research, and delivery of information and evaluations.

Faculty Development Within Reach of All

In 1997, the New England Assembly of School Faculty looked into this exact idea. (The New England Assembly of School Faculty is a regional advisory committee from the New England area, New York, and New Jersey made up of all directors, representative educational members from our programs, a student representative, and a public member.) Nurse anesthesia programs had been expanding; new ones were opening and some of the existing structures were changing as they signed on affiliates, both academic and clinical, or moved to academic settings. With these changes came many clinical practitioners who would assume the role of faculty to our students. These new faculty, as well as many of the existing faculty, looked to the program directors for guidance about how to best serve students and programs. It was with that impetus that the Assembly looked for ways to help them.

The AANA, in particular, the ASF, and Education Committee organizers provided the New England Assembly with the ideas for just this type of faculty development. The directors of the New England nurse anesthesia programs regularly attended the AANA Assembly of School Faculty meeting, but they questioned how to get this valuable information back to share with the clinical faculty at home. Many more clinical faculty now attend the ASF, but many are still unable to since they are staffing the operating rooms .The leaders and planners of the New England Assembly decided to take faculty development on the road. We organized a workshop with an educational theme: the New England Assembly Faculty Development Workshop. To fund this project, faculty in this group petitioned all of our schools, university and hospital-based, to contribute a modest amount. The first time it was held, we selected a speaker that many of the directors had heard at one of the annual meetings, who was positive, energetic, and motivated. She shared some pertinent information on effective communication, student motivation, and conflict resolution. Her presentation was relevant to our interaction with our students and our colleagues in the clinical sites. We selected the auditorium of a centrally located hospital that offered a low cost for our first workshop. We applied for six continuing education units for our all-day program and paid for the hospital cafeteria lunch for all who attended. We made name tags with every attendee's affiliation site to encourage networking between all in attendance. We called it the Faculty Appreciation Seminar. "If you build it (right), they will come" was our philosophy.

We sat back and waited, and they did come! Our objectives then were to provide a free workshop around educational issues, provide an opportunity for all of our faculty at both our academic and clinical sites to network and share concerns, and to provide a "thank you" to our most important colleagues — our clinical educators.

Our objectives have not changed to this day. We have been holding this workshop for 20 years now. We have expanded to a much nicer location, offered better food, opened the workshop (for a modest fee) to others outside our geographical area, and even won the Crystal Apple award for innovation in education in 2002. We still provide continuing education units and offer attendance to our own faculties for a very nominal sum. The program evaluations from participants then and now are very enlightening. Our faculties have told us what they need and want. We have taken their leads and designed programs to fulfill these areas where the need for knowledge of an educational nature is greatest.

Thus far, our programs have included topics on legal issues, dealing with the difficult students, conflict resolution, effective teaching methods, public speaking, management styles, evaluation, emotional intelligence and the role of doctoral education in promoting leaders, among others. We have used lecturers, interactive presentations, role-play, videos, trigger films, and discussion formats. With the changes available in technology now, this type of workshop can be available to all of our faculties even in the most remote areas. While the New England region is geographically small enough for attendees to return home the same day, individual states, no matter how large, can have workshops for a weekend in a central location or held in conjunction with one of the national meetings such as a pre-convention/post-convention workshop modeled after our regional breakout sessions. Workshops can be offered as a webinar or an on-line course. Faculty can pursue higher education, and are doing so in record numbers. On-line and hybrid programs are making this a reality. They are designed to be friendly to working CRNAs, and to promote and encourage them to adopt educator and leadership roles. Many of these courses include a course in educational leadership that will "teach us to teach."

Future (and Past) Thoughts on Faculty Development

The AANA has historically been involved in promoting faculty development and needs to continue to provide this support and opportunity to our programs. Clinical CRNAs and students need to be encouraged to become involved in education and to be comfortable in this role. Back in 2006, I wrote: "The CCNA (Council on Certification of Nurse Anesthetists) should highly encourage CRNAs to obtain a portion of their recertification continuing education credits in educational offerings (ie, evaluation etc.) if they are involved in the teaching of students." It was my wish then that this would occur and encourage us to become educators as well as the clinicians that we are upon graduation. This statement in my former chapter has come to light. AANA Learn offers the following programs:

- Educator Series: Didactic and Clinical Instruction
- Educator Series: Evaluation for Nurse Anesthesia Educators
- Educator Series: Principles and Goals of Writing Curriculum

All of the programs are worth one Class A credit, according to the new CPC program. The former CCNA is now NBCRNA. The new CPC program promotes teaching and learning to be an educator. Recognized as Class B credits are returning to school and taking courses; speaking at a conference; presenting a Journal Club or Grand Rounds; publishing, teaching, or supervising clinically; participating in advocacy both at the state and/or national level; conducting scholarly projects or publications; and, once again, taking life support courses. This in itself will promote faculty development in so many ways.

I wrote then that "CCNA should consider giving continuing education units for teaching in programs and mentoring students for CE credits, and that CRNA faculty who prepare and deliver lectures and/or coursework to our students should be eligible to receive continuing education credits." This, too, has come to pass and our teachers are encouraged to teach with full recognition and credits.

Summary

So much has changed in the past 10 years. We, as CRNAs, were trained to be clinicians first and foremost. The role of the educator has, for most of us, fallen on our shoulders. Some of us are natural teachers with the gift of patience, the knowledge to precept, and the ability to motivate; but, for the majority of us, we need the tools that good faculty development programs can provide.

This quote from the former website of a community college is just as relevant today as it was back when I wrote this chapter in 2006:

"Faculty is one of our greatest assets. A program of faculty development is therefore dedicated to aggressively supporting the ongoing personal and professional growth of faculty. By providing information, training, forums, connections, and activities, the program vitalizes the faculty, strengthens the program, improves the quality of instruction, and helps the school better serve the community."

References

1. Stanford Faculty Development Center for Medical Teachers. http://sfdc.stanford.edu. Accessed August 30, 2016.

2. Steinert Y, Mann K, Centeno A, et al. A systematic review of faculty development initiatives designed to improve teaching effectiveness in medical education: BEME Guide No. 8. *Med Teach*. 2006;28(6):497–526.

3. Lancaster J, Stein S, Garrelts MacLean L, et al. Faculty development program models to advance teaching and learning within health science programs. *Am J Pharm Educ*. June 17, 2014;78(5):99.

4. Faculty Focus. http://www.facultyfocus.com/free-reports/. Accessed July, 2016.

5. California Northstate University College of Medicine. http://medicine.cnsu.edu/faculty/faculty-development. Accessed August, 2016.

6. A Checklist for Effective Faculty Development Programs. Faculty Focus. http://www.facultyfocus.com/articles/faculty-development/a-checklist-for-effective-faculty-development-programs/. Accessed July, 2016.

7. Position on Doctoral Preparation of Nurse Anesthetists. Park Ridge, IL: American Association of Nurse Anesthetists; 2007.

8. Standards for Accreditation of Nurse Anesthesia Programs. Park Ridge, IL: American Association of Nurse Anesthetists; 2014.

9. Continued Professional Certification (CPC) Program Class B Requirements—Professional Development Activities and their Values Approved by the NBCRNA for Use with the CPC Program. Source: NBCRNA website: http://www.nbcrna.com/cpc/Documents/2016/CPC_Class_B_revised.pdf. Accessed August 31, 2016.

10. Nursing Faculty Shortage. American Association of Colleges of Nursing. http://www.aacn.nche.edu/media-relations/fact-sheets/nursing-faculty-shortage. Accessed July, 2016.

11. Jetha F, Boschma G, Clauson M. Professional development needs of novice nursing clinical teachers: a rapid evidence assessment. *Int J Nurs Educ Scholarsh*. 2016;13(1):1–10.

12. AANA Learn. American Association of Nurse Anesthetists. http://www.aana.com/ceandeducation/Pages/AANALearn-Landing-Page.aspx. Accessed September 2016.

13. Hartland W, Biddle C, Fallacaro M. Accessing the living laboratory: trigger films as an aid to developing, enabling, and assessing anesthesia clinical instructors. *AANA J*. 2003;71(4):287–291.

14. Skeff KM, Stratos GA, Bergen MR, et al. Regional teaching improvement programs for community-based teachers. *Am J Med*. 1999;106(1):76–80.

15. Yelon S, Ford K, Anderson W. Twelve tips for increasing transfer of training from faculty development programs. *Med Teach*. 2014;36:945–950.

16. The Standards and Guidelines: Council on Accreditation of Nurse Anesthesia Educational Programs. Park Ridge, IL: American Association of Nurse Anesthetists; 2013.

CHAPTER 14

Simulation in Nurse Anesthesia Education

John M. O'Donnell, DrPH, MSN, CRNA
Paul E. Phrampus, MD, FACEP, FSSH

Keywords: Assessment, best practices, debriefing, scenario design, simulation education, translational science.

Key Concepts

- Simulation is now accepted across the entire health care industry as an important component of provider preparation and safety and has moved from a focus on computerized mannequins to include a spectrum of activities and applications ranging from simple task trainers to virtual environments.
- Simulation can be used as a primary approach or supplemental activity.
- Common uses for simulation in nurse anesthesia education include development of skills in procedures; crisis management; management of common clinical events; nontechnical domains (patient and provider communication, team skills, professionalism); decision making; competence verification; science concept reinforcement; preparation for specific clinical activities; and remediation of deficits.
- Simulations should be designed with the learner level and educational objectives as a foundation.
- The purpose of any simulation is creation of activities and environments that are real enough to allow performance improvements to transfer from the simulation lab environment to the patient care environment.
- Faculty preparation is critical for effective simulation with a wide array of resources available including best practices, assessment instruments, standards, terminology dictionaries, and regulatory body recommendations.
- Scenario topic selection derived from needs assessment and linked to specific educational objectives is ideal. Adherence to strict development pathways will result in efficient development of effective scenarios that can be deployed reliably by prepared instructors.
- Faculty should resist the lure to introduce unnecessary complexity during scenario design. Extraneous scenario details, unnecessary equipment or unfocused debriefing points can increase student cognitive load, which can impair the learning process.
- Post-simulation debriefing should be structured, allow student input, and ensure that educational objectives are met.

Worldwide Adoption of Simulation

Simulation has been defined as "a technique, not a technology, to replace or amplify real experiences with guided experiences that evoke or replicate substantial aspects of the real world in a fully interactive manner."[1] Simulated educational approaches are now embedded in health care professional training programs across the world, and the methodology involved has been described as one of the most important innovations in health care education over the last 25 years.[2–6] Simulation can be used in all phases of a nurse anesthesia curriculum to reinforce concepts of basic science, help students prepare for entry into clinical practice, evaluate new devices, enhance professionalism skills, develop teamwork skills, and augment real clinical experiences (through rare event training and crisis resource management).[2,7–20]

The use of simulation as either a primary educational approach (simulation-based medical or nursing education) or as a supplement for both didactic teaching and clinical experience (simulation augmentation) are now well-described and accepted educational methods with a growing literature and evidence base. As of 2013, more than 10,900 papers had been published with this large body of literature reinforcing that simulation educational methods are now deeply embedded across a wide spectrum of health care education and research applications.[21] Simulation literature is available in journals throughout the health professions and in education-specific publications as well as the lay literature. Areas of research and educational focus are as diverse as the health care professions themselves with the prospect of providing students with experiences in a non-clinical environment that are real enough that the learnings acquired will translate to improvement in preparation for actual clinical care. This prospect is especially appealing to both students and faculty. Further, there are now a number of meta-analyses and systematic reviews that have been conducted looking at educational practices and conditions of teaching and learning, as well as a wide variety of outcomes.[21–31] This approach offers the opportunity to prepare students for aspects of clinical care that are less common, but critical to practice such as fires, anaphylaxis, and hemorrhage, etc.[8,15,18,32] These targets include high-risk procedures (central venous catheter placement), rare event management (malignant hyperthermia), and teamwork skill development.[16,33–38]

The 2011 Research Consensus Conference of the international Society for Simulation in Healthcare reviewed the available literature for evidence supporting a wide spectrum of educational and research applications including procedural skill training, instructional design, reporting findings, and describing a simulation translational science nomenclature.[39–43] This translational science nomenclature for simulation educational and research efforts is important because it can help nurse anesthesia educators to understand and frame their work. It is also useful in conceptualizing objectives for scenarios and the courses in which they exist. The traditional definition of translational science describes the process by which research moves from the laboratory or bench setting to the clinical area or bedside setting.[44,45] This process can be applied to nurse anesthesia simulation education and research efforts as the student anesthetist's knowledge, skill, and attitude outcomes gained in the simulation environment then translate into actual improvements in clinical skill with resultant improvement in their ability to care for our patients (**Table 14.1**).

Table 14.1 Translational Science Targets, Simulation Translational Science Targets, and a Potential Nurse Anesthesia Translational Science Target [60,131–134]

	Traditional translational science targets	Simulation translational science targets	Target audience	Setting	Potential nurse anesthesia translational science target
T1[a]	Basic science principles are translated to clinical application	Simulation educational laboratory improvement	Individuals and teams	Simulation lab	Airway training
T2	Evidence-based guidelines are developed and applied in clinical situations	Improved patient care practices	Individuals and teams	Clinical area or in-vitro simulation setting	Improved airway skill/ increased opportunity
T3	Evidence-based guidelines become accepted health care practice (HP)	Improved patient outcomes	Individuals/ patient cohorts	Clinical area/ facility	Decreased airway complication rates
T4	Outcomes research demonstrates the impact of the HP on population health	Improved population outcomes, cost savings, skill retention, systemic educational improvements	Patient population/ provider populations	Health care and educational systems	Reduction of costs related to airway complications

Abbreviation: T[a], translational phase.

Simulation Literature in Nurse Anesthesia

In nurse anesthesia education, simulation can be as simplistic as using a textbook to practice epidural catheter threading or a part-task trainer for spinal needle insertion (**Figures 14.1** and **14.2**, next page).

Figure 14.1

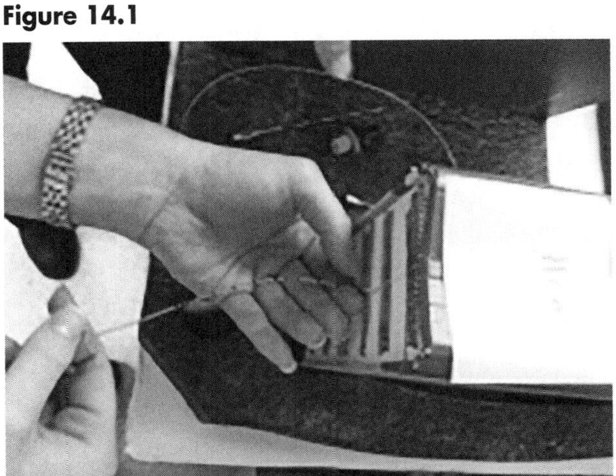

Use of a well-worn, outdated anesthesia textbook as a supplemental part-task simulator for deliberate practice of the advancement of an epidural catheter to a specific depth. Note: the magic marker stripes are meant to represent spinous processes.

Figure 14.2

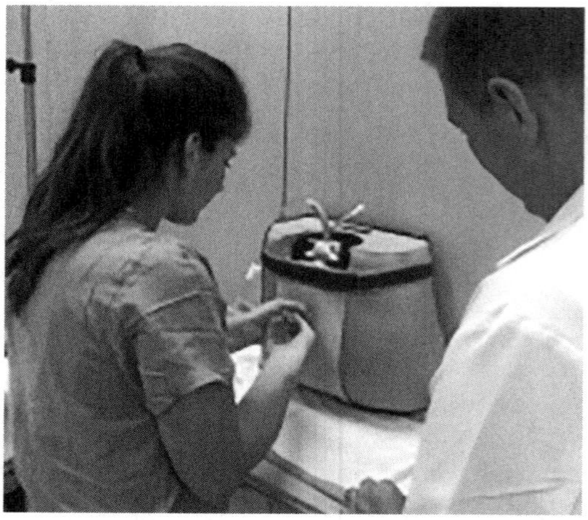

Student utilizing a part-task Nasco (Fort Atkinson, Wisconsin) Spinal Anesthesia Trainer. In this case the student is deliberately practicing the needle angle, insertion of the needle, hand position, dural puncture, and CSF return assessment. Later, the student will be asked to complete the entire technique with prepping, gloving, draping, and use of a kit as part of a scaffolded competency assessment.

Simulation can also be complex as with computerized mannequins that can respond to interventions with realistic physiologic and pharmacologic responses. According to the standards and guidelines of anesthesia educational programs, practice doctorate, "Simulated clinical experiences are learning experiences involving the imitation or representation of clinical activities that are designed for competency attainment, competency assessment, or competency maintenance."[46] While most anesthesia nursing educators have substantial exposure to some form of simulation through task training, Basic Life Support (BLS), Advanced Cardiac Life Support (ACLS), and Pediatric Life Support (PALS) certification, formal preparation in curriculum development and application of known best practices has been limited because these elements have not been a traditional component of nurse anesthesia educational curricula.

Simulation has been documented in nurse anesthesia educational approaches for more than 25 years. Use of high-fidelity patient simulators in nurse anesthesia education was first published by Fletcher at the University of Pittsburgh in 1995.[47] This *AANA Journal* Course review paper introduced the concept of patient simulation and the capabilities of simulators to the profession. Later that year, Fletcher and O'Donnell (University of Pittsburgh) conducted the first formal instructor training program for nurse anesthesia educators at the University of Buffalo in collaboration with educators from the University of Toronto. Also in 1995, the first simulation center in a school of nursing was opened at the Medical College of Georgia and the development was led by the program director Alfred Lupien.

In a follow-up publication, Fletcher described development of the ERR WATCH (Environment, Resources, Reevaluation, Workload, Attention, Teamwork, Communication, Help) acronym, which was used for nurse anesthesia student crisis management training at the University of Pittsburgh.[19] O'Donnell et al, described the development of the first anesthesia crisis resource management (ACRM) course for nurse anesthesia students in the United States.[18] This paper described course development and operational considerations, and provided a financial breakdown for the cost of course development in 1997 dollars.[18] Fallacaro surveyed anesthesia practitioner perceptions on the importance of training students to face untoward anesthetic events. Anesthetists were asked to report on how often they had experienced the events and also to judge the importance of training for them.[32] Hotchkiss and

Mendoza reported on the use of simulation to gain experience in malignant hyperthermia case management. These authors concluded that the ability to experience rare but critical events is a highly valuable application of the method.[16] Henrichs et al, conducted a qualitative study of nurse anesthesia student perceptions related to management of simple to complex problems during simulation. Students were interviewed after four training episodes that included simple to complex events.[17] Students reported experiencing apprehension and fear prior to events but identified multiple potential advantages including enhanced critical thinking and problem solving. Disadvantages identified by students included the lack of realism and issues around a lack of familiarity with the system.[17] Hotchkiss et al, looked specifically at the authenticity of the simulation experience for critical events management. This study included the use of videotaped clinical crisis vignettes or trigger films, which complemented simulation activities. Students were videotaped during short crisis events with videos rated by seasoned anesthetists. While the reviewers reported that the events appeared to be realistic, concerns regarding ability to mirror the actual operating room (OR) culture were noted. Participants were reported to be anxious, hypervigilant, and mechanical in some of their treatment. Concern was noted that the short length of scenarios contributed to the lack of realism.[15]

Hartland et al, used simulation-derived scenarios in working toward development of valid and reliable trigger films of various clinical events and student-instructor interactions. These researchers noted that the development of such films could represent a valuable approach to developing clinical instructors. Also in 2003, Register et al, reported on using a simulator and associated software as a supplemental educational tool for learning about management of patients with intra-pulmonary shunt. Both CRNAs and students were educated in the program.[13]

More recently, investigators have reported use of supplemental technologies to augment simulation training efforts for nurse anesthetists. These include multimedia augmentation (Chen et al),[48] hand-held computers in support of decision-making (Coopmans et al)[12] and video-facilitated feedback post simulation (Grant et al).[49,50]

Paige et al, reported on the use of simulation training for inter-professional training. Teamwork scales were used to determine performance among teams including nurse anesthesia students, nursing students, and medical students. Significant improvement was reported in team performance across two scenarios.[51] Lyk-Jensen et al, reported on the adaptation of the anesthesia non-technical skills (ANTS) tool for nurse anesthesia practitioners in the Netherlands. This tool is designed to provide information on key anesthesiologist nontechnical skills (communication, situational awareness, etc.). The authors reported successful modification with the development of a role-specific N-ANTS tool (nurse anesthesia ANTS).[52]

Airway and other procedural skills have been studied in nurse anesthesia education using a simulation model. Several investigators have looked at using simulation to teach resuscitation and airway skills for nurse anesthetists and students.[53,54] In a unique application, Sell and Palmer reported having nurse anesthesia students demonstrate airway skills to grade school children. A simulated OR and series of skill stations were set up in a disadvantaged grade school. Nurse anesthesia students met the Council on Accreditation (COA) requirement to teach others through this community outreach event.[55]

Cannon-Diehl et al, and Hawkins et al, reported on surveys conducted to assess CRNA perceptions regarding use of simulation in educational programs and for higher stakes evaluations including certification and recertification.[2,56] Cannon-Diehl et al, indicated that respondents were familiar with simulation and felt that ACLS, anesthesia machine issues, and malignant hyperthermia management would be valuable for continuing education efforts. However, while respondents valued simulation as a competency assessment, they had mixed-responses with higher stakes assessment such as recertification.[2] Hawkins et al, conducted a pilot study that included survey and experiential activities. A consensus of practicing CRNAs surveyed (n =378) felt that simulation should be used within nurse anesthesia educational programs with more than 85% believing it should also be used for initial certification; however, only 52.9% agreed that simulation should be required as a continuing education component for recertification.[56]

In order to use simulation methodology for high stakes exams in nurse anesthesia, it is critical to develop valid and reliable assessment instruments that are able to capture performance. Henrichs et al, reported on a head-to-head comparison of CRNAs (n=26) vs. anesthesiologists' (n=35) performance on management of intraoperative emergency events. The purpose of the study was to determine if differences in performance between the two providers could be quantified in the simulated environment. It was reported that the overall average score of CRNA participants was slightly lower (59.9% vs. 66.6%). No attempt was made to establish a passing standard; however, the authors concluded that the wide variability of performance within both groups was concerning and suggested that clinical skill training using simulation could potentially be used to improve the level of preparation across their community.[57]

Paige et al, at Florida International University (FIU) report on the use of objective, structured, clinical exams (OSCEs) in nurse anesthesia education. These exams range across the entire seven-term curriculum and are parallel with well-established educational methods from other health care disciplines. Both formative and summative evaluation components were included in the OSCE process with students required to demonstrate specific competencies across a range of skills and behaviors. The work was conducted in the FIU Simulation Training Assessment and Research (STAR) center and utilized Laerdal 3G (Stavengar, Norway) simulators.[51] Overstreet et al, also reported on the use of simulation in assessment of competence among nurse anesthesia students. These authors advocated that simple assessment checklists should be replaced by more complex rubrics to reduce subjectivity.[7]

Terminology, Best Practices, Accreditation, Certification

Older simulation literature is filled with unclear terminology and outdated terms. In 2016, the International Society for Simulation in Healthcare published the *Healthcare Simulation Dictionary*.[58] This dictionary, along with the recently published International Nursing Association for Clinical Simulation and Learning (INACSL) terminology (Standard I), promises to enhance communications among educators and also to standardize reporting of education and research findings within the field.[59]

Best practices for simulation educators have been reviewed in a number of systematic reviews with simulation societies and regulatory bodies such as the National Councils of State Boards of Nursing weighing in to identify educational approaches which are thought to represent best practices[59–71] (**Table 14.2**).

Table 14.2 Systematic Review Best Practices Results, INACSL Standards, and National Council of State Boards of Nursing Guidelines for Pre-Licensure Programs and Faculty Preparation Checklist

Issenberg et al., Systematic Review (2005)[63]	McGaghie et al., Systematic Review (2010)[60]	INACSL Standards of Best Practice in Simulation Education (2013–2015)[65–71]	Alexander et al., NCSBN Guidelines, Pre-licensure Programs, Faculty Checklist (2015)[64]	Alexander et al., NCSBN Guidelines- Pre-licensure Programs, Faculty Checklist (2015)[64]
Feedback	Feedback	Terminology	Institutional commitment	Theory-based
Repetitive practice	Deliberate practice	Professional integrity (of participants)	Appropriate facilities	Adhere to INACSL Standards of Best Practice
Curriculum integration	Curriculum integration	Participant objectives	Resources: educational, technology, equipment to meet objectives	Evaluation tool design is based on INACSL standards
Practice with increasing level of difficulty	Outcome measurement	Facilitation	Lead faculty/sim personnel are qualified	Outcomes/objectives communicated to students prior to simulation
Use of multiple learning strategies	Simulation fidelity	Facilitator	Faculty are prepared to lead simulations	Establish a supportive environment encouraging: • active listening • repetitive practice • reflection
Provide for clinical variation	Skill acquisition & maintenance	Debriefing process	Programmatic understanding of policies and processes supporting simulation experiences	Appropriate facilitation methods
Controlled environment	Mastery learning	Participation assessment and evaluation		Standardized method of debriefing
Provide for individualized (in addition to team) learning	Transfer to practice	Simulation enhanced inter-professional education		Rubric for evaluation of KSA developed
Clearly defined learner outcomes & benchmarks	Team training	Simulation design		Method established for sharing student performance with clinical faculty
Ensure the simulator is a valid learning tool	High stakes testing			Collect and retain evaluation data: • facilitators/facilitation • simulation experience
	Instructor training			Faculty members have opportunity for professional development
	Educational and professional context			

The literature reviewing the impact of specific simulation elements on positive learning outcomes continues to emerge. Technology-enhanced simulation training for team performance, technical skills across health care disciplines, and for improvements in patient care shows moderate-to-large effect when compared with no intervention.[21,25,29,30,72–87] When compared head-to-head with other educational approaches, the effects are smaller or less clear, although many reviews acknowledge a lack of evidence or poor methodology in the available studies.

Simulation substitution for actual clinical practice hours and experiences is controversial. In 2012, a landmark longitudinal study was funded by the National Council of State Boards of Nursing (NCSBN) in partnership with the National League for Nursing (NLN). This study recruited subjects from a total of 10 pre-licensure schools of nursing including both two- and four-year programs, and compared replacement of 10% (control) vs. 25% vs. 50% of actual clinical experience with scenario-based simulation activities. Outcomes were favorable with no statistical difference in National Council Licensure Examination (NCLEX) board pass rates, employment, clinical skills, knowledge level or attitudes.[62] The subjects were followed for six months post-graduation, again with no difference noted in performance in the work setting.[62] This work has impacted regulation at the state level with two follow-up papers identifying individual and programmatic preparatory elements needed for high quality pre-licensure level simulation.[64,90] In a second follow-up survey by the NCSBN, 29/34 boards now allow simulation to replace clinical hours in pre-licensure education.[88]

In the nurse anesthesia profession, students are permitted to partially meet two clinical requirements with simulated experiences. However, COA accreditation standards are clear stating, "Simple models and simulated experiences may be used to satisfy part of this requirement. No clinical experiences can be obtained by simulation alone."[46] Further, the COA has emphasized that simulation is not an end unto itself and that activities should be designed to support student performance of the actual event in the clinical environment.

Accreditation is now available for simulation centers, and certification is available for simulation educators. The Society for Simulation in Healthcare (SSH) has established standards for accreditation of simulation centers with full accreditation being defined as meeting standards in four areas: research, teaching/education, assessment, and system integration.[89] Instructor certification of simulation educators at both basic and advanced levels is also available via SSH and, for undergraduate education, is being recommended as a best practice by the NCSBN.[64,90] The Certified Health Care Simulation Educator credential (CHSE) requires taking and passing a standardized certification examination with advanced certification requiring development of a professional portfolio and evidence of longstanding effort in the simulation educational domain.

The Spectrum of Simulation Devices and Approaches

Role-playing and other forms of nonpatient interaction have long been used in nursing and nurse anesthesia education. Early examples in nursing occurred with static mannequins, such as Mrs. Chase from the early 1900s, that foreshadowed the evolution of the current computer-controlled devices.[91] Widely available simulation began with the development of Resusci Annie in 1960 for use in CPR. The first computer-controlled patient simulators (Harvey Cardiopulmonary Simulator/Sim-One) were developed in the late 1960s,[92] with the modern era of simulation beginning in 1990 with the release of the anesthesia simulator consultant, a screen-based anesthesia simulator.

Simulators can be classified according to application. Examples include part or partial task trainers (for specific skills), computerized mannequins (Laerdal 3-G, CAE HPS, Gaumard Adult Simulator), screen-based software systems (serious games, avatar environments, augmented reality, and virtual reality systems including haptic interfaces). In many programs, modalities are strategically deployed in a manner designed to best meet student learning objectives. For example, at the Winter Institute for Simulation, Education and Research (WISER) at the University of Pittsburgh, there is a standardized central venous catheter training course for all practitioners who wish to become credentialed in placing central lines. This is based on the blended curriculum principle combining online learning activities with a hands-on simulation experience. Students review on-screen material (including video, interactive images, and anatomical renderings) in order to develop the requisite baseline knowledge. Scaffolded simulation activities are then used including ultrasound of human models, use of an ultra-soundable CVC simulator, use of a CVC partial task trainer (for needle location and aspiration), and use of a three-dimensionally printed model (printed in house) of a vessel for dilation and catheter insertion.

Emerging as an important supplemental application in nurse anesthesia education is the use of standardized patients (SPs) who can be deployed in both teaching and testing simulations. The individuals need special training and are often used in medicine for objective, structured clinical exams, which are a core component of the United States Medical Licensure Exam (USMLE) in the U.S and across the world.[93] Standardized patients present a variety of conditions in a standardized manner. They are also trained in providing feedback and student assessment. These SP evaluations can be more accurate than those of observing faculty. Examples of SP use include preoperative evaluation, head to toe physical assessment, demonstration of professional behaviors, and demonstration of effective patient communication.[94,95]

Barriers to Implementation of Simulation Efforts

There are host of impediments to the development of an effective simulation program; however, once a simulation program is up and running, some of the most common barriers are created unknowingly in the design process for simulation scenarios. Failing to recognize that there are many ways to conduct effective simulation and that a one-size-fits-all panacea does not exist, can allow for scenario design strategies to become bloated with unnecessary technology and complexity.

When considering potential barriers to simulation, it is necessary to step back and look at the overall cost picture (ie, net commitment of resources) of an educational encounter. Simulation efforts are scrutinized even more carefully than standard approaches because of the multi-resource commitment. Resources include, but are not limited to, the equipment, technical and administrative support, preparation time, breakdown time, cleanup time, and supplies (both fixed and consumable). Design considerations for any learning encounter should seriously consider these resource commitment factors at all levels of decision making.

There is a paucity of literature informing faculty of the ideal ways to develop a simulation encounter although, as noted, there are now some valuable guides (Table 14.3).

Table 14.3 Scenario Development and Testing Process Checklist

1. Identify topic	6. Compile comprehensive equipment lists
2. Determine learner level	7. Establish feedback/debriefing plan
3. Create specific learning objectives	8. Determine assessment strategy
4. Develop the story	9. Complete facilitation instructions
5. Develop flow of the scenario	10. Perform scenario testing (a,ß)

(Used by permission from the Winter Institute for Simulation, Education, and Research)

Unfortunately, there is a strong and persistent undercurrent of closely held myths influencing faculty decision-making during the design of simulation-based learning encounters. Blind adherence to these myths can manifest as hidden barriers that result in operational problems as well as faculty and student frustration when the educational activity is attempted. Faculty make literally hundreds of decisions during design and implementation of a simulation. Thoughtfulness, attention to detail, and adherence to accomplishing objectives while being as efficient as possible in the creation of relevant learning encounters are key concerns. The ultimate barrier for simulation-based learning is that if the costs outweigh the benefits simulation will be used sparingly or abandoned altogether.

The Fidelity (Realism) Barrier

As simulation devices have become more multifunctional and affordable, expectations for increased simulation training among stakeholders has increased substantially. This has, in large part, resulted in rapid growth of the simulation market which is now a multibillion dollar industry. As noted, there is a wide spectrum of devices on the market, but they often require substantial technical expertise to program and operate. Despite their complexity and cost, computerized mannequins continue to be the centerpiece of simulation training and education. One consequence of this focus on high-technology devices is the adoption of terminology attempting to accurately categorize how closely the simulator resembles a human being (and also how closely a simulation setting represents a real clinical setting). The most common descriptor for this "just like the real thing" ethic is fidelity. Fidelity is often described along a continuum (low, medium, high) with high-fidelity simulators being touted as superior training devices by advocates of the terminology.[51,96–98] Unfortunately, this quest for more fidelity is a design principle that contributes to increasing the complexity of simulation-based training encounters. This happens because we can, and not necessarily because it is in the interest of meeting the learning outcomes of the simulation.

In addition to the possibility of increasing confusion on the part of students, every element that is added to the simulated environment increases the time that must be allotted for set-up and clean-up of the scenario. The operational reality is that only so much time can be allotted to simulation during a training day and across an entire curriculum. Especially time-consuming is the extensive use of moulage and other mannequin treatments (eg, smells, vomit, spouting blood) designed to make the simulator appear real. Extensive moulage can add huge amounts of time and effort to set up and to freshen-up between scenarios. This can greatly decrease the total amount of student learning time in a given program.

While so-called high-fidelity devices are computerized and technologically sophisticated, and moulage can look and feel and smell like real body excrescences, it is ludicrous to suggest that highly intelligent and clinically sophisticated nurse anesthesia students believe that these representations are actually real or are just like clinical situations. Further, maintaining a significant focus on fidelity can lead to faulty decision-making in scenario design. For example, when the design team attempts to increase the fidelity of a simulation scenario without an understanding of the impact, it introduces complexity for the student. This can lead to confusion in the student's interpretation of the environment, misunderstanding as to the intention of the learning activity, and an increase in cognitive load similar to what occurs during high-stress events in an operating room.[99–101] While there may be some benefit to enhancing stress load (eustress), students already enter the simulated environment with a sense of hypervigilance and try to immediately react to what is happening. Any simulator feature, piece of equipment, or supply introduced into the context of the learning encounter will be integrated into the participant's perception and evaluated by them to determine if it is a critical element or clue to a successful simulation performance. Further, faculty facilitators must keep track of these elements as well. Thus, add-on details in pursuit of the high-fidelity myth can tax available resources, elevate overall expense, and introduce additional student and faculty cognitive load,[100,102,103] decisions that add complexity without value.

As an alternative, we make the case for relevance over realism. We concur with the opinion of Hamstra et al, that attempting to argue that the simulator (or environment) exactly replicates a real human (or clinical situation) may not be productive. We join these authors in advocating that the term fidelity should be abandoned.[76] Device choice should be driven by informed educators rather than inaccurate labels. It is far more useful during curricular and research design to focus on learner engagement, alignment of the activity with learner-specific objectives, and on how the simulator functions. These items are real enough for trainees to improve and, hopefully, transfer their newly acquired skill to clinical care. Describing mannequins with respect to the level of technology incorporated and the features available and relevant to actual care is an accurate and clear pathway to discuss their integration into training designs. The fidelity terminology has the potential to create a false sense of value and motivates novice instructors in the use of complex devices for simple training (eg, computerized simulator used for basic intubation practice) with resultant reduction in the lifespan of more expensive devices.

The Video Barrier

Another design element that adds to the total time and complexity of the simulation is the routine use of video recording and playback. Unfortunately, there is a pervasive belief that the use of video is inextricably linked to high quality simulation-based learning and debriefing. Similar to the fidelity discussion above, there is no conclusive evidence that video playback and/or review results in superior learning outcomes in simulation.[49,104] While outcomes may not be improved, the routine use of video collection, playback, and review will increase the cost, resource allocation, and time allotted to a simulation event. Further, if not used tactically and thoughtfully, it has the potential to transform the debriefing experience from an active to a passive learning experience. Additionally, use of video recording has been identified by Decarlo et al, as the most important pervasive factor contributing to the reluctance of participants to engage in simulation based learning encounters.[105]

This discussion is not meant as a rebuke of video use and review, but more to encourage the questioning of its routine use. In fact, multiple authors have reported positive outcomes when video is used for the purposes of answering specific research questions or for the training of teams where the team is encouraged to actively participate in the analysis of the videotaped performance(s).[50,106–112] Instead of assuming that video needs to be used in all cases, an active evaluation of the strengths, weaknesses, and true costs of video should be conducted as part of the design process. This will allow a critical evaluation of the use of the technology to ensure that learning outcome benefits outweigh the costs, complexities, and student reluctance to be on video.

The Faculty Preparation Barrier

No discussion of barriers to simulation in nurse anesthesia education would be complete without discussing the lack of available faculty development programs specific to the nurse anesthesia profession. It is important to understand that we are by no means alone in this need. The imperative that the next generation of health care educators receive formalized training in educational methods in general and in use of simulation techniques in particular is a topic of active discussion around the world. As such, it was an area of specific focus at the 2011 Research Consensus Conference of the Society for Simulation in Healthcare (SSH) and remains an ongoing challenge for educational program administrators who are responsible for assuring faculty member competence and readiness to engage in simulation and other forms of immersive education.[113–115]

Multiple authors have noted that faculty preparation is critical to the success of any simulation program.[61,116] Sometimes this issue can be lost in the many variables that challenge administrators in the development and implementation of a simulation program (**Figure 14.3**).

Figure 14.3 Variables to be Considered in Development and Implementation of an Effective Simulation Program

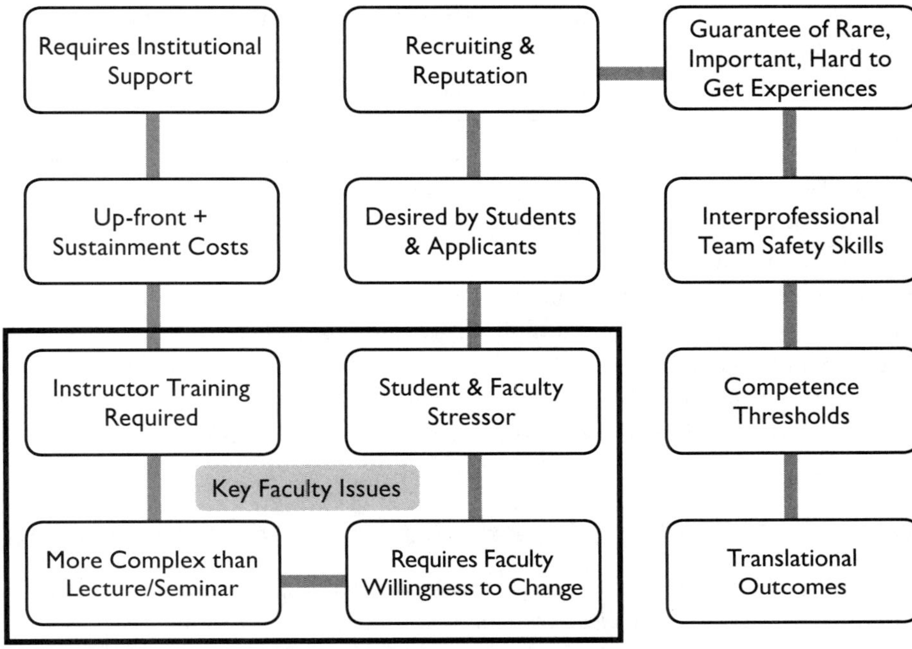

Note the box indicating the importance of faculty preparation, support, and involvement.

Faculty who have not had the advantage of focused development in simulation methodology are far more likely to design and implement inefficient and costly simulations. While it is not necessary for every faculty member utilizing simulation to become an expert, there are significant advantages for the development of core competencies in the areas of facilitation and debriefing (**Table 14.4**).

Table 14.4 Core Faculty Competencies Required of Simulation Educators[4,30,60–71]

- Engage in strategy for curricular integration
- Develop curricular materials (objectives, scenarios, equipment lists, faculty instructions, assessment, and evaluation instruments)
- Engage in curricular quality improvement
- Effectively direct a simulation scenario/event
- Utilize facilitation skills (coaching, cueing, prompting)
- Provide effective feedback
- Implement pre-briefing/debriefing/co-debriefing
- Engage in data analysis and interpretation
- Demonstrate effective use of technologies (simulators, AV, LMS, data management)

These faculty competencies are considered to be best practices that are likely to enhance student learning outcomes. Those faculty members who undergo more formal training and begin to develop a full range of expertise are more likely to create simulations using efficient design processes that result in better outcomes.

A challenging problem is that faculty may be reluctant to engage as simulation educators for a wide variety of reasons including, but not limited to, the need for change, lack of comfort with technology, or possibly the fact that most faculty do not have a formal educational component in their professional training[61,116–118] (Figure 14.3). This concept of a lack of formal educator preparedness has now made its way into the Council on Accreditation of Nurse Anesthesia Programs standards and guidelines, practice doctorate.[46] The applicable area is B. Faculty Standard, CRNA Faculty, 17: "Core CRNA program faculty, including the program administrator, assistant program administrator, and course directors, have formal instruction in curriculum, evaluation, and instruction." The areas required are certainly applicable to developing simulation curriculum, but are probably insufficient for full simulation faculty readiness. This is because the skill sets required of simulation educators are broad and include becoming familiar with a variety of low- to high-technology simulation devices as well as developing at least a working understanding of how activities can be integrated smoothly into an overall curriculum (Table 14.4).

Effective Practices in Scenario Design and Topic Selection

Use of a structured design process integrating best practice simulation methods will assist in the efficiency and the effectiveness of the integration of simulation-based education into existing nurse anesthesia curricula. This standardization of the design process has multiple benefits. First, it streamlines the development process within a group of faculty; second, it can ensure consistency in areas such as running and facilitating scenarios; third, it can ensure a smoother process especially as new faculty are oriented to the simulation program. We have found that the use of agreed-upon templates for every step of the process is critical. Recognizing that not every faculty member is interested in developing a full simulation competency set, lead faculty can develop curricula in consultation with subject matter experts (SMEs). The scenarios and curriculum developed are created in the standardized process which results in parallel student instructional and faculty support materials. Thus, all faculty participants have access to an expert level curriculum and become skilled in deploying it. This approach is known as the expert-curriculum, competent-facilitator model of curriculum design and has been implemented at WISER, University of Pittsburgh, as well as in simulation centers across the world.

The focus of most simulation experiences is a clinically oriented story. This story serves as a call to action for participants and is known as a simulation scenario. Scenarios are a powerful tool to ensure participants understand the relevance of the simulation-based educational exercise to their current and future practice as a nurse anesthetist. Attention to scenario detail will assist in helping participants understand that their engagement with simulation-based learning is directly relevant and likely to be important to their future practice. Expertly developed scenario-based education can be used to shorten the learning curve for complex skills, enhance competence, and allow participants to envision how a particular skill can be applied in the clinical learning environment. It is also likely that simulation harbors the ability to speed the transition to independent practice from the role of a senior student to an entry-level practitioner.

Scenario Development and Testing Process

We will describe a scenario development pathway that attempts to adhere to best simulation education principles and has been used successfully in creation of hundreds of scenarios at WISER (**Figure 14.4**).

Figure 14.4 The Anatomy of a Scenario Development Pathway Dissected Into Key Components

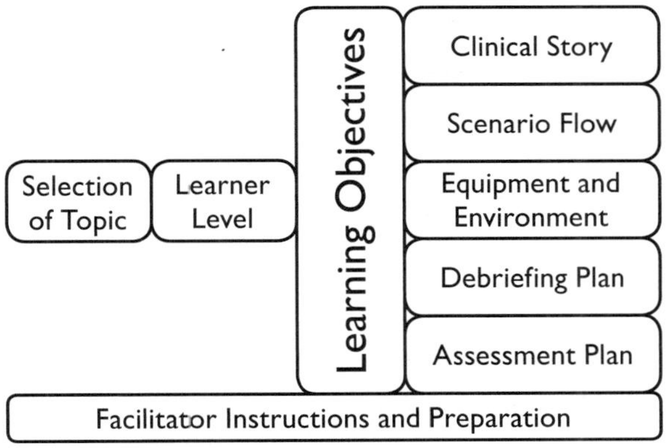

Step 1: Identify Topic

Topic selection drives the entire process and is an important first step. The overall topic will ideally be determined from a needs analysis of the curriculum that would benefit from simulation-based education. For nurse anesthesia educators, scenario topics are likely to correspond with clinical supplementation or augmentation needs, or a desire to evaluate specific competencies. Typically, topics will involve aspects of patient assessment, critical thinking, clinical judgments, or the development and execution of an anesthetic plan.

Step 2: Determine Learner Level

The next step is to clearly align the learner level with the challenge of the scenario. Clearly, a scenario designed for a student in the first week of the program would look quite different than for a senior with pregraduate status. A clear understanding of learner level will drive development of objectives, performance expectations, amount of available assistance, and debriefing approach.

Step 3: Create Specific Learning Objectives

The development of learning objectives is the foundational bedrock of decision-making for the design of any scenario in simulation-based learning. Our experience is that even senior educators struggle to write clear, detailed, level-appropriate objectives. Detailed learning objectives facilitate faculty efficiency in developing an effective scenario. For example, a learning objective such as "correctly provide general anesthesia for a patient with asthma" contains too much subjectivity relative to supporting scenario design. A better learning objective might read, "At the conclusion of this scenario, the third rotation student registered nurse anesthetist (SRNA) will demonstrate the ability to initiate two treatment interventions for a patient experiencing hypotension under general endotracheal anesthesia during a 15-minute lunch break."

This objective adheres to the SMART (specific, measurable, achievable, relevant, time-bound) principle for objective development and is used for evaluating the quality of learning objectives[119] (**Figure 14.5**).

Figure 14.5 SMART Acronym for Quality Evaluation in Objective Formation

- S { • Specific
- M { • Measurable
- A { • Achievable
- R { • Realistic
- T { • Time Bound

Depending on the level and number of participants and the complexity of the scenario, between four and six objectives are easily achievable in a 15–20 minute simulation encounter.

Step 4: Develop the Story

The next step in scenario development is to create a clinically relevant story that will serve as a call to action for participants to engage in a simulation. The story serves as a supporting element for accomplishment of learning objectives during a simulation session. The story is typically divided into three sections. The first section is commonly referred to as the stem and is a sentence or two designed to engage the student into the scenario. The second phase is termed information offered (IO) and represents information that is freely available on the chart or during hand-off. The third phase is termed information elicited (IE) and represents information that must be gathered through questioning or critical observation (**Figure 14.6**).

Figure 14.6 A Simple Clinical Scenario Separated into Three Phases: Stem, Information Offered, and Information Elicited

The student is freely offered information in phase 2.
He or she must request or gather the information in phase 3.

Stem	• You are assigned to relieve your CRNA colleague for lunch. Mrs. Smith is 65 years old and having right total hip arthroplasty with general anesthesia.
Information Offered	• Allergy history, last oral intake, anesthetic agents used, airway, co-morbid condition, fluid status, baseline vital signs
Information Elicited	• Blood loss, coagulation status, use of bone cement, vasopressors administered, current vital signs

Actual cases that can be replicated or adapted are preferred because an understanding that they are managing a case which actually occurred conveys the relevance of the experience to learners. It is important to minimize design to the specific level needed to support the learning objectives of the target learning group. If an actual case is being replicated, reduce the details of the case and include only those that are directly relevant.

Step 5: Develop Flow of the Scenario

Developing the flow of the scenario involves mapping out projected clinical outcomes for the patient. Specific branch or trigger points must be planned with anticipation of changes in feedback flow to the participants after correct or incorrect actions (eg, physiology change with improvement or deterioration, cueing or prompting from facilitator, etc.). It is important to attempt to condense the scenario flow into essential core elements so that progress can be made in addressing each learning objective. Changes of physiology or patient status that are not related to the learning objectives can increase the chance that the participant(s) will veer off on an undesired tangent. As noted, added detail with introduction of minutia will increase complexity and decrease the reliability of how the scenario runs.

Step 6: Compile Comprehensive Equipment List

Developing a comprehensive equipment list is part and parcel of scenario development in simulation-based education. Every essential piece of equipment needed to ensure the scenario runs well must be on the list. Incomplete equipment lists lead to mid-event scenario failures with loss of student confidence or a sense of confusion as they may believe that the failure is part of the scenario. Like other aspects of scenario design, the equipment list should be distilled to what is absolutely necessary to meet the learning objectives. As with other design features, additional elements introduced in an attempt to enhance realism/mimic reality can lead to greater complexity, student confusion, and increased cost.

Step 7: Establish Feedback/Debriefing Plan

A plan for feedback and debriefing should be included in the design of any scenario. As noted, feedback can include simulator responses, monitor responses, facilitator cues/prompts, standardized patient responses, or the combination. Debriefing is a form of specialized feedback and represents an opportunity to release emotion, analyze and consolidate understanding of performance, create reflection, and summarize key learning points.[120–124] There are multiple decisions that need to be made related to developing a debriefing plan (**Figure 14.7**).

Figure 14.7 Factors To Be Considered When Developing a Feedback and Debriefing Plan for a Simulation Encounter

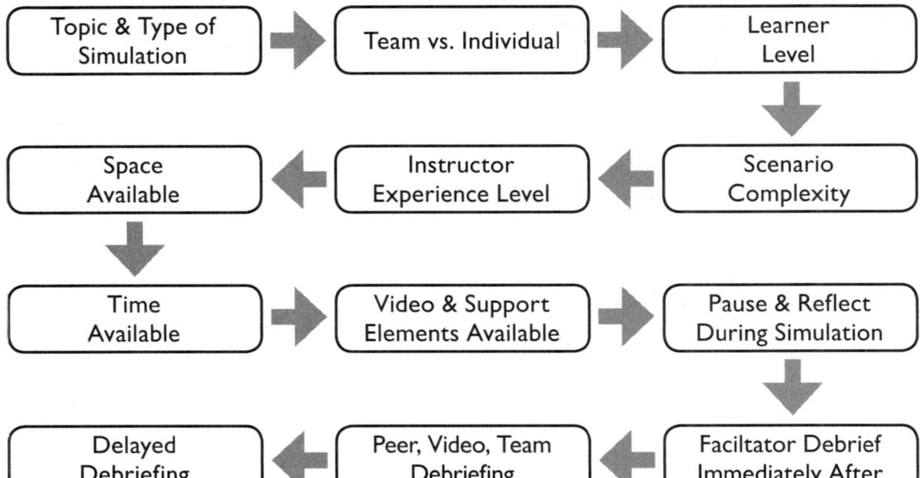

From a logistical standpoint, time allotted, space available, and support infrastructure will drive some of these decisions. From an educational standpoint, there are many other variables that affect these decisions, including whether the scenario was stressful, the need for equipment/technique demonstration, and the simulation experience of the facilitators.

It is critical that time allocated for the debriefing be part of the plan and that the plan include a list of topics or points (mapped to learning objectives) that must be covered for a given scenario. Debriefing points and learning objectives should be aligned. If they are not, a redesign of one or the other is necessary. Debriefing sessions are notorious for introduction of extraneous content by faculty members. This can reduce efficiency, increase cognitive load, and become confusing for the students. Additionally, for reliable performance of a given simulation across a curriculum, it is critical that debriefing content be consistent.

Step 8: Determine Assessment Strategy

Best practices in the design of simulation scenarios include the development of an assessment plan. Assessment can range from purely formative to purely summative with well-designed and efficient programs, including a mixed modality. Part of the plan must include development of (or adaptation of existing) assessment tools. The plan should also include faculty training and directions for use. Checklists, anchored rating scales, global rating scales, or combinations constructed as rubrics are typical in simulation evaluation. In many cases, the assessment plan may be a list of expected actions that the participant should perform in sequence during the scenario and is not what would be classically described as a formal assessment tool. Such a list is used to help inform the debriefing activity, and can be incorporated with other debriefing points. Any assessment plan should also map back to the learning objectives in a similar manner to the debriefing points. Assessment elements that are not included in the learning objectives should either be removed, or consideration given to align the learning objectives with the assessment plan.

Step 9: Complete Facilitation Instructions

Designing comprehensive facilitation instructions will enhance the ability of a scenario to be implemented smoothly, especially by faculty who did not participate in the original design. Specific instructions should be included so that the facilitator knows how to execute the scenario. Environment setup, equipment use, room setup, scenario objectives, scenario flows, debriefing plan, assessment plan, and assessment tool instructions are examples of items to be included in this step. Describing participant orientation, environmental briefing, or pre-briefing of clinical roles prior to the scenario should be indicated. This facilitator section should also include any specific nuances related to the technology utilized during the scenario, including computerized simulators, audiovisual equipment and other supporting materials that require operator familiarization. It is helpful to provide an approximation for times to set up, run, debrief, and reset each scenario. If the involved technology in a given program is complex, a separate technology plan should be included in the scenario.

Step 10: Perform Scenario Testing (α, ß)

We suggest a two-phase alpha and beta testing process for any new scenario prior to implementation of the scenario on actual students. The alpha (*α*) test phase is when members of the design team of the scenario play the role of students and undergo a dress rehearsal from beginning to end. This includes assembly of all equipment, full environmental setup, and a dry run of the scenario. The alpha test phase allows for identification of missing equipment and will point out scenario design flaws. It also will help to establish general time estimates for the scenario. The alpha phase is limited by the fact that the group of people involved in design often share a mental model of the way the scenario should flow. Thus, a beta phase of testing is needed.

The beta (*ß*) phase includes participants with at least requisite knowledge of the level of students for whom the scenario is designed, but who are not involved in the design process. Senior SRNAs can be used for new SRNA scenarios and CRNAs for senior SRNA scenarios. Participants undergo the same dress rehearsal process. The beta phase will uncover additional scenario design flaws and may also identify missing equipment and elements of the story that need to be refined. Finally, the beta phase can be used to develop a more accurate estimate of scenario time frames.

The Importance of Debriefing

Debriefing is recognized by multiple researchers, systematic reviews, standards, and regulatory bodies as a best practice in simulation education.[75,120,122,124–128] Debriefing of a simulation encounter does not occur by accident. It is a deliberate conversation that faculty members initiate in order to help their participants think about and reflect on what happened during the simulation. Key questions that should be answered include: What happened? When did key events occur? Why did participants act in a certain way or initiate interventions? What did participants do in response to events and what was the outcome of participant actions (positive or negative)?

The well-executed debriefing is a controlled conversation that maintains a steady focus on the debriefing plan points. Harmonizing the learning that occurs as a result of the simulation activity is possible through debriefing by use of communication techniques (both verbal and non-verbal) that facilitate active reflection of the event and assist the participants in self-discovery as to whether learning goals were attained.

Structuring the debriefing conversation in a way that focuses on the specific learning objectives of the simulation encounter does several things that are valuable. First, it is an opportunity to hear participants reveal their opinions on how successful they were in managing events, decisions, and other aspects within the scenario. Second, it allows the faculty to probe depth of underlying knowledge and reveal critical thought processes that were employed to manage the scenario. This important exploration of understanding extends to aspects of the management of the scenario that were successful as well as those areas needing improvement. Third, the use of supporting elements such as graphics, media, standard references, and algorithms provide a near real-time comparison of best practices and processes with the simulation performance. This can help to solidify knowledge and understanding. Asking participants to compare the simulation experience with similar clinical events (normalizing) can lead participants to understanding connections to future challenges in simulation as well as in the clinical environment. The debriefing is used to recap the major learning points that were realized (or not) as a result of participation in the simulated encounter. This is critical to ensure learning as there is likely a finite amount of knowledge that is carried forward from any individual learning encounter. An overall synthesis of the key learning objectives provides clarity to participants, helps them understand the relative importance of events, and gives them a clear understanding of what the faculty member prioritized as the most valuable aspects. Creating a binary type of packaging such as "What was effective?" and "What should be changed?" can clarify the key takeaways.

Another priority for facilitators is careful observation of participant actions and performance during the scenario with formation of professional opinions. A key task during the debriefing is to reveal participant perception in order to compare it with your opinion (**Figure 14.8**).

Figure 14.8 Gap Analysis Matrix Representing the Intersection of Facilitator and Participants' Summative Opinions Regarding Performance at the End of a Simulation Session

Notice that the performance opinions exist on a continuum (poor to good). During the debriefing conversation, the facilitator assesses whether his or her perceptions and those of participants are aligned. This will help to determine the debriefing strategy.

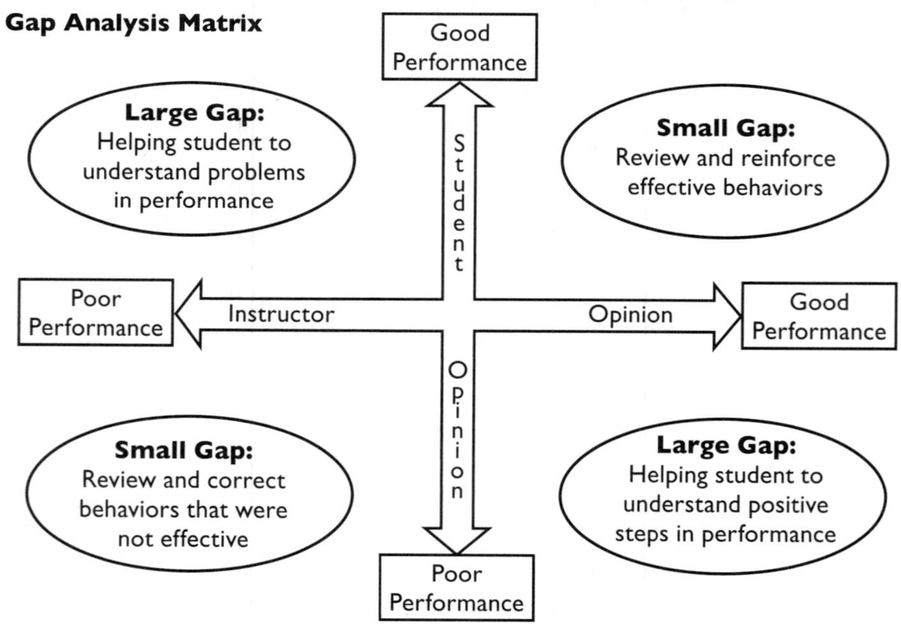

(Used by permission from the Winter Institute for Simulation, Education, and Research)

Faculty members running a debriefing have the obligation to share professional judgments formed by observing the simulation encounter; however, it is important not to reveal your opinion early in the debriefing session as this may bias participant responses. By employing a series of probing questions, the facilitator can elicit initial participant beliefs about what occurred and how they did. Objectives should be covered, but the length of time spent reviewing each objective is up to the faculty member and depends on participant performance. The debriefing session is also a time for expression of emotions engendered by the simulation event and to relieve the stress of having their performance closely scrutinized in an artificial environment.

Debriefing Models

It is important that busy faculty rapidly gain skills necessary to conduct an effective debriefing. In 2007, Fanning and Gaba noted: "*There are surprisingly few papers in the peer-reviewed literature to illustrate how to debrief, how to teach or learn to debrief, what methods of debriefing exist and how effective they are at achieving learning objectives and goals.*"[129] While there are now a multitude of models and more than 100 papers published regarding simulation debriefing, this statement remains true. In a recent critical review of health care simulation debriefing methods, Sawyer et al, examined debriefing timing, facilitation, conversation structures, and process elements that have been reported in the literature. They noted a wide variety of methods with no clear conclusions with respect to what works in specific situations or simulation types. They did, however, note that one commonly identified value theme was that a structured approach is important. Further, they noted that most debriefing structures include at minimum an opening phase, a review of simulation events, and a concluding phase. They also were able to synthesize three areas of emphasis during their review. They termed these "phases" and indicated they include "essential elements, conversational techniques/educational strategies and debriefing adjuncts."[120] These authors acknowledge that there is not a one-size-fits-all debriefing model or any scholarly work that lends superiority or inferiority to any one model. In fact, there is no empirical evidence that the adoption of any one model improves learning outcomes relative to any other model. We would be remiss, however, if we did not acknowledge the importance of debriefing relative to simulation outcomes. Two recent reviews by Levett-Jones and Cook (who included debriefing as a form of feedback) reported that a critical synthesis of the literature reveals a significant impact of debriefing on a variety of performance outcomes.[30,75]

The selection and adoption of a debriefing model within a nurse anesthesia faculty makes practical, operational sense. Standardization of faculty training, quality assurance, and efficiency in programmatic execution are a few examples. Adoption of a single model can expedite the onboarding of new faculty members as the opportunities for mentoring and support in training with the model will be increased. The selection of a particular model of debriefing has to consider ease of adoption, cost for training, and scalability. The level of the learners, the program mission for simulation, time in simulation, and the available supporting technologies are also variables to be considered in the final selection process. Additionally, the number of faculty needing training and the simulation competence of experienced faculty will play a critical role.

The Structured and Support Debriefing Model (SSD)

The Structured and Supported Debriefing (SSD) model was the result of a collaboration between WISER and the American Heart Association (AHA) and was carried out to develop a method that would support ACLS and PALS instructor training. Further modification of the final WISER-AHA collaboration product has resulted in a scalable and generalizable debriefing model designed to meet the needs of most health care simulation educators.[124,128] One big advantage of the model for the AHA was that it could be learned rapidly and, thus, could be scaled for ACLS and PALS training across the world. The model has been successfully deployed in a number of languages and regions of the world and is integrated into the AHA core instructor curriculum.

The SSD model reflects two core components. Structured refers to a three-phase approach to debriefing with the goals and objectives of each phase being clearly outlined. The operationalization of the SSD model of debriefing centers around the use of a job aid with the acronym GAS. The GAS acronym is descriptive of the three phases of the SSD method which are known as gather, analyze, and summarize.[124,128] Each phase includes defined goals, responsibilities, and recommendations for conversational phrasing to assist in the process (**Figure 14.9**).

Figure 14.9 The GAS Job Aid of the Structured and Supported Debriefing Model

Phase	Goal	Actions	Sample Questions	Time
Gather	Listen to participants to understand what they think & how they feel about session	• Request narrative from team leader • Request clarifying or supplemental information from team	All: How do you feel? Team Leader: Can you tell us what happened? Team Members: Can you add to the account?	25%
Analyze	Facilitate participants reflection **on** & analysis **of** their actions	• Review of accurate record of events • Report observation (correct & incorrect steps) • Ask a series of questions to reveal participants' thinking processes • Assist participants to reflect on their performance • Direct/redirect participants to assure continuous focus on session objectives	• I noticed... • Tell me more about... • How did you feel about... • What were you thinking when... • I understand, however, tell me about "X" ___ aspect of the scenario... • Conflict resolution: Let's refocus—"what's important is not who is right but what is right for the patient..."	50%
Summarize	Facilitate identification & review of lessons learned	• Participants identify positive aspects of team or individual behaviors & behaviors that require change • Summary of comments or statements	• List two actions or events that you felt were effective or well done • Describe two areas that you think you/team need to work on...	25%

(Used by permission from Winter Institute for Simulation, Education, and Research)

The term "supported" refers to two central tenets. The first involves support of the participant. This requires observation of the student's emotional readiness and well-being after the simulation. Second, "supported" refers to use of external references, algorithms, or best practices in support of learning objective. These should be routinely incorporated into the debriefing. This reduces tension within a debriefing and allows instructors to guide students to review the objective material in comparison to their own performance. It also helps to reduce instructor stress because having direct conversations with participants concerning performance deficiencies can be challenging and uncomfortable. One trap that should be avoided is to give learners the mistaken impression that suboptimal performance is okay. Use of support materials also helps to refocus students on the patient-centric aspect of simulation education, and reminds them that because simulation learning can be more permanent understanding correct approaches is critical. In fact, trainees often report that they very clearly recall their simulation experiences when confronted with the actual clinical situation even years later. Reinforce to participants that this is a safe environment where they can develop and gain new or different skills without patient risk.

As noted, there are many variables that need to be considered when planning a debriefing session. Some are predictable and can be used upfront to guide debriefing decisions. In general, your objectives, learner level, and faculty experience with debriefing are important first considerations. The more objectives included in the scenario, the longer the debriefing is likely to take. Novice learners may require longer debriefing explanations than experts. Instructors with little experience with debriefing are likely to take longer. Further, team events, more complex events, and scenario-based types of training take more time to debrief than do clinical skill training events.

In GAS, the G or gather phase provides a mental transition from the simulated to the debriefing environment. The simulated environment can be emotionally charged and/or stressful and this phase allows decompression. The gather phase has three basic goals. The first is to actively assess the participants and their emotional readiness to continue into the debriefing conversation. Next, the facilitator should assist participant active recall of the scenario narrative. Encouraging all of the participants to add some aspect from their recollection promotes active mental processing, stimulates formation of a shared mental model, and helps participants understand that perceptions vary. Last, the G phase can be helpful for the facilitator to gain an understanding of the trainee performance perceptions and compare it with their own. Any divergence is known as a performance gap (Figure 14.8). In the G phase, it is not yet necessary to focus on or encourage the conversation in the direction of the learning objectives. Instead, recall and active reflection on scenario events should be encouraged.

The G phase can be initiated by observing something that acknowledges the state of the participant (or team) during the scenario. Consider something like, "That looked stressful, let's talk about it...." A natural transition would be to then ask the participant (or another member of the team if there was more than one) to give his or her account of scenario events. It is important to realize that when one team member begins to give an account of the scenario, everyone else begins to reflect on what happened and will be comparing their own recollection to what is being said. Thus, we are forcing active reflection across an entire learner group.

The analyze (A) phase is next. Consistent focus on accomplishment of learning objectives is the goal. Through a series of probing questions, we begin to lead the discussion in a way that allows the participants to actively discover what they performed correctly and what may need to be corrected for the future. During the A phase, it is helpful to introduce the objective supporting materials. Examples include a log file record of physiology, a short video clip, clinical pathways, algorithms, and hospital policies. During the A phase, the facilitator will ask questions that prompt thoughts and recollection about specific events as they relate to the learning objectives. Students are encouraged to form their own understanding of actions that were correct (for reinforcement) and incorrect (for correction). Let's consider the total hip arthroplasty case noted earlier (Figure 14.6). In this case, the two participants (P1 and P2) were asked to assume care for a patient who became hypotensive during a general anesthetic. They failed to appropriately treat the hypotension. The facilitator (F) might lead an analyze phase conversation in the following manner:

F: Let's take a look at the simulator log file. At three minutes into your lunch relief, what was the blood pressure?

P1: 90/50

F: Right, now look again 10 minutes into the case, what was the blood pressure at that point?

P2: Not much different, 92/50.

F: Exactly. Can you tell me two things that could have been done to improve the blood pressure during this timeframe?

P1: Absolutely. We talked about, but never gave a fluid bolus.

P2: That's right. Also, we should've considered a vasopressor such as ephedrine or phenylephrine. Looking at the high heart rate, I say phenylephrine.

F: Exactly, Great work. Now let's review this simple guideline for blood pressure management in such cases. (Now the facilitator directs the attention of the group to a poster [supporting element] of institutional care guidelines on the wall.)

What is important to realize in the above exchange is that the facilitator never indicated what the participants did was wrong; instead, they were allowed to discover the treatment error. By use of the supporting material (the simulator log file), there was an immediate deference to the supporting elements as a source of expertise. Second, the care guidelines served as a second supporting element. This allowed the source of the correction of their errors to be an objective expert source, and the facilitator was in a less confrontational role. This process of identifying topics for discussion, creating active reflection, and promoting discovery will continue until the facilitator is comfortable that all of the learning objectives for the scenario have been covered.

While the S or summarize phase seems to be self-explanatory, it is one of the areas that even experienced debriefers describe as challenging. In the S phase, the facilitator deliberately concludes the session and seeks to clear up any confusion that may have arisen during the analysis. Given the recent scenario and the array of topics covered in the first two phases of the debriefing, there is likely a significant amount of information that must be cognitively digested. Creating a clear summary allows the facilitator to focus on just a couple of the most important takeaway points that should be absorbed and carried into future practice. We have deliberately incorporated a Plus-Delta technique of after-action debriefing into the S phase. Participants are asked to state one or two actions that each, as an individual, or the team, performed that were effective. This is the plus (+) component. Participants are then asked to identify two areas for change (delta = $\triangle$) in order to improve for the next time. The use of the numeric two (or a number of your choice) is important for both the plus and the delta aspects. Psychologically, participants will attempt to meet the stated numeric; thus, it represents a very effective psychological forcing function to move the conversation forward. Because participants often recall the last aspects of an educational encounter (the so-called recency effect[130]), we suggest ending each debriefing with the delta discussion. We believe that this is important for ongoing professional self-improvement in both simulation and in subsequent professional activities.

Summary

Over the past two decades, nursing and nurse anesthesia education has undergone a remarkable evolution. Technological innovation has driven change with the advent of learning management systems, wireless networks, and a wide variety of sophisticated adjuncts available to the educator. Simulation educational methods have allowed a shift from instructor-centric, static, lecture-based activities to incorporate experiential learning activities which are student- and, thus, patient-centric and designed to fully engage the participant. Simulation educational methodology is now understood as all activities in which faculty design objectives and activities that allow students to engage in experiential learning and become more ready for real clinical events. In simulation, this spectrum includes role-play, part-task specific skill training, use of standardized patient encounters, and OSCEs and computerized simulations.

Leaders in nurse anesthesia education are now fully embracing these advances and are seeking new and better practices for integrating simulation-based educational activities within the nurse anesthesia curricula. Best practices, standards, and regulatory changes promulgated by state boards of nursing, consumer demand, and an evolving understanding that simulation methods are (head-to-head) superior to traditional educational approaches in the areas of knowledge, skill, and attitude change in the simulation lab (T1 effect) have helped to solidify the place of simulation within nurse anesthesia education. Further, the increasingly solid evidence in the broader simulation literature that translation to improved clinical care processes and patient outcomes can be demonstrated will continue to reinforce use of these approaches. The evidence also suggests that simulation can be employed to effectively supplement clinical experiences and, thus, augment development of clinical skills.

Perhaps the most important questions to be answered by nurse anesthesia simulation educators are those posed by the British epidemiologist Archie Cochrane (1909–1988) for whom the Cochrane Reviews are named. Cochrane posed his questions in relation to health care interventions when discussing methods to determine whether interventions can work (efficacy), whether they also work in the real world (effectiveness), and whether there is a favorable cost-benefit relationship (efficiency)[131,132] (**Figure 14.10**).

Figure 14.10 The Cochrane Efficacy, Effectiveness, Efficiency Continuum

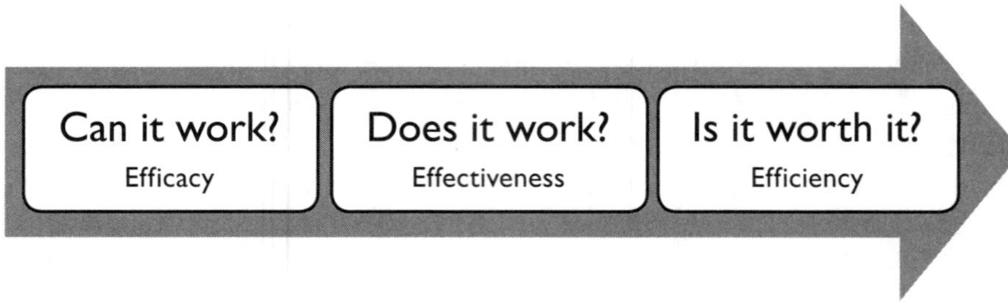
Can it work?
Efficacy
Does it work?
Effectiveness
Is it worth it?
Efficiency

More recent work in this area has focused on providing methods that clearly distinguish between efficacy and effectiveness research.[133,134] We would argue that a similar approach would benefit nurse anesthesia education for both SRNAs and CRNAs and, thus, the overall profession. Through sharing of our collective experience, it is critical that we identify which simulation educational interventions produce the best outcomes in the lab and which interventions translate learning from the lab (efficacy studies) to clinical areas across the United States (effectiveness studies). Finally, we need to clearly describe how the substantial educational investment represented by engaging in simulation education results in returns for our institutions, our colleagues, our students, and, ultimately, our patients.

References

1. Gaba D. The future vision of simulation in health care. *Qua Saf Health Care.* 2004;13 Suppl 1:i2–i10.

2. Cannon-Diehl MR, Rugari SM, Jones TS. High-fidelity simulation for continuing education in nurse anesthesia. *AANA J.* 2012;80(3):191–196.

3. Cannon-Diehl MR. Simulation in healthcare and nursing: state of the science. *Crit Care Nurs Q.* 2009;32(2):128–136.

4. Lopreiato JO, Sawyer T. Simulation-based medical education in pediatrics. *Acad Pediatr.* 2015;15(2):134–142.

5. Cheng A, Hunt EA, Donoghue A, et al. Examining pediatric resuscitation education using simulation and scripted debriefing: a multicenter randomized trial. *JAMA pediatrics.* 2013;167(6):528–536.

6. Kelly MA, Berragan E, Husebo SE, Orr F. Simulation in nursing education-international perspectives and contemporary scope of practice. *J Nurs Scholarsh.* 2016;48(3):312–321.

7. Overstreet M, McCarver L, Shields J, Patterson J. Simulation and rubrics: technology and grading student performance in nurse anesthesia education. *Nurs Clin North Am.* 2015;50(2):347–365.

8. Garbee DD, Paige J, Barrier K, et al. Interprofessional teamwork among students in simulated codes: a quasi-experimental study. *Nurs Educ Perspect.* 2013;34(5):339–344.

9. Penprase B, Mileto L, Bittinger A, et al. The use of high-fidelity simulation in the admissions process: one nurse anesthesia program's experience. *AANA J.* 2012;80(1):43–48.

10. Jones T, Goss S, Weeks B, Miura H, Bassandeh D, Cheek DJ. The effects of high-fidelity simulation on salivary cortisol levels in SRNA students: a pilot study. *Scientific World J.* 2011;11:86–92.

11. Turcato N, Roberson C, Covert K. Simulation-based education: what's in it for nurse anesthesia educators? *AANA J.* 2008;76(4):257–262.

12. Coopmans VC, Biddle C. CRNA performance using a handheld, computerized, decision-making aid during critical events in a simulated environment: a methodologic inquiry. *AANA J.* 2008;76(1):29–35.

13. Register M, Graham-Garcia J, Haas R. The use of simulation to demonstrate hemodynamic response to varying degrees of intrapulmonary shunt. *AANA J.* 2003;71(4):277–284.

14. Hartland W, Biddle C, Fallacaro M. Accessing the living laboratory: trigger films as an aid to developing, enabling, and assessing anesthesia clinical instructors. *AANA J.* 2003;71(4):287–291.

15. Hotchkiss MA, Biddle C, Fallacaro M. Assessing the authenticity of the human simulation experience in anesthesiology. *AANA J.* 2002;70(6):470–473.

16. Hotchkiss MA, Mendoza SN. *AANA Journal* Course: Update for nurse anesthetists full-body patient simulation technology: gaining experience using a malignant hyperthermia model. *AANA J.* 2001;69(1):59–65.

17. Henrichs B. The Perceptions of Student Registered Nurse Anesthetists of the Anesthesia Patient Simulator Experience. Presented at: Technology for the Next Century; 2000; Orlando, FL.

18. O'Donnell JM, Fletcher J, Dixon B, Palmer L. Planning and implementing an anesthesia crisis resource management course for student nurse anesthetists. *CRNA.* 1998;9(2):50–58.

19. Fletcher J. *AANA Journal* course: Update for nurse anesthetists ERR WATCH: anesthesia crisis resource management from the nurse anesthetist's perspective. *AANA J.* 1998;66(6):595–602.

20. Fletcher JL. *AANA Journal* course: Update for nurse anesthetists anesthesia simulation: a tool for learning and research. *AANA J.* 1995;63(1):61–67.

21. Cook DA, Hatala R, Brydges R, et al. Technology-enhanced simulation for health professions education: a systematic review and meta-analysis. *JAMA.* 2011;306(9):978–988.

22. Shin S, Park JH, Kim JH. Effectiveness of patient simulation in nursing education: meta-analysis. *Nurse Educ Today.* 2015;35(1):176–182.

23. Oh PJ, Jeon KD, Koh MS. The effects of simulation-based learning using standardized patients in nursing students: a meta-analysis. *Nurse Educ Today.* 2015;35(5):e6–e15.

24. Lee J, Oh PJ. Effects of the use of high-fidelity human simulation in nursing education: a meta-analysis. *J Nurs Educ.* 2015;54(9):501–507.

25. Cheng A, Lockey A, Bhanji F, Lin Y, Hunt EA, Lang E. The use of high-fidelity manikins for advanced life support training a systematic review and meta-analysis. *Resuscitation.* 2015;93:142–149.

26. Brydges R, Manzone J, Shanks D, et al. Self-regulated learning in simulation-based training: a systematic review and meta-analysis. *Med Educ.* 2015;49(4):368–378.

27. Cook DA. How much evidence does it take? A cumulative meta-analysis of outcomes of simulation-based education. *Med Educ.* 2014;48(8):750–760.

28. Cheng A, Lang TR, Starr SR, Pusic M, Cook DA. Technology-enhanced simulation and pediatric education: a meta-analysis. *Pediatrics.* 2014;133(5):e1313–1323.

29. Lorello GR, Cook DA, Johnson RL, Brydges R. Simulation-based training in anaesthesiology: a systematic review and meta-analysis. *British Journal of Anaesthesia.* 2014;112(2):231–245.

30. Cook DA, Hamstra SJ, Brydges R, et al. Comparative effectiveness of instructional design features in simulation-based education: systematic review and meta-analysis. *Med Teach.* 2013;35(1):e867–898.

31. Salas E, DiazGranados D, Klein C, et al. Does team training improve team performance? A meta-analysis. *Hum Factors.* 2008;50(6):903–933.

32. Fallacaro MD. Untoward pathophysiological events: simulation as an experiential learning option to prepare anesthesia providers. *CRNA.* 2000;11(3):138–143.

33. Barsuk JH, Cohen ER, Nguyen D, et al. Attending physician adherence to a 29-component central venous catheter bundle checklist during simulated procedures. *Crit Care Med.* 2016;44(10):1871–1881.

34. Mok M, Ker J. Developing clinical skills bundles. *Clin Teach.* 2015;12(6):403–407.

35. Craft C, Feldon DF, Brown EA. Instructional design affects the efficacy of simulation-based training in central venous catheterization. *Am J Surg.* 2014;207(5):782–789.

36. Barsuk JH, Cohen ER, Potts S, et al. Dissemination of a simulation-based mastery learning intervention reduces central line-associated bloodstream infections. *BMJ Qual Saf.* 2014;23(9):749–756.

37. Cain CL, Riess ML, Gettrust L, Novalija J. Malignant hyperthermia crisis: optimizing patient outcomes through simulation and interdisciplinary collaboration. *AORN J.* 2014;99(2):301–308.

38. Schwid HA, O'Donnell D. Educational computer simulation of malignant hyperthermia. *J Clin Monit.* 1992;8(3):201–208.

39. Kardong-Edgren S, Gaba D, Dieckmann P, Cook DA. Reporting inquiry in simulation. *Simul Healthc.* 2011;Suppl 6:S63–66.

40. McGaghie WC, Draycott TJ, Dunn WF, Lopez CM, Stefanidis D. Evaluating the impact of simulation on translational patient outcomes. *Simul Healthc.* 2011;Suppl 6:S42–47.

41. Nestel D, Groom J, Eikeland-Husebo S, O'Donnell JM. Simulation for learning and teaching procedural skills: the state of the science. *Simul Healthc.* 2011;Suppl 6:S10–13.

42. Scerbo MW, Murray WB, Alinier G, et al. A path to better healthcare simulation systems: leveraging the integrated systems design approach. *Simul Healthc.* 2011;Suppl 6:S20–23.

43. Schaefer JJ III, Vanderbilt AA, Cason CL, et al. Literature review: instructional design and pedagogy science in healthcare simulation. *Simul Healthc.* 2011;Suppl 6:S30–41.

44. McGaghie WC, Issenberg SB, Barsuk JH, Wayne DB. A critical review of simulation-based mastery learning with translational outcomes. *Med Educ.* 2014;48(4):375–385.

45. Callard F, Rose D, Wykes T. Close to the bench as well as at the bedside: involving service users in all phases of translational research. *Health Expect.* 2012;15(4):389-400.

46. Programs CCoAoNAE. Standards and Guidelines, DNP Entry. Park Ridge, IL: American Association of Nurse Anesthetists; 2016.

47. Fletcher JL. *AANA Journal* Course: Update for nurse anesthetists Anesthesia simulation: A tool for learning and research. *AANA J.* 1995;63:61–67.

48. Chen PT, Cheng HW, Yen CR, et al. Instructor-based real-time multimedia medical simulation to update concepts of difficult airway management for experienced airway practitioners. *J Chin Med Assoc.* 2008;71(4):174–179.

49. Grant JS, Dawkins D, Molhook L, Keltner NL, Vance DE. Comparing the effectiveness of video-assisted oral debriefing and oral debriefing alone on behaviors by undergraduate nursing students during high-fidelity simulation. *Nurse Educ Pract.* 2014;14(5):479–484.

50. Grant JS, Moss J, Epps C, Watts P. Using video-facilitated feedback to improve student performance following high-fidelity simulation. *Clin Simul Nurs.* 2010;6(5):e177–e184.

51. Paige JT, Garbee DD, Kozmenko V, et al. Getting a head start: high-fidelity, simulation-based operating room team training of interprofessional students. *J Am Coll Surg.* 2014;218(1):140–149.

52. Lyk-Jensen HT, Jepsen RM, Spanager L, Dieckmann P, Ostergaard D. Assessing nurse anaesthetists' non-technical skills in the operating room. *Acta Anaesthesiol Scand.* 2014;58(7):794–801.

53. Long RE. Using simulation to teach resuscitation: an important patient safety tool. *Crit Care Nurs Clin North Am.* 2005;17(1):1–8, ix.

54. Boonmak P, Boonmak S, Srichaipanha S, Poomsawat S. Knowledge and skill after brief ACLS training. *J Med Assoc Thai.* 2004;87(11):1311–1314.

55. Sell S, Palmer L. Community initiative: elementary and middle school students a creative approach. *AANA J.* 2004;72(2):107–113.

56. Hawkins R, Bendickson L, Benson P, et al. A pilot study evaluating the perceptions of Certified Registered Nurse Anesthetists toward human patient simulation. *AANA J.* 2014;82(5):375–384.

57. Henrichs BM, Avidan MS, Murray DJ, et al. Performance of Certified Registered Nurse Anesthetists and anesthesiologists in a simulation-based skills assessment. *Anesth Analg.* 2009;108(1):255–262.

58. Lopreiato J, Downing D, Gammon W, et al. Healthcare Simulation Dictionary. http://www.ssih.org/dictionary. 2016. Accessed July, 25, 2016.

59. International Nursing Association for Clinical Simulation and Learning. INACSL Board of Directors. Standard I: Terminology. *Clin Simul Nurs.* 2011;7(4):S3–S7.

60. McGaghie WC, Issenberg SB, Petrusa ER, Scalese RJ. A critical review of simulation-based medical education research: 2003–2009. *Med Educ.* 2010;44(1):50–63.

61. Motola I, Devine LA, Chung HS, Sullivan JE, Issenberg SB. Simulation in healthcare education: a best evidence practical guide. AMEE Guide No. 82. *Medical Teacher.* 2013;35(10):e1511–1530.

62. Hayden JK, Smiley RA, Alexander M, Kardong-Edgren S, Jeffries PR. The NCSBN national simulation study: a longitudinal, randomized, controlled study replacing clinical hours with simulation in prelicensure nursing education. *J Nurs Regul.* 2014;5 Suppl 2:S1–41.

63. Issenberg SB, McGaghie WC. Features and uses of high-fidelity medical simulations that can lead to effective learning: A BEME systematic review. *Med Teach.* 2005;27(1):110–28.

64. Alexander M, Durham CF, Hooper JI, et al. NCSBN Simulation Guidelines for Prelicensure Nursing Programs. *Jour Nurs Regul.* 2015;6(3):39–42.

65. International Nursing Association for Clinical Simulation and Learning. INACSL Board of Directors. Standards of Best Practice: Simulation. *Clin Simul Nurs.* 2013;9(6):Sii–Siii.

66. International Nursing Association for Clinical Simulation and Learning. INACSL Board of Direcors. Standard IV: Facilitation Methods. *Clin Simul Nurs.* 2011;7(4):S12–S13.

67. International Nursing Association for Clinical Simulation and Learning.INACSL Board of Directors. Standard V: Simulation Facilitator. *Clin Simul Nurs.* 2011;7(4):S14–S15.

68. International Nursing Association for Clinical Simulation and Learning. INACSL Board of Directors. Standard VI: The Debriefing Process. *Clin Simul Nurs.* 2011;7(4):S16–S17.

69. International Nursing Association for Clinical Simulation and Learning. INACSL Board of Directors. Standard II: Professional Integrity of Participant. *Clin Simul Nurs.* 2011;7(4):S8–S9.

70. International Nursing Association for Clinical Simulation and Learning. INACSL Board of Directors. Standard VII: Evaluation of Expected Outcomes. *Clin Simul Nurs.* 2011;7(4):S18–S19.

71. International Nursing Association for Clinical Simulation and Learning. INACSL Board of Directors. Standard III: Participant Objectives. *Clin Simul Nurs.* 2011;7(4):S10–S11.

72. O'Leary JA, Nash R, Lewis PA. High fidelity patient simulation as an educational tool in paediatric intensive care: a systematic review. *Nurse Educ Today.* 2015;35(10):e8–e12.

73. Garden AL, Le Fevre DM, Waddington HL, Weller JM. Debriefing after simulation-based non-technical skill training in healthcare: a systematic review of effective practice. *Anaesth Intensive Care.* 2015;43(3):300–308.

74. Brydges R, Hatala R, Zendejas B, Erwin PJ, Cook DA. Linking simulation-based educational assessments and patient-related outcomes: a systematic review and meta-analysis. *Acad Med.* 2015;90(2):246–256.

75. Levett-Jones T, Lapkin S. A systematic review of the effectiveness of simulation debriefing in health professional education. *Nurse Educ Today.* 2014;34(6):e58–63.

76. Hamstra SJ, Brydges R, Hatala R, Zendejas B, Cook DA. Reconsidering fidelity in simulation-based training. *Acad Med.* 2014;89(3):387–392.

77. Gjeraa K, Moller TP, Ostergaard D. Efficacy of simulation-based trauma team training of non-technical skills. A systematic review. *Acta Anaesthesiol Scand.* 2014;58(7):775–787.

78. Dawe SR, Pena GN, Windsor JA, et al. Systematic review of skills transfer after surgical simulation-based training. *Br J Surg.* 2014;101(9):1063–1076.

79. Zendejas B, Brydges R, Wang AT, Cook DA. Patient outcomes in simulation-based medical education: a systematic review. *J Gen Intern Med.* 2013;28(8):1078–1089.

80. Mundell WC, Kennedy CC, Szostek JH, Cook DA. Simulation technology for resuscitation training: a systematic review and meta-analysis. *Resuscitation.* 2013;84(9):1174–1183.

81. McKinney J, Cook DA, Wood D, Hatala R. Simulation-based training for cardiac auscultation skills: systematic review and meta-analysis. *J Gen Intern Med.* 2013;28(2):283–291.

82. Kennedy CC, Maldonado F, Cook DA. Simulation-based bronchoscopy training: systematic review and meta-analysis. *Chest.* 2013;144(1):183–192.

83. Ilgen JS, Sherbino J, Cook DA. Technology-enhanced simulation in emergency medicine: a systematic review and meta-analysis. *Acad Emerg Med.* 2013;20(2):117–127.

84. Cumin D, Boyd MJ, Webster CS, Weller JM. A systematic review of simulation for multidisciplinary team training in operating rooms. *Simul Healthc.* 2013;8(3):171–179.

85. Cook DA, Brydges R, Zendejas B, Hamstra SJ, Hatala R. Technology-enhanced simulation to assess health professionals: a systematic review of validity evidence, research methods, and reporting quality. *Acad Med.* 2013;88(6):872–883.

86. Cook DA, Brydges R, Zendejas B, Hamstra SJ, Hatala R. Mastery learning for health professionals using technology-enhanced simulation: a systematic review and meta-analysis. *Acad Med.* 2013;88(8):1178–1186.

87. Norman J. Systematic review of the literature on simulation in nursing education. *ABNF J.* 2012;23(2):24–28.

88. Rutherford-Hemming T, Lioce L, Kardong-Edgren SS, Jeffries PR, Sittner B. After the National Council of State Boards of Nursing simulation study recommendations and next steps. *Clin Simul Nurs.* 2016;12(1):2–7.

89. Society for Simulation in Healthcare. Full Accreditation. http://www.ssih.org/Accreditation/Full-Accreditation. Accessed September 5, 2016.

90. Society for Simulation in Healthcare. SSH Certification Programs. http://www.ssih.org/Certification. Accessed September 5, 2016.

91. Herrmann EK. Mrs. Chase: a noble and enduring figure. *Am J Nurs.* 1981;81(10):1836.

92. Rosen RK. The history of medical simulation. In: Loyd GE, Lake CL, Greenberg RB, eds. *Practical health care simulations.* Philadelphia: Elsevier Mosby; 2004:3–26.

93. Peitzman SJ, Cuddy MM. Performance in physical examination on the USMLE step 2 clinical skills examination. *Acad Med.* 2015;90(2):209–213.

94. Turner TR, Scerbo MW, Gliva-McConvey GA, Wallace AM. Standardized patient encounters: periodic versus postencounter evaluation of nontechnical clinical performance. *Simul Healthc.* 2016;11(3):164–172.

95. Plaksin J, Nicholson J, Kundrod S, Zabar S, Kalet A, Altshuler L. The benefits and risks of being a standardized patient: a narrative review of the literature. *Patient.* 2016:9(1):15–25.

96. Lee J, Cheng A, Angelski C, Allain D, Ali S. High-fidelity simulation in pediatric emergency medicine: a national survey of facilitator comfort and practice. *Pediatr Emerg Care.* 2015;31(4):260–265.

97. Ignacio J, Dolmans D, Scherpbier A, Rethans JJ, Chan S, Liaw SY. Comparison of standardized patients with high-fidelity simulators for managing stress and improving performance in clinical deterioration: A mixed methods study. *Nurse Educ Today.* 2015;35(12):1161–1168.

98. Schulz CM, Skrzypczak M, Raith S, et al. High-fidelity human patient simulators compared with human actors in an unannounced mass-casualty exercise. *Prehosp Disaster Med.* 2014;29(2):176–182.

99. Davis DH, Oliver M, Byrne AJ. A novel method of measuring the mental workload of anaesthetists during simulated practice. *Br J Anaesth.* 2009;103(5):665–669.

100. Haji FA, Rojas D, Childs R, de Ribaupierre S, Dubrowski A. Measuring cognitive load: performance, mental effort and simulation task complexity. *Med Educ.* 2015;49(8):815–827.

101. Chen R, Grierson LE, Norman GR. Evaluating the impact of high- and low-fidelity instruction in the development of auscultation skills. *Med Educ.* 2015;49(3):276–285.

102. Naismith LM, Cheung JJ, Ringsted C, Cavalcanti RB. Limitations of subjective cognitive load measures in simulation-based procedural training. *Med Educ.* 2015;49(8):805–814.

103. Fraser KL, Ayres P, Sweller J. Cognitive load theory for the design of medical simulations. *Simul Healthc.* 2015;10(5):295–307.

104. Byrne AJ, Sellen AJ, Jones JG, et al. Effect of videotape feedback on anaesthetists' performance while managing simulated anaesthetic crises: a multicentre study. *Anaesthesia.* 2002;57(2):176–179.

105. Decarlo D, Collingridge DS, Grant C, Ventre KM. Factors Influencing Nurses' Attitudes Toward Simulation-Based Education. *Simul Healthc.* 2008;3(2):90–96.

106. Maignan M, Koch FX, Chaix J, et al. Team Emergency Assessment Measure (TEAM) for the assessment of non-technical skills during resuscitation: validation of the French version. *Resuscitation.* 2016;101:115–120.

107. Gormley GJ, Fenwick T. Learning to manage complexity through simulation: students' challenges and possible strategies. *Perspect Med Educ.* 2016;5(3):138–146.

108. Tully J, Dameff C, Kaib S, Moffitt M. Recording medical students' encounters with standardized patients using Google Glass: providing end-of-life clinical education. *Acad Med.* 2015;90(3):314–316.

109. Nguyen LN, Tardioli K, Roberts M, Watterson J. Development and incorporation of hybrid simulation OSCE into in-training examinations to assess multiple CanMEDS competencies in urologic trainees. *Can Urol Assoc J.* 2015;9(1–2):32–36.

110. Kiesewetter J, Fischer MR. The teamwork assessment scale: a novel instrument to assess quality of undergraduate medical students' teamwork using the example of simulation-based ward-rounds. *GMS Z Med Ausbild.* 2015;32(2):Doc19.

111. Hu YY, Parker SH, Lipsitz SR, et al. Surgeons' leadership styles and team behavior in the operating room. *J Am Coll Surg.* 2016;222(1):41–51.

112. DeVita MA, Schaefer J, Lutz J, Wang H, Dongilli T. Improving medical emergency team (MET) performance using a novel curriculum and a computerized human patient simulator. *Qual Saf Health Care.* 2005;14(5):326–331.

113. George BC, Teitelbaum EN, Darosa DA, et al. Duration of faculty training needed to ensure reliable or performance ratings. *J Surg Educ.* 2013;70(6):703–708.

114. Hallmark BF. Faculty development in simulation education. *Nurs Clin North Am.* 2015;50(2):389–397.

115. Locatis C, Weisberg M. Strategies contributing to effectiveness of health science faculty training. *J Biocommun.* 1981;8(1):4–9.

116. Issenberg SB, Scalese RJ. Simulation in health care education. *Perspectives Biol Med.* 2008;51(1):31–46.

117. Jansen DA, Berry C, Brenner GH, Johnson N, Larson G. A collaborative project to influence nursing faculty interest in simulation. *Clin SimulNurs.* 6(6):e223–e229.

118. Talcott K, O'Donnell JM, Burns HK. Technology and the nurse educator: are you ELITE? *Nurse Educ.* 2013;38(3):126–131.

119. Doran GT. There's a S.M.A.R.T. way to write management's goals and objectives. *Manag Rev.* 1981;70(11):35–36.

120. Sawyer T, Eppich W, Brett-Fleegler M, Grant V, Cheng A. More than one way to debrief: a critical review of healthcare simulation debriefing methods. *Simul Healthc.* 2016;11(3):209–217.

121. Boet S, Pigford AA, Fitzsimmons A, Reeves S, Triby E, Bould MD. Interprofessional team debriefings with or without an instructor after a simulated crisis scenario: an exploratory case study. *J Interprof Care.* 2016:1–9.

122. Paige JT, Arora S, Fernandez G, Seymour N. Debriefing 101: training faculty to promote learning in simulation-based training. *Am J Surg.* 2015;209(1):126–131.

123. Eppich WJ, Hunt EA, Duval-Arnould JM, Siddall VJ, Cheng A. Structuring feedback and debriefing to achieve mastery learning goals. *Acad Med.* 2015;90(1):1501–1508.

124. Phrampus PE, O'Donnell J M. Debriefing: using a structured and supported approach. In: Levine A, ed. *The Comprehensive Textbook of Healthcare Simulation.* Vol 1. New York, NY: Springer; 2013:73–84.

125. Cheng A, Palaganas J, Eppich W, Rudolph J, Robinson T, Grant V. Co-debriefing for simulation-based education: a primer for facilitators. *Simul Healthc.* 2015;10(2):69–75.

126. Cheng A, Grant V, Dieckmann P, Arora S, Robinson T, Eppich W. Faculty development for simulation programs: five issues for the future of debriefing training. *Simul Healthc.* 2015;10(4):217–222.

127. Decker S, Fey M, Sideras S, et al. Standards of best practice: simulation standard VI: the debriefing process. *Clin Simul Nurs.* 2014;9(6):S26–S29.

128. O'Donnell JM, Rodgers D, Lee W, et al. *Structured and Supported Debriefing* [interactive multimedia program], Dallas, TX.: American Heart Association; 2009.

129. Fanning RM, Gaba DM. The role of debriefing in simulation-based learning. *Simul.* 2007;2(2):115–125.

130. Greene, RL. Sources of recency effects in free recall. *Psychol Bull.* 1986;99(2):221–228.

131. Cochrane AL. *Effectiveness and Efficiency: Random Reflections on Health Services.* London, UK: The Nuffield Hospitals Trust; 1972.

132. Haynes B. Can it work? Does it work? Is it worth it? The testing of healthcare interventions is evolving. *BMJ.* 1999;319(7211):652–653.

133. Gartlehner G, Hansen RA, Nissman D, Lohr KN, Carey TS. A simple and valid tool distinguished efficacy from effectiveness studies. *J Clin Epidemiol.* 2006;59(10):1040–1048.

134. Kim SY. Efficacy versus Effectiveness. *Korean J Fam Med.* 2013;34(4):227.

CHAPTER 15

Teaching Psychomotor Skills and the Administration of Regional Anesthesia

Charles A. Reese, PhD, CRNA

Keywords: Cognitive skills, educational taxonomy, epidural blocks, peripheral nerve blocks, psychomotor skills, regional anesthesia, subarachnoid blocks, technical skills.

Key Concepts

- Training in regional anesthesia requires mastery of both cognitive and technical skills.
- The number of regional anesthetics performed for surgery and pain control continues to increase.
- Student competence in the clinical environment does not correlate with performance on standard paper tests and assignment work.
- Educational taxonomies may be used to develop improved methods to train and assess anesthetists in regional anesthesia techniques. They provide guidance for the design, delivery, and evaluation of learning experiences as well as a simple, quick, and easy checklist for planning and executing learning episodes.
- It may be reasonable to expect students to achieve a high level of proficiency with common blocks (ie, spinal, epidural) for healthy patients during training; however, achieving the same proficiency with blocks in patients with significant surgical comorbidities or anatomical anomalies (ie, scoliosis, ankylosing spondylitis) may be beyond the scope of basic clinical training. It is unlikely that students will have the opportunity to become proficient in the intermediate and more advanced techniques during basic training.
- A regional anesthesia-specific adaptation of the psychomotor domain is provided.
- Training must include experiences with emerging technologies, including ultrasound guidance.

Introduction

The role of graduate-level education in nurse anesthesia is to provide practitioners a degree of proficiency and comfort in the profession. In this context, "proficiency" can be defined as "advancement in knowledge." When learning to perform regional anesthesia techniques, the student must develop specific, and often unique, skills working with the tangible materials and tools related to the technique.

In addition to cognitive skills, training in regional anesthesia requires mastery of technical skills as well. As the student must personally perform the work, it is necessary for him or her to have appropriately developed psychomotor skills to be able to recognize and manage the various components and the equipment used to perform the techniques in an appropriate manner and order. The student must also learn to appreciate the potential difficulties and dangers associated with the performance of the tasks.

This is a general discussion of learning taxonomy, offering a unique hierarchical taxonomy of psychomotor skills relevant to the practice of regional anesthesia.These skills are discussed specifically from the viewpoint of the needs of student registered nurse anesthetists (SRNAs). The discussion ends with a consideration of emerging technology: ultrasound guidance.

The number and variety of regional anesthetics performed for surgery and pain control has increased substantially over the past several decades. Regional anesthesia techniques provide excellent analgesia or anesthesia and are cost-effective. There is an ever-increasing demand for regional anesthesia by both surgeons and patients. Their use avoids manipulation of the airway and significant hemodynamic consequences often associated with general anesthesia. While serious, poor outcomes are rare, they are possible. When they do occur, they may be catastrophic.

As with all clinical procedures, proper training is paramount to safe practice. Most complications appear to be related to poor fundamental technique and lack of essential precautions that should have been inculcated during the clinician's primary training. Although peripheral nerve blocks have been greatly refined by the adaptation of the peripheral nerve stimulator and ultrasound, they still require a comprehensive appreciation of anatomy and significant dexterity.

During more than four decades of mentoring students, I have observed that student competence in the clinical environment does not correlate with performance in standard paper tests and assignment work. There is little guidance for clinical instructors about how to safely and effectively teach regional anesthesia techniques. There is a paucity of research on educational methods for such training; thus, the genesis of this attempt is to offer thoughts regarding teaching the psychomotor components of regional anesthesia.

Regardless of the formal structure of their curriculum, SRNA learners have already been exposed to the first two elements of learning taxonomy (ie, affective and cognitive domains) by the time they are introduced into the clinical learning environment (ie, psychomotor domain). During their initial clinical practicums, most special equipment and processes, including regional anesthesia, are unfamiliar to the student.

As nurse anesthesia educational programs (NAEPs) have adapted to the graduate education framework, in most instances, time committed to didactic endeavors has reduced the actual time students physically spend in their clinical experience. Perhaps the transition to doctoral-level preparation will further erode the critical clinical component. In addition, access to clinical resources, particularly regional anesthesia appropriate cases, is often highly competitive. This may be especially evident in programs that coexist with anesthesiology residency programs. Therefore, it is imperative to develop a clear, substantial educational justification of the clinical activities students are required to perform in order to justify the amount of clinical material and associated resources provided students as part of this aspect of their education. This raises the concern of just what clinical experiences should be expected of students and what they should be expected to learn (ie, learning objectives) as a result of those experiences. With a clear understanding of what should be learned through a particular teaching and learning activity, it becomes possible to design the activity in a manner which best focuses on the learning of that particular outcome or combination of outcomes.

Consumers and government regulatory organizations are becoming more focused on "competency" among health care providers. Although how to accurately define competency in regional anesthesia is unclear, educators and accreditation organizations need to establish ways to identify, measure, and evaluate those less well-defined cognitive and psychomotor skills that are necessary for the safe and efficient practice of regional anesthesia.

Anesthesiology Resident Training

Due to lack of extensive evidence-based data for SRNAs, one must extrapolate available anesthesiology residency data. Intuitively, if anesthesiology residents are not performing regional techniques, it is reasonable to assume that SRNAs are not either.

In 1986, anesthesiology residencies were increased from two to three year's duration. In 1989, the length was again increased, from three to four years, including internship. Concurrently, numerous extended specialty specific postgraduate fellowship programs emerged, including regional anesthesia. More recently these have advanced to include the evolving ultrasound guided regional anesthesia techniques.

Several studies of anesthesia residencies (U.S.) revealed interesting, albeit disappointing, information regarding the administration of regional anesthesia. In 1980, among responding training programs, regional anesthesia was used in only 21% of all cases (range: 2.8-55.7%).[1] This data also suggested that some residency programs failed to provide even a minimal exposure in the most basic regional techniques, and that there was wide interprogram variability.-

A follow-up survey in 1990 showed an increase in regional cases (30%), attributed mostly to an increase in the use of epidurals in obstetrics and pain management; however, interprogram variability persisted (2.8-58.5%).[2] A most extreme example cited was spinal anesthetics; depending on the program, a resident in even well-respected programs could complete his or her four-year education having performed as few as 3 or as many as 387 techniques. Interestingly, the residency review committee (RRC) for anesthesiology of the Accreditation Council for Graduate Medical Education (ACGME) has considered increasing the numbers of blocks that residents must perform during their residency program. Given current case statistics, doing so will no doubt further reduce the availability of clinical material for other learners.

In 1996, the RRC began requiring a graduate to have performed a minimum of 40 spinals and 50 epidurals (type not specified) in order to qualify to write his or her board examination. While not required, the RRC also suggested performance of 40 peripheral nerve blocks for surgery and 25 for pain management to achieve competency; however, the types of these blocks were not specified. This lack of specificity may contribute to the aforementioned disparity in training statistics. Performing 40 of the same technique may satisfy the RRC requirements, but fails to encourage competency across the spectrum of techniques.

The most recent data showed that resident experiences in spinals and epidurals increased slightly, and that interprogram variability was narrowing. However, resident experiences with peripheral nerve blocks continued to be problematic as 40 percent of residents still did not attain the suggested minimal experiences for peripheral nerve blocks.[3]

The RRC's requirement of only 40 unspecified peripheral nerve blocks has been questioned as possibly not providing enough experience for an individual to develop expertise in regional anesthesia.[4] Rosenblatt et al., reported that only 50% of residents were able to perform an interscalene block autonomously after experience with 7–9 cases. When their experience exceeded 15 cases, 87.5% reported autonomous success. Of these, 96.3% of blocks were reported as adequate for surgery. Clearly, it is unlikely that practitioners not confident in a particular block will use that block in their future practice. Worse yet, they may attempt to provide blocks without the necessary skills and experience. Current requirements may be insufficient for graduates to approach competency. This is not only concerning from an educator's view; it may be considered a patient safety issue.

Studies addressing clinical competence in regional anesthesia suggest it may take 60-90 supervised procedures to master lumbar epidural technique with an adequate success rate.[5] Kopacz and colleagues[6] suggest that 45 spinal and 60 epidural procedures must be done to achieve a 90% success rate. These figures are similar to mastery of frequently used technical procedures in other specialties (ie, flexible fiberoptic sigmoidoscopy by family practice residents); however, these are aggregate statistics and likely underestimate the needs of some students.

Intuitively, it seems it would take considerably more experience to attain success in peripheral nerve block techniques, particularly those of the lower extremity. Rosenblatt and associates[4] showed that more than 10 interscalene blocks must be accomplished before the student attains even 50% autonomy. Konrad and coworkers have shown that at least 70 axillary block experiences are required before a success rate of 85% can be achieved. Thus, when compared to available data, it is very unlikely that anesthesia students are performing enough peripheral nerve blocks to develop a requisite proficiency.

Establishing general numerical minimums does not assess students' technical or clinical competence. Rather than attempt to provide a full range of experiences to learners, with limited opportunities for each, perhaps they would be better served by concentrating on a core group of commonly applicable and relatively simple nerve blocks.[8]

Students must also develop nontechnical proficiency, such as patient selection and perioperative management of regionally anesthetized patients, including the associated physiologic and pharmacologic changes. Experience must be gained with the management of intraoperative sedation as well as awareness and management of complications. The ability to analyze and apply outcomes data is also important to one's overall practice.

Student Registered Nurse Anesthetist Training

Success by graduate registered nurse anesthetists on the national board on certification and recertification of nurse anesthetists' certification examination suggests only that the graduates' theoretical (ie, cognitive) knowledge is adequate for entry level to practice. As with all written examinations, it is silent on the objective evaluation of their regional anesthesia clinical skills.

The history of regional anesthesia training of student registered nurse anesthetists mostly parallels that of anesthesiology residents. That the RRC is concerned about the adequacy of resident training in regional anesthesia should be a harbinger of concern for the Council on Accreditation of Nurse Anesthesia Educational Programs (COANAEP) as well. While statistics are not available for NAEPs, it should be fair to assume that considerable discrepancies exist between programs in the quantity, and quality, of training in regional anesthesia. One can only speculate that access to clinical material and interprogram variability is similarly problematic. This may be particularly so in programs collocated with anesthesiology residencies where access to clinical cases is highly competitive.

While formal course work focused on regional anesthesia has a long tradition in didactic curriculums, inclusion of regional anesthesia in NAEP clinical curriculums has been measured. In 1990, the COANAEP outlined the requirement for administration and/or maintenance of 30 regional cases. Actual administration was strongly encouraged.[9] In 1994, the COANAEP informed NAEPs that "Administration of regional anesthetics ... will be required by the year 2000."[10] In 1999, the COANAEP began requiring administration of a minimum of 25 regional cases, including 5 spinal, 5 epidural, and 5 peripheral blocks (type not specified).[11] A footnote advised that the number of spinals and epidurals was to increase to 15 each by 2003. In 2004, the total number of regional cases required remained the same, but the specific stipulations by technique were removed.[12]

Most recent data (2014), as reported by NAEP directors, indicates that graduating students (N=1855) report an average of 106 (±58) actual administrations of regional anesthesia techniques. These include 42 (±25) spinal, 39 (±28) epidural, and 25(±28) peripheral blocks during their training. Management of regional techniques fares better in that graduates report an average of 112 (±58) cases.[13]

[Note: As with all statistics, caution must be used when drawing conclusions or implying correlations from data. This is especially true in that some of the studies mentioned previously state only "regional anesthesia" and did not classify by type of technique or patient population. Care must be taken when comparing statistics as anesthesiology residencies are 48 months' duration, not including fellowships, and are almost exclusively clinically based, while NAEPs average 28 months' duration and include a substantial amount of didactic education as well as clinical experiences.

The 2012 American Association of Nurse Anesthetists (AANA) Practice Profile Survey states that the following percentages reflect full-time CRNAs (N=6,112) performing the following as part of their current practice: spinal, 72.9%; epidural, 53.6%; 23.1%; pain management, 15.4%; and ophthalmologic block, 6.4%. Regarding brachial plexus block (N=1,924): axillary, 68.1%; interscalene 83.9%; subclavian 20.5%, reported by AANA in 2012.

Scope of Practice

Given the fact that, in addition to spinal and epidural techniques, there are more than 40 different combined and peripheral nerve block techniques, it is understandable that a student is not likely to become proficient with any specific procedure during his or her basic training experience. This lack of proficiency is further aggravated by the numerous technical variations introduced by different anesthesiologist and CRNA clinical instructors.

In which techniques should a graduate SRNA be proficient? Hadzic[14] offers an attractive approach. He divides more than 40 common techniques into three categories, ranked by degree of difficulty, time required to master, and potential for complications (See **Figure 15.1**). The student is introduced first to the essential (basic) techniques, then to the more complex (intermediate), and finally, to the advanced techniques. Critical to this approach, of course, is the availability of and access to clinical material at each of these levels.

Figure 15.1 Regional Anesthesia Techniques, Ranked by Degree of Difficulty, Time Required to Master, and Potential for Complications

Basic Techniques	Intermediate Techniques	Advanced Techniques
• Superficial cervical plexus block • Axillary brachial plexus block[a] • Intravenous regional anesthesia (Bier block)[a] • Wrist block • Digital nerve block • Intercostobrachial nerve block • Saphenous nerve block[b] • Ankle block[b] • Spinal anesthesia[a] • Lumbar epidural anesthesia[a] • Combined spinal-epidural anesthesia[a] • Femoral nerve block[b]	Deep cervical plexus block • Interscalene block[b] • Supraclavicular block[b] • Infraclavicular block[b] • Sciatic nerve block: posterior approach • Genitofemoral nerve block • Popliteal block: all approaches • Suprascapular nerve block • Intercostal nerve block • Thoracic epidural anesthesia: single injection or continuous • Lumbar plexus block[b] • Combined lumbarplexus/ sciatic block • Continuous femoral nerve block[b] • Sciatic nerve block: anterior approach and parafemoral technique • Obturator nerve block • Continuous sciatic nerve block[b] • Continuous popliteal block: all approaches • Cervical epidural anesthesia • Cervical paravertebral block • Maxillary nerve block • Mandibular nerve block • Retrobulbar and peribulbar nerve block	• Continuous interscalene brachial plexus block[b] • Continuous infraclavicular brachial plexus block[b] • Thoracic paravertebral block: single-injection, continuous • Thoracolumbar paravertebral block • Combined lumbar plexus/ sciatic blocks • Lumbar plexus block • Continuous femoral nerve block[b] • Sciatic nerve block: anterior approach • Anterior sciatic nerve block: para femoral technique • Obturator block • Continuous sciatic block: posterior approach • Continuous popliteal nerve block: intertendinous and lateral approaches

Adapted from Hadzic A, Vloka JD. *Peripheral Nerve Blocks: Principles and Practice.* New York, NY: McGraw Hill Professional; 2004.

[a] The author's opinion of techniques that student registered nurse anesthetists should demonstrate competency in prior to graduation.

[b] The author's opinion of techniques that student registered nurse anesthetists should receive significant exposure to prior to graduation.

It may be reasonable to expect students to achieve a high level of proficiency with common blocks (ie, spinal, epidural) in a normal population of patients during their basic training experience; however, a high degree of success in patients with significant surgical co-morbidities or anatomical anomalies (ie, scoliosis, ankylosing spondylitis) may be beyond this scope. It is unlikely that students will have the opportunity to become proficient in the intermediate and more advanced techniques during their basic training. As mentioned previously, reduction of clinical working hours for SRNAs and competition for clinical cases may severely limit SRNAs' opportunities for all but the most basic spinal and epidural techniques.

Even if cases are available, students should not attempt more advanced techniques until they have demonstrated proficiency with the basic techniques. To have students try, and fail, at a more complex technique when they are not ready may deter their use of regional anesthesia in the future.

Taxonomy-Learning Domains

The problem of rote learning by students has been recognized for more than four centuries.[15] Educators universally agree that the learning process must not only provide knowledge about things, it must provide the capability and competence of the student to actually do things. This quandary was addressed by the development of educational theories that provided an approach to the development of educational objectives based on the behaviorist perspective of identifying what the student is able to do as a result of the educational activity.[16,17]

Dr Benjamin Bloom's taxonomy, or variations thereof, continues to be the most widely used framework of its kind in education and training. This is largely due to its simplicity, clarity, and effectiveness for explaining and applying learning objectives and teaching methods, and for measuring learning outcomes. Bloom's work, known as Bloom's taxonomy of learning domains, or Bloom's taxonomy of educational objectives, was introduced in 1956 to assist in the design and assessment of learning activities.[18] His original work introduced and discussed two unique domains, the cognitive and the affective. Numerous authors, adding more relevance to the field of academic education, have expanded his seminal work by introducing a third domain, psychomotor.

Definition of Taxonomy

Taxonomy provides a coherent structure for planning, designing, assessing, and for evaluating training and its overall learning effectiveness. Models serve as a kind of checklist by which one can ensure that teaching is planned in such a manner as to deliver the necessary learner development. They provide a template by which the validity and coverage of training can be assessed.

More often than not, training is limited to nonparticipative, unfeeling attempts to transfer knowledge. Recognizing that such teaching is focused on fact transfer and rote recall of information (the lowest level of learning), Bloom felt that learning should focus on mastery of subjects and the promotion of higher forms of thinking, rather than simply transferring facts. He attempted to establish a system of developing educational learning objectives that could be properly measured in order to assure mastery of a subject. Thus, elements of the domains within his taxonomy are structured from the very simple (ie, memorizing facts) to the more complex (ie, analyzing or evaluating information). The complete Bloom's taxonomy comprises a structure of three overlapping domains. Depending on the publication referenced, the details of these domains may vary, particularly the third domain.

Given that Bloom was a behaviorist, it is not surprising that his taxonomy is a structured hierarchy which assumes a cumulative nature of learning: that student advancement to the next level of learning is dependent on previous success in the lower level. However, taken from a cognitivist's view, the outcome of an educational experience should ultimately focus on the modification of the students' ability to do certain things. In this context, Bloom's taxonomy of educational objectives could more appropriately be entitled taxonomy of cognitive abilities of the graduate.

Those new to clinical education need not be threatened by the academic jargon or the seeming complexity of taxonomies. Academics write for other academics; thus, at first look, their terminology and processes may appear complex. They truly are relatively simple and logical models.

Taxonomy can be defined as a structure, or a plan, used to help the teacher in planning to cover each developmental stage of a student's growth. Domain can be defined as a category. While domains often appear in shorthand forms such as KSA (knowledge-skills-attitude) or do-think-feel, etc., Bloom's original terminology included:

- Cognitive domain: intellectual capability (ie, knowledge, or ability to think). This relates to the intellectual or rational dimension of a student's experience.
- Affective domain: feelings, emotions and behavior (ie, attitude, or ability to feel). This relates to the emotional or feeling dimension of a student's experience.
- Psychomotor domain: learning of manual and physical skills (ie, the ability to move, act, or manipulate the body in order to perform a physical movement; the ability to do). This relates to the bodily movement associated with pre-conscious cognitive functioning.

From the perspective of the health sciences, the three domains may be seen as:

- Cognitive domain (knowing): the knowledge of and ability to work with information and ideas. Relates to the acquisition of knowledge, intellectual skills, and abilities (ie, diagnosis of disease, and developing strategies for treatment options).
- Affective domain (feeling): the ability to organize, articulate, live, and work by a coherent value system germane to the capabilities achieved through education. Relates to the ability to deal with feelings, emotions, mindsets, and values. This includes the nurturing of desirable attitudes for personal and professional development (ie, allaying the concerns and fears of patients and their families as they experience surgery, displaying mutual trust and respect in working with members of the health care team, upholding high ethical standards in practice).
- Psychomotor domain (doing): relates to the acquisition of skills that require varying levels of well-coordinated physical activity and precise manipulative procedures (ie, selection of anesthesia equipment, performing a specific regional anesthetic technique).

Effective learning, particularly when training is expected to result in measurable behaviors, should touch on all levels of each of the domains where relevant to the student. In this instance, the student is expected to demonstrate knowledge and intellect (cognitive domain); attitude and beliefs (affective domain); and the ability to effect physical and bodily skills to act (psychomotor domain).

The domains are traditionally represented in matrix form, creating a checklist or template for designing learning programs or lesson plans. Within the domains, categories (or levels) are organized in order of complexity. An essential premise of Bloom's taxonomy is that each level must be mastered before progressing to the next, and that one must assume mastery of the simpler form before progressing to more complex levels. Thus, the categories within a domain are considered increasingly complex levels of learning development (See **Figure 15.2**). In this regard, the psychomotor domain may perhaps be the most versatile to maneuver within when planning and providing clinical training.

Figure 15.2 Domains of Bloom's Taxonomy

Level	Cognitive Domain	Affective Domain	Psychomotor Domain[1]
	Knowledge	Attitude	Skills
1	Recall data	Receive (awareness)	Imitation (copy) (see then do)
2	Understand	Respond (react)	Manipulation (follow instructions) (hands-on practice)
3	Apply (use)	Value (understand and act)	Develop precision (practice, practice, practice)
4	Analyze (structure/ elements)	Organize personal value system	Articulation (combine, integrate related skills) • Integration –Learner knows why –Learner knows when
5	Synthesize (create/ build)	Internalize value system (adopt behavior)	Naturalization (automate, become expert; learner can perform the skill while concurrently performing other tasks)
6	Evaluate (assess, judge in relational terms)		

[1] The psychomotor domain as discussed by R.H. Dave (a student of Bloom) in 1967.

Objectives and learning activities for an introductory course may be appropriately concentrated in the lower levels, while objectives and learning activities for a course in the later semesters will normally be concentrated in the upper levels. This does not imply, however, that teachers should only convey information to learners and expect only memorization from them in the lower levels. Analysis and evaluation of information are essential in the practice of anesthesia. It is imperative that higher order thinking skills are encouraged and taught even from the beginning.

The Psychomotor Domain

As the scope of this chapter is limited to a discussion of the acquisition of psychomotor skills, the reader is encouraged to seek more in-depth understanding of the cognitive and affective domains elsewhere.

Bloom's initial work focused on what he would call the cognitive domain.[18] His later work focused on the affective Domain.[19] Most recently, numerous authors have expanded Bloom's model to include a third domain, psychomotor or skills (See Figure 15.3).[20–22]

Figure 15.3 Comparison of Psychomotor Domains

	Dave	Simpson	Harrow
1	Imitation (copy)	Perception (awareness)	Reflex movement
2	Manipulation	Set	Basic fundamental movements
3	Develop precision	Guided response	Perceptual abilities
4	Articulation	Mechanism	Physical abilities
5	Naturalization	Complex overt response	Skilled movements
6	(None)	Adaptation	Non-discursive
7	(None)	Origination	(None)

Dave's adaptation is the simplest and easiest to apply in a corporate environment. Harrow's and Simpson's models of the psychomotor domain, which offer different advantages and emotional perspectives, are particularly useful for adults learning entirely new and challenging physical skills (ie, those requiring additional attention to awareness and sensory perception, and mental and emotional preparation).[21,22] This is especially true when students must step out of their comfort zone to address sensory, perception (and, by implication, attitudinal), and preparation issues (ie, a threatening task such as that first epidural!).

When taken collectively, taxonomy concepts are useful in the planning and design of the university-level educational process, including lesson plans and materials as well as the evaluation of learning. As educators, those of us involved in nurse anesthesia education should find taxonomies useful as a framework for ensuring we are utilizing the most appropriate type of learning required of our mission; however, we must remember that learning design and evaluation for a given learning event need not cover all aspects of a given taxonomy. Emphasis should be placed on only those aspects that are appropriate to that event.

When planning a learning activity, the teacher must decide which domain the desired learning best fits. When it was first introduced, the psychomotor domain addressed primarily physical movements. This domain has evolved to include other professional and social skills such as interpersonal communications (provider-to-provider, provider-to-patient, provider-to-family, telephone skills, public speaking, etc.) as well as manual tasks (ie, airway management, regional anesthesia techniques, computer keyboard skills), which are important in the field of anesthesiology.

Psychomotor skills may require speed, tools, or equipment; are not evaluated by written means; and must be performed and observed in order to determine the student's mastery of the skill. In our context, an example of a learning activity in the psychomotor domain is learning how to perform an epidural anesthetic technique. A non-example is identifying the various indications for performing an epidural.

Clinical Teaching/Learning

Clinical teaching is one of the most enriching activities a teacher can do. Opportunities for directly demonstrating procedures, observing and guiding learners' technical skills, and providing immediate substantive feedback to learners are without comparison in other teaching formats. Clinical teaching is a powerful personal and interpersonal experience. While complex, fundamental principles define the roles that learners and teachers assume.

Learning in the clinical anesthesia environment requires dynamic interpersonal communication between two people: a learner and a teacher. Considerable commitment and effort are required of both. Appreciating this relationship, the teacher must anticipate and consider the following:

The Role of the Teacher

The role of the teacher includes the knowledge, attitudes, and skills that he or she brings to the learning relationship. Too often, teachers in the health sciences feel they must be a font of knowledge and skills which they will impart to learners. We know from our own experiences (both as learners and as teachers) that this is an impossible feat. Certainly, knowledge of the material and ability to perform a task are necessary; however, they are not sufficient to guarantee successful learning. As clinical teachers, we assume multiple roles in our interactions with learners. Adapted from Ulian's work , most behaviors and characteristics of (perceived) excellent clinical teachers fall into four roles:[23]

- The anesthetist is the expert and primary source of knowledge. There is a substantial difference between the anesthetist's and learner's experience and knowledge of the profession; thus, the reason they are together. As a member of the profession and socializing agent, the anesthetist helps uphold professional standards and is ultimately responsible for evaluating the learner's competency.
- The teacher is aware of the needs and aspirations of the learner.
- The teacher listens and encourages learners, but is also aware that he or she will not be able to provide the learner with everything that is needed.
- As supervisor, the teacher demonstrates skills and procedures, provides the learner with opportunities for guided practice, observes and evaluates learner performance, and provides feedback.
- As a person, the teacher must nurture an atmosphere of trust in which learners are safe and comfortable offering their ideas, thoughts, and feelings. This does not necessarily require that the teacher like the learner, but he or she does

accept their needs. As a person, the teacher may provide significant personal support outside the clinical environment and may serve as a role model.

The Role of the Learner

The role of the learner includes the experiences and knowledge that the learner brings to the learning relationship. It is important that teachers be aware of the different types of learners in order to individualize their approach. Learners bring numerous needs, problems, and anxieties to the learning relationship. Teachers must realize they cannot be all things to all learners. Anesthesia learners may be categorized as:[24]

- The compliant learner is the typical good student. Compliant learners work hard, are task-oriented, show little emotional turmoil, and are primarily oriented toward truly understanding the material. They are generally compliant with the teacher's directions.
- Anesthesia students are often the anxious dependent learner. They are very dependent on the teacher for knowledge and support. They may be difficult to engage in discussion and prefer the lecture format with copious handouts/notes. They are overly concerned about grades and are anxious about being evaluated. Their feelings of incompetence and anxiety often inhibit learning.
- The independent student is generally older than his or her peers and may have completed previous graduate work. Independent students often appear confident and unthreatened by the teacher, attempting to form peer relationships with them. They approach material calmly, objectively, and often in creative ways.
- Due to their pessimism and low self-esteem, the sniper student often has trouble forming productive relationships with authority figures (ie, teachers). Sniper students are often elusive when confronted with issues and may become hostile when corrected or given negative feedback.
- The silent student is most noticeable by what he or she does not do, often feeling vulnerable and helpless. Interestingly, silent students typically do not exhibit the anxiety of the anxious dependent learner.

Conditions for Effective Learning

Teachers must be mindful of the conditions or external influences which influence the learning process. The study of nurse anesthesia requires maturity and discipline. Nurse anesthesia students are adult learners. Intuitively then, their clinical education should follow the doctrines of adult education. Unfortunately, this is not always the case as nurse anesthesia educators are frequently not aware of these tenets. Four of these principles are particularly noteworthy:

- Adult learners are normally anxious to apply what they learn as soon as possible. Thus, many find the front-loaded curriculum format frustrating. Teachers should strive to make all material presented somehow clinically relevant.
- Adult learners enjoy learning principles and concepts. They benefit from solving problems rather than simply learning facts. Unfortunately, due to the

sheer density and breadth of medical information, there are numerous facts that simply must be memorized. Nurse anesthesia learners have had a significant clinical experience (nonanesthesia) base prior to entering their course of study. It is wise to build on this clinical experience to emphasize application, rather than simple retention, as an underpinning for discussion and to enhance their clinical reasoning and problem-solving skills. Such discussions often take a "what-if" format.

- Adult learners enjoy active participation in the learning process. Incorporating them into the development of appropriate learning objectives is important. While it can be argued that learners do not know what they need to know, the knowledgeable teacher can guide and negotiate with learners as to what learning should take place, given the resources available. This generally leads to enhanced motivation and participation.
- Adult learners need to know about their progress. Formative feedback (ie, feedback intended for the sake of improving performance) will help them evaluate their own progress. The clinical environment provides numerous opportunities for the teacher to evaluate competence (ie, summative evaluation). Teacher's comments, particularly negative ones, play a critical role in helping a learner learn and perform a skill appropriately, make better decisions, and change his or her professional behavior. Timely, well-intentioned, and appropriate feedback is critical to instilling learner confidence in the learner-teacher relationship and enhancing progress toward the learning objective.

Principles of Clinical Teaching

Anesthesia expertise is a complex balance of both explicit and tacit knowledge.[25] Explicit knowledge is formal and specific. Such knowledge is gained from lectures, texts, and tutorials; however, this alone is not appropriate for acquiring regional anesthesia skills.

Tacit knowledge is gained through experience, is critical to learning and maintaining expertise, and is difficult to define, demonstrate, or measure.[26] Although experts demonstrate a high degree of tacit knowledge, it is not easy to transfer to learners in the clinical setting using the apprenticeship model. This is best acquired by close interaction between teachers and learners as well as independent clinical experience.[27] Teachers share tacit knowledge by describing elements as they perform a procedure. This should be done in a relaxed environment and is most successful with a good teacher-learner relationship. Unfortunately, this may be limited by time pressure to complete the task and by concerns with patient safety.

Learner training must be provided at an appropriate level. Enhanced learning takes place for adult learners when there is a degree of challenge. The learner's task should be complex enough that they can learn, while not being so complex that it is impossible to achieve. Initially, this should begin in non-threatening situations such as skills-laboratory settings. Once basic skills are acquired, the learner may be placed in more advanced clinical settings, such as supervised performance on actual patients.

Clinical anesthesia teaching generally takes place in an immediate preoperative preparation area, the surgical/obstetric suite, or immediate postoperative recovery area. These interactions provide the cornerstone for teaching/learning the knowledge, skills, and attitudes of anesthesia. Unique to this experience is the fact that the patient is present and an active participant. The teacher should assume control of the environment as well as the procedure, allowing the learner to concentrate on the specific skill being learned. In this context, the environment entails patient comfort, allows monitoring of sedation and physiological factors, and provides interaction with other members of the care team. The learner should be aware of the entire scope of patient care and not be lulled into a false sense that the task is the sole element. There are four fundamental objectives of these interactions:

- Teaching should be based on patient-related data and information. During clinical interactions, teaching focuses on the patient's history, physical examination, diagnostic study findings, and, often, procedures. Procedures, in particular, provide a unique opportunity to teach psychomotor skills as well as provide an opportunity to demonstrate appropriate anesthetist-patient interaction skills. During procedures, what the patient says and how he or she reacts must be incorporated into the activity and the learning process.
- Typically, patient data are reviewed with learners in the patient's absence prior to an actual encounter. The intent is to discuss relevant findings in order to prepare learners for the time actually spent with the patient. Aberrations in findings as well as the teacher's insights and previous experiences can be freely discussed. Time must be allowed for questions from the patient and family. Closure to the visit should focus on the patient's immediate concerns and ensuring that no confusion or ambiguity persists on the part of the provider or patient. It must be clear to all that the patient is of central importance throughout the encounter.
- Clinical teaching must respect the patient's dignity and comfort. This feature is paramount. When properly conducted, clinical learning encounters are positive experiences for both learners and patients. The patient, teacher, and learner must be comfortable during the interaction. Demonstrating concern and respect for the patient is reassuring and serves to minimize distress and anxiety regarding the medical situation and about any procedures he or she may be about to experience.

It is very important to introduce yourself and your role (the teacher should identify himself or herself and then introduce any learners). The teacher should clearly state the purpose of his or her being there and request permission of the patient (ie, "I'm here to discuss your anesthesia care but first I'd like to ask you a few questions about your medical history." or "Is it OK if I take a look at your epidural catheter?"). This is particularly important when the encounter will involve physically touching the patient for whatever reason. In some cases, it is helpful for the teacher to revisit the patient alone in order to clarify any misunderstandings.

Care must be taken to clearly, and in layman's terms, describe any technical procedure(s) one plans to perform. All communications, including technical discussions, are made in such a way as to make the patient feel included. As part of the problem-solving process, the patient should be encouraged to participate in the discussion with the teacher and learners. Conclusions and recommendations should be clearly communicated. Again, it may be helpful for the teacher to reiterate and summarize the key points of the discussion, particularly when an invasive procedure (ie, regional anesthesia) is planned. A parting optimistic statement to the patient (ie, "We'll take good care of you.") will serve to relieve anxieties.

- Psychomotor skills are best taught in the clinical environment. Performing a motor skill for the first time requires the learner to have a concept of the desired outcome. Clinical interactions allow the teacher to demonstrate (and learners to directly observe and practice) the technical elements of procedures as well as psychosocial aspects such as concern and caring. This is not taught by lecture but rather by example. In the clinical environment, the learning of psychomotor clinical skills is often personified by the saying, "See one, do one, teach one."

Clinical interactions are fundamental to teaching/learning psychomotor skills in anesthesia. Decreasing time and volume of clinical experiences in nurse anesthesia educational programs (NAEPs) should be of concern. In addition to diagnostic and therapeutic procedures, physical examination and problem-solving skills are best learned in this environment. Once the fundamentals of technical skills are mastered, emphasis should be focused on problem solving. When the patient is made aware that the discussion of what-ifs is a learning encounter, he or she is generally reassured and may actively engage in the discussion.

As previously discussed, central to the basis of most taxonomies of learning psychomotor skills is a clearly organized series of steps, building on one another until the skill is properly learned and executed. Care must be taken as didactic information can overload the learner's cognitive capacity. The overall skill is broken into discrete components and presented/learned sequentially until the entire skill is mastered. It is generally best for the teacher to initially present (actually perform) the overall skill set in its entirety, discuss/demonstrate its components, and then have the learner attempt the skill with close supervision. The initial demonstration provides the boundaries of what is acceptable and a sense of desired outcome. Remember, motivated learners are highly observant—what they do may be more influential that what they teach! For this to be effective, teachers must remember that they are the experts and can likely perform the demonstrated skill in their sleep. Indeed, this is a hallmark of mastery. For the teacher providing guidance, the task may be easier done than said. However, when teaching new skills (ie, regional anesthesia techniques), the learner, more often than not, does not know what he or she doesn't know. Enhanced learning takes place when complex skills are deconstructed into individual processes and decisions. The effective teacher closely monitors learners' level of comprehension and ability and matches teaching to that level. For example, a student registered nurse anesthetist may need to first be made aware that an epidural is an appropriate technique for a given patient situation. This is followed by a review of the proper equipment and pharmaceuticals and then an overview and demonstration of the technical aspects. The learner then begins to appreciate what he or she does not know and hopefully anticipates learning more. It should be evident to the reader that these steps parallel those of taxonomies previously described.

- Clinical teaching is a unique opportunity to provide learners feedback. Teacher evaluation of learners is perhaps most effective when done during clinical interactions. Both formative and summative feedback are valuable. In educational vernacular, feedback refers to the process of sharing information with learners about their current performance with the intent that they may improve it with future experiences. Such feedback may be negative or positive. Negative feedback is given in the hopes of changing unacceptable behavior, while positive feedback is given to strengthen appropriate behavior.

Criticisms are intended to make the learner feel bad; they are not negative feedback. Compliments are meant to make the learner feel good; they are not positive feedback. Neither is helpful in improving performance. Feedback, rather, should be informative, consisting of observations and judgments intended to help the learner improve. Ideally, feedback will be limited to two or three specific points of the task being learned. This feedback may be constructive criticism, identification of weaknesses, problem-solving, or positive reinforcement.

Poor performance may be the result of the learner's lack of appreciation of the value of the task or not understanding the teacher's expectations. Feedback can enforce why the skill is important or the rationale for specific elements as the teacher desires. When a knowledge deficit is identified, the teachers can use this opportunity to offer guidance as to recommended resources.

Rather than evaluative, feedback should be descriptive. For example, while observing a learner attempt an epidural placement, a teacher's comment, "Geez, you really are clumsy!" would be evaluative and of little support. A more descriptive (and less pejorative) feedback statement would be, "Perhaps next time you should try holding the Tuohy needle like this … ." Such descriptive feedback is unambiguous and provides clear suggestions for improvement.

Feedback should be targeted and as specific to the task as possible. For example, if a learner has properly performed a preoperative evaluation a teacher's compliment, such as "Nice job," does not reinforce the learner's specific favorable behavior. A more helpful statement would be, "I am particularly pleased with your interview technique and your ability to focus on that patient's concerns with spinal anesthesia. I think she now better understands what happened with her previous experience and what to expect today."

Timing of feedback is critical. It should be provided as soon after the experience as practical. A singular summative evaluation after a week or month of clinical experiences does not provide learners with the opportunity to adjust behaviors in response to the feedback. Indeed, it is likely they do not even remember the events being evaluated.

Learning Alternatives

The time-honored process of teaching regional anesthesia directly on preoperative patients is less than ideal. Fundamental to anesthesia training is an adequate and appropriate patient case load and acuity mix. Learning regional anesthesia, particularly peripheral nerve blocks, is greatly enhanced when separate, properly equipped anesthetizing locations are used prior to entering the surgical theater. Adequate staffing to allow the learner adequate time to prepare and perform the technique is critical as well. When a learner will be mentored by multiple teachers, it is best for the teaching staff to have previously come to an agreement on one best way. This minimizes unnecessary stress on the learner; they do not have to learn his or her way in addition to the fundamentals of the skill being learned.

Numerous methods have been described to teach regional anesthesia:

Audiovisual

Electronic media-based interactive educational programs have proliferated in recent years. Many have been adapted to personal handheld devices, allowing the anesthetist to review information immediately before performing a technique.[28] Realistic graphics enhance many of these offerings.

3-D Animation

Some are incorporating the use of virtual-reality models for teaching peripheral nerve and plexus blocks. One such model incorporates clear schematic drawings, relevant video clips, and live demonstrations. Others have used short three-dimensional virtual-reality animations to demonstrate the steps in performing peripheral nerve block. Animation allows the superficial anatomy to appear transparent while showing landmarks and geometry of needle placement.

Cadaver/Animal Models

Cadaver preparations allow an in-depth review of relevant anatomy and geometry associated with blocks. Blocks on anesthetized animals provided real time experience with enhanced feel of tissue planes. The latter is particularly useful when learning perineural catheter techniques.

One group has described a unique embalming method which more closely mimics tissue conditions of living patients (ie, color, soft consistency, and movability) while allowing flap dissection to demonstrate anatomical planes. They also describe simulation of pulsatile landmarks by implanting latex tubing along peripheral arterial routes in the extremity of cadavers.[29,30]

Supplemental Equipment

Use of the peripheral nerve stimulation has long allowed visual confirmation of needle placement. More recently, ultrasound-guided needle placement has gained considerable popularity.[31] (More complete discussion follows.)

Videotape-feedback

Videotaping a learner while performing a technique provides the opportunity for timely critique by both teacher and learner as well as opportune feedback.[32] Unfortunately, this does not evaluate learners' cognitive skills.

Web-based Education

Many NAEPs incorporate a high percentage of web-based teaching modules. While not shown to be superior to textbook/lecture learning, practical benefits include the ability to standardize content, build learning progressions, incorporate multimedia technology, and provide flexibility in terms of location, time, pace, and repetition.[33,34]

Although SRNAs are accustomed to this approach and enjoy having off-hour (nonclassroom) access, it has not been shown that it justifies the time and expense of developing complex regional anesthesia case-based modules. While there may be practical advantages of web-based teaching, regional anesthesia educators should be cautious about developing such curriculums based primarily on faculty or student preference.[35]

Simulation

When possible, demonstration and practice on task-specific simulation models allows the learner the opportunity to see and get a feel for the technique before actually attempting it on a live patient. In addition to commercial products, numerous green-grocer models have been described using various types of commonly available produce such as oranges, bananas, bread, etc.[36] Each type of vegetable or fruit mimics the various human tissue layers.

Virtual Model

At least one innovative company, Energid Technologies has described its efforts to develop a localized virtual patient model for regional anesthesia simulation training.[37] The company's model reportedly captures the reflexive responses during nerve block stimulation by combining advanced technologies in tissue deformation, motor nerve stimulation model, and haptic feedback rendering. Currently, fiscal considerations limit the availability of such devices.

Personal Experience

Certainly, one's personal experience with the anesthesia/surgery process can be informative. One interesting report discusses residents' responses following the experience of receiving regional techniques themselves (compensated volunteers).[38] They reported that they learned to be more sensitive to patient concerns and to communicate better with their patients about the anesthetic plan. They also came to appreciate the value of sedation, and the discomfort associated with local anesthetic infiltration, paresthesias, and nerve stimulators.

Regional Block Rotation

The paucity of exposure to peripheral nerve block techniques has given rise to unique methods for teaching. In that consistency is helpful, it would be ideal if learners were allowed a defined rotation during which they were assigned only to cases that had a high likelihood of receiving regional techniques. This may provide the learner an opportunity to perform several blocks per day under direct mentorship. This repetition of techniques, particularly peripheral nerve blocks, in a short period of time, is designed to increase the learner's awareness of the role of regional applications and personal confidence in selecting these techniques as part of their anesthesia care plan as well as enhancing their technical skills. Clearly this is an ideal situation which currently exists in a few NAEPs, most notably the military programs. From personal experience, this is likewise uncommon in many anesthesiology residencies.

Using such a system, Duke University Health System anesthesia residents increased their experience with spinal blocks from a median of 66 (59–74) to 107 (92–123), and epidural blocks from a median of 133 (127–142) to 233 (221–241).[39] Their exposure to peripheral nerve blocks increased even more dramatically from a median of 80 (58–105) to 350 (237–408). One must keep in mind, however, that these numbers were gained over a four-year residency period and numerous perioperative area assignments.

While this approach was encouraging for one teaching program, a national survey in the same year showed less favorable results.[40] Fifty-eight percent of responding anesthesiology residencies offered a specific peripheral nerve block rotation. Sixty-one percent of these rotations were one month's duration. Sixty-nine percent of these provided formal didactic instruction during the rotation. Interestingly, multimedia, mannequins, and cadaver dissection were used infrequently (13–25%), suggesting these were strictly clinical experiences. Surprisingly, on average, residents performed only 2 supraclavicular and 10 axillary brachial plexus techniques. Perhaps this was due to the fact that 48% of the time, these blocks were performed in the operating room and not a specific regional anesthetizing area (ie, block room).

A significant disadvantage to this approach is that, once blocked, learners turn over the intraoperative management to another anesthesia provider, and thus may not appreciate that there is more to regional anesthesia than needle placement. They do not follow their blocks into the operating room and do not manage their blocks intraoperatively. Therefore, they do not learn to anticipate, recognize, and manage the failed or partial block or the complications and side effects associated with their blocks. The interpersonal relationship between the provider and patient, which is very important to the overall success of blocks in the awake patient, may be diminished by this approach as well.

Although most adverse events during a regional anesthetic are benign (but not unimportant), such as the patient moving during surgery or otherwise harmless physiologic alterations, they do require a degree of experience and finesse to manage. In other situations, complications (ie, bradycardia, hypotension, seizure, airway difficulties) may be devastating.[41]

Regional Anesthesia Fellowship

Fellowship programs offer anesthesiology residents the greatest opportunity to become highly skilled in regional anesthesia. In 2005, approximately 12 active fellowship programs existed in the United States and Canada.[42] To minimize the differences in the quality and quantity of regional anesthesia experience in these fellowships, program directors have recently published consensus-based guidelines for regional anesthesia fellowships in North America.[43]

It is suggested that the AANA should closely watch the development of regional anesthesiology fellowship training and, in those instances where possible, partner with them to provide regional experiences for SRNAs. A fundamental tenet of a professional is one's ability to pass on (teach) information to others. Regional anesthesia fellows should be encouraged to mentor other learners as part of their educational process.

Continuing Education Opportunities

Continuing education meetings, such as regional anesthesia hands-on workshops, serve a valuable purpose by providing didactic information and limited demonstrations of evolving techniques, and the opportunity for learners to communicate directly with experts in the field as well as with learner colleagues. Workshops also enhance learning at both the entry level and for learners desiring to update their skills.

As the technology becomes available, we can expect to find more computer-based high-fidelity learning opportunities. Virtual reality applications will enhance the anatomical and technical manipulations associated with various techniques. As the cost of electronic imaging technology decreases, as we experienced with noninvasive blood pressure monitoring and pulse oximetry, we will undoubtedly see an increase in its clinical use.

Hands-on Workshops

The AANA regional anesthesia workshops (spinal/epidural and upper/lower extremity) have consistently had maximum attendance since their inception in the early 1990s. Participants in these workshops are CRNAs who did not have the opportunity to learn regional in their generic programs, had didactic but limited clinical experience, and, in both situations, have not practiced regional anesthesia consistently since graduation and wish to update and enhance their knowledge and skills.

Regardless of format, it appears SRNA/CRNAs are high-functioning learners who, although having various learner preferences, are capable of learning regardless of the educational format. Learning styles may not correlate with knowledge acquisition. Studies have failed to demonstrate the influence of learning style on knowledge development.[44,45]

The Instructional Process

Regardless of the domain, there are fundamental steps in the overall instructional process. The following is an example of a lesson plan adapting Dave's psychomotor domain to teach the physical skills associated with placing an epidural anesthetic.

Learning objective: Learner will demonstrate basic skills of placing an epidural anesthetic (**Tables 15.1** and **15.2**, next page).

Table 15.1 Steps to the Instructional Process

Steps	Instructor	Learner	Type of Instruction
Imitation	• Provide content knowledge • Demonstrate the entire skill, including all steps, without interruption • Provide learner opportunity to imitate the skill	• Learner listens to and observes instructor • Learner imitates instructor	• Explanation • Demonstration • Guided practice
Manipulation	• Reduce skill into essential steps/actions; explain each step/action (ie, opening kit, preparing drugs and equipment, patient positioning, technique, patient aftercare) • Provide learner opportunity to imitate each step • Provide learner opportunity to imitate entire skill	• Learner repetitively attempts specific steps • Learner attempts entire skill	• Guided practice • Feedback

Adapted from Romiszowski, A. The development of physical skills: instruction in the psychomotor domain. In: Reigeluth CM, ed. *Instructional-Design Theories and Models: A New Paradigm of Instructional Theory, Volume II.* Mahwah, NJ: Lawrence Erlbaum Associates; 1999:457–482.

Table 15.2 Lesson Plan Example

Steps	Instructor	Learner	Type of Instruction
Imitation	• Provide content knowledge • Demonstrate the entire skill, including all steps, without interruption • Provide learner opportunity to imitate the skill	• Learner listens to and observes instructor • Learner imitates instructor	• Explanation • Demonstration • Guided practice
Manipulation	• Reduce skill into essential steps and actions; explain each step/action • Provide learner opportunity to imitate each step • Provide learner opportunity to imitate entire skill	• Learner repetitively attempts specific steps • Learner attempts entire skill	• Guided practice • Feedback
Precision	• Provide learner time to practice independently	• Learner practices until able to perform with no mistakes • Learner increases speed of performing skill	• Independent practice
Articulation	• Provide learner time to practice independently	• Learner fine-tunes ability to perform skill	• Independent practice
Naturalization	• Evaluate learner's entire performance	• Learner performs skill with only minimal supervision	• Evaluation

Adapted from Romiszowski, A. The development of physical skills: instruction in the psychomotor domain. In: Reigeluth CM, ed. *Instructional-Design Theories and Models: A New Paradigm of Instructional Theory, Volume II*. Mahwah, NJ: Lawrence Erlbaum Associates; 1999:457–482.

Proposed Regional Anesthesia-Specific Psychomotor Domain Taxonomy

Technical procedures such as regional anesthesia should be analyzed to determine the skills necessary to perform them appropriately and safely. A regional anesthesia-specific adaptation of the psychomotor domain is modeled in part after a presentation by Ferris and Aziz.[46] The example used is for epidural anesthesia, but can be easily adapted for any technique.

This hierarchy builds on the fundamental recognition of the equipment and materials required of the skills of regional anesthesia; through several levels of the skill in handling and using the materials and to achieve desirable outcomes; followed by the ability to create and execute a plan which will achieve a desirable result and ending in a means to evaluate the results and plan for improvements in outcomes.

1. Recognition of the equipment and materials used in the epidural anesthesia technique

The fundamental practical skill competence in regional anesthesia is the ability to recognize the materials and tools of the trade. This is essential for both an effective technique as well as personal and patient safety. For example, the learner must know and appreciate the various components of an epidural technique, such as the unique design of the tip; the association of the hub notch to the tip orifice; the significance of the markings on the shaft of the needle; the various markings on the epidural catheter; and the purpose and function of the luer hub, etc. This level of competence involves learning how to recognize the equipment and materials associated with the technique to be performed.

2. Proper care and handling of equipment and materials used in regional anesthesia techniques

Our tools must be handled appropriately. In addition to sterility, personal safety (ie, needle sticks) and patient safety (ie, correct drugs) must be paramount. Learners must be properly instructed and observed using acceptable techniques throughout procedures so that these risks can be identified and pre-empted. This level of competence involves learning how to care for and safely handle equipment and materials.

3. Basic operation of equipment and materials used in regional anesthesia techniques

Basic to the epidural technique is the learners' ability to properly hold and put to use the necessary equipment: prepping solutions, draping materials, the epidural needle, various syringes, the epidural catheter and luer adapter, and taping materials. These tasks, when accomplished in a sequence, should result in the completion of a universally acceptable technique. This is not the time for clinical instructors to offer their pearls of wisdom, but rather offer a most basic unitary technique. This level of competence involves learning how to operate equipment and materials while incorporating elements of safety associated with their use.

4. Competent operation of equipment and materials used in regional anesthesia techniques

At this level, the learner is becoming confident and competent with the equipment and materials of epidural anesthesia. This level builds upon the previous level in that the learner is now able to perform the complete sequence of tasks associated with the epidural technique in an acceptable manner. For example, the learner can appropriately set up the epidural kit, prepare the patient, perform the loss of resistance technique, place the epidural catheter, and prepare and tape the catheter. This level of competence involves the ability to consistently and safely perform the technique in an acceptable manner.

5. Expert operation of equipment and materials

This level is identified by the learner's ability to repetitively use equipment and materials in a rapid, efficient, effective, and safe manner. The learner is now able to perform the tasks with the correct outcome in the broader context of the technique's application rather than simply on the narrow context of placing the needle/catheter. An example of his or her level of competence would be the learner's ability to appropriately perform epidural techniques in a series of multiple patients in a safe and fluid manner.

6. Planning the work process

At this level, the learner is able to analyze system requirements in order to prioritize work to be done. The process of work planning requires an intimate understanding of surgical/obstetrical schedule requirements, patient information, and anesthesia provider availability/capability. This may require the ability to discern the order of operations in order to effectively and efficiently produce the desired outcomes. An example of his level of competence would be a learner's ability to prioritize and then appropriately perform epidural techniques in a series of multiple patients in a safe and fluid manner.

7. Evaluation of patient outcomes and implementation of improvements

At this level, the learner is able to review the overall quality of the epidural technique and process and identify deficiencies and actions which could be taken to either correct or prevent the faults through appropriate planning. This level of competence represents the highest level of achievement and is highlighted by the ability to critically review previous actions.

Evolving Technology: Future Directions

Since its introduction in the 1880s, regional anesthesia has become an indispensable method of providing perioperative pain control. The practice of regional anesthesia is dynamic. The increasing demand by surgeons and patients, as well as the rapid development of newer pharmacologic preparations, continuous catheter techniques, and, most recently, ultrasound-enhanced techniques, require that all anesthesia providers become more adept in a variety of regional anesthesia techniques. Advances in student training in regional anesthesia have been slow but steady. It is best to develop a solid base of knowledge and competency during the formative training years and a desire to continue learning post-graduation.

General anesthesia has made exponential advances in safety, due largely to advancements in noninvasive objective (real-time) patient monitoring technologies. Until recently, such monitoring during placement of peripheral nerve and central neuraxial regional techniques has not enjoyed the same capabilities. Consequently, regional techniques have largely been the purview of only a few highly skilled enthusiasts.

From their inception, regional anesthesia techniques have relied on indirect identification of target nerves derived from collateral osseous and/or vascular structures and mapping of surface landmarks. This assumes minimal morphometric variation among individuals. The growing trend in patient obesity further confounds this approach. While the use of electrical nerve stimulation to isolate peripheral nerves prior to injection has gained wide favor and technical sophistication, it still relies largely on clinicians' ability to identify elusive topical and structural landmarks.

By any measure, regional anesthesia is experiencing a renaissance due largely to direct visualization: adapting noninvasive ultrasound technology to enhance nerve block techniques. The acronym UgRA (ultrasound guided regional anesthesia) is commonly used to describe this clinical practice. The rapid development of quality task-specific technology is decreasing its cost, making regional anesthesia available to a wider populace of providers and patients. This evolution is rapidly creating a new gold standard in the specialty. A 2009 study of members of the American Society of Regional Anesthesia and Pain Medicine members found that 67% (of 583 respondents) routinely used use UgRA. Undoubtedly, this percentage has improved.[47] The adjunct use of this technology to facilitate peripheral and central neuraxis blocks is consistent with the scope of practice of CRNAs appropriately trained in regional anesthesia techniques.

Presumed advantages of UgRA include direct visualization of relevant adjacent anatomical structures adjacent to target nerves (ie, vessels, bones, tendons, muscles, or pleura). Real-time visualization of the needle (ie, hyperechoic image and tissue movement) allows enhanced precision of needle trajectory. Development of needles with greater echogenicity has been rapid. This allows placement of reduced volumes of local anesthetic agent in close proximity to nerves which, in turn, minimizes the prospect for systemic toxicity, enhances onset and duration, and may reduce incidence of complications. However, as the present occurrence of poor outcomes is exceedingly low, the latter remains more intuitive than documented. Not surprisingly, ultrasound imaging has confirmed that anatomy is highly variable, explaining, in part, historically poor success rates and reproducibly of some techniques. Continued advancements in probe and display technology will further enhance this capability.

Experience suggests the actual distribution of injected local anesthetic is likewise variable, refuting the maxim that just get close with a needle will suffice. Indeed, direct observation of the distribution of injected local anesthetic is the foremost advantage of UgRA. If distribution of local anesthetic is inadequate, visualized needle replacement is possible in order to enhance the block.

Additionally, placement of local anesthetic in close proximity to nerves, independent of the volume used, hastens its onset time and extends its duration significantly. This reduction in required volume (to as little as 20%-30% of previous recommendations) reduces the likelihood of intravenous/systemic toxicity. Low-volume blocks may provide an enhanced opportunity to provide peripheral blocks for patients with impaired cardiovascular function or for children who may have increased incidence of local anesthetic toxicity due to low levels of binding proteins.

Perhaps the most challenging obstacle to the adoption of UgRA is provider resistance! This seems particularly true for seasoned clinicians who feel they are adept with topographical landmarks and/or electrical stimulation and are skeptical of emerging techniques. This cadre adapts slowly and often cites experience vs. evidence-based practice. Currently, most UgRA literature is experiential case reports and is inconclusive. There are few large randomized studies comparing advantages or complications of UgRA with other techniques. Given the extremely low incidence of complications, it is unlikely any such studies of sufficient statistical power will be forthcoming.

Adverse work conditions strongly affect the occurrence of errors. Production pressure (ie, room turn overtime) is a prime example; however, more subtle and insidious factors may prevail. When adapting to UgRA, one is cautioned to not become so engrossed in the technology so as to drift or deviate from guidelines leading to unsafe risky practices. Examples include personal adaptions from accepted techniques, lapses in sterile technique, failure to fractionate dosing or observe total dosing, etc. Such drift is commonly slow and subtle.

Given its emerging popularity, how does one go about attaining this new expertise? In addition to specific manual skills, UGRA requires knowledge and application of rapidly evolving technology. The paradigm "see one, do one" is obsolete for teaching clinical mastery of complex procedures.[48]

Optimally, learners should have an opportunity to acquire didactic knowledge and perform task elements of a procedure prior to actual patient clinical application. This process should include deliberate practice, guidance, informative feedback, repetition, and correction of errors.[49] This entails several learning components:

- Cognitive knowledge about the specific procedure, including its steps (and their order) must be achieved prior to any task learning. During this phase, learners lack situational awareness as they tend to focus entirely on the necessary sequence of tasks or their previous errors.
- Scanning technique involves basic knowledge of ultrasound physics, machine component function and manipulation, and acquisition of images.
- Sono anatomy includes recognition of relevant anatomy of the block to be performed and interpretation of the anatomic structures displayed as images on an ultrasound monitor.
- Needle guidance involves the coordinated hand-eye skills necessary to simultaneously advance the injection needle to the target tissue.

Regional anesthesia techniques are complex. The addition of ultrasonography has added to this complexity. Hierarchical task analysis has identified 256 specific tasks associated with the safe and effective performance of ultrasound-guided axillary brachial plexus block. Two hundred-twelve of these tasks are considered at risk of error of differing degrees.[50]

Fundamental technical skills of UgRA include the ability to:

- (1) visualize a needle and, specifically, the needle tip as it is being advanced toward the target nerve(s);
- (2) maintain the needle in the appropriate axial view (ie, in-plane);
- (3) adjust the needle trajectory; and
- (4) observe the distribution of local anesthetic during injection.[51]

Fortunately, anesthesia learners, even those with limited experience, seem adept in rapidly acquiring these skills.[52]

Highly illustrated texts and digital media by experienced clinicians that demonstrate practical techniques are affordable basic prerequisites. Obviously, close supervision by an experienced provider is ideal; however, a cadre of highly experienced clinicians available and capable of supervising such learning often does not exist. Even if so, expense and credentialing obstacles would inhibit their ability to provide such teaching in the learner's clinical environment; thus, learners are left to wing-it on their own.

Professional organizations offer focused hands-on workshops. Such venues are noticeably limited by not providing actual patient experiences and can only offer acknowledgment of attendance, which may not be recognized by institutional credentialing committees.[53]

Formal recommendations for education and training in UgRA recommend that learners practice probe handling and actual needle insertion techniques using simulators and phantoms.[43] Real-time haptic (tactile, sense of touch, feel) feedback including hand-eye coordination of probe/needle manipulation is paramount. Indeed, two fundamental mistakes learners make in their early attempts are failure to visualize the needle before/during advancement and unintentional probe movement, both of which can be improved with preclinical simulation training.[54]

Simulation has been shown to improve personal confidence as well as familiarity with equipment and achievement of technical skills before attempting on actual patients. Proficiency and retention of knowledge are likewise enhanced. Indeed, many learners now expect simulation experiences. In some instances, simulation is used to assess performance.[55] High-fidelity and partial-task simulators are both commonplace; however, no difference in learning between these levels of simulation has been shown.[56]

Noteworthy improvement in speed and accuracy has been shown in teaching ultrasonography to neophyte clinicians using simulated/phantom models such as gelatin/plastic gel, cadaver tissue, animal meat, and a variety of grocery products (including tofu!). Unfortunately, needle tracks do not seal when the needle is removed from plastic gel models leaving persistent hyperechoic artifact which obscures the practice site. Unfortunately, tissue/vegetable models are rapidly perishable.[57]

A novel homemade model, incorporating pork shoulders with bovine tendons inserted into them, provides haptic feedback when crossing tissue planes and ultrasound practice with needle visualization, and hydrodissection when injecting local anesthetic comparable with human tissue. Needle tracking artifact as seen with gel models is minimal.[58]

Even when supervised and provided timely and appropriate feedback, the number of simulated blocks necessary to attain proficiency is highly variable with the complexity of the task being learned and among learners.[56]

With experience, procedural time is decreased and learner's ability to efficiently identify and inject neural structures is improved. Unfortunately, the volume and complexity of experiences necessary for even a minimal level of competency often exceeds the opportunities available of many learners.

In addition to technical practice, mentored simulated experiences with regional anesthesia crisis (ie, local anesthesia toxicity) may enhance providers' ability to recognize and implement corrective measures. This experience may also serve to reinforce fundamental preventive measures (ie, test dose and fractionating dosing).[59] Promising work is under way in the areas of radiation force sonography (allowing quality images of deeper structures), artificial intelligence, impedance neurography, and three-dimensional ultrasound.[60]

Professional organizations are actively working to define training criteria and educational standards. Perhaps this will include some form of formal provider assessment and/or credentialing. Interested learners are encouraged to become familiar with the anesthesia and pain therapy joint committee's recommendations for education and training in ultrasound-guided regional anesthesia.[51] This joint committee was established to recommend the scope of practice, teaching curriculum, and options for implementing the practice of UgRA.

This seminal document clearly defines and structures common tasks used when performing an ultrasound-guided nerve block, articulates the core competencies and skill sets associated with UgRA, advocates training processes for both established practitioners and students in training, and recommends the establishment of a quality improvement process for UgRA. Learners are advised that evolving knowledge will update (and may make obsolete) some of this material. Familiarization of current literature is required.

Summary

Ideally, SRNA learners would be independently proficient in basic regional anesthesia techniques upon graduation. This ideal is not currently being accomplished. More highly skilled clinical instructors and increased access to clinical patient opportunities are needed. True mastery would perhaps best be accomplished by the establishment of postgraduate fellowship programs modeled after, or perhaps integrated with, those of physician anesthesiologists. Until that time, nurse anesthesia educators must develop methodologies for teaching regional anesthesia which not only emphasize technical skills, but also overall patient management and evaluation of learner competency.

Educational taxonomies may be used to develop improved methods to train and assess anesthetists in regional anesthesia techniques. They provide guidance for the design, delivery, and evaluation of learning experiences when planning and executing learning episodes. They encourage a variety of teaching and learning methods.

Despite criticism, Bloom's (and others') taxonomy of educational outcomes remains influential in the development of educational programs. The use of taxonomies in the first two domains (cognitive and affective) has been used extensively in primary and secondary education where educators generally have an extensive theoretical background in education. Clinical educators in the health sciences have historically had little formal training in the concepts that underlie the educational process.

Although the latest addition to taxonomies, the psychomotor domain, seems to have been developed for the primary and secondary educational levels, where learners have a significant need to develop the elements of psychomotor skills it also has meaningful application for higher education where competence in the physical motor skills associated with the performance of the professional practice (ie, regional anesthesia) are to be mastered.

How a taxonomy is applied will differ depending on the educational level of the learners. Professional education, such as nurse anesthesia, is generally consumed by young adults with a strong academic background and a high degree of previous sophisticated clinical experience. Thus, their educational experience focuses on the need to develop knowledge, attitudes and skills pertaining to the specific practices of anesthesiology.

The intent of this discussion has been to guide clinical instructors in their quest to establish a rational process of educational activities leading to planned outcomes. It is hoped that clinical instructors will be better able to develop graduate anesthetists with a coherent set of practical skills that lead to appropriate levels of competence in regional anesthesia.

A reasoned design in developing clinical practicums should enable more efficient use of equipment and instructor resources as the kind and amount of experience provided will be targeted to gain the maximum effect. A further benefit of planning clinical practicums around logical objectives should be the ability to design formal assessment of the learners' practical skills and overall patient care.

Regional anesthesia has become a popular method of providing anesthesia and analgesia for numerous surgical and obstetrical procedures. The ultimate success in performing regional anesthesia techniques lies in clinicians' innate ability to use appropriate psychomotor skills. The current focus solely on recording the number of regional techniques performed during a generic program is inadequate as it does not address:

- How is competency defined?
- How many of a specific nerve block is enough to establish competency?
- How do learners become skilled in overall patient care?

Performance of techniques is not enough. Care of the patient throughout his or her regional anesthetic experience is necessary to learn pharmacology, complications, and regional anesthesia-related outcomes.

References

1. Bridenbaugh LD. Are anesthesia resident programs failing regional anesthesia? *Reg Anesth*. 1982;7(1):26–28.

2. Kopacz DJ, Bridenbaugh LD. Are anesthesia residency programs failing regional anesthesia? The past, present, and future. *Reg Anesth*. 1993;18(2):84–87.

3. Kopacz DJ, Neal JM. Regional anesthesia and pain medicine: residency training—the year 2000. *Reg Anesth Pain Med*. 2002;27(1):9–14.

4. Rosenblatt MA, Fishkind D. Proficiency in interscalene anesthesia-how many blocks are necessary? *J Clin Anesth*. 2003;15(4):285–288.

5. Schuepfer G, Konrad C, Schmeck J, Poortmans G, Staffelbach B, Jöhr M. Generating a learning curve for pediatric caudal epidural blocks: an empirical evaluation of technical skills in novice and experienced anesthetists. *Reg Anesth Pain Med*. 2000;25(4):385–388.

6. Kopacz DJ, Neal JM, Pollock JE. The regional anesthesia "learning curve." What is the minimum number of epidural and spinal blocks to reach consistency? *Reg Anesth*. 1996;21(3):182–190.

7. Konrad C, Schuepfer G, Wietlisbach M, Gerber H. Learning manual skills in anesthesiology. Is there a recommended number of cases for anesthetic procedures? *Anesth Analg*. 1998;86(3):635–639.

8. Hadzic A, Vloka JD, Koenigsamen J. Training requirements for peripheral nerve blocks. *Current Opinion in Anaesthesiology*: 2002;15(6):669–673.

9. Standards and Guidelines for Accreditation of Nurse Anesthesia Educational Programs. Council on Accreditation of Nurse Anesthesia Educational Programs. Park Ridge, IL: American Association of Nurse Anesthetists; 1990.

10. Standards and Guidelines for Accreditation of Nurse Anesthesia Educational Programs. Council on Accreditation of Nurse Anesthesia Educational Programs. Park Ridge, IL: American Association of Nurse Anesthetists; 1994.

11. Standards and Guidelines for Accreditation of Nurse Anesthesia Educational Programs. Council on Accreditation of Nurse Anesthesia Educational Programs. Park Ridge, IL: American Association of Nurse Anesthetists; 1999.

12. Standards and Guidelines for Accreditation of Nurse Anesthesia Educational Programs. Council on Accreditation of Nurse Anesthesia Educational Programs. Park Ridge, IL: American Association of Nurse Anesthetists; 2004.

13. National Board on Certification and Recertification of Nurse Anesthetists. Summary of NCE and Self-Evaluation Exam SEE Performance and Clinical Experience, September 1, 2013 through August 31, 2014. Chicago, IL: NBCRNA; 2014.

14. Hadzic A, Vloka JD. *Peripheral Nerve Blocks: Principles and Practice*. New York, NY: McGraw Hill Professional; 2004.

15. Butterfield S. *Educational Objectives and National Assessment*. Philadelphia, PA: Open University Press; 1995.

16. Airasian PW. The impact of the taxonomy on testing and evaluation. In: Anderson LW, Sosniak LA, eds. *Bloom's Taxonomy of Educational Objectives: A Forty-year Retrospective.* Chicago, IL: The National Society for the Study of Education; 1994:82–102.

17. Rohwer WDJ, Sloane K. Psychological perspectives. In: Anderson LW, Sosniak LA, eds. *Bloom's Taxonomy of Educational Objectives: A Forty-year Retrospective.* Chicago, IL: The National Society for the Study of Education; 1994:41–63.

18. Bloom BS. *Taxonomy of Educational Objectives: Book 1: Cognitive Domain.* White Plains, NY: Longman; 1956:94–97

19. Krathwohl DR, Bloom BS, Masia BB. *Taxonomy of Educational Objectives Book 2: Affective Domain.* White Plains, NY: Longman; 192–197.

20. Dave RH. Psychomotor Levels. In Developing and Writing Behavioral Objectives, ed. Robert J. Armstrong. Tucson AZ: Educational Innovators Press; 1970:20–21.

21. Simpson EJ. *The Classification of Educational Objectives in the Psychomotor Domain.* Vol. 3. Washington, DC: Gryphon House; 1972.

22. Harrow A. *A Taxonomy of the Psychomotor Domain. A Guide for Developing Behavioral Objectives.* New York, NY: David McKay Co; 1972.

23. Ullian JA. National Society for Performance and Instruction. Medical student and resident perceptions of clinical teaching. *Healthcare Chapter News.* 1986;1(4):4–5.

24. Mann RD, Arnold S, Binder J, et al. *The College Classroom: Conflict, Change and Learning.* New York, NY: John Wiley; 1970:288–291.

25. Smith A, Goodwin D, Mort M, Pope C. Expertise in practice: an ethnographic study exploring acquisition and use of knowledge in anaesthesia. *Br J Anaesth.* 2003;91(3):319–328.

26. Pope C, Smith A, Goodwin D, Mort M. Passing on tacit knowledge in anaesthesia: a qualitative study. *Med Educ.* 2003;37:650–655.

27. Smith AF, Pope C, Goodwin D, Mort M. What defines expertise in regional anaesthesia? An observational analysis of practice. *Br J Anaesth.* 2006;97(3):40l–407.

28. Delbos A, Eisenbach JC, Albert N, et al. *Peripheral Nerve Blocks on DVD: Upper and Lower Limb Package.* Version 2.0. [DVD] New York, NY: Lippincott Williams & Wilkins; 2005.

29. Schwarz G, Feigl G, Kleinert R, et al. Pneumatic pulse simulation for teaching peripheral plexus blocks in cadavers. *Anesth Anal.* 2002;95(6):1822–1823.

30. Feigl G, Anderhuber F, Schwarz G, Dorn C, Fasel J, Likar R. Training methods for regional anaesthesia. evaluation and comparison. [in German]. *Der Anaesthetist.* 2007;56(5):437–443.

31. Grau T, Bartusseck E, Conradi R, et al. Ultrasound imaging improves learning curves in obstetric epidural anesthesia: a preliminary study. *Can J Anaesth.* 2003;50(10):1047–1050.

32. Birnbach DJ, Santos AC, Bourlier RA, et al. The effectiveness of video technology as an adjunct to teach and evaluate epidural anesthesia performance skills. *Anesthesiology.* 2002;96(1):5–9.

33. Chumley-Jones HS, Dobbie A, Alford CL. Web-based learning: sound educational method or hype? A review of the evaluation literature. *Acad Med.* 2002;77(Suppl 10):S86–S93.

34. Cook DA. The research we still are not doing: an agenda for the study of computer-based learning. *Acad Med.* 2005;80:541–548.

35. Kopp, SL, Smith, HM. Developing effective web-based regional anesthesia education: a randomized study evaluating case-based versus non-case-based module design. *Reg Anesth Pain Med.* 2011;36:336–342.

36. Leighton BL. A greengrocer's model of the epidural space. *Anesthesiology.* 1989:70(2):368–369.

37. Hu J, Lim YJ, Tardella N, Chang C, Warren L. Localized virtual patient model for regional anesthesia simulation training system. *Stud Health Technol Inform.* 2007;125:185–190.

38. McDonald SB, Thompson GE. "See one, do one, teach one, have one": a novel variation on regional anesthesia training. *Reg Anesth Pain Med.* 2002;27(5):456–459.

39. Martin G, Lineberger CK, MacLeod DB, et al. A new teaching model for resident training in regional anesthesia. *Anesth Analg.* 2002;95(5):1423–1427.

40. Chelly JE, Greger J, Gebhard R, Hagberg CA, Al-Samsam T, Khan A. Training of residents in peripheral nerve blocks during anesthesiology residency. *J Clin Anesth.* 2002;14(8):584–588.

41. Liguori GA, Kahn RL, Gordon J, et al. The use of metoprolol and glycopyrrolate to prevent hypotensive/bradycardic events during shoulder arthroscopy in the sitting position under interscalene block. *Anesth Analg.* 1998;87(6):1320–1325.

42. Neal JM, Kopacz DJ, Liguori GA, Beckman JD, Hargett MJ. The training and careers of regional anesthesia fellows—1983–2002. *Reg Anesth Pain Med.* 2005;30(3):226–232.

43. Hargett, MJ, Beckman, JD, Liguori, GA, Neal, JM. Guidelines for regional anesthesia fellowship training, *Reg Anesth Pain Med.* 2005;30(3): 218–225.

44. Cook DA, Thompson WG, Thomas KG, Thomas MR, Pankratz VS. Impact of self-assessment questions and learning styles in Web-based learning: a randomized, controlled, crossover trial. *Acad Med.* 2006;8193:231–238.

45. Cook DA, Thompson WG, Thomas KG, Thomas MR. Lack of interaction between sensing-intuitive learning styles and problem-first versus information-first instruction: a randomized crossover trial. *Adv Health Sci Educ Theory Pract.* 2009;14(1):79–90.

46. Ferris TLJ, Aziz SM. A psychomotor skills extension to Bloom's taxonomy of education objectives for engineering education. Presented at: Exploring Innovation in Education and Research; March 1–5, 2005; Tainan, Taiwan.

47. Ramlogan R, Manickam B, Chan VWS, et al. Challenges and training tools associated with the practice of ultrasound-guided regional anesthesia: a survey of the American Society of Regional Anesthesia and Pain Medicine. *Reg Anesth Pain Med.* 2010;35:224–226.

48. Choy I, Okrainec A. Simulation in surgery: perfecting the practice. *Surg Clin North Am.* 2010;90:457–473.

49. Ericsson KA, Krampe R, Tesch-Romer C. The role of deliberate practice in the acquisition of expert performance. *Psychol Rev.* 1993;100(3):363–406.

50. O'Sullivan O, Aboulafia A, Iohom G, O'Donnell BD, Shorten GD. Proactive error analysis of ultrasound-guided axillary brachial plexus block performance. *Reg Anesth Pain Med.* 2011;36(5):502–507.

51. Sites BD, Chan VW, Neal JM, et al. The American Society of Regional Anesthesia and Pain Medicine and the European Society of Regional Anaesthesia and Pain Therapy Joint Committee recommendations for education and training in ultrasound-guided regional anesthesia. *Reg Anesth Pain Med.* 2009;34(1):40–46.

52. Sites BD, Gallagher JD, Cravero J, Lundberg J, Blike G. The learning curve associated with a simulated ultrasound-guided interventional task by inexperienced anesthesia residents. *Reg Anesth Pain Med.* 2004;29:544–548.

53. Rosenberg AD, Cuff GC, Albert DB, Marshall MH, Kim IT. Value of workshops on ultrasound-guided regional anesthesia including hands-on simulator experience. In: Proceedings of the 2010 Annual Meeting of the American Society Anesthesiologists. 2010; San Diego, CA.

54. Sites BD, Spence BC, Gallagher JD, et al. Characterizing novice behavior associated with learning ultrasound-guided peripheral regional anesthesia. *Reg Anesth Pain Med.* 2007;32(2):107–115.

55. Waldrop WB, Murray DJ, Boulet JR, Kras JF. Management of anesthesia equipment failure: a simulation-based resident skill assessment. *Anesth Analg.* 2009;109:426–433.

56. Friedman Z, Siddiqui N, Katznelson R, et al. Clinical impact of epidural anesthesia simulation on short- and long-term learning curve: high- versus low-fidelity model training. *Reg Anesth Pain Med.* 2009;34:229–232.

57. Niazi AU, Ramlogan R, Prasad A, Chan VW. A new simulation model for ultrasound-aided regional anesthesia. *Reg Anesth Pain Med.* 2010;35:320–321.

58. Hocking G, Hebard S, Mitchell C. A review of the benefits and pitfalls of phantoms in ultrasound-guided regional anesthesia. *RegAnesth Pain Med.* 2011;36(2):162–170.

59. Gaba DM, Howard SK, Flanagan B, Smith BE, Fish KJ, Botney R. Assessment of clinical performance during simulated crises using both technical and behavioral ratings. *Anesthesiology.* 1998;89:8–18.

60. Boulet JR, Murray DJ. Simulation-based assessment in anesthesiology: requirements for practical implementation. *Anesthesiology.* 2010;112(4):1041–1052.

CHAPTER 16

Professionalism in Nurse Anesthesia Education

Bernadette Henrichs, PhD, CRNA, CCRN

Keywords: Code of ethics, expert, leader, mentor, nurturer, practice standards, professionalism, social media, teacher, vigilance.

Key Concepts

- Nurse anesthesia is a profession and its members are considered professionals.
- Certified Registered Nurse Anesthetists (CRNAs) should display positive attributes of a professional.
- CRNAs have a code of ethics that must be adhered to.
- Practice standards should be followed as CRNAs care for their patients.
- Behaviors that distract from patient care and vigilance during the administration of an anesthetic are not acceptable.
- Posting on social media should be carefully thought out and avoided if it risks confidentiality.
- CRNAs should be role models for nurse anesthesia students to show them how to grow as professionals.
- Mentoring is vital to the growth and development of our students, both professionally and personally.
- Mentoring involves many attributes to be effective.
- Lifelong learning must be part of a CRNA's professionalism.
- Being a member of the professional organization instills professionalism in an individual.

Definition of a Profession and Professionalism

Is nursing considered a profession? Is nurse anesthesia considered a profession? In the past, nursing focused on caring for the patient without any academic consideration. In the Florence Nightingale era, nurses were viewed as "attendants of the sick."[1] This was their calling; however, that has changed over the past few decades. The modernization of nursing careers emerged from Scotland "as a way of preparing nurses as academic as well as clinical leaders in contemporary health care."[2] Nursing must not only be clinically competent, but also academically successful to be recognized as a profession and as a successful career.

It is important for nursing to be looked upon as a profession. The nursing profession can no longer dwell in "the gray margins that exist between vocational and professional status."[2] Nurses must be looked upon, not only as clinical caregivers, but also as successful researchers and scholars. Emphasis is now placed on autonomy in the clinical field along with membership in a professional organization.[3] Nurse anesthetists must now be fully engaged in research, teaching, and practice. This is what contributes to our existence as professionals. Nurse anesthetists must build relationships that include mutual trust and respect with other health care professionals where decisions about patient care can be discussed and shared, and where prestige is brought to the profession.

Professionalism is defined as "the body of qualities or features characteristic of a profession."[4(p.129)] These qualities include a "high degree of skill and knowledge that is applied to the practice."[4(p.129)] Although other occupations have high degrees of skill, professions differ in that they "not only carry out the work, but also prescribe the work, which they then carry out."[4(p.129)] Professional practice includes professional values, core competencies, core knowledge, and role development.[5] Thus, professionals work autonomously in a competent fashion and are looked upon by society as being skilled and trustworthy. Professionals must meet the expectations of society as they serve and care for the members of the community. Codes of conduct help guide how the profession is expressed.

Professionalism is reflective of the distance taken to reach the status of the profession.[6] Wynd found that professionalism correlates to several factors, including years of experience, higher graduate educational degrees, membership and serving as officers in organizations, and certification in nursing specialty areas such as nurse anesthesia.[3] Benefits of certification may include recognition of expertise, higher salaries, increased potential for promotion, job security, and greater professional credibility due to increased confidence in specialty skills and knowledge.[7] Being a member of an organization, such as the American Association of Nurse Anesthetists (AANA), is important as a professional. Those who join professional organizations perceive themselves as more professional than those who do not join professional organizations.[3] The members help to strengthen the organization and, thus, help grow the profession. The more members a professional organization has, the stronger the organization it becomes. Aspects of professionalism, according to Shaw et al,[4] include:

- Putting patients' interests first and acting to protect them
- Respecting patients' dignity and choices
- Protecting the confidentiality of patients' information

- Cooperating with team members, along with other health care colleagues, in the interest of patients
- Maintaining professional knowledge and competence
- Being trustworthy

The word profession can be defined as public avowal.[8(p.530)] A profession has obligations to the community at large. Welie explains: "A profession is a collective of expert service providers who have jointly and publicly committed to always give priority to the existential needs and interests of the public they serve above their own interests, and in turn are trusted by the public to do so."[8] Thus, professionals selflessly protect the public whom they serve. In the nurse anesthesia profession, CRNAs vow to protect their patients as they administer anesthesia while a patient undergoes surgery, being an advocate and watchdog for them while they are under anesthesia.

Code of Ethics for the Certified Registered Nurse Anesthetist (CRNA)

The AANA has a code of ethics for the CRNA and also for nurse anesthesia students that serves to guide its members in fulfilling their obligations as professionals.[9] According to the AANA, the responsibilities of a professional include being accountable and responsible for our services and actions while administering anesthesia. These responsibilities, according to the AANA, include:

- The CRNA, as an independently licensed professional, is responsible and accountable for judgments made and actions taken in his or her professional practice. Neither physician orders nor institutional policies relieve the CRNA of responsibility for his or her judgments made or actions taken.
- The CRNA practices in accordance with the professional practice standards established by the profession.
- The CRNA participates in activities that contribute to the ongoing development of the profession and its body of knowledge.
- The CRNA is responsible and accountable for his or her conduct in maintaining the dignity and integrity of the profession.
- The CRNA collaborates and cooperates with other health care providers involved in a patient's care.
- The CRNA respects the expertise and responsibility of all health care providers involved in providing services to patients.
- The CRNA is responsible and accountable for his or her actions, including self-awareness and assessment of fitness for duty.

The professional nurse anesthetist should have the "incentive to attain the highest possible degree of ethical conduct."[10] By being professional in this manner, respect and confidence will be achieved in both the CRNA and also by the members of the profession, and accorded by the members of the society in which they serve.

Attributes and Qualities of a Professional

The attributes and qualities of a professional include a long list of powerful themes, including altruism, accountability, autonomy, punctuality, dependability, empathy, kindness, consideration, community service, compassion, competence, continuing education, excellence, honesty, integrity, self-regulation, increase in scientific knowledge, knowledge of ethical standards, moral reasoning, participation in professional organizations, reflection, research, respect, self-awareness, self-motivation (particularly in respect to life-long learning), a sense of calling, trustworthiness, and working with others,[11,12] Celik[6] sums up this list in a collective fashion, and describes the following, more focused list describing professionalism:

1. Autonomy
2. High-level scientific knowledge
3. Participation in professional organizations
4. Research
5. Community service
6. Competence and continuing education
7. A code for nurses

Walker, Clendon, and Walton conducted a study to discover nurses' attitudes to professionalism. The researchers were seeking to find out how much the nurses knew about professionalism, its requirements, and how it affects patient care.[13] The researchers asked the nurses what they considered to be the personal attitudes, attributes, and values that make up professionalism. A total of 245 nurses participated in the survey and focus groups, reflecting New Zealand's nursing organization membership. The attributes were ranked in order of importance from the top by 25 nurses in two focus groups (**Table 16.1**).

Table 16.1 Professional Attributes, Ranked by Order of Importance

1. Adherence to a code of conduct
2. Integrity, trust, honesty, and ethical behavior
3. Keeping focus on the patient
4. Owning up to mistakes
5. Maintaining patient confidentiality
6. Boundaries and the need to limit self-disclosure
7. Commitment to cultural safety
8. Empathy, caring, and compassion
9. Good communication and interpersonal skills
10. Self-awareness, remaining non-judgmental
11. Showing knowledge and technical competence
12. Commitment to ongoing education and updating nursing knowledge
13. Work ethic, conscientiousness and time management
14. Supporting other nurses
15. Personal values and morality
16. Modeling dignity and respect
17. Being open and honest with communication
18. Having and inspiring confidence
19. Maintaining positive attitudes
20. Kindness, patience, and endurance
21. Commitment to insightful reflection on practice
22. Giving and accepting honest peer assessment
23. Appearance: standard of dress

Used by permission from Walker L, Clendon J, Walton J. What nurses think about professionalism. *Nurs N Z.* 2015;21(1):12–13.[13]

Although this study was conducted in New Zealand, it can be applied to U.S. professional nurses.

Unprofessional Behavior and Barriers to Professionalism

A nurse anesthetist or nurse anesthesia student should display academic integrity and ethical and professional conduct. Being cognizant of the qualities and attributes of a professional is important, but it is also important to be aware of qualities and attributes that reflect negative characteristics of a professional. Unprofessional behavior of a health care worker can be defined as conduct that "demonstrates disrespect or a lack of compassion, lack of commitment to ethical principles, or a lack of integrity or accountability toward patients or coworkers.[14] Professional misconduct includes violations of professional standards. In the clinical area, this behavior has been associated with preventable error and threats to patient safety.[15] In other words, lack of professionalism can lead to errors in one's practice that could have been prevented. It can also lead to patient harm. Such negative activity is unbefitting of a professional. Students entering the profession must be scrutinized for breaches in professional misconduct that can lead to lack of academic integrity. These breaches may be demonstrated by plagiarism, cheating, inaccurate reporting of clinical hours, false documentation, illegal drug possession or diversion of medications, forging a signature, incivility, aggression in the classroom or clinical area, inaccurate information on resumes, or covering up or not reporting medication errors.[15]

Unprofessionalism that may affect patient safety include improper sterile technique, poor hand hygiene, and inadequate handoff to another health care professional.[14] Other unprofessional behavior includes bullying, improper use of phones in the operating room, dressing unprofessionally, inappropriate postings on social media, or displaying a negative attitude to patients and faculty/staff by not showing kindness, empathy and patience (**Table 16.2**, next page). All of these unacceptable actions have legal ramifications and the program must follow due process when conducting an investigation to protect the rights of the patients. When a student reports unprofessional behavior by another member of the health care team, his or her rights within the academic institution must also be protected in a delicate, legal manner.[15]

Table 16.2 Unprofessional Behavior

- Not adhering to the AANA Code of Ethics or the AANA Standards for Nurse Anesthesia Practice
- Plagiarism
- Cheating (student)
- Inaccurate reporting of clinical hours (student)
- Possession of illegal drugs
- Diversion of medications
- Forging a signature
- Incivility
- Aggression (classroom or clinical area)
- Inaccurate information on resume
- Not reporting medication errors
- Bullying
- Improper use of cell phones in the OR
- Inappropriate posting on social media
- Having a negative attitude to patients and/or faculty and staff
- Lack of vigilance
- Showing a lack of kindness, empathy, patience
- Dressing unprofessionally; unprofessional appearance (tattoos, piercings)

When unprofessionalism is noted, it may be difficult to call attention to the behavior. It may be looked upon as being confrontational or unacceptable, especially if one is a student. Although difficult to do, as professionals, it is our duty to speak up and report unprofessional behaviors of students and/or colleagues. In some situations, this may prevent the patient's safety from being jeopardized.[14] It is important for faculty to encourage students to speak up if they believe someone is acting unprofessionally, especially if the patient's safety is jeopardized.

Nurse anesthesia program administrators and instructors must assure that students are familiar with the AANA's Code of Ethics and its Practice Standards.[16] The AANA Standards for Nurse Anesthesia Practice are published on the AANA website (http://www.aana.com) and describe minimum standards that professional CRNAs should follow as they administer anesthesia. These important documents must become very familiar to CRNAs and nurse anesthesia students starting on day one of the program. Assuring that students are aware of these documents may decrease the incidence of unprofessional behavior that occurs when not following such standards and expectations of a professional. Student evaluations should contain an assessment of professionalism. Clinical preceptors have an obligation to make these assessments part of the student's daily clinical review. Didactic instructors must also assess professionalism and provide feedback to the student.

Reading for Pleasure/Improper Use of Smartphone in the Operating Room

Exemplifying professionalism includes being empathetic and caring to patients and giving them the most vigilant care possible. This is vital since CRNAs and student registered nurse anesthetists (SRNAs) become the watchdogs when patients are being administered anesthesia. Thus, demonstrating a lack of vigilance in the operating room by reading a magazine or newspaper or by sending or reading texts on a personal phone demonstrate unprofessional behavior. Each patient should be cared for as if he or she were a loved one. Reading for pleasure in the operating room or being on a personal phone is unacceptable, whether one is playing electronic games or checking emails. A patient should be assured of 100 percent attention from the anesthesia provider while being administered anesthesia.

Social Media

Social media has its advantages in controlled situations and is even used by the nurse anesthesia professional organization to communicate with its members. Posting on a social media site can serve as a real-time method to communicate with a target audience such as family and friends. It can also be used as a method for organizations to communicate with its members. Social media can facilitate medical discussions, increase awareness of health issues by posting factual information, educate consumers, improve communication with the public, or serve as a marketing and recruiting tool.[17] Social media sites can be successful avenues to communicate and can be conducted without a direct cost to the person.

Social media has its disadvantages and CRNAs and nurse anesthesia students must use caution in posting to social media sites. They must remember that what is posted is considered published. If unprofessional or ethically inappropriate content is posted, this can reflect poorly on the person, the profession, and the employing institution or nurse anesthesia program.[18] Patient information should never be posted due to patient confidentiality. Even if a patient's name is never used, patients should not be discussed on such sites. This is a violation of HIPAA (Health Information Portability and Accountability Act) and failure to comply with HIPAA can result in civil and criminal penalties.[19] Once the information is posted, a "visible electronic 'footprint' is made with the potential for unintended and/or negative consequences". Nurse anesthesia program administrators and instructors must assure that students are educated and aware of the program's or institution's policies regarding social media, and they must assure that students realize the consequences of violating such policies. The following tips will help the student and CRNA know how to best manage their online reputation by understanding the benefits and risks of social media:[17(pp.42–43)]

- Take advantage of the privacy protections and settings that are available on each social media website. Review your settings routinely as privacy settings and terms/conditions can change regularly.
- Remember that anything posted should be considered public, and could be misconstrued, misinterpreted, or taken out of context. This may potentially be accessible for the rest of one's career.
- Realize that postings exist forever, even if one uses the most secure privacy settings. They are never anonymous, may exist in different forms, and are indexed by Google.
- Remember that subpoenas can be issued which may require internet service providers, social networking companies, and websites to produce IP addresses or email addresses that will identify the source of the content.
- Realize that pictures and comments posted online may be misinterpreted.

- Routinely monitor one's online presence and reputation to watch for possible hacking of the site, which could lead to spam being on that website. Spam on the website may lead to inaccurate or inappropriate postings.
- Ensure that one is complying with regulatory agency standards and employer policies, and that the person is up-to-date with privacy and confidentiality laws. Descriptions of a specific case or the patient's history without using the patient's name or identifier number can potentially identify a patient and violate privacy and confidentiality laws.
- Be compliant with institutional and employer policies and procedures.
- Realize that copyright, trade slander, and libel laws apply to content posted online.
- Respect and maintain the professional boundaries of the health care provider and patient relationship in accordance with professional ethical guidelines.
- Keep personal and professional content separate. For example, one can use Facebook for personal friends and family and a professional page such as LinkedIn for professional relationships.
- Do not post content outside your area of expertise and keep the focus on general information, assuring that no patients are identified.

In addition to these guidelines, the AANA also has social media guidelines posted on its website.[20] As a professional, CRNAs and nurse anesthesia students should be aware of such guidelines and follow them accordingly.

Can Professionalism Be Taught and Learned?

How is professionalism learned? Can nurse anesthesia students be taught how to become a professional CRNA? Teaching students how to become professionals begins with didactic and clinical faculty and instructors serving as role models and mentors to the students.[21] Learning the role of professionalism begins in the classroom and continues into the clinical area. It begins on day one and continues throughout the program. A formal course on professionalism should be included in the curriculum, possibly in a professional aspects course. Topics may include, but are not limited, to:

- Understanding the professional code of conduct and standards
- Identifying the role of an SRNA and CRNA
- Being successful as a CRNA
- Building a positive reputation
- Identifying appropriate and inappropriate behavior of a professional
- Conveying a professional image, including dress, make-up, hairstyle, piercings, and tattoos
- Getting along with coworkers, supervisors, and subordinates
- Avoiding conflict in the anesthesia community
- Using proper verbal and nonverbal etiquette

Along with a formal course on professionalism, informal or hidden curriculums play a critical role in the students' knowledge about professionalism.[22] Professionalism is "more than learning and application of technical skills."[22] Professionalism involves a social, moral, and political contract with its members and the public. The CRNA has a contract to put the patients first and provide anesthesia to them in a vigilant manner. By providing safe anesthesia, the patients put their trust in the CRNAs and in the nurse anesthesia profession.[23] Thus, CRNAs have an "obligation to be deserving of the trust that the public at large and each and every individual patient or client vests in the profession at large and in each and every member of the profession."[23(p.600)]

CRNAs have values, attitudes, and behaviors that guide us in maintaining our scruples and doing what is right for the patient and the profession, morally and politically. The CRNA, as part of a culture of anesthesia providers, will teach the student how to be a professional through role modeling and mentoring.

Didactic faculty members teach the concepts of anesthesiology, including physiology and pathophysiology; however, students must be able to apply this knowledge in the clinical area as they give hands-on care to patients. The clinical instructor plays a major role in helping the student grow into a professional by demonstrating the attributes of a professional. The CRNA serves as a role model and a mentor to the student.

Simulation as a Tool for Teaching

Simulation may be a helpful tool to becoming a CRNA and behaving as a professional. The technology of the patient simulator may appeal to contemporary learners who are computer savvy. Generation X and Generation Y students have grown up with computers, electronic games, and the Internet. Students from these generations "typically possess a natural attraction to technology.".[21(p.126)] Simulation can help the student respond to a clinical situation that may rarely be seen in the real operating room, and the faculty member can provide a structured learning lesson on how to manage the scenario in a safe, controlled environment. Simulation can also help the student see the big picture, improving critical thinking skills.[21(p.126)] Students can learn the role of a professional by acting out the role in the simulated operating room and receiving the guidance of the instructor on ethical and legal situations, leadership roles, and team-building scenarios; thus, professional behavior can be taught through the use of simulation.

Mentoring: Promoting Professionalism With CRNAs

Clinical and didactic faculty should serve as role models and mentors to nurse anesthesia students. Being a positive role model is "the single, most important effective component of learning professionalism" in a person's career.[24] The mentor as a role model has a powerful influence on the development of the student becoming a professional.[11]

Mentoring can be defined as someone with a higher rank or achievement who teaches or gives help and advice to a less experienced person, facilitating professional development. It is a symbolic relationship between a novice and an expert.[25] The mentoring relationship may include "role modeling, professional development, and emotional and psychological support."[26] It may also involve counseling and guiding one through an educational experience.

Mentoring often involves the association of an experienced and an inexperienced member of a specific organization. In anesthesia, the CRNA takes an active role in helping the protégé, the inexperienced nurse anesthesia student, to develop professionally and personally in the field. "The mentor plots the course; the protégé makes the journey."[27]

Mentoring is different from precepting. Precepting occurs when a CRNA is assigned to a nurse anesthesia student on a specific day and helps the student with his or her clinical skills, and evaluates the progress at the end of the day. Mentoring is a professional relationship between the CRNA and the nurse anesthesia student that spans over the course of the student's training, and sometimes extends over a lifetime. Mentoring can "improve professional satisfaction and provides a sense of giving back to one's profession."[25]

Mentors are considered clinical experts in their field. Clinical expertise, according to Fagerlund, "has been the primary strength of nurse anesthetists and the focus of nurse anesthesia educational programs."[28] Nurse anesthetists who are willing to teach will "probably find they are able to have more influence on the changes taking place within health care than are the individuals who have not developed these skills."[28]

The process of mentoring starts while one is still a student, and is also present during the development of one's profession; mentoring a student is not a short-lived task. A mutually supportive, open, and trusting relationship can develop between the student and the faculty member that may potentially continue throughout a lifetime.

Roles and Responsibilities of a Mentor

What are the roles and responsibilities of a mentor? A true mentor serves several roles. This person should instruct and guide the student in developing intellectual and technical skills. He or she should provide information and advice to the student and guide and encourage the student to engage in safe, clinical practice. A mentor should not only educate the student on how to perform clinical tasks, such as inserting an endotracheal tube, but also provide social support. The mentor should help the student develop professionally into a new career. A mentor will "model, inform, confirm or disconfirm, prescribe, or question."[29] A mentor will also "protect, promote and support . . . act as a counselor, providing advice, guidance, oral support and nurturing."[29]

Mentoring "demands hard work, discipline, rigor, creativity, honesty and integrity."[30] Not only does it require effort by both individuals, but it must also take into consideration the various personalities of people and their different learning styles.[30] The mentor should constantly strive to determine the most effective manner by which the student learns, and then adjust the teaching style to fulfill these goals.

An effective mentor has strong leadership qualities. A leader is "visible, committed, and knowledgeable" and is "calm, confident, and predictable."[27] The leaders of the anesthesia community should step forward to mentor inexperienced nurse anesthesia students. As a mentor, he or she may not only serve as a teacher, but also as a "coach, positive role model, developer of talent, opener of doors to opportunity, protector, sponsor, and successful leader."[27] Because of such leadership characteristics, the nurse anesthetist leader has the capability to make the mentoring process a successful venture.

A strong leader will take on the role of helping others to mold their professional roles by guiding them through the process. A leader will "*intentionally* influence another individual or a group in order to accomplish a goal."[31] A charismatic leader will motivate, excite, and move individuals to reach their goals; thus, a person with strong leadership abilities should not waste such talent and should mentor those around him or her. The mentor should "give the protégé the authority to set goals, dream, grow, and surpass the achievements of the teacher."[31]

The mentor must take on several roles in order to assist the student. The mentor must be a teacher and a role model for the student. In order to carry out these tasks, the mentor should be a well-respected expert in the field. Mentoring involves mutual respect between the mentor and the student. Successful mentoring requires the mentor to listen more than talk as he or she works with the student.

The student should feel comfortable asking questions to the mentor in a non-threatening manner. The student should never feel that the question is a "stupid one." The mentor should be knowledgeable in answering the questions.This will occur if the mentor is an expert, the best of the best in the role as an instructor in anesthesia. If the mentor does not know an answer, he or she should feel comfortable in putting pride aside and state that he or she does not know the answer. Together, the two can then seek to find the answer to the question in an informational manner. Thus, mentoring can become a learning experience for both the student and the instructor since learning is truly a lifelong experience that should never end.

A CRNA has the opportunity to mentor a student throughout the educational period. If achieved, the student will be successfully molded into his or her role in such a manner that it will positively affect his or her future career. Mentoring can have such a lasting influence on the student that the student may decide to serve as a mentor later on once his or her career has been established. The process can then continue with each new group of students, making the role of becoming a CRNA less stressful and more successful.

Evaluating the Success of Mentoring a Student

Mentors can help students learn their role professionally, master the clinical tasks, be knowledgeable, and make wise decisions in the delivery of anesthesia. Mentors can respond to the students' calls for help, share strategies for handling difficulties, and help them look at things in a positive fashion, all the while encouraging success. "Anesthetists who fail to mentor their junior colleagues jeopardize the future of nurse anesthesia and do a disservice to their patients, their communities, and their profession."[27]

With mentoring, not only does the student grow and develop throughout the educational experience, but so does the mentor. Learning never stops, despite the vast amount of information that one gains and the experience that one achieves with time. Not only does the process assist in role modeling, but it may also assist the nurse anesthesia student to reach professional excellence in nurse anesthesia. Mentoring can play an important role in the decision to enter and remain in an academic career. It is associated with higher career satisfaction and research success. It can also play a role in providing a sense of professional identity and enhanced commitment to the profession.[26] It is not only rewarding for the student, but also for the CRNA, as it can provide a feeling of emotional satisfaction and professionalism. Not only does the student grow and develop professionally, but so does the mentor. Learning never stops, despite the vast amount of information that one gains and the experience that one achieves with time. The mentor helps lay the path for the student to take and professionally grow. The relationship can open doors to future possibilities in one's professional career.

Mentoring can mold the student into a successful leader in his or her field. Once the student completes training and looks for employment, improved job satisfaction, with intent to stay at that institution where the training was conducted, is a satisfying outcome of the experience.[32]

Mentoring can be described as being similar to parenting. It is an investment in "the future of the nursing profession, just as parenting is an investment in the future of the human race."[33] Thus, the future of our profession depends highly on the success of having CRNAs serve as mentors for our nurse anesthesia students!

Examples of Mentoring Programs

A mentoring program can be as simple as pairing a senior student with a junior student. The older student is instructed to call the newer students at the start of the program to offer support and guidance. The senior student helps to answer any questions the new students may have, including those related to housing and transportation.

The senior student gives advice, answers didactic and clinical questions, and helps the student move through the program. Throughout the program, the senior student serves as a resource for any questions the newer student may have, including questions about academic courses, clinical rotations, the rules and regulations of the program, and social activities such as the yearly welcome picnic or the graduation ceremony.

At a more advanced level, mentoring may include the pairing of a CRNA, who serves as a positive role model, with a nurse anesthesia student who has a similar personality or similar interests. They may have common concerns such as small children, or they both may be single parents, or they both may be new to the area, having moved due to enrollment into the program. Having similar backgrounds or similar interests will help the CRNA provide support to the nurse anesthesia student and hopefully strengthen the bond between the two individuals.

If the match between the student and the CRNA is not a good fit, a different CRNA should be paired with the student. It is important that both the student and the CRNA get along well with each other, so that they feel comfortable sharing their thoughts and concerns and their relationship possibly develops into a strong working, lifelong bond.

During the first few weeks of clinical experience in the operating room when the education and training can become very stressful, the student is encouraged to ask his or her mentor for guidance about the clinical experience. The student should feel comfortable reaching out for support and encouragement. Informal meetings between the mentor and the student are encouraged, along with phone calls and emails. Since students are encouraged to be honest when they talk to their mentors about their clinical experience, it is vital that discussions remain confidential in order to build trust between the student and mentor. The mentor is encouraged to provide guidance, understanding, and support to the student throughout the length of the nurse anesthesia program. Many lasting friendships have been formed from this early association and former students often volunteer to serve as mentors to new students once they become CRNAs.

Mentoring may also involve a nurse anesthesia student or a CRNA being paired with an undergraduate nursing student, guiding the undergraduate student along the path to becoming a CRNA in the future. All of these mentoring relationships can help the student professionally develop into the role of a CRNA and "instill a strong sense of professionalism."[25(p.35)]

In summary, a CRNA who professionally serves as a role model and mentors a nurse anesthesia student will display core values of compassion, empathy, integrity, respect, altruism, patience, calmness, and confidence. Mentoring can be a rewarding experience, not only for the CRNA, but also for the nurse anesthesia student. Successful mentoring can result in a successful, positive outcome for the profession of nurse anesthesia as a whole. Qualities of mentoring are listed below:

- Mentoring involves taking an active role in helping the inexperienced nurse anesthesia student to develop into a CRNA, both professionally and personally.
- A mentor serves as a protector, supporter, teacher, counselor, advisor, leader, role model, nurturer, listener, sponsor, promoter, and a friend to the student.
- Mentoring involves work, dedication, determination, time, discipline, honesty, creativity, a positive attitude, and a sense of humor.
- Mentoring a student should include the task of obtaining specific goals. These goals should be established by the mentor and the student at the beginning of the learning process and should include both long-term and short-term tasks.
- Goals should be broad but also specific.
- Mentoring can be a rewarding experience for both the mentor and the student.

Professionalism and Appearance

Consider two students arriving at the hospital from home or school to check assignments for the next day or to interview an inpatient preoperatively or postoperatively. The first student is wearing a pair of dress pants and button-down shirt and may also be wearing a white lab coat over the dress apparel. The second student is wearing a pair of shorts, a T-shirt, and flip flops. Which student is dressed professionally? One may make the description even more interesting by picturing the student wearing heavy make-up, having a colorful tattoo over the entire length of his or her arm, and with multiple piercings. First impressions matter when one is trying to build a trusting relationship with a patient as our society seems to value physical appearance.[5] Appearance not only plays a role in developing a trusting relationship, but it also has an impact on whether or not the patient will feel confident with that anesthesia provider.

Appearance is known to affect the patient-provider relationship.[5] First impressions really do matter when one is trying to build confidence and trust with a patient. First impressions are an important foundation in "building a trusting relationship in a society that values physical appearance."[34(p.63)] The professional attire of the anesthesia provider can also affect the anxiety and comfort level of the patient.[5,35] Lehna and colleagues state that "professionalism and attire are intimately connected with the notion of competency."[36(p.97)]

Dress code is a significant part of one's professional image.[37] Students must be informed by their program director that their personal attire may display how professional they look. Professionalism can be described in relationship to image and conduct.[5] If the anesthesia provider is professional looking, the patient will be less anxious, more comfortable, and trusting that the anesthesia provider is competent to deliver the anesthetic care.[5] Nurse anesthetists and nurse anesthesia students should wear business clothes or business casual clothing. Overdressing is better than underdressing professionally as "it never hurts to overdress slightly."[38]

Clothing should be conservative (no short dresses or shorts) and should not be trendy.[38] It should be clean and should not show wear and tear. The clothes should fit properly and not be too tight or too loose.

Tattoos and body piercings have increased in the past few years and policies should be written that address what should be acceptable and unacceptable for the anesthesia provider. It is important to realize that tattoos and body piercings are considered a reflection of that person's expression of art; they express uniqueness and individuality. People with tattoos and body piercings are normally proud of their tattoos and piercings and normally want to display them to others; however, professionalism must be considered when caring for patients. The literature reports that health care providers with visible tattoos and body piercings are viewed negatively by others, including patients.[5(p.194)] Coincidentally, physicians and nurses, especially females without body art, tend to look less favorably at those with body art.[39]

If the tattoo can be covered, then it may be best to cover it with clothing. If not covered, it may affect one's professional image in a negative manner.[5(p.193)] Although body piercings may be visible, they can be removed and, thus, should be removed before caring for a patient in the clinical area. Hair should be combed and tidy. Make-up should be light and cologne, if worn, should be minimal as a strong, powerful smell may make a patient feel nauseated. With jewelry, less is more. Dressing appropriately improves one's image professionally and builds confidence and rapport with patients.[38]

A name badge should always be worn in the clinical area and should include the provider's name and title. The anesthesia provider should introduce himself or herself with confidence. For example, "My name is______. I am a Certified Registered Nurse Anesthetist" or, for the student, "I am a registered nurse who is now a student studying nurse anesthesia."

Along with dress code monitoring, tardiness and attendance of students in the clinical area should also be monitored. Showing up late or not showing up at all can affect the overall image of a professional and should be monitored by program directors.[5] Nurse anesthesia programs must develop policies, not only on dress code, but also on attendance, tardiness, and absenteeism. The policies should be fair and consistently enforced so that the student is aware of the consequences if not followed. These policies can help form the professional behavior of the future CRNA. Both tardiness and absenteeism are important topics that must be adhered to. This will help to shape the professional image of the profession.

Importance of a Positive Attitude

Developing a positive attitude toward any field of learning in education is just as important as learning about that field or teaching in that field.[6(p.497)] Negative attitudes will limit one's ability not only to learn, but also to teach. Thus, anesthesia providers must strive for a positive attitude toward nursing, especially when they are teaching and serving as role models to students.

Membership in a Professional Organization

A true professional engages in its professional organization and gets involved in committees and tasks. More than 90 percent of CRNAs are members of the AANA. This is due to the members' commitments to professional development and advancement of the profession. Overall, nurse anesthetists strive for excellence in providing safe anesthesia to their patients. They also strive to continue as a profession, supporting the organization and its members. Nurse anesthetists "want to excel, and as a result, embrace things that are in themselves most excellent, including membership."[40(p.41)] "Actively involved CRNAs are engaged in a great cause: moving our profession forward so that we can continue to serve and care for the human race."[41(p.24)]

Participation in professional activities and commitment to the organization will enhance the profession and is "essential for maintaining a desirable practice environment."[42(p.101)] Those who are active members of the profession's organization will help the future of nurse anesthesia continue as an excellent profession. Actively involved CRNAs are on a journey of continued growth and development throughout their lifetime as they pursue excellence. One of the ways this is performed, along with participating in professional organizations, is through continuing education. CRNAs are required to obtain continuing education units, whether through face-to-face conference attendance or by reading a publication/journal article and then taking an examination to demonstrate that learning occurred. Lifelong learning is a major part of the nurse anesthesia profession.

Considering Professionalism With Applicant Selection

Should professionalism be considered when choosing an applicant for a position in a nurse anesthesia program? Professionalism is a key component of a CRNA's qualities and should be considered when choosing an applicant for a position in a nurse anesthesia program. A CRNA is expected to do more than provide anesthesia once his or her educational training has concluded. A CRNA is expected to embrace leadership and be an advocate for the profession. As a registered nurse, an applicant will hopefully have leadership qualities and professional attributes that will make him or her a highly respected CRNA in the future. This is an important aspect of a professional. These professional values and beliefs should continue as a CRNA for the rest of one's life.

By choosing applicants who demonstrate leadership qualities and display professional values, including emotional intelligence, the profession will gain future nurse anesthetists who will become leaders in the field of nurse anesthesia. Important attributes that should be considered in selecting applicants and assessing professionalism include: dress, body language, timeliness, demeanor, professional verbiage, and a positive attitude.

Summary

How can professionalism be assessed or displayed in an individual's personality? Development and assessment of a professional can be applied to an adaptation of the classic Miller's pyramid of progression from knowledge to competence, as described by Consorti.[43] Initially, the student learns the traits of becoming a professional (*knowledge*). Later, the student learns how to act like a professional (*knows how*). As the student develops in his or her career, the student will begin to act like a professional and display and show professional attributes (*shows*). Finally, the student will develop into a nurse anesthesia professional by actually "doing,", in other words, by practicing as a safe, competent CRNA and by becoming a leader in the nurse anesthesia professional (*does*). Thus, a CRNA must rise above and be viewed as a true leader in the profession of nursing. As nurse anesthesia educators, we must be role models to nurse anesthesia students and help them to achieve these same goals. We must help them to grow and become the professionals that CRNAs are!

References

1. Keeling J, Templeman J. An exploratory study: student nurses' perceptions of professionalism. *Nurse Educ Prac.* 2013;13(1):18–22.

2. Andrew N. Professional identity in nursing: are we there yet? *Nurse Educ Today.* 2012;32(8):846–849.

3. Wynd CA. Current factors contributing to professionalism in nursing. *J Prof Nurs.* 2003;19(5):251–261.

4. Zijlstra-Shaw S, Robinson PG, Roberts T. Assessing professionalism within dental education; the need for a definition. *Eur J Dent Educ.* 2012;16(1):e128–e136.

5. Rizk K, Bofinger R. Florence Nightingale versus Dennis Rodman: evaluating professional image in the modern world. In: Oermann M, ed. *Annual Review of Nursing Education.* Vol.6. New York, NY: Springer; 2008:189–204.

6. Celik B, Karadag A, Hisar F. Instrument of professional attitude for student nurses (IPASN): a confirmatory factor analytic study. *Nurse Educ Today.* 2012;32(5): 497–500.

7. Cary AH. Certified registered nurses: results of the study of the certified workforce. *Amer J Nurs.* 2001;101(1):44–52.

8. Welie JV Is dentistry a profession? Part 1. Professionalism defined. *J Can Dent Assoc.* 2004;70(8):529–532.

9. Code of Ethics for the Certified Registered Nurse Anesthetist. American Association of Nurse Anesthetists. http://www.aana.com/resources2/professionalpractice/Documents/PPM%20Code%20of%20Ethics.pdf. Accessed July 26, 2015.

10. Mannino MJ. The AANA code of ethics. *AANA J.* 1986;54(6):473–475.

11. Elliott, D., May W, Schaff, P, et al. Shaping professionalism in pre-clinical medical students: professionalsim and the practice of medicine. *Med Teach.* 2009;31(7):e295–e302.

12. Leger C. The value of professionalism in nurse anesthesia. *American Association of Nurse Anesthetists News Bulletin.* 2012; January 3:31.

13. Walker L, Clendon J, Walton J. What nurses think about professionalism. *Kai Tiaki Nursing New Zealand.* 2015;21(1):12–13.

14. Martinez W, Etchegaray JM, Thomas EJ, et al. 'Speaking up' about patient safety concerns and unprofessional behavior among residents: validation of two scales. *BMJ Qual Saf.* 2015;24(11):671–680.

15. Anselmi K, Glasgow M, Gambescia S. Using a nursing student conduct committee to foster professionalism among nursing students. *J Prof Nurs.* 2014;30(6):481–485.

16. AANA Standards for Nurse Anesthesia Practice. American Association of Nurse Anesthetists. http://www.aana.com/resources2/professionalpractice/Documents/PPM%20Standards%20for%20Nurse%20Anesthesia%20Practice.pdf. Accessed July 26, 2015.

17. Leiker M. When to 'friend' a patient: social media tips for health care professionals. *Wis Med J.* 2011;110(1):42–43.

18. Cleary M, Ferguson C, Jackson D, Watson R. Editorial: Social media and the new e-professionalism. *Contemp Nurse.* 2013;45(2):152–154.

19. HIPAA: Health insurance portability and accountability act. American Medical Association. http://www.ama-assn.org/ama/pub/physician-resources/solutions-managing-your-practice/coding-billing-insurance/hipaahealth-insurance-portability-accountability-act.page? Accessed July 26, 2015.

20. AANA social media guidelines. American Association of Nurse Anesthetists: http://www.aana.com/myaana/Advocacy/stategovtaffairs/stateassociationresources/Documents/SMA%20Documents/AANA%20Social%20Media%20Guidelines%20Dec%202014.pdf.

21. Duphily NH. Simulation education: a primer for professionalism. *Teaching and Learning in Nursing.* 2014;9:126–128.

22. Baingana R, Nakasujja N, Galukande M, Omona K, Mafigiri D, Sewankambo NK. Learning health professionalism at Makerere University: an exploratory study amongst undergraduate students. *BMC Medical Education.* 2010;10(76):1–10.

23. Welie, J. Is dentistry a profession? Part 2. The hallmarks of professionalism. *J Can Den Assoc.* 2004;70(9):599–602.

24. Byszewski A, Hendelman W, McGuinty C, Moineau G. Wanted: Role models medical students' perceptions of professionalism. *BMC Medical Education.* 2012;12(115):1–9.

25. Grost E, Brooks A. From SRNA to CRNA: Why mentoring matters. *AANA News Bulletin.* March 2013:34–35.

26. Bryant A, Brody A, Perez A, et al. Development and implementation of a peer mentoring program for early career gerontological faculty. *J Nurs Scholarsh.* 2015;47(3):258–266.

27. Pollock, GS. We are all leaders. *AANA J.* 1996;64(3):225–227.

28. Fagerlund K, Kusy M. Teaching, learning, and leading. *AANA J.* 1999;67(1):45–47.

29. Walker WO, Kelly PC, Hume R. Mentoring for the new millennium. http://med-ed-online.org/f0000038.htm. Accessed December 20, 2007.

30. Centeno AM. How to enjoy your mentee's success and learn from it. *MedEduc.* 2002;36(12):1214–1215.

31. Faut-Callahan M. Mentoring: A call to professional responsibility. *AANA J.* 2001;69(4):248–251.

32. Stachura LM, Hoff J. Toward achievement of mentoring for nurses. *NursAdm Q.* 1990;15(1):56–62.

33. Brown BJ. Comments from the editor. *Nurs Adm Q.* 1990;15(1):vii–viii.

34. LaSala K, Nelson J. What contributes to professionalism? *Medsurg Nursing.* 2005;14(1):63–67.

35. Brosky ME, Keefer OA, Hodges JS, Pesun IJ, Cook G. Patient perceptions of professionalism in dentistry. *J Dent Educ.* 2003;67(8):909–915.

36. Lehna C, Pfoutz S, Peterson T, et al. Nursing attire: Indicators of professionalism? *J Prof Nurs.* 1999;15(3):192–199.

37. Nihalani N, Kunwar A, Staller J, Lamberti J. How should psychiatrists dress?—A survey. *Community Ment Health J.* 2006;42(3):291–302.

38. Yankee S. Dress rehearsal. *ProQuest Nursing & Allied Health Source.* 2005;18(8):31.

39. Rooks JK, Roberts, DJ, Scheltema K. Tattoos: their relationship to trauma, psychopathology, and other myths. *Minn Med.* 2000;83:24–27.

40. Overdiek R. Learning the value of membership. *AANA News Bulletin.* 2007;61(3):41.

41. Overdiek R. Traveling the road to "Anesthesia Excellence." *AANA News Bulletin.* 2007;61(9):24.

42. Faut-Callahan M. Graduate education for nurse anesthetists: master's versus a clinical doctorate. *AANA J.* 1992;60(1):98–103.

43. Consorti F, Notarangelo M, Potasso L, Toscano E. Developing professionalism in Italian medical students: an educational framework. *Adv Med Educ Prac.* 2012;3:55–50.

CHAPTER 17

Student Evaluation in the Clinical Area

John C. Preston, DNSc, CRNA, FNAP, APN
James R. Halliburton, DNSc, CRNA, APRN

Keywords: Clinical faculty, clinical practice, nurse anesthesia educational program, reflective learning, student clinical evaluations.

Key Concepts

- The assessment of *quality* is easily confused with *satisfaction*. While related, they are distinct and very different concepts.
- There are different types of evaluations, each serving a specific, and sometimes overlapping purpose.
- Types of evaluation are varied and have specific goals that need to be accomplished.
- Reflective learning is a key feature of assisting the clinical student to progress and self-evaluation is an essential component of this process.
- Good documentation for poor performance is critical in assisting both the student and the program in formulating a specific plan of remediation.

Introduction

There are a variety of purposes for clinical evaluation in nurse anesthesia education. Although not an exhaustive listing, they include evaluating that student clinical practice: complies with educational accreditation requirements, is safe and does not threaten the public's safety, meets institutional standards, satisfies student (consumer) expectation, evidences the quality of the faculty instruction and also meets accreditation standards. Accreditation types of evaluation are varied and have specific goals that need to be accomplished. An evaluation should be clear, specific and tied to the level of proficiency expected and being evaluated. Reflective learning is a key feature of assisting the clinical student to progress and self-evaluation is an essential component of this process. The instrument used to evaluate clinical performance should be competency based. Good documentation for poor performance is critical in assisting both the student and the program in formulating a specific plan of remediation. In the event that remediation fails, good documentation serves as a tool to substantiate dismissal from the program.

Quality vs. Satisfaction

What are some of the impediments to accurate evaluation? Avedis Donabedian, physician and the founder of the study of quality in health care, is possibly best known for creating the Donabedian Model of Care that represented the three types of interconnected information needed to evaluate care quality in any setting: structure, process and outcome.[1] Avedis Donabedian, were he alive today, would likely remind us that while we may be seeking to identify student performance "quality" through our evaluation methods, what in actuality may be collected, is information on the evaluator's personal "satisfaction" with a student's performance. Quality and satisfaction, while frequently and intimately interrelated, are two completely divergent concepts. Something can be satisfactory to us, and yet be of poor quality. Likewise, something can be extremely high quality, and yet not be assessed to be at all satisfactory. First, therefore, it is essential that we acknowledge this limitation. Even our best laid evaluation plans, programs, processes and tools are not perfect and require careful oversight and cautious attention paid to the data they provide.

Second, an evaluation, even when "properly performed," is an attempt at making a subjective process into an objective one. Regardless of our work and the purity of our motivation, subjectivity is still inherent in any evaluation – both the evaluation process and the outcome of that process. It is this subjectivity that causes many of the challenges associated with the data yielded by evaluation within the context of the educational environment.

The evaluation of students by faculty and preceptors is high stakes, because the result of that evaluation can negatively impact the ability of the student to progress or ultimately be successful in their goal of programmatic completion. When challenges to evaluation occur, they principally involve the student's sense of a violation of fairness. These challenges can arise from many foci, but frequently and typically fall into the categories of: (1) accuracy of the evaluation; (2) generalizability of isolated evaluative findings to overall performance; (3) failure of the program to link defined competences to evaluation findings; and (4) failure of the program to support and uphold defined due process in their use of the evaluative data.

No matter that these limitations exist, evaluation is an essential component of health profession's education. The responsibility is not to perfection, but rather it is to do one's best, acknowledge their potential for subjective influence and use the data cautiously, always seeking to verify, validate and when necessary correct the final impression in light of additional input. The purpose here is that the highest quality determinations can be derived from the result of any evaluation. Possibly the best quote that speaks to this effort was from Vince Lombardi who said "Perfection is not attainable, but if we chase perfection we can catch excellence."

Purposes for Clinical Evaluation

The evaluation of student clinical practice serves several objectives, including: protecting the public, satisfying student expectation, meeting institutional requirements, and complying with the standards of educational accreditors (foremost the Council on Accreditation of Nurse Anesthesia Educational Programs–the COA). The accreditation programs are designed to promote quality in education and thereby support quality in professional practice and place ongoing comprehensive programmatic assessment at the core of their expectations. In nurse anesthesia education, student clinical evaluation not only serves the program's need for assessment of its effectiveness to impart knowledge and skills as well as the student's effectiveness at attaining the knowledge, skills and abilities requisite for entry to practice, but can also serve as a guide for employer evaluation of the newly hired CRNA.

The questions of "how much evaluation is enough" and "how often to evaluate" have certainly been uttered by more than one nurse anesthesia program administrator. Unfortunately, there is no one answer to this question. Rather it depends on whether your evaluation data demonstrates whether the program is going in the right direction, or not. Often, the frequency of evaluation may be, at least in part, determined by the academic unit in which the nurse anesthesia program is housed (ie, a College of Nursing), which has policies governing student evaluation. In addition, the graduate school of a particular university may have requirements for the frequency of evaluation of courses and the individual components within a course. It is not unusual for larger universities to have divisions or departments of "Institutional Success," and these units may take responsibility for academic evaluation programs including frequency, tool construction, and data collection. Ultimately, an educational program must develop, implement, and then utilize the data received from a self-constructed and comprehensive evaluation program for ongoing purposeful programmatic improvement. To accomplish this is to address the expectation of the COA and all other educational accrediting bodies.

The data from student and program evaluation evidences the quality of the faculty instruction, and it is this instruction that supports the ongoing development and advancement of the nurse anesthesia profession through the generation of new practitioners who continue to fulfill the professions' responsibilities. It is therefore through the function of clinical evaluation that the foundational educational efforts of the mission of the American Association of Nurse Anesthetists are perpetuated. Education is both the alpha and omega components of the nurse anesthesia profession. The evaluation of that education is of paramount importance to individuals, academic institutions, professional associations and the public that utilizes the care the members of the profession provide.

Public accountability has become a major factor in both clinical practice and clinical education. Today's health care consumer has access to a wide variety of information regarding the quality of available health care. One such resource is the Institute of Medicine (IOM). The IOM released a landmark report on April 8, 2003 entitled "Health Professions Education: A Bridge to Quality." This document calls for nursing practice education "that prepares individuals with interdisciplinary, information systems, quality improvement and patient safety skills and expertise."[2] Other areas of emphasis in the IOM's report that can be linked to clinical evaluation of performance include practicing evidence-based medicine and delivering care that is patient centered. In addition to publications by the IOM, the public has access to state health department's documents, articles in journals, magazines and newspapers, as well as the internet. The easy availability of information has led to a more educated consumer who demands accountability from all aspects of the health care system, including the educational components.

In October of 2010, the IOM released another pivotal publication, "The Future of Nursing: Leading Change, Advancing Health." Among many important recommendations, the report emphasized that "...nurses need to attain requisite competencies to deliver high-quality care."[3] Critical to the determination of any educational program's success at achieving this goal would be the careful and comprehensive evaluation of the students who are enrolled in nursing education programs. As the clinical component of a nurse anesthesia educational program is the locus where didactic learning is translated into care delivery, clinical evaluation serves as a vital backbone of educational quality assessment.

Students' expectations regarding evaluation of clinical practice usually center around specific tasks and outcomes. This is especially true in the early part of their clinical experience. Frequently, students' expectations of experiences they should have and tasks they wish to master are unrealistic based on their didactic knowledge and previous skill achievements. At that stage, they perform best when demonstrating technical skills comprised of specific objectives. They want to know exactly what is expected of them and how each task will be graded. As they progress through the program, students' expectations evolve to include a desire to be assessed on the correlation of clinical performance with didactic knowledge.

Interwoven throughout students' expectations is a desire to be appraised as to how well their performance has prepared them for the certification examination and the "real world." Institutions set forth performance benchmarks for programs and students. A minimally acceptable grade is part of an academic institution's policies for progression. This information is typically published in general information documents, the student handbook and the institution's website. Programs are typically required to post students' grades to the registrar's office at regular intervals, usually by academic term. All of these sources of data help generate the figurative measuring stick that is used to assess acceptable progression, knowledge attainment and skill development necessary for successful program completion.

Finally, the evaluation of students provides an indirect ability to assess the depth, breadth and quality of instruction and guidance provided to the student by the faculty. Even the most motivated and engaged student will not properly progress without faculty guidance and input. Regardless of the situation, an essential component of every program's review of student evaluative data should include an element of reflection on the instruction provided to the students under evaluation. Both successes and struggles should initially be considered to be a shared result until ruled-in or ruled-out through a thorough assessment of the evaluative data under consideration. Thus, clinical evaluation is critical for the collection of necessary data to support the quality and effectiveness of the faculty who interface with our students.

Influences of Accreditation

Institutions of higher learning have to maintain their compliance with a collection of academic accreditors. These range from regional institutional accreditation agencies, to college/discipline-specific accrediting groups and finally in the case of nurse anesthesia education, programmatic (or specialized) accreditation by the Council on Accreditation of Nurse Anesthesia Educational Programs (COA). The COA is the only national recognized accrediting body authorized by the United States Department of Education to approve nurse anesthesia educational programs. The COA exists to help ensure the academic quality of educational offerings of nurse anesthesia programs. This is done by the promulgation of standards that educational programs must meet in order to be accredited. This process is outlined in Chapter 5. At the core of the maintenance of educational quality is the need for planned and purposeful change. This change needs to be based on data, and that data is obtained through an organized plan of continuous programmatic evaluation. Several of the COA's standards and/or criteria (in both the Master's Standards and the Practice Doctoral Standards) address the need for clinical evaluation of students. These standards and criteria are identified in the following sections and should serve educators as an overview, and not an exclusive listing, of the standards/criteria that may be cited as having significance for clinical education.

In the COA's current "master's standards," multiple criteria clearly relate to the evaluation of clinical education and performance. In *Standard III: Program of Study* this includes C12. In *Standard IV: Program Effectiveness* of the clinical component includes D1a, D1b, D1d, D2, D3a, D4a, D4b, D4d.[4] *Standard IV* addresses principles that examine the quality of student enhancement of the educational process. Specifically, criteria D4a and D4b require formative, summative and student self-evaluation.[4] It is this evaluation that forms the backbone of the clinical evaluation plan each program must develop, implement and evaluate the results for continuous quality improvement of the clinical education component.

Likewise, the following COA's Practice Doctoral Standards should be carefully assessed for their relationship to the evaluation of the clinical component of all practice doctoral programs, and the associated programmatic elements: E2, E3, H1.1, H2.2, H2.3.[5] The aspects of evaluation delineated in this section encompasses professional socialization, certification, competency, safety, call experience, perianesthesia continuum, critical thinking, communication skills and professional responsibility, all essential elements of any nurse anesthesia educational program's clinical component.

The COA's *Standard V: Accountability* in the "master's standards" mandates that programs be responsible to its communities of interest. Specifically, Criteria E7 requires cumulative records of educational activities (which should directly and/or indirectly include evaluative materials) while Criteria E13 addresses clinical supervision ratios as it relates to patient safety and student knowledge and ability.[4] The same requirement is reflected in the COA's Practice Doctoral Standards, G1.[5] Of note, is the fact that the COA considers a program's community of interest the same stakeholders identified by this author as being concerned with student clinical evaluation. Additionally, this is a program indicator of compliance with COA Standards.

While these specific criteria have been culled for the reader's attention, depending on the situation many more components of the COA Standards can be related to clinical evaluation, so the reader should not take this list to be exclusive or all encompassing. It is beyond the scope of this chapter to detail the specific relevancies of these identified standards/criteria, but educators are nonetheless directed to familiarize themselves with all of the COA Standards that apply to their educational program and to yield acute attention to these elements specifically as they relate to the evaluation of students and the program with respect to clinical education.

Types of Clinical Evaluations

There are several different types of evaluations which may be used when assessing the clinical performance of learners. Each type serves a specific purpose. Akin to individual pearls, while each form of evaluation is valuable on its own merit, the maximum effect and value to the program is obtained when all of the evaluation components are strung together as a whole (like a pearl necklace) in a comprehensive and purposeful plan of systematic educational evaluation. Two examples of evaluation data source external to the currently enrolled students, but equally important in the overall evaluation of the clinical component of any program, are the employers of the program graduates and the alumni of the program.

Nurse anesthesia educational programs survey employers of recent graduates to determine if the graduate received appropriate didactic and clinical knowledge and experience necessary to prepare them to function as safe, competent practitioners. Although this is not clinical evaluation of individual students per se, it is one indicator of the quality of the program's clinical education.

Alumni of nurse anesthesia educational programs are also typically surveyed approximately one year after completion of their program. One-year alumni evaluation of a program provides invaluable insight into the outcome effectiveness of an educational program. These evaluations should include inquiry about all components of the program including the clinical portion. These evaluations serve a dual role of assessing the consumers of the educational program and as well as the products of the educational environment. While much of the evaluation of learners conducted while the student is in progress with their education is focused on satisfaction, post-graduation evaluation allows for retrospective assessment of educational and learning effectiveness from the individuals who are actively required to apply their knowledge on a daily basis. Once again this assists the programs in evaluating the appropriateness and scope of the clinical experience they provide to students. It can also indicate clinical experiences needing more emphasis or exposure.

Formative Evaluations

Formative evaluations are used to provide an ongoing assessment of performance. It is these individual "evaluative pixels" that, over time, enable a larger picture of performance to be built. A classic example of a formative evaluation from the clinical environment is the written daily clinical evaluation. The evaluation is used to motivate learners, diagnose their strengths and weaknesses, and provide feedback to help them develop self-awareness. Reflective learning should be included as part of the formative evaluation. An example of a daily clinical formative evaluation tool is presented in **Figure 17.1** on the next page. It is important to note that while this has been included for the reader's consideration, it is only an exemplar and can/should be improved to meet the exact needs of any program that utilizes it.

The utilization of formative evaluation should consist of both a written and verbal component. Many preceptors delay giving the student a written evaluation at the end of a clinical day, and frequently may not provide written feedback for a number of days. Many reasons are given for this practice. They include the fact that it's late and both the student and preceptor are tired. The preceptor, the student or both may have commitments that preclude taking the time for immediately composing a written evaluation. A simple method for introducing the student to reflective learning in the clinical area, while giving verbal feedback, is the use of a brief post-clinical conference at the end of a clinical day. The preceptor can ask the student a few leading questions such as: "What do you feel that you did well today? What could you have done better?" Following the disclosure of self-evaluation information, the preceptor can then give specific, pertinent, objective-based feedback. The written formative evaluation should follow the same criteria used during the verbal exchange and should aim to capture what was discussed. While additional information may be identified upon reflection and should be documented in the evaluation, there should be no wholesale surprises in the written evaluation.

Figure 17.1 is an example of an objective based daily clinical self-evaluation currently in use in a nurse anesthesia educational program. This form is used for the first 9 months of an 18-month clinical program component, and again, has been included only as an exemplar. Programs should always carefully assess if any evaluation tool needs modification to meet the specific needs of that program's students, faculty and accreditation requirements in effect at the time of usage. The two page document indicates student's name and site/rotation specific demographic information and defines the evaluative categories that were consistent with the most current COA outcome criteria enforced at the time of publication. Page one also provides sections for specific comments about achievements and areas needing improvement.

Figure 17.1 Example of a Daily Clinical Student Self-Evaluation Tool

XXXXXXXXXX UNIVERSITY
DEPARTMENT OF NURSE ANESTHESIA
STUDENT CLINICAL PERFORMANCE EVALUATION (Months 1–9)

Student: ______________________ Date: ______________

Clinical Site: ______________________ Rotation Type: ______________

Scheduled Clinical Time: ____________ Actual Clinical Hours Worked: ____________

AM____ PM____ Call time: ______________

Student Self-Evaluation of Knowledge/Skills/Abilities			
Patient Safety	**Met**	**Unmet**	**N/A**
Practices precautions to blood-borne pathogens			
Familiar with operation of all anesthesia equipment			
Maintain work area with drugs and supplies appropriate for the day's cases			
Maintain accurate and legible anesthesia record in a timely manner			
Skillfully participates in patient positioning to optimize patient outcomes			
Individualized Perianesthetic Management	**Met**	**Unmet**	**N/A**
Demonstrates skill in anticipation of needs for holistic patient management and choosing appropriate intervention			
Perform skillfully in emergency and non-emergency situations			
Performs technical skills with speed and dexterity			
Demonstrates ability to administer a variety of anesthetic techniques			
Plans emergence with completion of surgical procedure			
Treats complications associated with emergence and extubation			
Provides optimum patient comfort and status upon arrival to PACU			
Critical Thinking	**Met**	**Unmet**	**N/A**
Provide nurse anesthesia care based on sound principles and evidence based research			
Formulates plans for all patient, considering medical history, procedure and position			
Demonstrates skill in assessing complex patient needs and choosing important intervention			
Chooses technique in accordance with optimizing patient condition postoperatively			
Continually assesses data and patient response and revises anesthetic appropriately			
Identify and take appropriate action when confronted with anesthetic equipment-related malfunctions			

1

Student Self-Evaluation of Knowledge/Skills/Abilities			
Communication Skill	**Met**	**Unmet**	**N/A**
Demonstrate qualities of patient advocacy			
Accepts constructive instruction easily			
Exhibit dignity and respect when communicating with all individuals			
Use appropriate verbal, nonverbal, and written communication in the delivery of perianesthetic care			
Communicates status upon arrival to PACU			
Professional Role	**Met**	**Unmet**	**N/A**
Instills confidence in team by demonstrating anesthetic skills and knowledge			
Assumes the qualities and role of patient advocate			
Exhibits confidence as an independent practitioner			
Situationally aware of skills and abilities			
Demonstrates qualities of professionalism and is acceptable as a colleague in anesthesia department			

Student Comments
I did very well on:
I need improvement on:
I intitiated the following topics to increase my knowledge:

Student Signature & Date: ______________________________

2

A parallel document accompanies this form for clinical preceptor evaluation of student performance (**Figure 17.2**, next page). This document uses the same criteria as the student self-evaluation and provides the preceptor the opportunity to identify their assessed strengths and areas for improvement, as well as their identification of the teaching topics discussed during the course of the clinical experience.

Figure 17.2 Example of a Daily Clinical Preceptor Evaluation Tool

XXXXXXXXXX UNIVERSITY
DEPARTMENT OF NURSE ANESTHESIA
PRECEPTOR CLINICAL PERFORMANCE EVALUATION (Months 1–9)

Student: ______________________ Date: ______________

At the **END** of this semester, the student will:

Knowledge Base: Synthesize the anesthetic process using analytical judgment for all types of patients within the life span.

Skill Base: Perform safely, accurately, and appropriately using knowledge base and acquired technical skills.

Application and performance: Demonstrate self-direction using appropriate consultation. Formulate and implement an appropriate anesthetic without supporting cues. Demonstrate complex time and case management skills.

Preceptor Evaluation of Technical Skills			
Patient Safety	**Met**	**Unmet**	**N/A**
Practices precautions to blood-borne pathogens			
Familiar with operation of all anesthesia equipment			
Maintain work area with drugs and supplies appropriate for the day's cases			
Maintain accurate and legible anesthesia record in a timely manner			
Skillfully participates in patient positioning to optimize patient outcomes			
Individualized Perianesthetic Management	**Met**	**Unmet**	**N/A**
Demonstrates skill in anticipation of needs for holistic patient management and choosing appropriate intervention			
Perform skillfully in emergency and non-emergency situation			
Performs technical skills with speed and dexterity			
Demonstrates ability to administer a variety of anesthetic techniques			
Plans emergence with completion of surgical procedure			
Treats complications associated with emergence and extubation			
Provides optimum patient comfort and status upon arrival to PACU			
Critical Thinking	**Met**	**Unmet**	**N/A**
Provide nurse anesthesia care based on sound principles and evidence based research			
Formulates plans for all patient, considering medical history, procedure and position			
Demonstrates skill in assessing complex patient needs and choosing important intervention			
Chooses technique in accordance with optimizing patient condition postoperatively			
Continually assesses data and patient response and revises anesthetic appropriately			
Identify and take appropriate action when confronted with anesthetic equipment-related malfunctions			

1

Preceptor Evaluation of Technical Skills			
Communication Skill	**Met**	**Unmet**	**N/A**
Demonstrate qualities of patient advocacy			
Accepts constructive instruction easily			
Exhibit dignity and respect when communicating with all individuals			
Use appropriate verbal, nonverbal, and written communication in the delivery of perianesthetic care			
Communicates status upon arrival to PACU			
Professional Role	**Met**	**Unmet**	**N/A**
Instills confidence in team by demonstrating anesthetic skills and knowledge			
Assumes the qualities and role of patient advocate			
Exhibits confidence as an independent practitioner			
Situationally aware of skills and abilities			
Demonstrates qualities of professionalism and is acceptable as a colleague in anesthesia department			

Preceptor Comments
The student did well on:
The student needs improvement on:
Teaching topics discussed were:

Preceptor Signature & Date: ______________________________

2

Summative Evaluation

Summative evaluations serve an associated, but different purpose than formative evaluations. Summative evaluations are built upon the foundation established by the formative evaluations, but with one very important difference. The summative evaluation established the attainment of knowledge, skill and/or ability needed to progress to the next stage or phase of the clinical education.[6] The classic example of a summative clinical evaluation is the "end of semester" evaluation or "end of rotation" evaluation. These evaluations should clearly identify the specific objectives that the learner is to obtain and an assessment of their performance relative to each one identified. Each clinical component (quarter, semester, etc.) should have a corresponding summative evaluation specific for that point in the program. Depending on how the evaluation is composed, the objectives may be different from evaluation to evaluation (building in number and complexity with each subsequent summative evaluation) or be the same for all or many of the evaluations, but clearly identifying the need for ever-increasing demonstration of sophistication relative to the learner's application and performance relative to these objectives. The exact construction is not as important as the ability of the tools and process to identify progress (or the lack of progress) as the student moves through their clinical education component.

Terminal Evaluation

Terminal evaluations are given at the completion of a nurse anesthesia educational program. Two purposes served by these evaluations: First they help to assure adequate clinical skills and the ability to apply those skills in the delivery of anesthesia care required for practice. Educational programs have the responsibility to only release those individuals who can demonstrate the attainment of the COAs graduate competencies. The terminal evaluation provides a mechanism to, at least in part, assess and document these competencies.[7]

Second, the flip side of evaluation is an opportunity for programs to evaluate their success at adequately preparing individuals to enter their profession. No student is allowed to complete an accredited nurse anesthesia program without the attestation by the program administrator that they are adequately prepared and ready to end their studies. The terminal evaluation process provides the program a final opportunity for comprehensive assessment needed to ensure compliance with this requirement. It is the final gate-keeping safeguard for the program, and ultimately for the profession.

Task Specific Evaluation

Task specific evaluations are useful during specific situations. A classic example is the evaluation focused on a simulation exercise. These are typically used to measure mastery of certain psychomotor skills such as intubation or insertion of a central line. When developing task specific evaluations, it is usually necessary to break down a complex skill into smaller logical steps. These steps often must occur (or be demonstrated) in a specified order. Most ideally, each objective should include a range of acceptable performance for both each step of the task as well as for the task performance as whole.

360° Evaluation

The 360-degree performance evaluation is based on feedback from every individual who comes in contact with the one being evaluated.[8] In the case of a nurse anesthesia student in the clinical area, this would most likely include, at a minimum, the clinical instructor (CRNA and/or anesthesiologist), the surgeon, and facility staff (such as nurses and scrub technicians). Although many of these individuals would be willing to verbally give input as to a student's performance, it would be labor intensive to routinely seek to obtain evaluative feedback in writing from many of these individuals. While not likely practical for routine clinical evaluation, it is potentially useful in isolated and specific cases where a high-stakes evaluative assessment is needed to determine, as example, programmatic progression. The caution with which this process should be considered for nurse anesthesia education is that while this may be helpful as a supplement to the established routine evaluative processes, it should most likely not be utilized in isolation. Should any of the participants not be familiar with the objectives they are evaluating the individual on, the validity of the process could be called into question and provide grounds for judicial dismissal of the actions based upon the evaluation. For a multitude of reasons, therefore, the traditional 360-degree evaluation is not typically part of a nurse anesthesia program's comprehensive clinical evaluation plan. In addition, this type of evaluations is not mandated by the Council on Accreditation.

Self-evaluation

A critically essential component of the clinical evaluation process is the learner student's self-evaluation. Such evaluation is mandated by the COA as well as most other educational accrediting agencies. Even in the absence of any mandate, reflective self-evaluation is an essential component of growth and development and should be employed, both formally and informally, throughout the student's program. Adult learners derive significant benefit from self-evaluation and it should be modeled by faculty as well as incorporated at every phase of instruction.

Most students have a realistic assessment of their progress. While all educational institutions should require students to complete a formal self-evaluation at the completion of each clinical term (or rotation), frequent informal reflective self-evaluation should optimally be completed on a daily basis. Learners should be encouraged to be specific and to delineate achievements. In formal self-evaluation, the objectives delineated on the self-evaluation form completed by the student should be directly linked (if not identical) to the objectives listed on the summative evaluation form for that clinical term (or rotation).

Clinical Faculty & Clinical Site Evaluation

Students should have the opportunity to evaluate all aspects of their nurse anesthesia educational program and that includes the clinical components. At a minimum, this should include clinical faculty, the clinical coordinators and the clinical sites. The frequency of this evaluation should be spelled-out in the program's comprehensive evaluation plan, but programs should consider this to be at least an annually performed evaluation.

Elements of Clinical Evaluations

Clinical evaluations should be based on objectives appropriate to the level of proficiency expected and observed. Specific behaviors in relation to clinical performance, which encompass the affective, cognitive and psychomotor domains should be assessed. Values such as work ethic, civility and professionalism should also be included.

The Affective domain is concerned with objectives pertaining to appreciations, attitude, emotions and values.[9] An example of an objective meeting this criterion is: identification of bio-psychosocial problems that might affect the anesthetic management of the patient.

The Cognitive domain looks at objectives related to knowledge or information.[9] Objectives that evaluate a student's ability to synthesize a patient's history and laboratory results to develop a plan of care would fall into this category.

The Psychomotor domain is the easiest to evaluate in the clinical area. It is comprised of objectives assessing basic motor skill and physical movement.[9] The student's ability to insert an intravenous catheter would be a skill defined as within the psychomotor domain.

Assessing values such as work ethic can easily become subjective unless explicitly defined. Including definitions in clinical syllabi makes it clear to the student what values are expected and will be evaluated.

Additional components of a clinical evaluation include the fact that it should be factual, descriptive, clear, concise and constructive, as well as timely. The evaluation needs to be behaviorally directed and based on changeable items. For example, if a student is having difficulty with performing intubations, a written observation may include the fact that, today while attempting laryngoscopy, the student did not sweep the blade to move the tongue out of the way. Such a critique clearly and concisely delineates, in a timely manner, the fact that the student is not using proper technique to accomplish a specific task.

The Instrument

The instrument used to evaluate clinical performance needs to be competency based. The skill set needed for safe anesthesia practice should form the matrix of the summative and terminal evaluations. Working backwards from those criteria, performance objectives should be developed to test a student's clinical proficiency based on didactic knowledge, clinical experience and length in the program. The instrument must be reliable. Reliability means the repeatability of your measurement.[10] Will each student who successfully performs a task receive the same grade? Additionally, if one student performs the same task in the same manner, will he receive the same grade?

A valid instrument has a strength of conclusion, inference or proposition.[10] An example of validity would be testing the accuracy of charting on the anesthesia record after the important items were reviewed in conference. Research continues to validate the clinical evaluation instrument. Clinical evaluation instruments of nurse anesthesia programs are not standardized among programs, which suggests a lack of instrument validity. This is especially important when the results of an evaluation, or a collections of evaluations, are to be utilized as part of the evidence for a student dismissal.[11] Research continues to identify and define key concepts that need to be measured and create a clinical evaluation instrument that will validly measure the defined constructs.

A grading scale that is simple, consistent and easy to interpret should be a part of the instrument. The scale should be consistent with university/program criteria. If it varies from the university's/program's scale, that fact should be published in the clinical syllabus. It should be clearly defined how many evaluations below standard are allowed and what the consequence of receiving multiple poor evaluations will be.

Barriers to Effective Evaluations

Several barriers to effective evaluations exist. Principally, clinical faculty ocasionally do not fill out evaluations. This may especially be true if a student has not performed well. Reasons given for not documenting poor performance include not wanting to be the "bad guy" or "everyone else says what a great job he/she is doing," or "doing well with everyone else—so it must just be me," or "it's the first time, I'll see if it happens again," and occasionally "I don't want to get involved because I'm afraid of litigation." Whatever the reason, if providing information or reassurance does not help, it may be a challenge to get the most helpful evaluative information regardless of your tools and plan.

Another discrepancy exists when a CRNA tells the student what a great job he's done and then writes an observation of poor performance. Such a situation may require the program faculty to educate the clinical instructor as to how this sends mixed messages to the student and is not conducive to improving performance. In addition, the evaluation in question may need to receive a faculty generated addendum and may also create the need for a student-faculty conversation about the evaluation and their progress. Without this type of intervention, it is likely that the student will use (or try to use) the evaluative disconnect as leverage should their overall performance not be deemed acceptable.

A third barrier is the clinical faculty member who always gives only positive feedback. This is usually done because the clinical faculty is by nature a kind individual and does not want the student to suffer any negative evaluative effects that could prevent their progression. This behavior, however, can create significant problems for an educational program. It is to be expected that, should the student be deemed to not be progressing adequately, that they will produce those acceptable evaluations as evidence to support their position for retention or progression. If explanation of the consequences does not convince the faculty member to fairly evaluate both the good and the bad in every student every time, it unfortunately may be necessary to remove this instructor from engaging with the student in question until a decision can be made as to their progress. At a minimum, a faculty addendum to the evaluation and a carefully documented and witnessed conversation with the student about their progress is in order in these types of situations.

A phenomenon that can also occur with a student who has performed poorly on a few occasions is faculty group-think, or what has been classified by some as "ganging up." In this situation, in addition to giving evaluations based on previous performance, a group of anesthesia practitioners discuss the student and decide as a group how the student executes clinical tasks. While in some instances group-think can be productive and helpful in the identification of specific deficits that a student can work on to improve their performance, in many situations it results in a negative conclusion and blocks opportunity for improvement. Again, this type of situation needs immediate administrative faculty intervention. Frequently it can be corrected or contained through faculty-to-faculty conversation and intervention. Should that not prove successful, it may be necessary to remove the student from the clinical setting in favor of another clinical assignment for a time, or potentially permanently.

Evaluation Pitfalls

If evaluations are consistently being filled out incorrectly or the clinical faculty puts little effort into making meaningful observations, program faculty needs to examine the situation. At faculty business meetings, an in-service on current clinical objectives and expectations can go a long way toward improving documentation of clinical performance.

If a program has multiple distant clinical sites, a process for delivering summative evaluations to students off campus should be in place. If this does not (or cannot) include a face-to-face meeting on campus, two viable options are via computer webinar or through a telephone call or conference call if multiple individuals need to participate.

If the return rate of evaluations is the source of challenge, the first and possibly the simplest step to improve evaluation return rate is to critically assess your evaluation tool. Balancing the desire to have a comprehensive tool with a format that is easy to complete and understand has the potential to significantly and positively improve participation and return rate. This holds true not only for faculty evaluation of students, but also for student self-evaluation.

Addressing Unacceptable Evaluations

First and foremost, unacceptable performance should never come as a surprise to any student. Whether it is an individual case that did not go as well as it could have, a collective day of unacceptable performance or an entire term of sub-par performance, every student should be aware of their performance at all times. By utilizing both formative and summative evaluation strategies, progress can be communicated in every situation from matriculation to gradation.

When everything is going well, there is really nothing complex about clinical evaluation. Everyone is happy and the learner's progress is smooth and unchallenged. The challenge frequently occurs when the results of evaluation indicate unacceptable behavior, knowledge or performance. The actions necessary to successfully address unacceptable behavior are, in reality, straight forward. The challenge for some is properly implementing and following through with the actions indicated by the evaluation. The key is knowing what your evaluation plan is, knowing what the due process in your institution and/or program is, making sure that all students know or have access to this same information, and then following the process without disruption or deviation, unless that deviation is mutually agreed-upon by all parties involved and affected by the change. If you don't know your due process by heart, you should diagram it out so that it is clear for you and your faculty and then have your diagram verified and validated by the most senior academic official higher up than you in your educational environment (academic unit). Due process is the most important governor that will guide your management of unacceptable evaluation. While intricate adherence to your published due process will not preclude unsatisfied students from challenging your evaluative decisions, it will almost certainly make the difference between being successful in upholding your decisions and having your decisions overturned upon appeal. Timing is everything when you are dealing with evaluation. As much as possible, the shortest time period that can be adhered to between the incidence of unacceptable performance and the reporting to the student of their unacceptable performance should be the rule. Of course, you want to have the facts and clearly understand the situation, but delaying conversation and intervention evaporates valuable time for dealing with the situation.

With the rare exception of criminal behavior, most instances of unacceptable evaluation warrant a conversation with the student, identification of the problem or unacceptable behavior or performance, and exploration of the expected behavior or performance along with the identification of the necessary remediation needed to resolve the situation. If there is a knowledge deficit, then more studying may be at the heart of the remediation. If the evaluation identifies a skill deficit, independent study in a skills lab or simulation center may be called for to bring about correction. If that is not a possibility, more observation and progression in a step-wise manner towards a more complex skill may be the plan. If ability is central to the unacceptable evaluative finding, it may be beyond the ability of the program to address the situation and referral to external experts may be necessary for evaluation and input.

Whatever the case or cause, it is essential that the unacceptable evaluation be directly tied to the program's published performance expectations, and those expectations should have been what were deemed to be unacceptable in the evaluation. These must be the expectations that all students are held to, and that includes the student that is evaluated as unacceptable. Unacceptable has to mean, to everyone who reviews the situation, that they are not meeting the published standard—nothing more, nothing less.

Whenever you have to address unacceptable evaluation, there is almost always a degree of emotion involved and usually it is on both sides. Enter into these situations as committed to be devoid of emotion as possible. Emotion has no place in an objective and fair evaluation, whether it is positive or negative. Even if the other party(s) is/are highly emotionally charged, work to diffuse their emotion and to not reflect it. If the individual has been involved from the very beginning of their evaluation process, and you have attempted remediation, and you are evaluating based on more than one observation, and you are utilizing the published standards for performance, you will be much more likely to be able to control any emotional influence from the program's side of the situation.

Summary

Evaluation of clinical performance is an integral part of a nurse anesthesia educational program. This chapter has listed objectives for developing clinical evaluations. The reasons for evaluating clinical performance were delineated. Types and elements of clinical evaluations have been discussed. The components of an instrument for evaluating clinical performance were iterated. Barriers and pitfalls of evaluating in the clinical setting were enumerated. An overview of COA expectation for evaluation was also addressed.

The practice of nurse anesthesia is both clinically intensive and incredibly rewarding. In many regulatory realms, nurse anesthesia as a professional discipline is identified as the "gold standard," to which all the rest of advanced practice nursing is compared. In concert with our didactic preparation, it is our clinical education that develops and molds the members of our profession. Central to that effective core of education is the need to properly and thoroughly evaluate, and continually improve based upon the results of that evaluation, the development of the members of our profession.

References

1. Donabedian A. The quality of care: how can it be assessed? *JAMA.* 1988;260(12):1743–1748.

2. The Institute of Medicine. Health Professions Education: A Bridge to Quality. Available at: https://www.ncbi.nlm.nih.gov/pubmed/25057657.

3. *The Future of Nursing: Leading Change, Advancing Health.* Washington, DC: The National Academies Press; 2011.

4. Council on Accreditation of Nurse Anesthesia Educational Programs. *Standards for Accreditation of Nurse Anesthesia Educational Programs,* revised 6/3/2016.

5. Council on Accreditation of Nurse Anesthesia Educational Programs. *Standards for Accreditation of Nurse Anesthesia Educational Programs,* Practice Doctorate, 1/23/2015, revised 6/3/2016.

6. Gulikers JTM, Harm JA, Biemans, Wesselink R, van der Wel M. Aligning formative and summative assessments: a collaborative action research challenging teacher conceptions. *Studies in Educational Evaluation.* 2013;39(2):116–124, ISSN 0191–491X.

7. Skager R. Defining and Assessing Specified Educational Goals in Formative and Summative Evaluation. Chapter 3: Lifelong Education and Evaluation Practice. In: *Advances in Lifelong Education.* Amsterdam, Netherlands: Pergamon; 1978:53–87.

8. Assess Pros and Cons of 360-Degree Performance Appraisal. Taylor, S., Society for Human Resource Management, 7-12-2011, accessible at https://www.shrm.org/resourcesandtools/hr-topics/employee-relations/pages/360degreeperformance.aspx.

9. Planning for Instruction–Classifying Objectives. http://edtech2.tennessee.edu/projects/bobannon/classifications.html. Accessed April 23, 2016.

10. Brink Y, Louw QA. Clinical instruments: reliability and validity critical appraisal. *J Eval Clin Pract.* 2012;18(2):1126–1132.

11. Collins S, Callahan MF. A call for change: clinical evaluation of student registered nurse anesthetists. *AANA J.* 2014;82:65–72.

CHAPTER 18

From Novice to Expert: How RNs Become CRNAs

Elizabeth Seibert, PhD, CRNA

Keywords: Clinical instruction, experiential learning, novice-to-expert theory, nurse anesthesia education.

Key Concepts

- The novice-to-expert model provides one way of assessing a student registered nurse anesthetist's (SRNA's) clinical growth and development.
- Five levels of practice—novice, advanced beginner, competent, proficient, and expert—are distinguished in the novice-to-expert model.
- Movement from one stage to another and maturation as a nurse anesthetist are evidenced by changes in behaviors, not the passage of time.
- Novice SRNAs have critical care skills but need new rules to guide their performance because they lack experience in the anesthetic environment.
- Advanced beginners have few technical skills, an elementary knowledge of anesthetic management, a low level of comfort with complex situations, and the ability to manage simple cases with close supervision.
- Competent students demonstrate greater confidence because of improved situational awareness and technical and organizational skills that enable them to prioritize and respond more quickly to complex situations.
- Proficient students are able to perform safely and appropriately in myriad, challenging anesthetic situations. The proficient graduate SRNA becomes a competent entry-level practitioner.
- The expert level of practice is unlikely to be attained by SRNAs because it requires a tremendous amount of experience in a variety of situations and development of an intuitive ability to solve problems. Transition to the expert role is not guaranteed as years of experience do not guarantee the development of expertise.

Introduction

Registered nurses (RNs) entering a nurse anesthesia program often believe they understand what it takes to become a CRNA, but soon find that their perceptions underestimate the reality of the process. Having lived the experience, Certified Registered Nurse Anesthetists (CRNAs) are aware that becoming a nurse anesthetist is transformational and involves more than simply acquiring new knowledge and skills. CRNA clinical preceptors can ease the student registered nurse anesthetist's (SRNA's) transition from RN to CRNA by providing guidance and mentoring as the SRNA grows from a novice to a competent, entry-level practitioner.

Although experts at providing patient care, most CRNA preceptors have not received instruction in how to guide SRNAs through this developmental process. Other than abstract educational theories, their own experiences as learners, and suggestions made by seasoned clinical instructors, little information is available to guide the novice CRNA preceptor. Therefore, identifying patterns of learning and behavior that SRNAs exhibit at various stages of their training may be useful for clinical instructors. The validity of clinical evaluation also may be improved if behaviors that students commonly exhibit as they evolve into competent entry-level practitioners can be identified.[1] The purpose of this chapter is to briefly review one theory of how beginners learn to become competent health care providers and to identify characteristics of SRNAs at various stages in the clinical practicum.

Like all adult learners, student registered nurse anesthetists enter a new learning situation with well-established identities as capable, competent adults, and in the case of SRNAs, as successful critical care nurses. The process of becoming a CRNA challenges students' existing knowledge and skills as well as their images of themselves as expert nurses and leaders within their units. To achieve success and graduate from a nurse anesthesia program, students must construct a new personal and professional identity as CRNAs.[2]

Surprisingly little information is available about how RNs become CRNAs. Although undergraduate grade point average and science grade point average are acknowledged as factors contributing to successful academic outcomes,[3] studies have not identified other factors that lead to achievement of clinical competence as a nurse anesthetist. Surveys of nurse anesthesia educators and practitioners describe a core set of knowledge and skills that CRNAs need,[4] and personality characteristics that may predict safe practitioners,[5] but other than the National Certification Examination, valid methods for demonstrating competence in these areas are not available.[1] Experienced CRNAs learn to incorporate new knowledge into practice by first learning basic principles, then by trying out the new information in practice situations, and finally, by accumulating enough experience in various situations to place the knowledge in context.[6] Student registered nurse anesthetists may learn in a similar manner, but specific learning processes of SRNAs have not been described. Nurse anesthesia clinical instructors must look to the general educational and nursing education literature for suggestions about how students acquire new knowledge and skills.

The practice of nurse anesthesia, like many other health professions, involves both science and art. Course work in anatomy, physiology, chemistry, pharmacology, and other sciences augmented with instruction in technological aspects of anesthesia management provides the scientific basis of the profession; however, the mere acquisition of knowledge is not sufficient to ensure competent practice. The true art of the profession lies in the ability to organize knowledge so that it may be applied to specific patients in specific situations. This is the crux of the issue: What differentiates expert practitioners from novices or those who are merely competent?

Benner's Novice-to-Expert Framework

Patricia Benner's landmark study of practicing nurses described how clinicians learn and accrue knowledge through experience in a variety of situations. Using a qualitative, phenomenological approach, Benner sought to capture the knowledge embedded in nursing practice and identify differences between theoretical and practical knowledge. Basing her work on the Dreyfus Model of Skill Acquisition, Benner distinguished five levels of nursing practice—novice, advanced beginner, competent, proficient, and expert—and described common features of each level as well as implications for teaching and learning.[7–9]

Benner recognized that although nursing has a theoretical base, skilled practice does not rely on knowledge alone.[10] The distinction between theoretical and practical knowledge is described as the difference between "knowing that" and "knowing how." "Knowing that" refers to an individual's knowledge base and the ability to recall facts and rules, but "knowing how" refers to the incorporation of knowledge and experience into innate knowledge so a practitioner can make decisions intuitively.[11] The difference between "knowing how" and "knowing that" can be explained by a simple scenario: A CRNA may have a gut feeling that something is wrong with a patient and then respond reflexively to intervene. A student observing the CRNA's performance will ask for the CRNA's reasons and rationale, only to be frustrated when the CRNA cannot provide a ready answer or states that he or she "just knows." Students want solutions or knowledge (knowing that) while expert CRNAs "know how" from the experience of repeatedly applying knowledge and judgment in patient care situations.[7]

Benner's model is only one perspective on how individuals achieve expertise; however, the novice-to-expert model has relevance for CRNA clinical instructors for several reasons. First, much of nurse anesthesia education occurs in patient care situations, not in the classroom. Theoretical knowledge provides a foundation for practice but must be interpreted in the context of the clinical situation. Practitioners develop expertise through repeatedly encountering real-life situations. As a result, CRNAs develop situational awareness or an ability to respond to multiple inputs in complex environments.[12] Clinical instructors have the situational awareness that SRNAs lack and, thus, can guide SRNAs' development. Second, the various stages of the model are identified with different learning needs, providing a guideline for structuring learning activities to meet the needs of students in each stage. Third, the model lends itself to the development of evaluation tools. Since nurse anesthesia programs are expected to graduate competent entry-level practitioners, the model can help educators determine acceptable performance characteristics that SRNAs should achieve at different stages of training.[7,8] Finally, the model may help CRNAs recognize their own level of clinical prowess, appreciate the mastery they have attained, and identify areas for further growth.

The remainder of this chapter describes characteristics of each stage of the model, followed by examples of behaviors an SRNA might exhibit at that level. I have incorporated suggestions for clinical instruction throughout each section. Readers should understand that these descriptions are not the result of research, but are based on my observations of student registered nurse anesthetists in clinical settings, from discussions with clinical and didactic faculty, and from listening to students describe the joys and frustrations of their clinical journeys. A number of student readers have stated that they have found the information helpful and reassuring in evaluating their personal progress through their programs.

The Novice Student

The novice-to-expert model assumes that although beginners have certain basic abilities, they lack experience in the new role and situations where they must act.[7,13] Learning must begin somewhere.[10] To provide some context, novices are given rules and cues in the form of theoretical knowledge to guide their actions. Although they provide structure, rules also limit the novice because rules cannot cover all possible situations or actions. Rules may limit flexibility because of their prescriptive nature and because the student must remember the rule and how to apply it. Thus, the novice SRNA must take classroom knowledge and previous nursing experience and begin to apply it to new situations.

Nearly all SRNAs are unfamiliar with the operating room environment because most nursing programs do not include operating room experience in their curricula. The first step in helping the novice SRNA feel comfortable in his or her new role is an adequate orientation to the physical structure of the operating room (OR) and anesthesia department, the roles of key personnel, and pertinent policies and procedures. Today, many programs are able to ease students' transition to the OR by offering basic skills training in laboratory settings. SRNAs can learn and practice basic airway management and the sequence of anesthetic induction with task trainers or the human patient simulator. Instruction in a simulated operating room is extremely helpful in familiarizing the novice SRNA with technical aspects of the OR, such as operating the OR table and its attachments, checking the anesthesia machine, and preparing anesthetic equipment and drugs. Lessons on proper sterile technique for opening trays and gowning and gloving can also be incorporated at this time.

Most students entering the operating room for the first time are eager, enthusiastic, motivated, and anxious. Although they are impatient to immerse themselves in clinical experiences, students are also afraid of making mistakes, hurting patients, and being embarrassed by their lack of knowledge and skills. The whole process of anesthesia administration is mysterious, because most SRNAs have not seen a complete general anesthetic from induction through emergence. The fact that there are many ways to achieve the same goal in anesthesia is frustrating for novice SRNAs, who crave the structure offered by definitive guidelines, rules, and procedures that are more common in nursing practice.

Knowledge and skills acquired in critical care nursing are thought to best prepare SRNAs for nurse anesthesia practice, although little evidence exists to support this assumption. Accreditation standards for nurse anesthesia educational programs require that applicants have at least one year of critical care experience defined as work in which the RN "...has developed critical decision-making and psychomotor skills, competency in patient assessment, and the ability to use and interpret advanced monitoring techniques."[14(pp 29–30)] Applicants are expected to "...demonstrate competence with managing unstable patients, invasive monitoring, ventilators, and critical care pharmacology."[14(p.30)] Quantifying applicants' skills in these areas has been difficult for most nurse anesthesia programs, and little relationship has been found between years of critical care experience and the ability to automatically perform in routine situations.[12] Indeed, evaluating the SRNA's ability to perform effectively in clinical practice is an issue in most nurse anesthesia programs.

Clinical instructors may assume that all beginning SRNAs have a similar background or that the SRNA has intensive care unit experience similar to the preceptor's own. However, differences in acute care unit acuity and autonomy, years of experience, and basic nursing preparation mean that novice SRNAs vary greatly in their ability to use and interpret basic monitors, titrate vasoactive and sedative drugs, and apply knowledge to practice. The nurse anesthesia program's structure also impacts the novice SRNA's performance. Some programs are front-loaded and provide one or more semesters of classroom instruction before SRNAs enter the clinical arena. Others introduce students into clinical with only a few weeks of didactic instruction. Programs also vary in their ability to prepare SRNAs through simulated clinical experiences. The CRNA preceptor is then faced with identifying the strengths and weaknesses of the novice SRNA's basic knowledge and skills.

The novice stage is characterized by uncertainty and frustration. Students are unsure what to do and when to do it because they lack context for their actions. Although novice SRNAs may have dealt with events like hypotension, hypoxia, and sepsis as critical care nurses, the context in which these situations occur in the operating room is poles apart from their previous experience and requires different actions. Clinical instructors must identify pertinent features of anesthesia for novice SRNAs so they can learn which events are expected and which are not. For instance, beginners learn about the induction, maintenance, and emergence phases of anesthesia in the classroom. A novice may observe these events in a patient, but is unable to recognize characteristics of each stage because he or she has not been immersed in the experience before. Preceptors can help place the events in context by pointing out cardinal signs of each stage and discussing how these may be differentiated from other similar events.

A great source of student frustration is the result of unclear guidelines and practices among instructors. For example, beginning students are often frustrated when trying to organize their equipment set up and medications when CRNAs in a department do not agree on a common setup. When each CRNA prepares equipment and drugs differently, students feel compelled to learn individual preferences rather than a routine. Since most CRNAs are creatures of habit, they expect students to set up their way and are annoyed when students do not. Nothing disconcerts a novice more than starting the day with a disgruntled instructor; the novice feels he or she can do nothing right and performance rapidly deteriorates. As a result, learning anesthesia is overshadowed by pleasing the preceptor.

Student anxiety is decreased when instructors set clear expectations. Anxiety is common among new students, and miscommunication can occur if preceptors assume that novice students understand what they are saying. Beginning students are frequently overwhelmed by the complexity and rapidity of events in the operating room and are unable to concentrate on what is important, particularly during induction and emergence. Therefore, preceptors should discuss their expectations of the student's role and responsibilities *before* the patient is seen or arrives in the operating room. For example, if the instructor says, "I want you to focus on airway management," the student may assume that he or she will also give the drugs and watch the monitors while managing the airway. Since novices need rules, preceptors should be explicit about who will do what: "Once the monitors are on, you can start preoxygenating the patient. After you've preoxygenated for three minutes or the end-tidal oxygen is greater than 90%, I'll give the induction drugs. After the patient is asleep, check the lash reflex and then try to ventilate. I want you to use your precordial stethoscope so you can tell if you're ventilating or if the airway is obstructed." A less prescriptive technique is to ask students to describe what they intend to do and ascertain their understanding of their role.

An old adage states that a child must crawl before walking. Similarly, novice SRNAs must acquire a core set of knowledge, skills, and attitudes before advancing to more difficult tasks. Knowledge, skills, and attitudes correspond to Bloom's cognitive, psychomotor, and affective domains of learning.[15] In each domain, learning progresses from simple to complex. Understanding these basic concepts can help preceptors identify and design learning experiences that help students acquire new skills and progress to more difficult concepts.

Preceptors should direct novice students toward learning the basic psychomotor skills of the profession. Generally, instructors will have no problem achieving this goal because novice students perceive these tasks as what a nurse anesthetist does.[2] Basic skills that novices must learn include preparation of the anesthesia machine, drugs, and equipment; performing a preoperative history and physical assessment including listening to heart and lung sounds and evaluating the airway; establishing venous access; applying and using basic monitors; establishing and maintaining the airway using a bag and mask; performing LMA insertion and endotracheal intubation; and completing medical records. Frequently, the novice SRNA is so focused on intubation that the preceptor must remind him or her to attach the circuit and ventilate the patient, check the breath sounds, and turn on volatile agents. Students may find that preparing a detailed list of the steps involved in the induction process helps organize their thinking.

Novice SRNAs need guidance in organizing tasks to develop routines that provide structure and, ultimately, become habits. Basic monitoring with the senses (look, listen, feel) should be encouraged because novices often are more intent on watching the monitors or automated medical records system than observing the patient. Instructors can give guidance on developing scanning techniques for surveying the patient, surgical field, and monitors. Preceptors should require that novices use a consistent method for setting up equipment and drugs. Just as pilots use preprinted checkout forms, students should be encouraged to develop and use checklists or notes to guide them through the set-up process. CRNAs should share any "pearls" or mnemonics they have found useful such as MSMAID (machine, suction, monitors, airway, IV, drugs).

The anesthesia care plan is another area in which beginners often struggle. Programs have varying requirements for the number and frequency of care plans and whether they must be written or oral. The ability to rapidly develop an individualized plan of care is a crucial task for CRNAs. Novices' care plans frequently take a cookbook approach, miss important patient or surgical issues, and show lack of individualization. They frequently give little attention to different techniques of airway management, use of alternative drugs for induction or maintenance, or techniques other than general anesthesia. In addition, novices' care plans often show limited understanding of physiology, pharmacology, and potential implications of the surgical procedure.

Preceptors should take time to read and comment on written care plans, especially since students spend considerable time developing them. While understanding that at this point students are trying to learn the basics, preceptors can help SRNAs develop good care plans by asking them to prioritize the patient's problems and potential surgical issues, identify the anesthetic implications of each, propose interventions where needed, and provide a rationale for the intervention. Instructors will find that some students fail to recognize the importance of the care plan to learning and dismiss it as busy work. With these students, preceptors can emphasize the role of repetition in buttressing knowledge, and they can reinforce expectations for written care plans.

Students use a variety of sources to develop care plans, including the internet. Several SRNA-oriented websites offer numerous care plans for various surgical procedures. While certainly time-saving from the student's point of view, these care plans are not a shortcut to learning and the quality can vary greatly. Typewritten care plans should alert the CRNA to care plans that may not be original and prompt the preceptor to thoroughly evaluate the SRNA's knowledge during the case.

In summary, novice SRNAs begin to identify with their new role through repeated performance and accomplishment of recognizable tasks of nurse anesthesia practice. As students gain confidence in their ability to execute basic psychomotor skills, they are able to more fully participate in more demanding aspects of patient care such as planning and implementing an individualized anesthetic for each patient, making interventions in response to changes in physiologic parameters, and recognizing the stages of anesthesia. Most beginners progress from the novice to advanced beginner stage within a few months of entering clinical practice. How quickly an individual SRNA advances depends on the student's determination, the amount of time spent in clinical practice, the number and type of cases that the student is exposed to, and the willingness of instructors to allow students to gain necessary experiences.

The Advanced Beginner

Advanced beginner students have acquired enough experience to recognize important aspects of situations (ie, attributes of a patient or situation that require previous experience to recognize) and are beginning to feel somewhat comfortable in the clinical area.[7] According to Benner, advanced beginners "demonstrate marginally acceptable performance."[7] Although the advanced beginner is still focused on tasks, the student does not feel as overwhelmed by the environment, begins to place situations in context from participating in similar events, can identify situational cues as a result, and is able to make some interventions based on previous experiences.

In contrast to novice SRNAs, advanced beginners have achieved certain milestones. They are able to perform routine preparation of the anesthesia machine, basic airway equipment, and drugs in about 30 minutes at the start of the day. Planning and preparation for successive cases begins to occur during the preceding case. Their psychomotor skills with venous access, airway management, and manipulation of the anesthesia machine are improving. Because less effort and energy is required to complete these technical tasks, students can concentrate on improving techniques, making interventions, and applying knowledge to practice.

Advanced beginner SRNAs continue to struggle with mask ventilation and will not always recognize airway obstruction or failure to ventilate. Although their intubation skills are improving, students often perceive "production pressure" and think laryngoscopy and intubation must be performed quickly. Because their skills are not yet well developed, rushing through intubation may lead to lip lacerations and chipped teeth. At this stage, students' attention should be directed toward good body mechanics and correct airway management techniques.

Many novice and advanced beginner SRNAs exhibit poor body mechanics while masking the patient or intubating, a practice that increases student fatigue and can lead to failure. One technique that can make mask ventilation less tiring for students is to lean back slightly while ventilating, using body weight as leverage rather than forearm or hand strength. Posture should be corrected if a student tends to bend over when ventilating or intubating. Simple techniques such as making sure the table is at the student's waist level and the patient's head is at the top of the bed may improve success with laryngoscopy. Very short students may need a platform if the table is too high or if the patient's head is elevated.

Preceptors can assist advanced beginner SRNAs with improving basic airway management techniques. During mask ventilation, instructors should help students recognize and correct airway obstruction. Although the precordial stethoscope appears out of favor as a monitoring device, its use can help students identify and correct airway obstruction. When intubation is planned, using nondepolarizing neuromuscular blocking agents to slow the pace of induction will give students a few minutes to practice mask ventilation while the paralytic is taking effect. The additional time may also allow students to relax a little before tackling intubation. The use of video-assisted laryngoscopes has made teaching intubation much easier for both SRNAs and preceptors. Although every CRNA has his or her favorite tricks of the trade, the need for good basic intubation practices such as sniffing position, sweeping the tongue, staying off the lips and teeth, and identifying pertinent anatomy should be reinforced at this point.

Advanced beginners are able to identify certain salient points of anesthesia, and they are starting to place them in context. Preceptors can guide SRNAs by providing cues or guidelines about what to look for or expect in a given situation. One such guideline might be that systolic pressure less than 20% to 25% of baseline is hypotension and should be treated by administering fluids, placing the patient in the head-down position, decreasing volatile agents, or administering vasopressors; however, this guideline does not distinguish subtle nuances of treating hypotension. Nuances are fine distinctions between situations that affect the decision or intervention made. For example, a CRNA discusses the need for preoxygenation of all patients before induction and describes methods to accomplish this. The student grasps the concept and decides that using four deep breaths is an effective way to achieve preoxygenation; however, the student fails to consider patient conditions such as morbid obesity that might require a different technique. The guideline was good, but the student lacks sufficient experience to interpret the rule in light of differences in patient pathophysiology. Instructors can help students identify distinctions of common anesthesia events and share their rationales for making decisions and instituting interventions.

Because the judgment necessary to recognize nuances comes from experience, advanced beginners are dependent on the instructor's knowledge. Although they want to assert their capability and judgment, advanced beginners are unsure and question their ability to make meaningful contributions to a case. At this point, SRNAs doubt their interpretation of events and are hesitant to voice their opinions because they are afraid that instructors will think they are inept or unknowledgeable. Because they are unsure, students will often ask for permission before making an intervention. For example, when a patient becomes hypotensive in the period between induction and incision, a student may cycle the blood pressure cuff several times to verify the correctness of his or her assessment. The preceptor who observes this behavior can ask the student what he or she is thinking about. The student may timidly suggest an intervention or ask permission to initiate a treatment: "Is it okay if I give 5 mg of ephedrine?" An SRNA who is very unsure may appear frozen and unable to act. This situation provides a good opportunity for the instructor to discuss alternative treatments or what the CRNA might do in a similar scenario. Conversely, some advanced beginner SRNAs will move assertively to intervene before verifying their observations and plan with the preceptor. In this situation, the instructor can remind the student to discuss his or her rationale with the CRNA before initiating treatment.

Advanced beginners are still anxious, especially when confronted with new or challenging clinical situations. Although anxiety may improve vigilance, anxiety may also limit learning and impede decision-making. Many novices and advanced beginners express the fear that they will be solely responsible for the patient's entire care. A closely aligned fear is that the instructor will leave the student's side, abandoning the student (and patient) to a variety of imagined perils. Students may think that the preceptor's primary role is as an instructor when that role is actually secondary to providing patient care. Advanced beginner SRNAs should be reassured that they will be allowed to participate in cases to the extent possible depending on their level of preparedness, the patient's acuity, and the complexity of the surgical procedure. Although the advanced beginner generally requires constant supervision, students should know how, when, and who to call for help if the CRNA must leave the room. To determine a student's capability for greater independence, an instructor can review possible scenarios that might occur during the CRNA's absence and ask how the student would manage each event.

Advanced beginners are still task- and procedure-oriented. They are trying hard to make sense of situations by developing routines. Even small deviations from routine may derail a student. Advanced beginner SRNAs often report that their day is "ruined" and their performance disintegrates after they miss an intubation or IV start, or forget a portion of the drug or airway setup. Because the student's focus is on personal ability to execute a task rather than on patient care, inability to perform a skill is perceived as personal failure. The advanced beginner quickly begins to doubt his or her ability, leading to a vicious cycle of performance anxiety, self-flagellation, and further failure. Kindness and tact are imperative when CRNA instructors assess the advanced beginner's performance because an SRNA's enthusiasm and spirit can easily be crushed by harsh criticism.

Prioritization is another area in which the advanced beginner SRNA needs support. Because guidelines are often generic, they do not help the student decide what to do first or when to do it. The student may know that a volatile agent must be turned on after endotracheal tube (ETT) placement is verified but may wait to do so until the ETT is secured, the ventilator is turned on, gas flows are adjusted, and esophageal stethoscope and airway or bite block are placed. Similarly, a student may focus on a task such as completing medical records and not notice alarms or changes in vital signs. Preceptors can redirect the student's attention by asking, "What's that noise?" or "What do you think that means?" while pointing out the alarm or vital sign change.

Advanced beginner SRNAs feel little accountability for patient care. This lack of ownership may stem from previous critical care experience in which nurses lacked autonomy and decisions were physician- or protocol-driven. Advanced beginners focus on performing tasks and developing routines and doubt their knowledge and abilities. Therefore, advanced beginners often feel that responsibility for decision-making rests with those who have superior knowledge and experience. In addition, students entering the profession may underestimate the amount of responsibility that nurse anesthetists assume for patient care. Clinical instructors may observe this lack of ownership when students assume that they can leave at 3 pm even though the case will finish at 3:30 pm. This perception can be reinforced when instructors are too prescriptive or take over case management from the student. To gain a sense of ownership and confidence, advanced beginners must start making interventions based on their assessments and then observe firsthand the results of their decisions. In other words, students must be allowed to make both good and bad decisions.

If advanced beginners are to develop competence, they must be allowed opportunities to work through new and challenging situations.[8] Student registered nurse anesthetists must learn to deal with the ambiguity of decision-making and take responsibility for the results of their decisions. Every CRNA can recall particular experiences that helped him or her grow as a practitioner and that honed judgment and skills. Benner calls these events "paradigm cases" because they make a major impact on the learner.[7] CRNAs often share their paradigm cases or "pearls" with students by telling stories of their experiences and what was learned as a result. Advanced beginner SRNAs must begin to compile their own know-how based on patient care issues that exemplify certain concepts and provide concrete guides for future actions. Because paradigm cases also reveal developing competencies, students should be encouraged to share their experiences with their peers or other anesthesia providers. Sharing can be done formally through M&M or clinical conferences or informally through blogs, list serves, or discussions in the lounge.

Preceptors should not assume that advanced beginner SRNAs have good rationale for their actions. Students at this level have limited knowledge, misunderstand concepts, or apply theoretical knowledge inappropriately. Instructors should attempt to elicit the depth of the student's knowledge. For example, when asked to describe succinylcholine, a student may appropriately respond that it is a depolarizing neuromuscular blocking agent but may be unable to explain the process of depolarization. The instructor can clarify or explain misunderstood or unknown concepts or direct the student to review the topic and return to the instructor with an answer. Nurse anesthetists who have been practicing for awhile may hesitate to ask questions because they have forgotten the information or because they fear that the student knows more than the preceptor. Instructors can overcome this anxiety by admitting that time has dimmed their theoretical knowledge and asking the student to refresh his or her memory. Another technique instructors can use is to develop several stock questions (and answers) to ask students. Alternatively, preceptors may wish to become a local expert on a certain topic or type of case. As students become aware that an instructor is knowledgeable on a subject, they will come to expect questions about this topic from the CRNA or will consult the CRNA for expertise.

Through continued practice and exposure to different patient conditions, surgical procedures, and anesthesia providers, the advanced beginner SRNA gradually develops competence. This is an incremental process that might be characterized as two steps forward, one step back. With repeated practice and over time, the student takes more steps forward and fewer steps back. Students graduate to the competent level when able to manage a general anesthetic with minimal assistance for a healthy patient (ASA physical status I or II) undergoing a simple surgical procedure (eg, a hysterectomy, laparoscopic cholecystectomy, laminectomy, or similar procedure). Although variations in nurse anesthesia educational programs prohibit generalizations about when an SRNA will achieve this milestone, a student should probably advance to the competent stage after participating in 150 to 200 anesthetics or six months of full-time clinical experience.

The Competent Student

Competent students demonstrate improved technical and organizational skills and increasing knowledge and awareness of clinical situations.[8] Although they still have much to learn, the competent SRNA is sufficiently familiar with a variety of basic anesthesia situations and can make appropriate decisions and function with less preceptor intervention. When faced with circumstances similar to previously encountered clinical events, competent SRNAs are able to identify significant aspects of a situation, eliminate those that are insignificant, and, most importantly, anticipate events that may occur. As a result, competent students can limit the range of possible choices that can be made and focus on what needs to be done.[8]

Improved organizational ability enables competent SRNAs to deal with complex situations more easily. Less time and effort are wasted on unnecessary tasks, and students are not as easily overwhelmed when things do not go perfectly. Because they are better organized, competent SRNAs function more calmly and efficiently. As an example, preoperative evaluation is more thorough, focused, and accomplished in less time. Patients are speedily transported to the operating room and induction is accomplished smoothly and proficiently. Competent students take great pride in their ability to multitask and often describe a day as going well when they skillfully manage numerous demands.[8]

The competent SRNA's organizational skills now extend to anticipatory planning.[8] The competent student plans ahead for the day rather than just the first case, anticipating what is needed and preparing equipment and supplies in advance. Not only can students complete tasks in a timely manner, they also plan for events that might occur with a patient or surgical procedure. Care plans are improved as a student anticipates what might happen when a patient's coexisting disease and the surgical procedure intersect. The morbidly obese patient, for example, is recognized as potentially having a difficult airway. Therefore, the student considers appropriate airway management techniques, has the necessary equipment available, positions the patient appropriately for intubation, and plans alternatives to the primary plan. Adverse intraoperative events that accompany specific procedures are expected, and the student will have a second IV, fluid warmer, central line, and vasoactive drugs prepared when large volume shifts or hemodynamic changes are expected.

Prioritization is also improved in competent students. Although advanced beginners might know what needs to be done, their actions are haphazard because students do first what they know best how to do.[8] Competent SRNAs are able to identify what is most important and do that first. The ability to prioritize implies that students are able to make better judgments about critical aspects of situations and use their time efficiently. As described in an earlier example, novice or advanced beginners focus on a task such as completing medical records while ignoring alarms or vital sign changes. The competent student can receive sensory input from numerous sources, identify changes needing intervention, and implement a treatment. Unlike the proficient student who functions seamlessly, the competent student must still analyze the possibilities of each situation and think through the options. The advanced beginner's grasp of a situation was limited by tunnel vision; the competent SRNA sees the big picture.

Compared with the advanced beginner, competent students' psychomotor skills are vastly improved, and their movements are smoother and more fluid. Competent students complete endotracheal intubations easily on the first attempt most of the time, even when the airway is somewhat difficult. Although able to accomplish intubation quickly, competent students realize the value of taking time to visualize structures, using the right hand to manipulate the larynx, and directing those present to assist them. Manual dexterity has improved to the point that the student does not need to think about each step as it is performed. Therefore, competent students are able to assess their own skills and consider alternative steps if what they are doing is not working.

Competent SRNAs are much more comfortable with their skills and abilities and, as a result, may settle into routine methods of delivering an anesthetic. Although this beginning mastery is to be appreciated, there is some danger that students will become complacent and that their growth will slow. Stagnation can be prevented by continuing to expose students to more challenging patients and procedures. Students usually need little encouragement to try different drugs and techniques, but instructors can stimulate experimentation by suggesting alternatives. Another way to broaden the student's horizon is to ask a student to teach the instructor something new. Getting out of one's comfort zone can be a growth experience for both student and instructor.

Competent SRNAs assume greater personal and ethical responsibility for patient care. Accountability is evident when a student carefully checks the patient's medical records for necessary diagnostic studies or requests additional studies, discusses a proposed anesthetic plan with the instructor and provides rationale for decisions, and accepts responsibility for making mistakes without being defensive. Students at this level are aware that their actions can sometimes cause harm to patients, and they feel devastated after making an error that might compromise a patient. The competent student is becoming a patient advocate, interceding with the surgeon or other team members when decisions might jeopardize patient safety. Advocacy may be seen when a student suggests the use of extra padding to protect a patient during positioning, asks a surgeon to stop manipulations that cause a vagal response, or questions whether a certain technique is appropriate based on the patient's coexisting diseases.

Procedural rules or guidelines are no longer necessary or relied on because some decisions are becoming internalized. Having gained sufficient experience with a variety of patients and surgical procedures, competent students have begun to develop their own rules for dealing with perioperative events.[8] The competent SRNA has internalized a basic plan for delivering an anesthetic and intervening when anticipated events occur. The SRNA has encountered enough situations that he or she is able to acknowledge the significance of various physiological changes and recognize deviations from normal. For example, the student acknowledges the potential for hypotension in the interval between induction and skin incision and will automatically adjust volatile agents and increase fluids when blood pressure begins to decrease rather than waiting for repeated measurements to confirm hypotension. Students now trust that their observations and judgment are accurate and do not need continual affirmation from instructors that their decisions are correct. Competent students are better able to make a case for what they want to do.[8]

Although the competent student has a basic action plan in place, he or she is also able to individualize the plan in regard to existing patient pathophysiology.[8] The competent student recognizes the implications of disease states and adjusts the anesthetic plan to avoid placing the patient at risk. Thus, the competent student understands that a systolic blood pressure of 90 mm Hg may be acceptable in a young, healthy patient but not in a patient with hypertension and coronary artery disease. When different or unusual situations occur, competent students can reason through potential interventions and request help if unsure what to do. Competent SRNAs also recognize areas in which their knowledge is limited and spend considerable time reviewing previously learned material or looking up new information.

Students at this level begin to doubt the knowledge and wisdom of their instructors and other members of the health care team.[8] Students previously perceived the knowledge of other clinicians as superior, but they now may become critical of CRNAs and anesthesiologists whose judgments or rationale they perceive as faulty or unreliable, particularly if a student has observed poor outcomes as a result of these decisions. Students questioning other providers' decisions is similar to teenagers challenging parental authority. While questioning can demonstrate a student's ability to compare the effectiveness of different courses of action, it may also reflect immaturity if done in a disrespectful manner. For example, a student may roll their eyes, do something he or she was instructed not to do, or even may refuse to carry out a direct order. Of course, this lack of respect for an instructor's knowledge, experience, and authority generally infuriates the instructor. Such behavior may even place the patient at risk while exposing the student's immaturity, overconfidence, lack of knowledge, and ability to accept instruction. If the situation is untenable, an insubordinate student should be dismissed from the case and program administrators made immediately aware of this behavior. Less egregious behavior can be resolved with a frank discussion of events after the case is finished. While making clear that such behavior is not acceptable, the clinical instructor should review the situation with the student and attempt to elicit the rationale for his or her questioning of authority. The CRNA can use this opportunity to coach the student in more appropriate ways to deal with conflict.

Competence as an SRNA should not be confused with competence in a new graduate of a nurse anesthesia program. The competent SRNA moves toward proficiency as he or she continues to gain further experience with demanding cases, encounters some infrequently occurring anesthetic situations, and manages more patients who deviate from the norm. Again, this transformation occurs incrementally. Students may demonstrate proficiency in some areas and, at the same time, exhibit competent or advanced beginner abilities in other areas. A student may be quite proficient with psychomotor or patient assessment skills and competent in managing most major general surgery cases but may appear at the advanced beginner stage when confronted with cardiac procedures, major trauma, or transplant cases. Moving to a new clinical site or rotation may cause students to temporarily regress while becoming familiar with the new situation. Instructors should remember that even experienced CRNAs revert to less competent stages when learning to use new drugs or techniques. According to Benner, "Change, not passage of time, is the defining characteristic of experience."[8] Therefore, proficiency is not necessarily related to the number of months that a student has been in clinical practice but to changes in behavior that indicate maturation of knowledge, skills, and behavior as a nurse anesthetist.

The Proficient Student

Students who are soon to graduate and meet all requirements for initial certification are competent entry-level practitioners. These students are at the proficient level of the novice-to-expert model. Students at this point are able to see situations as a whole because they are able to synthesize previous experiences and understand the meaning of an event without systematically analyzing each aspect.[7,8] The proficient SRNA understands normal responses to anesthesia and surgery and recognizes when events deviate from what is expected. Although deeply involved and connected to the patient when managing an anesthetic, proficient SRNAs have the ability to mentally step back and see the big picture in light of the patient's physiologic responses to intraoperative events. Proficient students are able to zero in on the most important aspects in a rapidly changing environment and make decisions without considering multiple options.

Proficient students recognize the relevance of subtle nuances that might have been overlooked by the competent student. Proficient students are able to place these nuances in context, recognize their implications, eliminate certain options, and generate an appropriate plan of action. For example, when a proficient student administers anesthesia to a patient with coronary artery disease undergoing a carotid endarterectomy, he or she develops a plan to avoid or minimize hypotension following induction. If hypotension does occur, the student quickly addresses potential causes, acknowledges ramifications for the patient, and initiates interventions to correct the problem. Having participated in enough similar cases and having confidence in his or her judgment, the student does not need to weigh and eliminate all possible causes of hypotension. The proficient performer is beginning to show signs of intuitive decision-making that epitomizes expert practice.

Proficient students are able to manage many types of patients and anesthetics with minimal supervision. At this point, clinical faculty function more as advisors or coaches than as instructors. The student about to graduate should be able to independently develop an individualized anesthetic management plan and safely and efficiently implement the plan in collaboration with other members of the surgical and anesthesia team.

A heightened sense of responsibility is characteristic of proficient student registered nurse anesthetists, who often think they must do everything themselves and do not take advantage of help offered by other clinicians. While outwardly acknowledging the need to function as part of the operating room and anesthesia teams, students may mistake the ability to manage all parts of an anesthetic without assistance as proficiency. In reality, this behavior demonstrates insecurity because more seasoned clinicians readily seek help, share tasks, and request consultation when needed. Failing to share responsibility for a patient may also contribute an unnecessary burden when adverse events occur. When students feel unrealistically responsible for a patient, they may blame themselves for events that were unforeseeable, unpredictable, and unpreventable.

The technical skills of proficient SRNAs are excellent. Students are adept at performing IV insertion, spinal or epidural blocks, and airway management with a variety of devices; however, they may still need experience with peripheral regional blocks or more advanced monitoring techniques. Unfortunately, students sometimes confuse mastery of these skills combined with admirable organizational and time management ability as indicative of expertise. Students may feel overly responsible or become overly confident, resulting in the potential for humbling errors.

Proficient students seek improved patient outcomes in their practice.[8] No longer content with merely performing tasks quickly and efficiently, they seek to prevent common problems and minimize adverse events. For the proficient student, emerging a patient no longer means recognizing when to remove the ETT. Instead, the proficient student plans the emergence so that the patient wakes up without coughing on the ETT; is free from nausea, vomiting, and excessive pain or sedation; and is able to be discharged from the recovery room in a short time.

Giving information to patients is one area where proficient students differ from those who are competent.[8] For instance, the competent student might recite a laundry list of all possible anesthetic complications when obtaining informed consent. The proficient student will adjust discussion of possible adverse anesthetic events based on his or her reading of the patient's and family's ability to understand and readiness to learn. The student does not withhold important information or try to deceive the patient but tailors the information to what the patient needs and wants to know.[8]

Proficient students may become complacent in expanding their knowledge base or feel that information learned in the classroom is not practical or useful.[7] Some students may think that they know it all because their knowledge is more current than their instructor's or may think that they have seen it all if their case numbers are high. Such students may begin demonstrating unprofessional behaviors such as wandering in late to clinical training, failing to call the instructor for induction or emergence, or refusing to consider the instructor's suggestions. Fortunately, most soon-to-graduate students do not fall into this category, but those who do can be challenging for the instructor.

Although they have not yet passed the National Certification Examination, proficient students have achieved identities as nurse anesthetists. Their ability to perform appropriately in myriad challenging anesthetic situations has been confirmed by instructors, surgeons, and other operating room personnel. Although still a little anxious in new situations, proficient students feel that they are able to meet clinical challenges because they have confidence in their own abilities. Since they are no longer deeply engaged in learning new skills and knowledge, proficient students are able to expand their view of the nurse anesthetist's role as a patient care advocate and member of the health care system. Students now begin to evaluate how different anesthesia practice models affect CRNA practice, to identify and discuss professional issues, and to consider involvement in state and local professional associations.

The Expert Practitioner

The expert practitioner is easy to recognize, but identifying attributes of the expert is more difficult. Experts have gained a tremendous amount of experience in a variety of situations and have developed an intuitive ability to accurately determine the most important aspects of a problem without needing to consider a range of alternatives. According to Benner, experts do what normally works in a situation.[7] This is not to say that an expert does not consider other possibilities, diagnoses, or interventions, but that the expert does not need to methodically evaluate each option to make a judgment. Experts have difficulty verbalizing how they make decisions or respond to specific events, often replying, "It depends," when asked what course of action they would take in a particular situation. This answer suggests that experts consider a broad range of choices based on ingrained theoretical and experiential knowledge.

Experts anticipate potential events that may occur with a given patient or situation and plan for them. Experts are prepared to deal with various possibilities and are flexible enough to rapidly switch courses of action. The expert recognizes subtle changes in a patient's condition and acts before a crisis occurs. Within their work settings, experts are those individuals consulted by their peers for their superior knowledge and ability—the go-to persons.

Experts can make wrong decisions or evaluations of a situation. In this case, experts revert to more analytic problem solving.[7] However, even expert practitioners revert to the novice role when confronted with a new drug, technique, or unfamiliar situation. Untoward events such as malignant hyperthermia, cardiac arrest, and anaphylaxis happen infrequently in anesthesia. Therefore, even experienced CRNAs may need rules or algorithms to guide their practice when these unique events occur. Simulation centers with whole body simulators are one way for practitioners to experience these rare occurrences and develop a degree of comfort in dealing with them.

In my estimation, SRNAs cannot achieve the expert level of practice. At a minimum, graduates of nurse anesthesia programs are expected to demonstrate the knowledge and skills deemed by the profession to represent entry-level competence; however, the majority of graduates have not had sufficient experience in a wide range of situations to develop the intuitive decision-making skills that characterize expert practice. Indeed, not all CRNAs reach the expert stage, but expertise is something all CRNAs can strive to achieve.

Summary

The novice-to-expert model provides one way of examining and assessing a student registered nurse anesthetist's clinical growth and development. The normal growth pattern for SRNAs demonstrates slow but steady progression with occasional hesitations along the way. As with normal human growth and development, students advance at different rates. Some students grow rapidly; others take longer to achieve the same growth milestones. All have periodic growth spurts when things suddenly come together (the "ah-ha" moment). However, a few students will not progress much beyond the advanced beginner stage, a condition I have dubbed "failure to thrive." These individuals may even perform competently in situations where cases are simple, patients are healthy, and adequate support or supervision is available. However, the student who is not growing and progressing does not adapt when confronted with more difficult cases or patients, unusual or emergent situations, or rapidly changing circumstances. The novice-to-expert model can help educators distinguish students who are meeting the expected growth trajectory from those who are not.

A limitation of the novice-to-expert model is that it fails to take into account the important role that clinical instructors play in modeling behavior. Students construct an image of the ideal qualities of a CRNA based on the admirable and not so admirable qualities of their clinical and didactic instructors.[2] Generally, students hold their instructors in high esteem and view them as mentors. Positive instructor traits might be making a difference in patient care, acting as a patient advocate, and possessing clinical acumen and excellent technical skills. However, none of these traits is important if an instructor makes a student feel humiliated, threatened, or unwelcome. Clinical preceptors must recognize the impact their actions have on students, and that an instructor can facilitate or hinder learning according to the value that the instructor places on certain knowledge or skills.[16] Students gain confidence in their skills and ability to function in a range of situations through repeated practice and confirmation by others that they are making progress.[2] Preceptors can facilitate a working relationship with students through a friendly and open demeanor, discussing their rationale for decision-making, and sharing clinical "pearls."

References

1. Collins, S. Callahan, MF. A call for change: clinical evaluation of student registered nurse anesthetists. *AANA J.* 2014;82(1):65–72.

2. Stockhausen LJ. Learning to become a nurse: students' reflections on their clinical experiences. *Aust J Adv Nurs.* 2005;22(3):8–14.

3. Burns, SM. Predicting academic progression for student registered nurse anesthetists. *AANA J.* 2011;79(3):193–201.

4. Muckle, TJ. Plaus, KA. Henderson, J. Waters, E. Professional practice analysis: determining job relatedness of the certification examination for nurse anesthetists. *J Nurs Regul.* 2012;3(3):1–7.

5. Wong, E. Faculty discernment of student registered nurse anesthetist's personality characteristics that contribute to safe and unsafe nurse anesthesia practice: metrics of excellence. *AANA J.* 2011;79(3):227–235.

6. Wren KR. Learning from a nurse anesthetist perspective: A qualitative study. *AANA J.* 2001;69(4):273–278.

7. Benner PA. *From Novice to Expert: Excellence and Power in Clinical Nursing Practice.* Commemorative ed. Upper Saddle River, NJ: Prentice-Hall, Inc.; 2001.

8. Benner PA, Tanner CA, Chesla CA. *Expertise in Nursing Practice: Caring, Clinical Judgment Ethics.* New York, NY: Springer Publishing Company, Inc.; 1996.

9. Altmann, TK. An evaluation of the seminal work of Patricia Benner: Theory or philosophy? *Contemp Nurse.* 2007;25(1–2):114–123.

10. O'Connor AB. *Clinical Instruction and Evaluation: A Teaching Resource.* Sudbury, MA: Jones and Bartlett Publishers; 2001.

11. Dreyfus HL, Dreyfus SE. *Mind Over Machine.* New York, NY: Free Press; 1986.

12. Wright, SM. Fallacaro, MD. Predictors of situation awareness in student registered nurse anesthetists. *AANA J.* 2011;79(6):484–490.

13. Dreyfus HL, Dreyfus SE. The Relationship of Theory and Practice in the Acquisition of Skill. In: Benner PA, Tanner CA, Chesla CA, eds. *Expertise in Nursing Practice: Caring Clinical Judgment & Ethics.* New York, NY: Springer Publishing Company, Inc.; 1996.

14. Council on Accreditation of Nurse Anesthesia Educational Programs. Standards for Accreditation of Nurse Anesthesia Educational Programs. Park Ridge, IL: COA; 2004 (rev. 2016). http://home.coa.us.com/accreditation/Pages/Accreditation-Policies-Procedures-and-Standards.aspx. Accessed 08/15/2016.

15. Clark DR. Bloom's Taxonomy of Learning Domains. http://www.nwlink.com/~donclark/hrd/bloom.html. Published June 5, 1999. Updated January 12, 2015. Accessed August 16, 2016.

16. Teunissen PW, Scheele F, Scherpbier AJ, et al. How residents learn: qualitative evidence for the pivotal role of clinical activities. *Med Educ.* 2007;41(8):763–770.

CHAPTER 19

Innovations in Teaching and Education

Karita Käck, DNAP, CRNA

Keywords: Education, innovation, serious games, technology.

Key Concepts

- There are many innovations in graduate-level teaching and learning that are suggestive or already applied to other graduate nursing education.
- Online courses have proven to be as effective as the traditional face-to-face classroom.
- Technology offers innovative methods in teaching and learning that supports critical thinking and collaboration. Wikis, blogs, and podcasts are creative ways to deliver content in nurse anesthesia education.
- The millennial generation is tech-savvy, multitasking, and, mainly, visual learners. The flipped classroom allows for creativity, collaboration, and engagement of both instructors and students.
- Serious games is an innovative next step in teaching anesthesia to a new generation of nurse anesthetists.

Introduction

Innovation in education can be defined as a spark of new concepts and inspiration that question the status quo and create new ideas in teaching. Innovation in any industry is often driven by a commitment to excellence and continuous advancement by a dedicated profession. The past decade has produced so many new innovations in teaching and education that even formal educators have been left scrambling to keep up. Nurse anesthesia programs are not excluded from these changes and, in fact, new innovations may have exceeded the capacity of the nurse anesthesia educators in many programs. This may partially be due to the movement toward a doctoral degree for nurse anesthetists by 2022, adding an influx of post-master's degree students and the added length of the post-baccalaureate program.

Many practicing nurse anesthetists were taught during the old regime of traditional classroom education where the teacher lectured for hours, often after a long day in clinical practice. Many can remember reaching that warm, fuzzy feeling of slowly drifting into an open-eyed snooze while the slides all blended together and the notes had fewer and fewer actual words in them. Luckily, some of the new innovations in education challenge both the educator and student alike. Many of the new trends and innovations are based on technology and involve different instructional techniques or delivery systems such as wikis, video podcast presentations, synchronous and asynchronous online delivery of classes, and the inverted, or flipped, classroom. This chapter will examine the current trends in nurse anesthesia education in the classroom and in the clinical arena.

Online Teaching and Learning: A New Standard?

Correspondence courses have been available for a long time and were first offered at the University of Chicago in the 1890s, but true online learning did not begin until the 1990s when the World Wide Web was developed.[1] The prevalence of online learning and teaching in higher education is growing, as indicated in a report submitted from the e-learning industry in 2014. The report also showed that 4.6 out of 10 college students are taking at least one online course, and the number of students taking courses online is expected to grow to roughly 50 percent by 2019.[2]

Online teaching and learning are still considered foreign concepts to many educators and students. There is an ongoing uncertainty of quality and outcomes from online learning, especially if both the instructor and student have never participated in online learning and course work. Online learning has matured over the years and is now offered using many different methods to achieve the goals of improved access, flexibility, and efficiency. As with any change, there are always advantages and disadvantages.

The greatest advantages of online education are the opportunities offered. Physical presence is no longer a necessity and a course can be taught anywhere in the world if a computer workstation and an Internet connection are available. There is no missed class time due to illness, public holidays, or inclement weather. There is the opportunity to work with cutting edge technologies to deliver instruction and creative interactive tools that are more interesting to the learner than simple PowerPoint lectures, which can often contain canned verbiage.[3,4]

The disadvantage of online teaching, and one often mentioned by faculty, is the gap between instructor and students in the online format. There is a lack of social presence and immediate feedback from the class. The sense of how students are receiving and processing the presented material is lost. Many faculty members feel pressured to teach in this format with little input and no formal instruction. Online teaching differs from the face-to-face classroom, and some skepticism may come from a misconception of what represents an effective online course, and the steps involved in making the course effective and interesting to the students.[4,5]

With the move to a doctoral degree in nurse anesthesia programs and the addition of the doctoral standards to the Council on Accreditation (COA), numerous changes are needed for programs to be accredited. Some of the courses included in the doctoral degree appear to fit the online environment and offer flexibility to both students and educators. Programs currently offering a post-master's degree DNP or doctor of nurse anesthesia practice (DNAP) for the practicing CRNA have adopted the online curriculum, and continue to develop and improve upon the delivery and outcomes of these courses.

Definition of Terms

There are central terms commonly used during discussions of online education; the definitions used in this chapter are provided in **Table 19.1**, next page. The definitions are adapted from the Online Learning Consortium and are representative of terms used in higher education in many institutions.[6] The COA defines distance education as "An educational process that is characterized by the separation, in time or place, between instructor and student, either synchronously or asynchronously. The term includes courses in which 50 percent or more of instruction is provided via communication technologies including internet courses both synchronous and asynchronous, two-way and one-way interactive video, audio conferencing, multimedia, compact disc, video cassette, and audio tape." The COA further defines a distance education course where 50 percent or more of the course is offered at a distance.[7]

Table 19.1 Definition of Terms

Classroom course (face-to-face)	The course activity is organized around scheduled class meetings and measured by hours spent with in-person meetings in a variety of formats.
Synchronous course (Web-assisted)	Web-based technologies are used to extend classroom lectures to students at remote locations or on campus while maintaining a regular schedule and a real-time component. These courses may mix on-campus and remote students in the same class.
Online course	All course activity is done online with no required face-to-face sessions and no on-campus requirements.
Web-enhanced course	Online course activities complement class sessions without reducing the number of required class meetings. The Internet-based work or activity is typically 20% or less. These courses are very similar to traditional courses but usually require additional student and faculty support, as well as additional technology.
Hybrid, or blended, classroom course	Online activities are mixed with classroom meetings, replacing a significant number of face-to-face meetings, but not all.
Hybrid, or blended, online course	Most course activities are done online with a few required face-to-face sessions. These courses may be categorized as online but do still include face-to-face work. The institution sets the threshold for required online activity.
Flexible mode course	This course offers different delivery modes, where students can choose which delivery model to use for instructional and learning purposes. One example: Students use a learning resource center with both online materials and on-demand personalized assistance.

Applying Best Practices to Distance Education

While online programs and courses continue to develop in nurse anesthesia education there is some skepticism of the quality and the efficacy of online models.[8] As with traditional classroom education, online education has its own concerns. By applying best practices and andragogy to teaching, online education can provide excellence and high-quality nurse anesthesia education. The advancement to doctoral education of nurse anesthetists graduating in 2022 and beyond will increase the need for online education because of such benefits as flexibility of time, decreased need for a designated space, and increased access. Online learning is already a permanent fixture on most university campuses and many doctoral nursing programs are using the method to educate their students.

The transition from face-to-face to online teaching is challenging and will require a significant shift in teaching strategies. The goal of online teaching is not simply to replicate classroom teaching to the Internet platform, but to create a virtual environment that stimulates and engages the student. The online teaching environment requires creative instructional skills, some knowledge in technology (although many universities have highly skilled technology and specific online staff available), and different sets of communication skills.[9]

Students in nurse anesthesia programs are adult learners who require a curriculum that is authentic and applicable to their practice and profession as a whole. For CRNAs who are already practicing and completing their DNP/DNAP online, there is often apprehension regarding new technology in education and the new student identity. Online content should be easy to navigate. Complicated links and graphics are best avoided since they can hinder access and distract the learner. This allows the student to concentrate on content rather than technology. The role of faculty in online courses becomes that of instructor and facilitator, rather than conductor and maestro.

Moving from face-to-face to online teaching presents challenges to the institution and to faculty. Nearly 70 percent of all higher education institutions report online learning as critical to their long-term strategic plan. How do faculty feel about online teaching? In its 10th annual report, *Changing course: Ten Years of Tracking Online Education in the United States*, Allen and Seaman surveyed chief academic officers in 2800 colleges and universities regarding the nature and extent of online education.[10] When asked to rate faculty acceptance of online education, academic leaders reported a decline in faculty acceptance of online education in 2012 (30.4%) for the first time since 2004 (30.2%). In comparison, a recent study conducted by Chiasson et al in 2015,[11] surveyed 10 university faculty members about their perception in transitioning from face-to-face to online learning. Faculty members developed and taught a course that originated from their recent course library taught in the traditional face-to-face classroom environment. All of the participants perceived the development of online courses as more time-intensive, and modifications were required while teaching the course based on student understanding and feedback. Although some faculty members had a difficult time letting go of the control they had in the classroom, they felt that students took more responsibility for their own learning. At the end of the study, faculty described themselves as more confident as instructors following the design and teaching of online courses.[11]

In applying best practices to online teaching, the literature and personal experience suggest that the instructor should allow a considerable amount of time to design and develop the course. This means that planning and designing of the course should begin well before the course is presented. It is reasonable to have the course ready several weeks prior to making it available to students. Material and instructions should be logical and self-contained since there are few opportunities to improvise in an online course. Technological knowledge is required and faculty should consult instructional designers, when available, to provide assistance in designing the course. They can identify appropriate technology that supports learning and the instructor's pedagogy. This will assure that the students can easily access the course and that all the information in the course is correctly placed.

How effective is online learning? The U.S. Department of Education performed a meta-analysis in 2009 to evaluate online learning.[12]

The study addressed four questions:

1. How does the effectiveness of online learning compare with face-to-face instruction?
2. Does supplementing face-to-face instruction with online instruction enhance learning?

3. What practices are associated with more effective online learning?
4. What conditions influence the effectiveness of online learning?

The meta-analysis examined published literature returned between 1996–2008; studies were chosen based on the criteria of research design, ability to contrast online to face-to-face conditions, and objectively measure learning outcomes. The learners were divided between K-12, college, and graduate levels receiving professional training. Medicine or health care were the most common subjects in the articles. The key findings of the study indicated that:

- Students who took all or part of their class online performed better than those taking the same course through traditional face-to-face instruction.
- Instruction combining online and face-to-face elements did better when compared to either alone.
- Students who spent more time on a task in the online environment experienced a greater benefit compared to students spending less time in the face-to-face setting.
- Online learning appeared to be an effective option for undergraduate, graduate, and professional students.
- Video or online quizzes do not appear to influence the amount that students learn in online classes.
- Online learning can be enhanced by giving students control of their interactions with media and by prompting reflection.

In conclusion, the analysis did not show online learning superior as a medium; the advantages of online learning were more dependent on time spent in the course, pedagogy, and curriculum. The analysis suggested that a "blended instruction model" with face-to-face classroom combined with online learning was more effective than online learning by itself.[12]

The main disadvantage of online instruction is the lack of face-to-face interaction that allows the instructor to get visual cues from students and redirect the delivery or the topic if needed.[4] There are no visual indications to indicate that a student is feverishly taking notes or is bored, frustrated or nodding off. Online communication connects the student and the instructor virtually, and the use of facial expressions and tone of voice no longer play a role. Instead, the instructions and feedback are often written or recorded at an earlier date. Many believe that the written nature of communication enhances the interaction between student-student and student-instructor by requiring a deeper level of thinking and a richer understanding. The online environment provides a safe place for every student to have his or her voice heard, and to express opinions without trepidation.

Since online learning lacks the social connection between students, and between student and instructor, creating a social presence helps students develop a sense of community.[8,13] Social presence can be attained by allowing the students to project their own personality in the course. This increases the sense of social connection and increases group cohesion. Many instructors choose to open online courses with a presentation of themselves and an opportunity for students to do the same. This can be part of the course and embedded in the first learning module where students can write a short autobiography and be given the option of posting pictures. This can also be accomplished as the first assignment in the form of a short PowerPoint presentation where the students introduce themselves, and state their interests, reasons for taking the course, and 3 to 4 objectives that they hope to complete in the course. These objectives help set goals for the course and can be revisited as the course progresses.[13,14]

Newly developed courses are often structured to contain modules that are made available to students at the same day and time of each week or every other week. Each module contains instructions, assigned readings, videos, and other material that will be utilized in the module. Each module should have easily retrieved links to material or clear instructions if the students are assigned to search for the material. This serves as the basis for a discussion board where one or more questions will guide the discussion. Students look for comments from the instructor as a way to feel connected and validated. This emphasizes the importance of prompt and individualized feedback provided within a set time frame.[15] If the instructor comments and participates in the discussion board on a regular basis, students feel as though they are sharing in something and tend to stay on track in the course.[16]

Feedback in online courses has shown to be important and fundamental to the process of learning. Feedback that is timely and frequent has shown to be an important factor in learning since it contributes to and strengthens the connection between the instructor and the student. There are various avenues for delivery of feedback in an online course: posting comments to the discussion board, audio feedback, feedback as a brief video clip, or feedback in a synchronous Web-based format. In all formats described, addressing the student by name helps personalize the communication. Feedback should be positive, informational, or instructional. Feedback in the form of supportive and thought-provoking questions promotes critical thinking and further strengthens the development of the learning process as well as the student-instructor relationship.[16,17]

What is a reasonable time frame for feedback? Online learners identify immediate feedback as between 24-48 hours after their own online post. This may not be possible for the instructor, depending on the number of students in the class and total faculty workload. A reasonable time for online feedback is within 72 hours of the due date, and with larger assignments, it's best if returned within a week of the due date. Some feedback time-saving tips are helpful since this process can become time-consuming for the instructor. Keeping a bank of frequently used feedback comments in a word document that can be retrieved during the course is helpful; this can help in making specific, positive feedback comments. Another time-saving tool is using voice technology to provide audio feedback.[17] Five minutes of audio feedback can pack a lot of punch and feels personal, particularly when all other communication is in the text format.

The evaluation process of online courses differs from traditional classroom teaching. Using the discussion board is usually given a substantial part of the total grade since this reflects participation in the course. It is common to assign 30-50 percent of the grade to discussion board participation. Some instructors grade each module weekly according to timely participation and the quality of posts. Papers and other assignments can be given the remaining percentage of the total grade, all specifically specified in the syllabus.

Evaluations are usually distributed via email to students at the end of the semester. The anonymity of online evaluations can sometimes open a Pandora's box, allowing for comments that normally would never otherwise be expressed. Participation from students in course evaluations is often sparse making it difficult to gauge if the course was well-received or needs redesign. Most courses need updates before the course goes live in a new semester. This is the time to update material such as articles, videos, and Camtasia presentations to give the course a fresh look for the new cohort of students.

The question remains: Are online courses better or equal to the traditional face-to-face classroom? There are numerous studies currently examining online learning. Cook et al conducted a meta-analysis of 201 studies looking at online education, and concluded that Internet-based learning is educationally beneficial, with results that are similar to traditional methods.[17] This fact should support nurse anesthesia educators looking to combine online courses with traditional classroom instruction in the DNP/DNAP programs.

Discussion Board: Etiquette and Netiquette

Discussion board is a general term for a virtual bulletin board where individuals with access can leave comments and expect an answer. Discussion board has become a common element in every classroom management system. Depending on the length and content of the course, the discussion board commonly is tied to a specific module in the course where content is either presented or researched. Parameters are set up as to how often students are expected to participate; if they can see their peers post before their own; the day and time when comments are due; and a rubric by which the discussion forum is graded. The syllabus should be clear about student expectations in the discussion forum. There commonly are rules as to day and time of the week when posts are due, the maximum length of a post, and how many of their peer's posts they have to comment on. This is all reflected in the grade of the discussion forum and should reflect quality, timeliness, mechanics, and evidence of knowledge of the concept.

The following question often surfaces among online teaching faculty: How often should I comment on discussion boards? There is an intricate balance between avoiding interference in peer discussions and interjecting relevance. As the instructor, it's important to resist responding too soon so that students have time to interact and create a dialogue.[17] Many online instructors are experts in their profession and have entered higher education as a secondary or supplemental career. Facilitating a discussion board can become frustrating and stressful for these instructors, who might have no formal education in teaching and pedagogy, yet are often expected to develop and teach online courses.

A simple and unique way of managing a discussion board is to compare it to a dinner party at your house. Think of the students as guests who have never been to your house before and don't know any of the other guests. Everyone is somewhat apprehensive about the discussion at the table, but excited to be invited. As the host, you are responsible for making sure that people are comfortable and this may begin with an introduction of yourself followed by the guests' introductions. During dinner, the guests are continually served something appealing and everybody has their moment in the conversation. The host guides any disagreements in a professional manner and makes sure the conversation continues and never gets stale. Make sure to continually attend to your guest's needs and at the end of the evening, make sure to invite them back.[18]

In attending to our dinner conversation, we should make sure that the dialogue is appropriate, civil, and courteous. The online conversation should follow the same standards and is commonly referred to as Netiquette. Netiquette is best described as network or cyberspace etiquette with a set of rules on how to properly behave and communicate while online. It is prudent to include these rules in syllabi for online courses. The following rules were written in 1994 by Virginia Shea,[19] and can serve as a guide to all online communication:

Rule 1: Remember the Human—there are real people out there—it's easy to misinterpret your correspondent's meaning.

Rule 2: Adhere to the same standards of behavior online that you follow in real life—if you encounter an ethical dilemma in cyberspace, consult the code you follow in real life.

Rule 3: Know where you are in cyberspace—When you enter a domain of cyberspace that's new to you, take a look around. Spend a while listening.

Rule 4: Respect other people's time and bandwidth—don't forget that other people have concerns other than yours. Before you copy people on your messages, ask yourself whether they really need to know.

Rule 5: Make yourself look good online—You will be judged by the quality of your writing. Pay attention to the content of your writing.

Rule 6: Share expert knowledge—Don't be afraid to share what you know. It's especially polite to share the results of your questions with others.

Rule 7: Help keep flame wars under control—series of angry comments can destroy the camaraderie of a discussion group.

Rule 8: Respect other people's privacy.

Rule 9: Don't abuse your power.

Rule 10: Be forgiving of other people's mistakes.

Wikis, Blogs, Podcasts

Today's educators are facing changes in teaching and learning due to the ever-changing landscape where technology has become a permanent fixture. Technology can be used as an instrument for innovation in teaching, but it is important that the tools are easy to use, reliable, and add to the learning experience. If the new tools are added to the already large workload without adequate training, the subsequent acceptance from faculty will be cautious at best. The stress that new technology creates requires providing support to allows faculty to concentrate on content instead of technology. Educational institutions offering online courses need dedicated technology staff who can facilitate design of courses and suggest appropriate technology that fits the specific program or course.

Wikis, blogs, and podcasts are popular tools used in online courses and examples of Web-based collaboration ware (also known as Web 2.0 tools). All of these tools offer advantages and have been adopted, mostly within the last decade, into health care education. Their relative ease of access and use are making these applications ideal for projects because editing can appear in real time. Wikis, blogs, and podcasts are so-called transparent technology because they are easy to use and allow the user to focus on content.[20,21] They can all be used collaboratively between students in both the didactic and clinical arenas, and to deliver new information when students are unable to attend class.

The first wikis appeared in the 1990s and were used by scientists and engineers to create and share knowledge. "Wiki" comes from the Hawaiian language and means "quick." It is a fitting name since a wiki is a piece of software that allows everybody with access the ability to create and edit content using any Web browser.[22] The newly edited or created content is then immediately available to everybody in the group. A wiki can be as long as a book or as short as one page. The three main uses are to view, edit, and contribute. The content is instantly published and can be used as a tool to collaborate between students or between students and instructor. This way of communicating provides a unique sense of connection between students in the same group and can also be a good learning resource of shared experiences. Putting thoughts into the written word sometimes clarifies ideas and difficult concepts.[23]

Wikis can be incorporated into any course by adding a URL and be password protected and private to a group. This makes wikis useful as a platform in health care education to deliver content such as video podcasts and pertinent articles. The content can be delivered at predetermined intervals by multiple authors. Since wikis are Web pages, adding audio, video, and links is easy. The instructor has the ability to see the process of any collaborative group work or research projects and can interact with guidance and suggestions as needed. Clinical instructors with access can add content and participate in discussions they otherwise may not have access to. Hosting a journal club as a wiki is one way to share thoughts and develop discussion if students are at their clinical sites and unable to share immediate thoughts and knowledge in class.[24] Another time-saving avenue for faculty is using wikis as a live signup board for advising, laboratory time, and meetings with faculty.

Much like a wiki, a blog is an example of a document that is constantly evolving and unfolding with the ability for students and faculty to post entries and comments. Blogs are webpages that can be password protected, making them available only to certain members. This is where the similarities to the wiki end. In a blog, only the owner of the blog can both edit and add content, while members can only add comments. The latest entry will appear first, and only one page is shown at a time. Blogs can become a resource for learning by containing links to other web sites about national trends and new techniques.[25] A blog can be used as a teaching supplement where invited members (adjunct faculty and clinical instructors) can add comments to complement the discussion. There are currently numerous blogs containing anesthesia-related information from universities all over the world that feature videos, lectures, and daily board review questions.[26]

Podcasting, also called mobile learning, is becoming a staple in the education of health care professionals and the public. Podcasting is a technology containing media files that can be audio, video, or both, and are available to be downloaded often with minimal or no cost. The advantage of podcasts is their convenience. They can be played back any time as long as the student has access to a digital media player. Podcasts allows for instructor flexibility since the video, and or audio, can be created ahead of time.

The advantage of audio is that it fits the auditory learner who needs to hear what others read to process the information. Although the meshing hypothesis, where providing instruction based on individuals' preferred learning styles improves learning, is currently challenged, offering audio in the form of a podcast offers an additional method of delivering material.[27] Audio can also be used to clarify instructions by allowing the instructor to emphasize important information utilizing his or her tone of voice. This is suitable for specific instructions or to clarify a difficult concept.

Camtasia (TechSmith Corp., Okemos, Michigan)[28] is a user-friendly software program, compatible with both Windows and Macintosh, that can be used to create asynchronous audio/video presentations. The presentation can be viewed by the student at any time and can include assignments, instructions, an overview of material such as the syllabus, or a complete lecture. During the recording, anything displayed on the presenter's computer screen, such as the cursor moving over a picture or table, is recorded. This allows the presenter to show pictures, slides, or demonstrations using onscreen instructions. A webcam can be used showing a demonstration while adding narration. Camtasia (most familiar to the author) allows for slides, video clips, and audio to be added via a microphone. The sound is typically of better quality if a separate microphone from the one on the computer is used. The recording can later be edited and reviewed before it's made available to students. Using Camtasia can be fun, creative, and save time in the classroom by providing basic information online to students in preparation for class. This allows the instructor to facilitate active discussion or problem-solving while in class.[29] Camtasia works very well for all those snow days and class cancelations. Make-up class time is no longer needed since the lecture is recorded and distributed to students electronically.

Who Are We Teaching and How Do They Learn?

The millennials presently entering nurse anesthesia programs have a unique learning style shaped by their views of the world. It is a different view from the generation teaching them, mostly baby boomers and Generation X. Teaching anesthesia has to mesh both with different learning styles, the difficulty of the topics, the volume of material, and time constraints of the program. Traditionally, and still in most academic settings, faculty teaching anesthesia are doing so based on their extensive experience and expertise. This means that the instructor was born in an earlier generation when the theories on learning and teaching were much different.

The millennial generation (also called Generation Y or Net Gen) was born after 1980. The term "millennial" comes from the notion that these individuals would turn 18 and enter the workforce at the turn of the millennium. Learning more about the millennial generation will help us understand their needs and characteristics. This generation is technologically savvy (20% percent began using computers between ages 5 and 8), multitasking, visual, and are better learners by actively doing and discovering in peer groups.[30,31] Personal connection, dialogue, cultural differences, and disruption are stimulating to this group. A quick insight into how well you know this generation can be accessed through The Pew Research Center online quiz from 2010: http://www.Pewresearch.Org/Quiz/How-Millennial-Are-You/)[32]

It is important to remember that the millennial learners are digital natives who constantly access technology and stay connected without constraint; they tend to live life in public. They communicate via technology with abbreviated text messages, pictures, or short videos. They grew up being able to Google anything for answers so facts and knowledge alone do not stimulate this group. They like collaboration, teamwork, and welcome a variety of active learning methods. They typically don't want to be lectured to, but like to engage both with their classmates and faculty. Although this group uses technology extensively, they think in terms of the activity that technology allows them to participate in. This generation feels that technology in education is offered as a convenience, but should not replace face-to-face interaction, which they like and expect.[31] They appreciate professors and instructors who show them the same interest as they have been receiving from their parents, which is important to remember during discussion boards when considering the frequency and amount of feedback given.

Millennials are visual learners. They retain only 10 percent of what they read but 20 to 30 percent of what they see.[33] First-year college students today have watched, on average, more than 15,000 hours of television. Add video games, iBooks, and other sophisticated technology and we can understand why they are visual learners.[34] Scanning web pages is different from reading paper text. Web pages are scanned rather than read using an "F" pattern where the top of the page is scanned followed by a look down the left column and once more to the right at the middle of the page.[35] Covering complex and large volumes of information, as needed in nurse anesthesia education, presents a challenge to this generation.

Flipping Generation Y

The flipped classroom model was introduced in 2000 by J. Wesley Baker and by Lage et al.[36,37] They proposed a model where traditional teacher-directed lectures were developed prior to class using recorded lectures and readings, leaving class time for problem-solving, hands-on activities, and group work presented by students. Since then the flipped classroom model has been incorporated into higher education including graduate nursing and medical schools.[38] Research conducted in the last decade evaluating the flipped classroom model found an advantage in the ability to cover more material, to accommodate students with different learning styles, and to increase student engagement.[39,40]

The flipped classroom teaching model is typically divided into two sections: material assigned to students before class, and material covered in class. The before class assignments are often used to teach lower-order cognitive skills, such as knowledge and comprehension.[41] It is important to remember that flipping the classroom does not have to involve technology in its delivery to be successful. The assignment may involve a book chapter with assigned questions, a recent article discussing new evidence-based practice, or a case report in the covered topic. It is beneficial to the students if basic information can be provided in multiple forms. This allows them to choose how to learn (audio, video, readings from books or online); choose a space to learn (commuting on the train, home, waiting in line, riding a stationary bike); and when to learn (day, evening, weekends) to best assimilate information.

Class time, or face-to-face time, is reserved for higher order cognitive skills such as application and analysis.[42] This could be accomplished through small group exercises to develop an anesthesia care plan, provide a short online quiz, open book problem-solve, facilitate discussion for article review, or review clinical scenarios. The pre-class assignment can include the development of presentations to their peers or presentation of research of a newly implemented anesthetic technique. It is important that the students receive clear objectives for each assignment and sufficient time to complete readings. Nurse anesthesia students are under time constraints from their clinical and didactic environments and need adequate time to access the preassigned material. One week is suggested to allow for pre-class assignments.[43]

Having students come prepared for class is one of the great challenges of the flipped classroom. Significant time and some creativity are required by the instructor before class to engage the students in the material. Having students write exam questions for each topic helps in understanding the difficulty of writing good exam questions and researching the material for answers. Distractors for multiple-choice questions engage students to examine details of the content. Listing priorities related to the anesthetic considerations of a condition or disease can be done in small groups initially and later presented as discussion of the best practices and plan of care. Remembering how this generation communicates and learns use short videos. They are a great way to trigger discussion.

Most faculty using the flipped classroom model would agree that it can encourage active learning and lead to increased student motivation, participation, and learning if prepared well. It is the students' responsibility to complete the assignment and come to class prepared. The preparation from faculty is necessary to accomplish "buy in" of the concept and can require plenty of marketing; the introduction is best done in small doses.[44] Clear objectives and instructions are other stepping stones to success. An important component to remember is that the adult learner needs to see relevance between pre-classroom assignments and classroom activities. If the material discussed in class does not match the assigned material, and the later content of exams, the students will reject this teaching tool and the flipped classroom model will most certainly flip.

As with mathematicians, a lot of our work as nurse anesthetists involves finding solutions to problems and complications that do not exist, or that we haven't experienced yet.[45] Knowing the material is important, but so is the problem-solving, research of best practices, engagement, team work, and resilience. Much of the time spent in graduate studies is a practice in teaching ourselves and researching new information. Fortunately, this mimics our professional lives as nurse anesthetists.

Playing Serious Games

Does playing video games in a class of graduate students sound far-fetched? Think again. How about assigning the students a video game before coming to class where the end result is recognition and treatment of malignant hyperthermia or anaphylactic shock? There's an idea. To the millennial learner, playing video games comes naturally and is a way to stay stimulated, challenged, and rewarded. Depending on the complexity of the game, advancement can demand both significant knowledge and critical thinking skills.[46] The remaining question to ask is: Should we utilize video games as a vehicle to deliver material in nurse anesthesia education?

Video games that are used for educational purposes are often referred to as "serious games" or games that serve a purpose.[47] Serious games are a form of computer-generated simulation that are often understood to include simulation, learning, and game. Serious games can be seen as an extension of simulation since they are generally not limited by certain rules or parameters and by being realistically dynamic and interactive. They keep students focused and engaged, which creates a potential conduit for enhanced learning.[48] The military is using games to train combat medics, and the aviation industry uses games to prepare pilots for emergencies. During the last decade, serious games have appeared in nursing, medicine, and health sciences to teach clinical reasoning, complex concepts, and technical skills.[49]

How can games assist in higher education? Many computer-based games take the participant through challenges with several levels of difficulty followed by rewards for advancing through the game. The game recognizes improvements, and more challenging scenarios are presented which motivates the participant to repeatedly go back to this simulated world full of stimulus, challenge, and reward. The game can be analyzed for actions and communication between participants, making evaluation, assessment, and debriefing possible.[50] Games could open up methods to engage and advance critical thinking in situations not often experienced in clinical practice, which might be important knowledge to retain for a specific patient condition or symptom.

Is this an effective way to learn? In a meta-analysis of recent studies assessing serious games as an effective educational tool, Girard et al examined 30 randomized controlled studies published between 2007–2011.[50] After applying all inclusion and exclusion criteria, nine studies remained. The authors concluded that although more empirical studies are needed, serious games can open new avenues for learning and provide access to conditions that can't be produced in real-world situations. Much of the conclusion was attributed to the effect of engagement the students show when learning through serious games.

Serious games are already being used to learn techniques and to assess critical patients and situations.[50] Games are being developed that allow the learner to change the course and outcome by changing direction. This allows for an unlimited number of outcomes and the learner advances to a higher level by completing skills and competencies that align with learning outcomes. In anesthesia, there are specific conditions, skills, and competencies that can't be practiced during students' clinical education, but still require specific knowledge and proficiency. Games can simulate these situations and allow the practitioner to refine the response, making critical decisions easier.

Summary

We are all lifelong learners. The way we teach and share our knowledge is changing with each new generation of students and new teaching methods. Being open to innovative and new ideas is already in our practice as nurse anesthetists. Our commitment to the profession and education keeps us inventive in creating new teaching methods for the next generations of nurse anesthetists.

References

1. Capra T. Special Focus: a consideration of online learning. *Thought & Action*. Fall 2014:111–120.

2. Pappas C. Top 10 E-Learning Statistics From 2014 You Need to Know. https://elearningindustry.com/top-10-e-learning-statistics-for-2014-you-need-to-know. December 1, 2013. Accessed May 17, 2016.

3. Prober CG, Heath C. Lecture halls without lectures—a proposal for medical education. *N Engl J Med*. 2012;366(18):1657–1659.

4. Esani M. Focus: Educational technology. Moving from face-to-face to online teaching. *Clin Lab Sci*. 2010;23(3):187–190.

5. Sherbino J, Chan T, Schiff K. The reverse classroom: lectures on your own and homework with faculty. *CJEM*. 2013;15(3):178–180.

6. Sener J. Definitions of E-Learning Courses and Programs Version 2.0. Online Learning Consortium. http://onlinelearningconsortium.org/updated-e-learning-definitions-2/. Published July 7, 2015. Accessed April 26, 2016.

7. Standards for Accreditation of Nurse Anesthesia Programs. Park Ridge, IL: Council on Accreditation of Nurse Anesthesia Programs; 2014.

8. Brewer PE, Brewer EC. Pedagogical perspectives for the online education skeptic. *J Excell Coll Teach*. 2015;26(1):29.

9. Fish WW, Wickersham LE. Best practices for online instructors: Reminders. *Quarterly Review of Distance Education*. 2009;10(3):279–284.

10. Allen IE, Seaman J. Changing Course: Ten Years of Tracking Online Education in the United States. Sloan Consortium. http://www.onlinelearningsurvey.com/reports/changingcourse.pdf. Published January, 2013. Accessed March 21, 2016.

11. Chiasson K, Terras K, Smart K. Faculty perceptions of moving: a face-to-face course to online instruction. *J Coll Teach Learn*. 2015;12(4):231–239.

12. Means B, Toyama Y, Murphy R, Bakia M, Jones K. Evaluation of evidence-based practices in online learning: a meta-analysis and review of online learning studies. U.S. Department of Education; 2009.

13. Pinchevsky-Font T, Dunbar S. Best practices for online teaching and learning in health care related programs. *Internet J Allied Health Sci Pract*. 2015;13(1):1–7.

14. Thiele JE. Learning patterns of online students. *J Nurs Educ*. 2003;42(8):364–366.

15. Edwards M, Perry B, Janzen K. The making of an exemplary online educator. *Dist Ed*. 2011;32(1):101–118.

16. Leibold N, Schwarz LM. The art of giving online feedback. *J Effect Teach*. 2015;15(1):34–46.

17. Cook DA, Levinson AJ, Garside S, Dupras DM, Erwin PJ, Montori VM. Internet-based learning in the health professions: a meta-analysis. *JAMA*. 2008;300(10):1181–1196.

18. Hayek C. How Many Faculty Discussion Posts Each Week? A Simply Delicious Answer. Faculty Focus. http://www.facultyfocus.com/articles/online-education/how-many-faculty-discussion-posts-each-week-a-simply-delicious-answer/. Published January 18, 2012. Accessed January 24, 2016.

19. Shea V, Shea C. *Netiquette*. San Francisco, CA: Albion Books; 1994.

20. Boulos MN, Maramba I, Wheeler S. Wikis, blogs and podcasts: a new generation of Web-based tools for virtual collaborative clinical practice and education. *BMC Med Educ*. 2006;6:41.

21. Wheeler S, Kelly P, Gale K. The influence of online problem-based learning on teachers' professional practice and identity. *ALT-J: Research in Learning Technology*. 2005;13(2):125–137.

22. 7 Things You Should Know About Wikis. Educause Library. https://library.educause.edu/resources/2005/7/7-things-you-should-know-about-wikis. Published July 15, 2005. Accessed March 12, 2016.

23. Sandars J. Twelve tips for using blogs and wikis in medical education. *Med Teach*. 2006;28(8):680–682.

24. Billings DM. Wikis and blogs: consider the possibilities for continuing nursing education. *J Contin Educ Nurs*. 2009;40(12):534–535.

25. Saichaie K, Benson J, Kumar AB. How we created a targeted teaching tool using blog architecture for anesthesia and critical care education—the A/e anesthesia exchange blog. *Med Teach*. 2014;36(8):675–679.

26. Chu LF, Young C, Zamora A, Kurup V, Macario A. Anesthesia 2.0: Internet-based information resources and Web 2.0 applications in anesthesia education. *Curr Opin Anaesthesiol*. 2010;23(2):218–227.

27. Rogowsky BA, Calhoun BM, Tallal P. Matching learning style to instructional method: effects on comprehension. *J Educ Psychol*. 2015;107(1):64–78.

28. TechSmith. Camtasia Studio, Version 8.6.0. Okemos, MI: TechSmith Corporation; 2002.

29. Schumacher G, Thurkettle MA. Camtasia studio: a teaching tool for academicians and clinicians. *Comput Inform Nurs*. 2007;25(3):130–134.

30. Oblinger D, Oblinger J. Is it age or IT: first steps toward understanding the net generation. In: Oblinger D, Oblinger J, eds. *Educating the Net Generation*. Educase; 2005:2.1–2.20.

31. Platt A. Teaching medicine to millennials. *J Physician Assist Edu*. 2010;21(2):42–44.

32. How Millennial Are You? Pew Research Center. http://www.pewresearch.org/quiz/how-millennial-are-you/. Published February 24, 2010. Accessed January 23, 2016.

33. Miller LK. Cooperative learning users groups: modeling cooperation. *Library of Oriental Service*. 1996:125–132.

34. Manuel K. Teaching information literacy to Generation Y. *J Libr Admin*. 2002;36(1/2):195–217.

35. Nielsen J. How Users Read on the Web. Jakob Nielsen's Alertbox. Nielsen Norman Group. https://www.nngroup.com/articles/how-users-read-on-the-web/. Published October 1,1997. Accessed January 24, 2016.

36. Baker J. The "Classroom Flip": Using Web Course Management Tools to Become The Guide By The Side. *Communication Faculty Publications*. Paper 15. http://digitalcommons.cedarville.edu/media_and_applied_communications_publications/15/. Published 2000. Accessed March 1, 2016.

37. Lage MJ, Platt GJ, Treglia M. Inverting the classroom: a gateway to creating an inclusive learning environment. *J Econ Educ*. 2000;31(1):30–43.

38. Critz CM, Knight D. Using the flipped classroom in graduate nursing education. *Nurse Educ*. 2013;38(5):210–213.

39. Kurup V, Hersey D. The changing landscape of anesthesia education: is Flipped Classroom the answer? *Curr Opin Anaesthesiol*. 2013;26(6):726–731.

40. Flipped Classroom Trends: A Survey Of College Faculty. Magna Publications. Faculty Focus. http://www.facultyfocus.com/free-reports/flipped-classroom-trends-a-survey-of-college-faculty/. Updated 2015. Accessed November 12, 2015.

41. Moffett J. Twelve tips for "flipping" the classroom. *Med Teach*. 2015;37(4):331–336.

42. Bristol T. Flipping the classroom 1. *Teaching and Learning in Nursing*. 2014;9(1):43–46.

43. Hawks SJ. The flipped classroom: now or never? *AANA J*. 2014;82(4):264–269.

44. McLaughlin JE, Roth MT, Glatt DM, et al. The flipped classroom: a course redesign to foster learning and engagement in a health professions school. *Acad Med*. 2014;89(2):236–243.

45. Demski J. 6 Expert Tips for Flipping the Classroom. Campus Technology. https://campustechnology.com/articles/2013/01/23/6-expert-tips-for-flipping-the-classroom.aspx. Published January 23, 2013. Accessed February 11, 2016.

46. Hahn J, Earle, Bartel C. Teaching gaming with technology in the classroom: so you want to be an educator? *Nurs Educ Perspect*. 2014;35(3):197–198.

47. Petit dit Dariel OJ, Raby T, Ravaut F, Rothan-Tondeur M. Developing the serious games potential in nursing education. *Nurse Educ Today*. 2013;33(12):1569–1575.

48. Breslin P, McGowan C, Pecheux B, Sudol R. Serious gaming. Advanced computer simulation games help to transform healthcare and disaster preparedness. *Health Manag Technol*. 2007;28(10):14.

49. Knight JF, Carley S, Tregunna B, et al. Serious gaming technology in major incident triage training: a pragmatic controlled trial. *Resuscitation*. 2010;81(9):1175–1179.

50. Girard C, Ecalle J, Magnan A. Serious games as new educational tools: how effective are they? A meta-analysis of recent studies. *J Comput Assist Learn*. 2013;29(3):207–219.

CHAPTER 20

Simulation-Based Education: Practical Approaches to Curriculum Integration

Celeste G. Villanueva, EdD, CRNA, FNAP

Keywords: Constructivism, experiential, interprofessional education, patient safety, simulation-based learning, simulation-based team training, TeamSTEPPS.

Key Concepts

- Advancing patient safety and quality of care are fundamental driving forces for simulation-based education (SBE).
- Simulation-based assessment as a component of certification and recertification of nurse anesthetists is a concept that is gaining acceptance.
- Constructivism, the overarching learning theory foundational to the intent and instructional design of simulation-based techniques, has multiple theories under its umbrella. Understanding how theories inform instructional design is essential to creating effective learning experiences.
- Curriculum designs for simulation integration that are longitudinal and integral to other curricular components enhance the effectiveness of SBE.
- Explicitly establishing and maintaining a safe psychological environment for learners throughout the entire curriculum contributes to transfer of learning.
- TeamSTEPPS is one example of a teamwork and communications framework that, when consistently integrated into simulation exercises, hones nontechnical skills.
- Artifacts from all simulation-based instructional techniques are useful as evidence of a program's educational effectiveness if explicit linkages between learning objectives of a simulation-based learning activity and the desired competencies are established.
- Simulation-based crew resource management and simulation-based team training are strategies that improve patient safety. All health care professional programs should have team-training elements in their curricula.
- Nurse anesthesia programs should strive to incorporate an anesthesia crisis resource management component into the curriculum, emphasizing development of anesthesia nontechnical skills.
- Collaborative efforts across programs will accelerate the development of standardized curricular components and centralized resources to assist educators in the development and maintenance of effective simulation programs.

Introduction

A provocative statement regarding simulation was published in 1992: "...no industry in which human lives depend on the skilled performance of responsible operators has waited for unequivocal proof of the benefits of simulation before embracing it.... Neither should anesthesiology."[1] That call to action spawned volumes of literature, countless hours of education and training using simulation, and many well-designed studies seeking the ultimate proof of its benefit. Yet in 2004, the same author continued musing whether or not the year 2025 would see simulation-based education inextricably woven into the fabric of our health care system.[2] It appears that we are on the right track—the worldwide adoption of health care simulation and the scientific literature that chronicles and supports this phenomenon are described by O'Donnell and Phrampus in Chapter 14. They provide a comprehensive overview of instructional design principles for simulation scenario development and outline what are considered best practices in the crucial practice of debriefing simulation activity. This chapter is intended to complement Chapter 14's content by providing information and resources to enhance effective integration of simulation-based education (SBE) into the nurse anesthetist's practice, whether that practice has an educational or clinical focus. That said, most of the information primarily applies to educators charged with developing or enhancing the simulation component of a program's curriculum. The goal is to offer information and ideas that lead to the creation of a cohesive set of simulation-based learning (SBL) activities that integrate it well with other academic and clinical components of a curriculum, resulting in a high-quality learning experience for students.

Driving Forces for Simulation-Based Education

The veritable explosion of interest and investment in simulation extends beyond the domains traditionally associated with health care, which include the core professions of medicine (allopathic, osteopathic, podiatric); nursing (all categories of licensure, practice, degree and discipline); pharmacy; and dentistry, as well as the plethora of allied health professions. Other major stakeholders in health care—certification/licensure entities; accrediting organizations; malpractice insurance companies; nongovernmental agencies (eg, the National Academy of Medicine, the Institute of Healthcare Improvement); international agencies, such as the World Health Organization; and health care consumers are included in the list of powerful forces that drive the continued evolution of SBE. Educators, especially the program administrators who interact with institutional decision makers, should be conversant in the origins and facts supporting the existence of these forces in preparation for making a case—business, strategic planning, or curricular—for a simulation-related project. The following section provides more detail on these driving forces.

Patient Safety and Quality of Care

It is widely acknowledged that a key driver—possibly the strongest driver—for the use of simulation-based techniques for health care education, practice, and research is patient safety.[3–10] The Institute of Medicine (IOM), now called the National Academy of Medicine (NAM), ignited the flame for an overhaul of the U.S. health care system at the beginning of the 21st century in their landmark report *To Err is Human*,[11] which had astonishing revelations about the number of patient deaths: up to 98,000 of them annually due to medical errors and major shortcomings in patient safety. In the report, simulation is specifically mentioned many times as an important component of patient safety initiatives but most notably as part of Recommendation 8.1: "Patient safety programs should...establish interdisciplinary team training programs for providers that incorporate proven methods of team training, such as simulation."[11(p.14)] Contemporary accounts of the history of medical simulation, especially those published in anesthesiology literature, often begin with events in the 1960s[12–15]; however, with the linkages between simulation and patient safety expressed more publicly and urgently,[16–18] and the expanded scope from *medical* simulation to *health care* simulation, the turn of the 21st century marks what has been called the simulation revolution.[19–21]

Nearly five years after the raft of patient safety initiatives launched as a result of the 2000 IOM report, Wachter, the project director in charge of the *Making Health Care Safer* report essentially gave the U.S. a report card on its progress toward improved patient safety in five broad categories (regulation, error-reporting systems, information technology, the malpractice system and other vehicles for accountability, and workforce and training issues).[22] His overall assessment was that little progress had been made, a lamentable perspective shared by many patient safety leaders at the time. However, in the category of workforce and training, Wachter stated that signs of progress were definitely evident and singled out simulation, specifically for the purposes of team training, as an area of great promise, whose evolution into a required element of health care professionals' education would be a welcome development.

Patient safety continues to be a powerful motivator for simulation integration into the lifelong education of health care professionals, into research agendas,[23–25] and into the fabric of the patient care delivery systems. This is true both in the U.S. and abroad, as Byrne[26] illustrates in his account of the current state of government regulatory influences on patient safety regulation in the United States, Canada, and the United Kingdom (UK). There is sparse literature on formal patient safety programs that involve the use of simulation in Asia, Africa, or South America, where there are growing numbers of simulation centers. A framework for patient safety research and improvement has been proposed by preeminent U.S. patient safety thought leaders; one recommendation made for future directions is, "Use simulation to: evaluate teamwork and technical work, train staff to translate evidence into practice, and to identify and mitigate hazards."[24(p.336)] One last indicator of how influential patient safety is as a factor for continued use of simulation is the existence of an ongoing, multimillion dollar portfolio of simulation research projects funded by the Agency for Healthcare Research and Quality (AHRQ). The AHRQ is a federal agency under the aegis of the U.S. Department of Health & Human Services whose mission is to produce the evidence to make health care safer; higher quality; more accessible, equitable, and affordable; and to work with multiple partner agencies to ensure that the scientific evidence is understood and applied in practice. Since 2007, AHRQ has funded well over $10 million in research to advance knowledge of how simulation can improve patient safety,[27] and their commitment to steady, robust support for advancing the evidence base for simulation, especially as it relates to patient safety, is ongoing.[28]

Simulation-Enhanced Interprofessional Education

There is a global movement taking place, parallel to the worldwide adoption of health care simulation, that is aimed at developing and strengthening the skills of health professions' students to more effectively communicate and collaborate in interprofessional health care teams.[29,30] Long before patient care was declared a team sport, and team training characterized as a national obsession,[31] an interprofessional group of health professions' educators presciently stated that it would be interdisciplinary team practice and community-responsive health care providers with strong teamwork skills who would play the critical roles in improving the health care system.[32] Since Connors made this prediction, significant, albeit slow, progress is evident, specifically in health professions' education, where systematic approaches to break down traditional professional silos and focus on collaborative, patient-centered care are the imperatives. A summary report of two international workshops hosted by NAM contains detailed, comprehensive examples of diverse approaches to interprofessional education (IPE) that focus on teamwork and collaboration.[33] This report provides evidence of the current surge of educational redesign efforts by educators of health professionals. A compelling key message brought to light in the NAM summary report is that students crave a more interprofessional approach to learning; furthermore, employers of health professionals (Veteran's Health Administration, Kaiser Permanente, and the National Health Service of the United Kingdom) are voicing concern that novice health professionals entering the present workforce generally do not possess the requisite skills to work in a collaborative environment.[34] These two points clearly indicate that there is much more to accomplish in terms of redesigning health professions' education so that the goal of collaborative practice is a more attainable reality.

The patient safety movement is yet another powerful driver for developing teamwork and communication skills in graduates of health professions programs (as well as in experienced health care providers), specifically as a strategy to reduce medical errors. The sobering reality is that the original statistic of 98,000 deaths cited by the 2000 IOM report[11] was a major underestimation, and that patient harm from human error continues to be a significant problem. In 2013, based on much more accurate data analysis, the number of premature deaths associated with preventable harm to patients in hospitals was estimated to be more than 400,000.[35] More recently, it was suggested that medical error ranks as the third most common cause of death, based on extrapolated human error study data gathered between 1999 and 2013.[36] The good news is that root causes for the human errors that result in patient harm have been well-studied—a key source of such root cause analysis data is the Joint Commission, which publishes annual data related to sentinel events. Joint Commission data from 2011–2014 consistently show that the top three root causes for sentinel events are: human factors, leadership, and communication.[37] This is consistent with Wachter's[38] reporting of the common etiologies of errors in health care. The burgeoning global movement promoting the adoption of TeamSTEPPS (Team Strategies and Tools to Enhance Performance and Patient Safety)[39,40] as the standard communication and teamwork framework for entire health care systems is founded on the premise that establishing and sustaining teams that engage in collaborative, interprofessional, patient-centered practice is a critical strategy for reducing the unacceptably high error rate in health care. The integration of TeamSTEPPS within our nurse anesthesia program curriculum is discussed later in this chapter.

The term simulation-based IPE (SBIPE) is used to refer to the use of any type of simulation technique to enhance IPE. Robertson and Bandali's call to "bridge the gap"[41(p.449)] between IPE and health care simulation makes strong arguments for building an evidence base for SBIPE using patient safety and the widespread efforts underway to redesign health professions' educational curricula as ammunition for their position. Their case is made more compelling by the addition of the organizational imperatives to eliminate silo mentality from institutional cultures, transforming them into truly interprofessional entities. They also bring to light that the vast majority of the SBIPE literature is centered about physicians and nurses, and call for a widening of the lenses used for scientific inquiry to include all health professions (ie, pharmacy) and all applied health professions (a term synonymous to allied health professions). Simulation-based IPE is the subject of two recent systematic reviews.[42,43] Each review used slightly different inclusion criteria but there are three commonalities in their conclusions worth noting. First, the vast majority of studies (76%[43]–91%[42]) were published in 2007 or later, indicating the nascent stage of the SBIPE domain. Second, both reviews found that greater than 50% of the studies involved the professions of medicine or nursing only. Small percentages (18%[42]–28%[43]) of the reviewed studies involved physicians, nurses, and at least one other professional group. This finding justifies the concern articulated by Robertson and Bandali about the lack of exploration around IPE, based on realistic compositions of health teams. In other words, studying groups of doctors and nurses (even if there are multiple disciplines of each) will not necessarily yield results that can be applied to the whole health care team. Third, studies with research questions related to SBIPE lack rigor in study design, data analysis, and presentation of findings. These shortcomings primarily reflect the individual complexity and dynamic nature of the topics (IPE and SBE) and the challenges of combining the two into a cogent line of inquiry.

Examples of current SBIPE programs that show promise in terms of meeting criteria for rigor in instructional design and program evaluation are showcased in a comprehensive report on IPE,[33] and a comprehensive simulation text.[44] Recent studies involving nurse anesthesia students[45,46] are other examples of an encouraging trend. Simulation-based IPE (also called simulation-enhanced IPE) has established itself as a newly emerged field with health care simulation becoming the "preferred vehicle for IPE."[47(p.114)] This notion is not confined to U.S. thought leaders. During a recent global forum on innovation in health professional education, the appeal of using simulation as an innovative pedagogical approach to IPE was reported as a key workshop finding. Despite the many barriers to its widespread adoption, "simulation is generally thought to be an important tool for interprofessional education."[33(p.71)]

Simulation and Certification

The provocative topic of incorporating simulation into high-stakes assessment for anesthesiologists and nurse anesthetists is often raised during discussions of SBE. This is a complex issue that is of intense interest, largely driven by the many forces—both internal and external to our discipline—that demand the demonstration and documentation of professional competence throughout a provider's practice lifetime. Many challenges to incorporating simulation into professional certification processes exist, not the least of which is the fact that unequivocal evidence linking simulation-based assessments to competency in the clinical setting is lacking.[48,49] Simulation-based performance assessment has been incorporated into anesthesiology board examinations by the Israeli Board of Anesthesiology Examination Committee since 2003.[50,51] The Israeli national program of simulation-based assessment, which includes, but is not limited to, standardized patients and highly realistic, immersive mannequin-based simulations (MBS), has been expanded to include certification of paramedics as well as certification for nurse specialists in 16 nursing professions.[52] To date, Israel appears to be the only country requiring the use of simulation for high-stakes assessment as the basis for professional specialty certification or licensure.

Since 2004, in the U.S. and Canada, high stakes assessment using the standardized patient simulation technique has been incorporated into the licensing exams required for entry into the medical profession: the United States Medical Licensing Exam, Step 2 Clinical Skills, and the Medical Council of Canada Qualifying Examination, Part II. The value of these exams (in identifying individuals with clinical skill deficiencies and promulgating educational activities focused on ensuring clinical competence) has been well-supported by research.[48] In 2010, the American Board of Anesthesiology (ABA) instituted a required simulation component into its Maintenance of Certification in Anesthesiology (MOCA), Part IV program. The requirement is not a high-stakes assessment; rather, ABA diplomats must attend and self-reflect upon a simulation-based course that has been approved by the American Society of Anesthesiologists' (ASA) Committee on Simulation Education.[53] Guidelines are established for simulation-based MOCA courses; however, the specific content and structure of a curriculum is determined by the individual simulation programs approved to provide MOCA Part IV courses. Analyses of the initial implementation years of simulation-based MOCA requirements have been published.[54,55] For the most part, the response of ABA diplomats who have completed a simulation-based continuing education course report that the experience had educational value and was clinically relevant.[54–56] Opposing perspectives to maintenance of certification requirements are also evident not just from anesthesiologists,[49] but also from representatives of other medical specialties.[57–59]

Certification and recertification requirements for nurse anesthetists, as currently overseen by the National Board of Certification & Recertification for Nurse Anesthetists, do not include a simulation-based activity. A new Continued Professional Certification Program (CPC) officially went into effect in August 2016. There is a call for a national dialogue among nurse anesthesia stakeholders focusing on this relatively new CPC.[60] These authors advocate considering alternative CPC processes, including integrating SBE and simulation-based assessment techniques into the certification process—I strongly support such a notion. The Council on Accreditation of Nurse Anesthesia Educational Programs (COA), in a position paper on the value of simulation in nurse anesthesia education,[61] calls out Standard E.11 of the *Standards for Accreditation of Nurse Anesthesia Programs—Practice Doctorate* requiring that "simulated clinical experiences are incorporated into the curriculum."[62] The COA also posits that SBE will eventually be a component of the lifelong educational spectrum of all students entering the health care professions, including certification/recertification components and certification for employment requirements. This bodes well for continued evolution of simulation-related standards, policies, and procedures specific to nurse anesthesia educational programs.

Most simulation experts concur on the notion that a wide spectrum of simulation-based assessment methods will almost certainly be a requirement for certification, re-certification, and continuing education across all medical subspecialties, and possibly across all health care disciplines.[52,56,63] Thus, it is essential that nurse anesthetists, as a group, are well-informed, credible in the delivery of SBE, and engaged in collaborative efforts when making critical decisions about simulation as it relates to certification and recertification.

Malpractice Premium Incentives

Another compelling fact supporting a case for aggressive simulation integration to educational programs is in the growing number of medical specialties that use simulation, specifically crew/crisis resource management (CRM) training, as a risk management strategy.[64,65] The Controlled Risk Insurance Company (CRICO), Risk Management Foundation (RMF) of the Harvard Medical Institutions, in collaboration with the Center for Medical Simulation (CMS) of Cambridge, Massachusetts, set the prototype for an incentive program for discounted malpractice insurance premiums. In 2001, anesthesiologists who completed an 8-hour CRM training course provided by CMS were given discounted premiums of 6% below the usual rate. CRICO's 2006 actuarial analysis compared the malpractice claims numbers of anesthesiologists who had undergone the CRM with those who had not completed the program. The decreased number of claims of those who had completed the program was significant enough for CRICO to increase the discount to 25% in 2006.[66] Data regarding results for insurance premium incentive programs through CRICO for Certified Registered Nurse Anesthetists employed by Harvard Medical Institutions has not been reported in the literature. In 2003, based on the success of the anesthesiology premium discount incentive program, CRICO launched a similar program for obstetricians and gynecologists with similar success patterns evident.[66–68] The model of simulation-based CRM (also referred to as simulation-based team training, SBTT) as a quality risk management strategy is gaining traction with other risk management companies and across multiple clinical specialties, although concrete data in the peer-reviewed literature is sparse. This observation is based on my personal observations in recent years as a presenter and attendee at annual conferences of the Society for Simulation in Healthcare. I am also the co-developer/lead faculty of the curriculum for the in situ (in hospital) SBTT component of a perinatal patient safety program (PPSP) implemented in 2013–2016 for a large health care system in Northern California. The health care system's insurance services company funded the multimillion dollar program as part of an obstetric safety/risk management initiative. A program evaluation study on the educational effectiveness of the simulation-based team training we offered during this PPSP is in progress.

Trends in Higher Education

A final category of current driving forces for SBE is related to the current climate and realities of higher education. Most students enrolled in nurse anesthesia education programs come from the generations identified as Generation X (born between 1965–1980) and Generation Y, most commonly referred to as millennials (born between 1981–1997).[69] Interestingly, these two generations, despite having age ranges less than two decades apart, have notably different sets of collective values and characteristics, and both generations have different value sets from the baby boomer generation, which comprises approximately 42% of practicing nurse anesthetists.[70] Members of Generation X and millennials have commonalities when it comes to technology and how it affects every aspect of their lives. Frand,[71] in describing their set of attitudes and aptitudes, refers to the information-age mindset, developed as a result of growing up in a culture described as globally connected, service and information intense, and digitally-based. The pedagogical implications of this mindset are further outlined; an important one being that students prefer—and learn more effectively—via experiential, interactive, and authentic learning methodologies.[72]

The findings and recommendations delineated in seminal reports on the medical and nursing education research studies funded by the Carnegie Foundation for the Advancement of Teaching[73,74] call for a radical redesign of education practices in both professions, in large part because of the significant changes in the nature of today's health care systems, and its demands on practitioners and the learners who are entering the professions. But despite the compelling case made for changes in education that reflect the generational and global contexts of our current century, faculty of the health professions, by and large, are still teaching primarily according to 20th and even 19th century paradigms. Recent literature looking specifically at the pedagogic approach and the teaching/learning skill sets of medical and nursing educators confirm the persistence of pre-21st century thinking. While academic faculty are generally aware of the critical need for health professions' educational programs to keep pace with the continuously accelerating speed of information management, emerging technologies (both for clinical practice and for education), new approaches to learning, and the need to scale up curricular delivery models to accommodate a wider scope of learners, as an aggregate, there is a significant gap between what is expected of faculty and what they are able to deliver.[75,76]

The SBL techniques and curricular characteristics described in the following section are ways to meet a distinct need—indeed, an expectation—of the students that enter our programs. Contemporary nurse anesthesia students not only tend to have the information-age mindset as previously described, they often have backgrounds that include the use of SBL either during their pre-licensure nursing programs or via hospital-based, point-of-care (in situ) simulations in which they have participated as registered nurses. Furthermore, based on recent surveys of practicing CRNAs,[77,78] it is evident that a significant majority of our colleagues appear to strongly favor the use of SBL in academic programs (89% in the Hawkins study[78]), and indicate positive views of a simulation component to certification and recertification. Potential nurse anesthesia students should not only expect an academic program to have access to a simulation facility, they should be confident that their education will include a well-designed, effective SBL component, which brings us to the core topic of this chapter: curriculum integration.

Curricular Integration of Simulation-Based Education

A common message that simulation experts repeatedly deliver when providing advice on the appropriate use of simulation technologies is "it's all about the curriculum."

Glavin[79] describes a curriculum as "a statement of how learners can achieve a prescribed set of abilities that will equip them to identify and solve the problems they will face after they complete their program of study." The value of any simulation technology purchased does not depend on how much it costs or even how well the user can operate it. It depends on how well the technology user understands the content and the logic of an educational program's curriculum and how it leverages the interactive nature of a simulator to accomplish the curricular goals. A simulation program that is well integrated into a curriculum optimally matches the functionality of a type of simulator and the design of a simulation to a specific set of learning objectives. Furthermore, those learning objectives should be aligned with the designated learning outcomes and competencies upon which a program curriculum is constructed. In this section, an exemplar of simulation integration into a nurse anesthesia educational curriculum is used as a practical point of reference for discussion of relevant concepts.

Where and how does one begin to infuse simulation-based methodologies into an established nurse anesthesia program curriculum? Much of the answer to this question depends on the range of the program's inventory of (or access to) simulators; the availability of facilities (eg, a simulation center or dedicated laboratory space for simulation) and infrastructure (eg, trained simulation technical staff, information technology, and audiovisual support staff); the number of nurse anesthesia faculty trained in simulation instructional methods; and the level of philosophical and fiscal support provided by institutional administrators from the program level through the higher administrative echelons of an academic or hospital institution. An essential first step is to identify and empower a designated simulation champion, described by Medley[80] as "a faculty member who believes in the technology, is informed and excited about its use, and has a 'contagious' effect on other faculty members." Program administrators would be wise to designate resources for such an individual or individuals and develop a strategic plan to establish a core group of faculty skilled in the implementation of simulation- based learning.

Faculty development in SBE is a topic beyond the scope of this chapter, though the importance of faculty competence in the pedagogical areas relevant to simulation cannot be stressed enough. Other authors have focused on this topic,[81–83] all of them reiterating the observation of McGaghie's group that the role of instructors responsible for delivering SBE is ill-defined, if not mysterious,[84] and considers training of instructors a great unmet need. Despite the literature gap in this area, there are guidelines for faculty development that are emerging. Jeffries' group describes what they discovered about faculty development while implementing the landmark, 10-site simulation study for the National Council of State Boards of Nursing.[85] A set of recommendations they make reflect strategies that are essential to the success of our institution's nurse anesthesia simulation program: the establishment of a simulation team (primarily comprising program graduates who experienced SBE as students and strongly believe in the power of learning using simulation); the appointment of a simulation coordinator (a CRNA faculty trained and experienced in SBE) who oversees the simulation team; and the presence of an institutional network of professionals with expertise in supporting teaching and learning. This network extends well beyond the expert faculty and staff of the simulation center—it includes instructional designers, multi-media specialists, and others skilled in the applications of learning technology.

Table 20.1 Program of Nurse Anesthesia Simulation-Based Learning Curriculum

Simulation-based learning (SBL) activity	Instructional method: Brief description	Curriculum placement (Integrated nurse anesthesia curriculum) • Semester/clinical phase in program (I-III); Title of course associated with activity • Primary goal of activity	Hours per student
1. Introduction to simulation concepts	Lecture/Discussion: Orientation to conceptual foundations of simulation, establishing expectations for a safe psychological environment during any simulation-based activity	• Semester I/Pre-clinical; Basic Principles I • Establish ground rules for SBL sessions, explain program philosophy, establish a relaxed alertness environment[a] and a safe container[b]	2
2. TeamSTEPPS (TS) Fundamentals Course[c]	Interactive seminar/small group activity: 4-hour TS training course equivalent to courses implemented for direct providers of clinical care; PNA faculty are TS Master Trainers	• Semester I/Pre-clinical; Basic Principles I • Provide foundational knowledge of a standardized, internationally recognized teamwork and communication framework; set expectation for students to apply the TS principles and tools in all settings (academic, clinical, simulation, personal)	4
3. Orientation to OR environment & induction sequence	Experiential: Orientation to OR work environment (all aspects) and online orientation to induction sequence	• Semester I/Pre-clinical; Basic Principles I • Establish sensory familiarity with the environment and general overview of team roles early in training	8
4. Introduction to positioning in the OR	Lecture/Discussion, followed by experiential (role-play/standardized patient): Orientation to positioning, padding, and patient movement onto and off the OR table	• Semester I/ Pre-clinical; Basic Principles I • Practice principles of safe positioning	4
5. Introduction to induction – general endotracheal anesthesia (GETA)	Demonstration with MBS[d]: Modeling by various faculty of proper sequencing, technique, decision-making	• Semester I/Pre-clinical; Basic Principles I • Provide exemplars for psychomotor, cognitive, and affective skills for basic induction	4
6. Preoperative planning sessions with supervised practice of GETA or GA with laryngeal mask airway (LMA)	Lecture/Discussion/Group Work/Role-play, followed by experiential with MBS: Series of 3 case-based lectures, each followed by mock preoperative assessment exercise; student develops anesthetic plan, presents plan to faculty (authentic preceptor), implements simulated induction under supervision; incrementally complex patients	• Semester I/Pre-clinical; Basic Principles I • Develop assessment and clinical reasoning skills; early bridging of theory to practice (actual implementation of a plan); deliberate practice opportunities provided outside course activity	12

7. Technical skills workshops (not a comprehensive listing of sessions)	Lecture/Discussion, followed by experiential: Didactic instruction followed by repetitive, supervised practice utilizing an array of task trainers/ simulators including: 1. Airway trainers (basic & difficult) 2. Back simulators 3. Central venous access/peripheral nerve block trainer (with ultrasound capability) 4. SimSuite: central venous access simulator for cardiology, housed in simulation center at clinical affiliate site 5. Task trainers for fiberoptic intubation skills development (including dexterity trainers) 6. Arterial line insertion task trainer	• Semester 1/Pre-clinical: Basic Principles I • Basic airway management	8
		• Semester 1/Pre-clinical: Basic Principles I • Advanced airway management	6
		• Semester 1/Pre-clinical: Basic Principles I • SAB/Epidural insertion/management (basics)	4
		• Semester 2/Clinical Phase I: Basic Principles II • SAB/Epidural insertion/management	4
		• Semester 2/Clinical Phase I: Basic Principles II • Peripheral nerve block insertion/management	12
		• Semester 2/Clinical Phase I: Basic Principles II • Arterial line insertion	1
		• Semester 3 or 4/Clinical Phase II: Advanced Principles I or II • Advanced airway management II (Difficult airway management and neonatal resuscitation program)	8
		• Semester 3/Clinical Phase I: Advanced Principles I • Thoracic anesthesia airway management	4
		• Semester 3, 4, or 5/Clinical Phase II: Advanced Principles I or II • Possible opportunity for simulated central line (CVC and PAC) insertion using SimSuite (through partnering simulation center)	4
8. Anesthesia machine seminars	• Lecture/Demonstration, followed by experiential: hands-on practice with machine check, troubleshooting during MBS scenarios • Computer-basedsimulation (IP)[e]	• Semester 1/Pre-clinical; Basic Principles I • Focus of initial seminars on basic competence and safety; all subsequent MBS scenarios reinforce competencies related to anesthesia machine operation and troubleshooting	16

Simulation-based learning (SBL) activity	Instructional method: Brief description	Curriculum placement	Hours per student
9. Advanced health assessment skills workshops	Lecture/Demonstration, followed by experiential using: 1. Harvey (cardiopulmonary simulator) 2. Standardized Patients, culminating in an OSCE[f]	• Semester I/Pre-clinical; Advanced Health Assessment course • Refinement of assessment skills (for both pre- and post-op patients)	
10. Clinical orientation workshop	Demonstration, followed by experiential: Series of hands-on workshops comprising teaching stations (with preceptors) dedicated to essential anesthetic tasks and skills: 1. Drug and equipment setup 2. Positioning and monitoring 3. Documentation 4. Sterile technique for neuraxial block placement 5. Malignant hyperthermia protocol 6. Basic pediatric drug/equipment setup 7. Bier blocks	• Semester I/Pre-clinical; Basic Principles I • Reinforcement of concepts from lectures and previous lab sessions to foster students' confidence and ability to practice safely during initiation to clinical residency; near-peer instruction used heavily.	4
11. Assessment of preparedness to enter clinical residency	Experiential (MBS): Student completes the following steps of a simulated basic case: 1. Preoperative assessment (on a standardized patient) 2. Presentation of plan to authentic CRNA preceptor 3. Pre-surgical briefings (Joint Commission protocols) 4. General anesthesia induction 5. General anesthesia emergence 6. Transition of care to PACU RN	• Semester I/Pre-clinical; Basic Principles I (end of semester) • Assessment of competency in essential knowledge, skills, and behaviors related to a basic induction of general anesthesia associated with a common post-induction/post-emergence anesthetic complication; foster student confidence and ability to practice safely during initiation to clinical residency • Students must attain a threshold numerical score on the assessment checklist in order to progress into the clinical curriculum; remediation opportunities are available	4

12. Pathophysiology integrative simulation sessions	• Experiential with highly realistic MBS: Two, 4-hour sessions in which student triads are presented with scenarios related to a pathophysiologic condition recently reviewed/studied in the associated course; teaching in action occurs; each student required to: 1. Plan for and implement preoperative patient preparation. 2. Implement a simulated induction, maintenance, and emergence phase of the anesthetic (GETA required) 3. Manage common complications (mild to severe degrees), related to the particular patient co-morbidity. • Experiential with computer-based simulation (IP)	• Semester 2/Clinical Phase I; Pathophysiology & Basic Principles II • Reinforcement of physiology and pathophysiology concepts gained via reading, lecture/discussions, and clinical experience and synthesis of cognitive and technical knowledge; clinical reasoning and decision-making also a focus	8
13. Pediatric GETA mock induction sessions	Lecture/Discussion, followed by experiential with MBS: Each student is required to prepare for and implement a GETA induction on an infant	• Semester 2/Clinical Phase I; Basic Principles II • Application of principles of pediatric anesthetic management to practice; foster student confidence and safe practice prior to first encounter with pediatric patient during clinical experience	4
14. Basic acute pain management: ultrasound guided regional block workshop	Experiential (task trainer and standardized patient (SP) simulation): Faculty supervised ultrasound guided regional anesthesia practicum using SPs, with emphasis on anatomical recognition of specific critical landmarks, as well as appropriate patient interaction during procedure; additional skills training accomplished and regional anesthesia insertion task trainer (SimuLab)	• Semester 2/Clinical Phase I; Advanced Principles of Anesthesia II • Reinforcement of ultrasound guided regional anesthesia principles obtained via coursework and in the clinical setting, with emphasis on clinical reasoning, decision-making, and image recognition; major concepts of anesthesia non-technical skills as related to ultrasound anesthesia	8
15. High-risk obstetric anesthesia simulation sessions (IP)	Experiential with MBS and standardized patients: seminar in ACRM-type[g] format with all scenarios related to high-risk obstetrical patients; designed as interprofessional learner sessions for nurse anesthesia students with pre-licensure nursing students enrolled in their maternal-child clinical rotation	• Semester 4/Clinical Phase II; Advanced Principles I • Reinforcement of obstetrical anesthesia management principles obtained via reading, lecture/discussions, and clinical experience, with emphasis on clinical reasoning and decision-making; major concepts of TeamSTEPPS	4

Simulation-based learning (SBL) activity	Instructional method: Brief description	Curriculum placement	Hours per student
16. Neuroanesthesia and trauma anesthesia simulation sessions (IP)	Experiential (MBS and standardized patients): seminar in ACRM-like format with all scenarios related either to neurosurgical or trauma patients; interprofessional learners will likely be present (varies according to ability to coordinate schedule availability of other learners)	• Semester 4/Clinical Phase II; Advanced Principles II • Reinforcement of neuroanesthesia and trauma anesthesia management principles obtained via reading, lecture/discussions, and clinical experience, with emphasis on clinical reasoning, decision-making, and continued development of TeamSTEPPS	4
17. Advanced acute & chronic pain management	Lecture/Discussion, followed by experiential (task trainers): Didactic followed by advanced techniques in acute & chronic ultrasound guided regional peripheral nerve blocks utilizing regional insertion task trainers	• Semester 6/Clinical Phase III; Advanced Acute & Chronic Pain Management • Reinforcement of acute and chronic pain management principles and clinical techniques	8
18. Anesthesia crisis resource management I	Lecture/Discussion, followed by experiential (MBS): sessions using the ACRM format (heavily based on the Gaba/Stanford model)[h] Six complex, highly realistic scenarios (adult and pediatric patients), situated in a variety of anesthetizing locations are presented to learners in groups of 6; sessions are 8 hours in duration; each student immersed in 2 scenarios throughout the 8-hr. session; a mandatory 4-hour preparatory seminar is provided prior to the ACRM I sessions	• Semester 6/Clinical Phase III; Component of Masters of Science in Nursing Synthesis requirement[i] • Build upon the teamwork and communication goals articulated in TeamSTEPPS; hone knowledge and skills required to manage perioperative crisis situations; practice using cognitive aids (checklists) in the management of critical events; this is classified as simulation-based team training (not interprofessional education)	12
19. Anesthesia crisis resource management II	Experiential with MBS: ACRM session as described above; scenarios are more complex and include 2 high-risk obstetric situations	• Semester 7/Clinical Phase III; Component of Master of Science in Nursing Synthesis requirement • Further refinement of all skills described for ACRM I with emphatic focus during scenario debriefings to bring the team training lessons into their clinical practice as Certified Registered Nurse Anesthetists	8

20. Interprofessional simulation sessions with podiatric medicine students (Selected students are provided this optional opportunity)	Experiential with MBS: student nurse anesthetists take the role of instructor for second-year podiatric medical students who are enrolled in a clinical rotation run entirely in the simulation center to prepare them for hospital and clinic rotations	• Semester 6 or 7/Clinical Phase III; Clinical Anesthesia V or VI • Primary goal for students: instruct podiatric peers in proper execution of pre-surgical briefings, and facilitate the development of interpersonal and communication skills between anesthetists and surgeons during a conscious sedation/local anesthetic case, and during an intraoperative crisis (eg, anaphylaxis)	(4)
21. Interprofessional team practice for error management (Elective interprofessional education course offered by SMU; a small number of second-year nurse anesthesia students voluntarily enroll in this course)	Experiential, using a unique combination of PBL and SBL (standardized patient encounters) plus multiple other modes of immersive instructional techniques; student nurse anesthetists are immersed in dynamic clinical situations as members of a health care team with students from other disciplines (medicine, pre-licensure RN, nurse practitioners, nurse case managers, physical therapy, occupational therapy)	• Semester 4 and 5/Clinical Phase II; Clinical Anesthesia III or IV • Primary goal for students: to learn how an interprofessional team of health care practitioners can effectively prevent, recognize, mitigate, manage and disclose errors that occur in clinical practice	(27)

a The optimal emotional state for learning as described by Caine's Brain-Based Learning Framework.Nummela Caine R, Caine G, McClintic C, Klimek KJ. *12 Brain/Mind Learning Principles in Action – Developing Executive Functions of the Human Brain,* 2nd ed. Thousand Oaks, CA: Corwin Press; 2009.

b See section in the text describing establishment of a psychologically safe environment (concept of a Safe Container).

c This course is a component of the open source TeamSTEPPS® (TS) curriculum provided by the Agency for Healthcare Research and Quality (AHRQ) and the Department of Defense. See text for explanation of the acronym, TeamSTEPPS®. TeamSTEPPS@SMU is a university-wide initiative initiated in 2014 with the goal to provide all faculty, staff, administrative leaders, and students with the recommended level of training in the TS teamwork and communication framework.

d MBS: Mannequin-based simulation. Throughout the curriculum, close attention is paid to aligning how much physical resemblance to clinical reality is required for each simulation session and how best to match the learning objectives with the technical sophistication of the full body mannequin. Levels of "fidelity" are not used to describe the type of mannequin used.

e IP: In progress Any learning activity marked with this indicator is in the process of being introduced or reintroduced into the curriculum after the purchase of a new or upgraded simulation product (subsequent to proper faculty training), or the approval of a curricular revision.

f OSCE: Objective Structured Clinical Examination

g ACRM: Anesthesia Crisis Resource Management, delineated in item 19. "ACRM-type" refers to the fact that the debriefing periods for these sessions have more of instructional teaching component (relative to the clinical topic of the scenarios) versus traditionally formatted ACRM sessions.

h Fanning, RM., et al. Crisis resource management. *The Comprehensive Textbook of Healthcare Simulation*. New York, NY: Springer; 2013: 95–109.

i The SMU Master of Science in Nursing Synthesis is a master's thesis equivalent—nurse anesthesia students meet this requirement via completion of the PNA Synthesis/Special Project Series which includes comprehensive exams (written and oral) and completion of ACRM I and II, as described in the table. PBL: Problem Based Learning

j The critical feature of PBL is that the learners work as members of a team and that every member of the team has shared responsibility for the learning of each member of the team has shared responsibility for the learning of each member of the team

The Samuel Merritt University (SMU) simulation curriculum presented in **Table 20.1** above represents a dynamic work in progress in which deliberate integration of different simulation modalities began approximately 15 years ago. Our faculty began incorporating simple mannequin-based simulation (MBS) techniques in 2001 in a small teaching space that was inconsistently accessible and was equipped with rudimentary audiovisual technology. In 2006, the approval of capital funding by our university (a private institution) and the garnering of philanthropic donations for the construction of our state-of-the-art simulation center was largely predicated on our program's success with curricular integration of simulation. I raise this point to state emphatically that an effective simulation curriculum can be delivered in a wide range of physical facilities with varying levels of technological sophistication. Key elements of success are clear and deliberate curricular planning by faculty, who are taking incremental steps in the implementation of plans and continually assessing the effectiveness of your efforts on student learning. Hopefully, the impact on learning is already an integral component of your institution's assessment paradigm. Developing a curricular plan begins with understanding educational concepts that provide a solid theoretical foundation for a simulation curriculum.

Learning Theories and Simulation

In the latter one-third of the 20th century, education thought leaders recognized that the traditional version of formal schooling in the U.S., developed primarily to prepare students for an industrialized society (as opposed to an agrarian society), is inadequate to prepare individuals to compete in and contribute to society in the digital age. Since then, the focus for both academics and practitioners of education from primary to postsecondary levels is students' learning, as opposed to knowledge acquisition of facts and procedures.[86,87] The science of learning has evolved into a complex and interdisciplinary field that encompasses cognitive science, educational psychology, anthropology, sociology, neuroscience, computer science, and other emerging knowledge domains.

Constructivism—The Umbrella Theory

Learner-centered teaching appears to be the new paradigm of formal education at all levels, around which many educators strive to structure their work and for which there is substantial evidence to justify its use.[88] This new paradigm has become the benchmark for medical education,[89,90] nursing education, and the allied health professions overall.[91–93] In her book, *Learning-Centered Teaching—Five Key Changes to Practice*, considered a landmark publication in the field of higher education, Weimer[88] clearly identifies *constructivism* as the overarching learning theory serving as the foundation for all learner-centered instructional methods. "Constructivist approaches emphasize learners' actively constructing their own knowledge rather than passively receiving information transmitted to them from teachers and textbooks. From a constructivist perspective, knowledge cannot simply be given to students: Students must construct their own meanings."[88,94] In one of the health care professions' education guides written under the auspices of the international Association for Medical Education in Europe, constructivism is characterized as a philosophical principle that acknowledges the presence of multiple competing truths; furthermore, that education and research adhering to the constructivist tradition aims to understand how people create different versions of reality.[95] These authors make the important point that the existence of multiple, differently constructed perspectives on truth and reality are particularly useful to inform problem-solving and decision-making in a health care context.

The research and scholarly writings of many psychologists and philosophers are foundational to constructivism, notably Piaget,[96] Dewey,[97] Bruner,[98] and Vygotsky.[96,99,100] The simulation literature has a growing number of publications focusing on the learning theories (and their founding theorists) upon which SBL is based, presumably due to the recognition that educators wishing to adopt SBL as an instructional modality must strive for a deep understanding of the conceptual basis for learner-centered approaches to teaching.

Experiential Learning Theories

While not specifically geared toward SBL, Yardley and colleagues'[95] extensive overview of experiential learning is aimed at providing a better understanding of this type of learning as it relates to the authentic clinical workplace (as opposed to the other types of experiential learning like problem-based learning and other classroom-based techniques). A strong argument can be made that highly realistic patient simulation is, in fact, a type of authentic clinical experience. Thus, Yardley's explanations of the following experiential learning theories (all of which have constructivist roots) apply to the foundational base of all simulation-based educational approaches: Kolb (Learning Cycle—see **Figure 20.1** below); Dewey (Educative Experience); Piaget (Learning as Schemata); Knowles (Adult Learning); Vygotsky (Socio-cultural Learning), and Engeström (Cultural Historical Activity Theory). Yardley articulates an apt summary of the common thread in the aforementioned theorists' work: "They locate learning in social milieus of which learners are part…Without denying the difference in expertise that exists between learners and practitioners, they are co-members of social groups, which mediate learning."[95(p.13)]

Figure 20.1 Kolb's Experiential Learning Model as it Relates to Simulation-based Learning

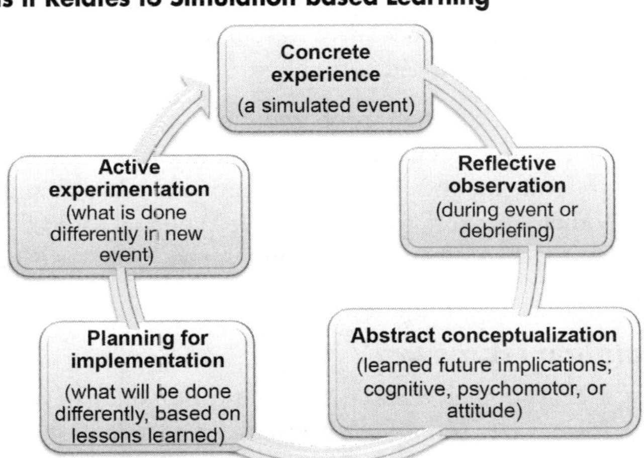

Adapted, with permission. Dunn, WF, ed. *Simulators in Critical Care Education and Beyond.* Des Plaines, IL; Society for Critical Care Medicine; 2004:17.

Other Theories Covered in the Simulation Literature

Other detailed overviews of learning theories and how they serve as the foundational underpinnings of SBL techniques are found in the literature.[101–103] These publications cover those theories placed under the umbrella of constructivism as listed in the previous paragraph as well as other theories/theorists that would be classified as constructivist: the novice to expert continuum;[103] situated [or situative] learning, as specifically defined by Lave and Wenger; reflective practice as articulated by Schön;[101] cognitive learning theory, cognitive load theory, observational learning according to Bandura; and collaborative learning.[102]

Related Theoretical Frameworks

Other learning theories not typically based in constructivist philosophical perspectives have also been deemed highly relevant to simulation instructional techniques: brain-based learning;[103] behaviorism and motor skills learning as defined by Fitts and Posner;[102] and deliberate practice as described by Ericcson.[104] The account of an international research summit focusing on simulation-based health care education specifically identifies the learning theories of Kolb, Vygotsky, Ericcson, and Fitz and Posner as having been particularly helpful to educators using simulation to create meaningful, theoretically grounded, learning activities.[23]

Seeking a Unified Theoretical Framework for SBL

Clearly, there are numerous theories that could be applied, in kaleidoscopic fashion, as a framework for activities that facilitate SBL. The selection is almost overwhelming and could be even more so if one considers the different conceptual frameworks underlying the domains, in addition to education, that are related to simulation: psychology, social science, human factors, and health care policy, to name only a few. Some argue that a singular theoretical framework of simulation should be developed. Kneebone[105] makes an argument for this:

> "A 'theory of simulation' is key to establishing a science, which allows us to formulate and test hypotheses, engaging critically with an evidence base, which transcends the accumulation of nuggets of knowledge. In this way, we will establish a creative, challenging yet mutually respectful alignment between our field and the sources of inspiration, which must feed it."[105(p.163)]

In a separate publication, Kneebone[104] proposed such a conceptual framework upon which to create, implement, and evaluate simulation exercises. His framework is specifically based upon the theories of Vygotsky, Lave and Wenger, and Ericcson. In similar fashion, other educators/researchers have explicitly based their work on frameworks rooted in Vygotskian theories and the works of Lave and Wenger, Ericcson ,and Kolb.[106,107]

Jeffries Simulation Framework

Perhaps the most widely adopted theoretical framework/model for SBL to date is the one created by Jeffries.[108] Her framework was initially intended for the design, implementation, and evaluation of simulation-based nursing education, but has since been used across many of the health care professions. The framework has roots in the constructivist family of theories and is distinguished by its wider scope and higher level of specificity than those frameworks previously mentioned. The Jeffries Simulation Framework (JSF) has five separate constructs (teacher, student, educational practice, simulation design characteristics, and outcomes) with established variables for each construct.

Five years after the introduction of the JSF, the National League for Nursing (NLN) funded the NLN-JSF project, which aimed at documenting the body of scientific evidence supporting the JSF, particularly the simulation design characteristics of the model.[109] The primary motivation for completing this project was to determine the degree to which current simulation education, practice, and research actually reflect the constructs of the JSF. This would be the first step in validating the JSF model as a possible guiding framework to adopt universally across the simulation community. The project—consisting of a systematic literature review and a consensus of expert opinions—determined that there is insufficient evidence currently available to warrant widespread adoption of the JSF. The strong recommendation by the NLN-JSF project team is for the explicit use of the JSF, (particularly the simulation design characteristics component of the model) by simulation practitioners to guide instructional design, research design and reporting, and scholarly work in general.

Learning Theories—Summary

Though the logic and value of widespread application of a single framework for SBL is intuitively reasonable, the multiprofessional, interprofessional, and international nature of health care simulation has made the realization of a standard, universally adopted, theoretical framework challenging and seemingly unattainable without significantly more research. The important message is that educators responsible for developing simulation-based curricular components should invest time investigating and developing an understanding of theoretical foundations of SBL and other immersive learning approaches.

Several recent systematic reviews of the efficacy of SBL stress the need for those of us who plan, design, implement, and assess simulation activities to no longer be asking whether or not learners are satisfied with their simulation experiences, or if they value simulation, or if they gain confidence after undergoing simulation. The evidence clearly supports affirmative answers to these early questions,[23,84,110] and the more pressing need is to buttress the growing literature base for SBL by answering more difficult questions like: How does simulation work (as a learning strategy)? What techniques are best to use for particular learning outcomes? What aspects of an instructional design make it more effective than another? What is the rationale for using a particular instructional design? Answering these higher-level questions requires an awareness of the vast selection of theoretical framework upon which to build a line of inquiry.

A Plan for Simulation Infusion Into a Curriculum

Please refer to Table 20.1 while considering the following curriculum features.

Distributed Curricular Design

Kozomenko[111] describes two major formats of a simulation-based curriculum: a brief, intensive course that spans a few weeks with daily sessions that last six to eight hours, or a longitudinal curriculum that provides for a distributed learning interval. The SMU simulation curriculum is based on a longitudinal format that spans the length of the 27-month program. Positive features of this "infusion" (vs. bolus) type of format are:

- It allows for a synchronized combination of didactic teaching and simulator-based activities.
- Each activity builds on the foundation of internalized experiences from previous learning activities.
- It allows for multiple repetitions of key themes in a curriculum.

Key examples of recurring themes throughout simulation activities are patient safety practices, teamwork, and communication strategies/skills. Most of our simulation scenarios, irrespective of complexity, contain some element reinforcing current safety practices expected of all anesthesia providers, for example, the Joint Commission Universal Protocol for Hospitals (pre-procedure verification process, mark the procedure site, time-out performance),[112] the use of checklists (also referred to as cognitive aids) during critical event management,[113,114] and the use of TeamSTEPPS strategies and tools.[39,115]

Inherent to the longitudinal nature of the curriculum is the fact that the SBL activities (see Table 20.1, left column) are constructed as a continuum where experiences from preceding activities are considered prerequisites for subsequent activities, the activities increase incrementally in complexity and challenge, and all activities are mandatory for proceeding from one to the other. This is referred to as scaffolding in the learning sciences.[86]

Simulation Is Defined Broadly

A common misperception among those relatively new to SBL is that simulation necessarily entails the use of highly sophisticated, computerized, full body mannequins. In Chapter 14, O'Donnell and Phrampus summarize the spectrum of simulator categories and, throughout their chapter, emphasize the need to match the instrument (ie, type of simulation) to the learning objective. Table 20.1 illustrates that our curriculum adheres to this principle: Each SBL activity is described in terms of the instructional modalities used and the specific type of simulator, if appropriate (second column), and the primary goal of the activity (third column). Note that for most of the SBL activities listed, there are multiple learning strategies used, an instructional feature of a simulation activity asserted as one of 10 that leads to effective learning.[116]

Many comprehensive textbooks and other types of publications are readily available as resources for simulation curriculum developers. The references cited here are recommended specifically to increase one's awareness of the various teaching strategies that best leverage the features of various simulation modalities.[117–125]

Establishing and Maintaining a Safe Psychological Environment

The simulation center at Samuel Merritt University serves 12 academic programs. Our faculty and staff adhere to the philosophy that, "Learning is active, learning is fun, and the Health Sciences Simulation Center is a safe place to learn." We are very committed to this philosophy, especially the commitment to providing a psychologically safe setting in which to learn. Therefore, we have adopted the concept of establishing a safe container described by Rudolph and colleagues[126] for every learner who engages in activity in our simulation center. There is a process that all faculty follow to establish and maintain a safe container every time a learner engages in SBL. That process (an interactive discussion using visual presentation aids) involves:

- Clarifying expectations for the learners
- Establishing a fiction contract with the learners
- Providing explicit logistical details for the simulation session/encounter
- Declaring and enacting a commitment to respect for learners and concern for their psychological safety

We require anyone who teaches at the simulation center, any standardized patient who is involved in a simulation session, and all learners to engage in our safe container talk ideally before every simulation session; in other words, the process is integral through the entire simulation curriculum of every program. Activity 1 in Table 20.1 happens early and often throughout the nurse anesthesia program and is one strategy to accomplish what Hamstra's group[127] delineates in its recommendation to focus on methods to enhance the transfer of learning.

Fiction Contract

The fiction contract (as defined in the simulation community) is a joint endeavor created between learners and faculty facilitators, especially those who debrief simulation sessions. In it, the instructor/faculty/facilitator acknowledges that the simulation cannot be exactly like real life but agrees to make the simulation as real as possible within resource and technology constraints. Participants agree to do their best to act as if everything were real.[128] This agreement is also referred to as a *suspension of disbelief.*

Commitment to Respect for Learners

To make this commitment explicit, we verbally declare the following statements as fundamental assumptions that we all operate under:

1. Everyone participating in a simulation:
    - is an intelligent, well-educated individual
    - cares about doing his or hr best
    - wants to improve
2. Mistakes are puzzles to be solved, not crimes to be punished.

Focus on Nontechnical Skills

Another term used synonymously with nontechnical skills is *human factors*, defined as "the way people think, feel, and interact with each other and with their environment."[129] Human factors are not necessarily to be construed as risk factors. Human factors can lie at the core of a major critical event or series of errors that may cascade into a bona fide crisis, but they are also the factors that often lie at the core of averting crises. The inclusion of human factors as a consistent theme within an anesthesiology curriculum is considered by some to represent a favorable paradigm shift away from the biomedical model to a more psychosocial one.[130] For the purposes of this chapter, the term nontechnical skills will be used, but realize that the related term human factors is widely used in the parlance of patient safety and simulation.

Anesthetist's Nontechnical Skills System

For the first 12 years of our program's SBL curricular integration, we adopted the Anaesthetist's Non-Technical Skills (ANTS)[131] system to foster an awareness of human factors in our students. The ANTS system has three levels of descriptions of nontechnical skills: categories, elements, and behavioral markers that are specifically defined. (See **Table 20.2** for a summary of the major levels.) A numerical rating scale is part of the system that, when used by trained individuals, has the potential to provide a metric that reflects the individual's nontechnical skills. The ANTS system was incorporated into the SMU simulation curriculum in the manner suggested by its authors—primarily as a tool for teaching or for structuring feedback to learners during debriefing, because of the absence of data indicating reliability and validity of the tool as a formal summative assessment instrument. Previous iterations of our simulation curriculum introduced the ANTS categories and elements during the second year of the curriculum to prepare students for their anesthesia crisis resource management (ACRM) sessions (described in a subsequent chapter section).

Table 20.2 Categories and Elements of the Anesthetists' Nontechnical Skills System

Category	Elements
Task management	Planning and preparing Prioritizing Providing and maintaining standards
Team working	Identifying and using resources [utilizing is what the authors use] Coordinating activities with team members Exchanging information Using authority and assertiveness Assessing capabilities Supporting others
Situation awareness	Gathering information Recognizing and understanding Anticipating
Decision making	Identifying options Balancing risks and selecting options Reevaluating

Adapted with permission.[131(p583)]

TeamSTEPPS: Institutional Adoption of a System

TeamSTEPPS, Team Strategies and Tools to Enhance Performance and Patient Safety, is the evidence-based teamwork system developed specifically for the health care domain by the Department of Defense (DoD) in partnership with the AHRQ.[39,132] It is also considered a comprehensive safety culture program for health care organizations. In 2012, Samuel Merritt University instituted a four-year, university-wide initiative aiming to train all faculty, staff, administrators, and students in the use of TeamSTEPPS. The Program of Nurse Anesthesia faculty were early adopters of the system and transitioned from ANTS to TeamSTEPPS in 2013.

The patient safety revolution catalyzed by the IOM's *To Err is Human* is credited as an initiating force for the TeamSTEPPS project.[39,133,134] **Figure 20.2** summarizes the system's framework of four core domains: leadership, mutual support, communication, and situation monitoring. A set of tools and strategies (in the form of recommended verbal and physical actions) is associated with each competency, designed to assist individuals in building proficiency with teamwork skills and for use during daily professional practice as part of active team building. There are 15 defined strategies, each one categorized as being most useful under one of the four competencies. In essence, the TeamSTEPPS system provides a common language and behaviors for team members to use when working together. A comparison of the elements within Table 20.2 and Figure 20.2 reveal commonalities between ANTS and TeamSTEPPS and no real discrepancies between the two exist. The rationale for our program transitioning to the latter is that TeamSTEPPS appears destined to be the most widely adopted teamwork and communication framework across all health care settings. The DoD and AHRQ consider TeamSTEPPS the national standard of team training programs.[39,134] Since its introduction to the U.S. health care community in 2006, the TeamSTEPPS initiative has achieved a global footprint, with diverse institutional implementations—the military and civilian hospitals, entire health care systems, independent clinics, and academic institutions.[39] Our hope is that our graduates will play a role in the dissemination of teamwork skills and behaviors, all in the name of patient safety and error reduction.

Figure 20.2 The TeamSTEPPS Framework for Communication and Teamwork

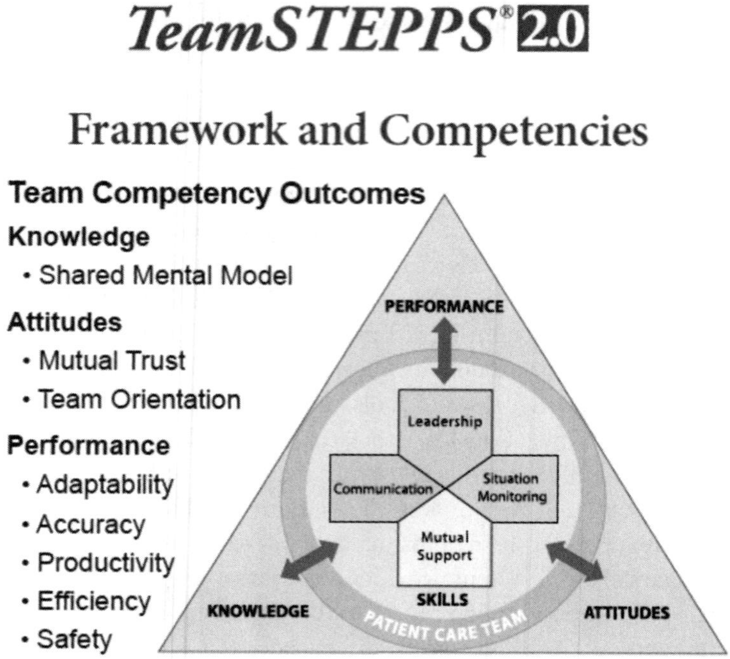

TeamSTEPPS has five key principles. It is based on team structure and four teachable-learnable skill domains, represented by the pentagons within the circle. Each domain is associated with specific tools and strategies. The points labeled in the three corners of the triangle represent the team outcomes gained with mastery of the tools within the domain.

Reprinted with permission of the Agency for Healthcare Research and Quality (AHRQ) from the *TeamSTEPPS 2.0 Pocket Guide* (December 2013). Team Strategies and Tools to Enhance Performance and Patient Safety 2.0 [TeamSTEPPS 2.0]. AHRQ; Rockville, MD (May 2015). Accessible at https://www.ahrq.gov/teamstepps/index.html.

Beginning with activity 2 (Table 20.1), students are indoctrinated early and often in TeamSTEPPS, which, as mentioned previously, is a recurrent theme built into our simulation scenarios. By the time they are engaged in activities 15, 16, 18, and 19, they are expected to demonstrate a high level of competence in the four teamwork domains.

Anesthesia Crisis Resource Management

The strong endorsement by the IOM in 1999 of the aviation industry's crew resource management (CRM) as a strategy to improve patient safety was mentioned earlier in this chapter. This was not a recommendation based on a passing trend. In his introduction to a critically acclaimed book on patient safety and quality care, Lucien Leape—renowned patient safety spokesman—stated that, despite the substantial work done to reduce human errors over the first decade of aggressive patient safety initiatives, the United States health care industry still has not established a culture of safety. Moreover, he characterized our health care system as dysfunctional.[135] Other patient safety experts concur with the persistence of our nation's challenges with human errors and a culture that allows them to persist.[136] Rigorously complied data continue to support the notion that the war against human error in health care is still an urgent need.[35,36] The compelling message is for all health care professions to use the safety-building strategies of the aviation industry, which include but are not limited to CRM, and to develop patient safety programs that are comprehensive, integrated, and span across the entirety of a professional's career.[137]

As indicated in SBL activities 15–16, 18–19 in Table 20.1, the SMU curriculum integrates ACRM concepts across several simulation modules. The SMU faculty incorporates discussions of ACRM principles (including the concepts fundamental to the ANTS system) and applications of TeamSTEPPS® tools and strategies into all their didactic courses where appropriate, as precursory to the formal ACRM sessions. Faculty are, of course, expected to model the behaviors and nontechnical skills in all settings. The learning activity described here is actually a hybrid of the CRM training that is integral to many anesthesia programs, and the team training promulgated by TeamSTEPPS (which may or may not have a simulation component). Put another way, our ACRM sessions are designed as CRM training using the TeamSTEPPS language. This approach is consistent with Gaba's statement that "[different approaches to teamwork training]...can largely be viewed as different paths to the same destination, and some are likely to be truly complementary to others."[137(p4)] An important distinction to make is that ACRM, constructed in its traditional format, is not interprofessional education (IPE). In an authentic simulation-based IPE activity, all participants would be learners, ideally learning while immersed in their own (future) professional role. In ACRM, the roles of the supporting team (surgeons, nurses, technicians, support staff) for the anesthetists who are actively involved in the simulated clinical action are generally not in the role of learner.

Data from a 2008 survey [138] indicated that principles of anesthesia crisis resource management (ACRM) were not formally integrated into the vast majority of nurse anesthesia educational curricula at the time. Moreover, many of the programs that did have an ACRM curricular component did not use MBS as a teaching technique specifically for ACRM. Accurate data related to the inclusion of ACRM training using a simulation-based approach in nurse anesthesia programs subsequent to the aforementioned survey has not been published, to my knowledge. Several nurse anesthesia programs do have a strong, simulation-based ACRM element integrated into their curricula. There is a wealth of resources available in our professional community that can be tapped by those educators seeking to incorporate or expand the ACRM component of their programs, using MBS. Anecdotally, and based on discussions during nurse anesthesia educator forums, there is a definite desire and need to establish mechanisms to share and access such resources. An important goal in including the topic of simulation into this book is to prompt more aggressive actions to meet that need.

Quantity of Simulation-based Learning

A question sometimes posed by educators developing a simulation program is, "How much simulation should be used in a curriculum?" There are no published standards or guidelines relative to the number of hours or percentage of curricular content that should incorporate simulation-based methodologies. McGaghie and colleagues[139] report the results of an analysis of 31 quantitative studies that sought to correlate the number of practice hours using simulation techniques to achievement of learning outcomes. Although the study results primarily bring to light the need for more rigorous methodology in this area of research, a notable principal finding is that, across all learner levels and clinical specialties such as medicine, nursing, and allied health, there is clear evidence that repetitive practice involving simulation techniques is associated with improved learner outcomes in a dose-response curve type of relationship.

An interesting, and not surprising, trend evident in the SMU program is that the paradigm for classroom teaching is definitely changing as a result of the aggressive growth of our simulation program. Once a faculty member experiences the overwhelmingly positive feedback of students (and faculty) to learner-centered, experiential activities incorporating simulation methodology, they become highly motivated to invest the time and energy to revise old lesson plans in favor of expanding their repertoire of innovative teaching strategies. One consequence of this is a steadily growing increase in hours using simulation-based and other experiential methods, with a concomitant decrease in the traditional didactic lecture style. This resonates well with our students, who personify the information-age mindset previously described. To date, this has not resulted in a downturn in metrics used to assess student performance in classroom activities.

On the contrary, the impact of using MBS has significantly improved the first-year student nurse anesthetists' level of skill, competence, and confidence before entering our clinical residency. Activities 1 through 11 listed in Table 20.1 describe an intense use of simulation-based techniques, particularly MBS, during semester 1. The impact on the knowledge, skill, attitude, and ability for safe practice has been similar, if not more effective, than that brought to light in two studies on first-year anesthesiology residents who experienced SBL. The purpose of each study was to evaluate the knowledge and confidence level of the residents (first study) and the level of competence and safe practice (second study). In the first study,[140] the first-year clinical anesthesiology residents were given an intense, three-day preparation course featuring basic airway management and operating room preparation, preparation for and completion of a general anesthesia/endotracheal tube induction, and transfer care of patient to the postoperative care unit, all on relatively healthy patients. In the second study,[141] the first-year clinical anesthesiology residents' group received MBS training over the first six weeks of their residency training in the basic management of intraoperative hypoxemia and hypotensive events. Both study results showed definite improvement over baseline and, by inference, improvement over groups that did not receive simulation-based preparation. It seems reasonable to infer that if the simulation-intense preparation extends over a 16-week period (one of our semesters) and includes significantly more content (eg, semester 1 activities in our program), increased competence and confidence would result. Our course evaluations bear this out, as do the informal reports that we receive from the clinical faculty on level of preparedness of first-year student nurse anesthetists. Anecdotally, clinical faculty have consistently indicated that our simulation curriculum has resulted in much better prepared students during first rotations, which allows them to focus earlier and more effectively on subjects not normally broached until well into that first rotation.

Aligning a Simulation Curriculum with Other Curriculum Components

Simulation-based instructional techniques are not touted to replace all other teaching methods incorporated into a curricular plan. Rather, they serve as an excellent adjunct to what already exists in most program blueprints. They definitely cannot replace actual clinical experience as the ultimate teaching method, assuming the experience meets accreditation and practice standards. Neither is simulation only applicable to teaching students; it is another technique for assessing whether or not a student accomplishes educational objectives. The use of simulation as an assessment strategy (formative or summative) is full of challenges,[142] and a comprehensive discussion of simulation as an assessment method is well beyond the scope of this chapter. Any discussion of simulation integration into a curriculum would not be complete without addressing, at even a basic level, how assessment of learning via simulation might be accomplished. Thus, the final section of this chapter will offer some insight into this topic, again using a component of the SMU curriculum as an example.

Simulation's Position in Miller's Pyramid

In the medical education literature, any discussion of curriculum components unfailingly calls up the framework for clinical assessment proposed by Miller[143] in 1990, often referred to as Miller's pyramid of assessment levels, which is built from the bottom up:

- *Knows* (knowledge) is the broad base of the pyramid and pertains to the recall of facts, principles, and theories and traditionally is assessed via written examinations, usually multiple-choice questions.
- *Knows How* (competence) refers to the ability of a practitioner to acquire information from a variety of sources, analyze the information, and then make rational judgments in the form of a diagnosis or a management plan; this is primarily assessed via case-based, problem-oriented essay examinations or oral examinations.
- *Shows How* (performance) was the innovative concept when Miller proposed his performance pyramid. How does one know what a practitioner will actually do in a realistic situation? Miller was a strong advocate of the widespread use of simulation via standardized patients in an objective structured clinical examination and opined that research should focus on providing concrete evidence in support of this educational and assessment methodology. His original discourse includes an observation about the "astonishing array of physical abnormalities [that] can be simulated"[143] and discusses how students' performance in such realistic situations is invaluable to assessing competency. Thus, it is reasonable to infer that Miller would have wholeheartedly supported the use of MBS simulation as a method to assess the *Shows how* level of competency.
- *Does* (action) is the top level of the pyramid and refers to assessment of a clinical practitioner when functioning independently (ie, without the presence of supervisory personnel); assessment at this level is currently approached via different techniques (eg, provider case records, multirater feedback), which usually are not (but may be) simulation-based.

Simulation's Role in Assessment of Core Competencies

Mannequin-based simulation learning activities fit well into a schema for assessing a student's attainment of an anesthesia program's educational outcomes, or at least their progress toward outcome attainment. Samuel Merritt University, like all institutions of higher education, requires each academic department to delineate a plan indicating how it measures and documents students' attainment of both the department's and the institution's established core competencies. A substantial component of the SMU Program of Nurse Anesthesia Core Competency Assessment Plan involves our SBL activities, which essentially addresses the *Shows How* level of assessment. **Figure 20.3** illustrates some of our assessment mechanisms for key program and institutional competencies, represented in the context of Miller's assessment pyramid. Specific metrics for each student are recorded for each of the assessment activities (eg, multiple-choice question examinations, the competency examination series, pharmacology comprehensive and oral comprehensive examinations, and the ACRM sessions in which the student was an active participant in the scenario). Additionally, an electronic portfolio can be compiled for each student, consisting of digitized recordings of key SBL activities throughout the curriculum, in particular items 6, 9 (OSCE), 11, 12, 13, 18, and 19 in Table 20.1. This provides a visual record of progress made throughout the course of the curriculum, especially since each recording is associated with a completed activity-specific assessment instrument.

Figure 20.3 Miller's Pyramid and the Role of Simulation in Competency Assessment

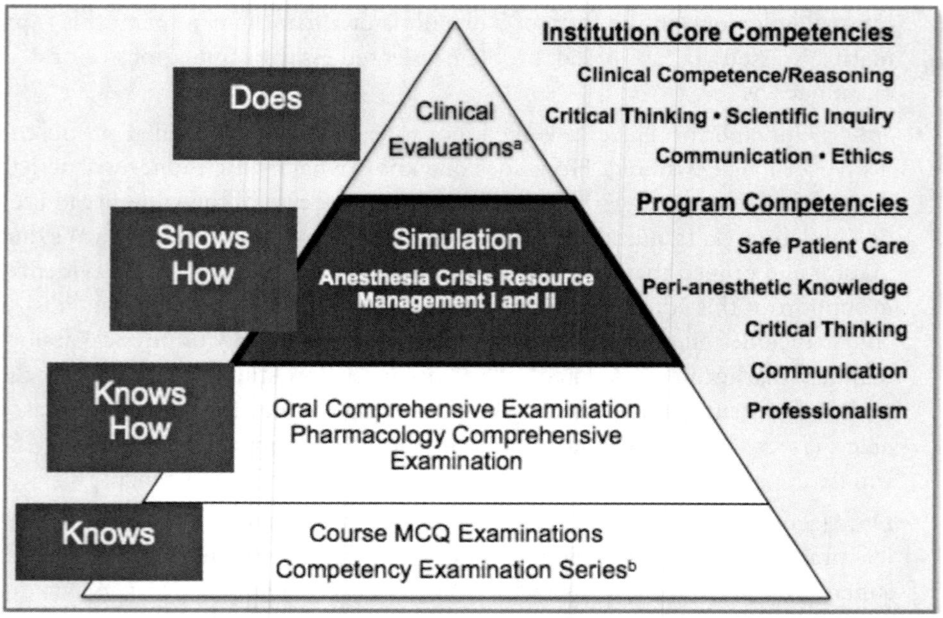

a Clinical evaluations refer to assessment of graduates. The *Does* level represents performance in the professional practice environment.

b Students utilize commercially available, online NCE preparatory programs/packages.

c Adapted with permission.[143(pS63)]

One final aspect of using simulation as an assessment strategy is the concept of linking learning objectives for an SBL activity to outcomes and competencies *up* through the curriculum. Ideally each objective of an activity (eg, an ACRM scenario) will logically link to a program outcome, which will subsequently link to a core university competency. **Figure 20.4** illustrates one set of hundreds of linkages that would exist throughout a simulation-based curriculum. Simulation techniques are powerful mechanisms in the academic setting, and they have the potential to provide compelling evidence of a program curriculum's effectiveness.

Figure 20.4 Mapping of Linkages Between the Learning Objectives at the Simulation Scenario Level up to Higher-Level Program and University Learning Outcomes

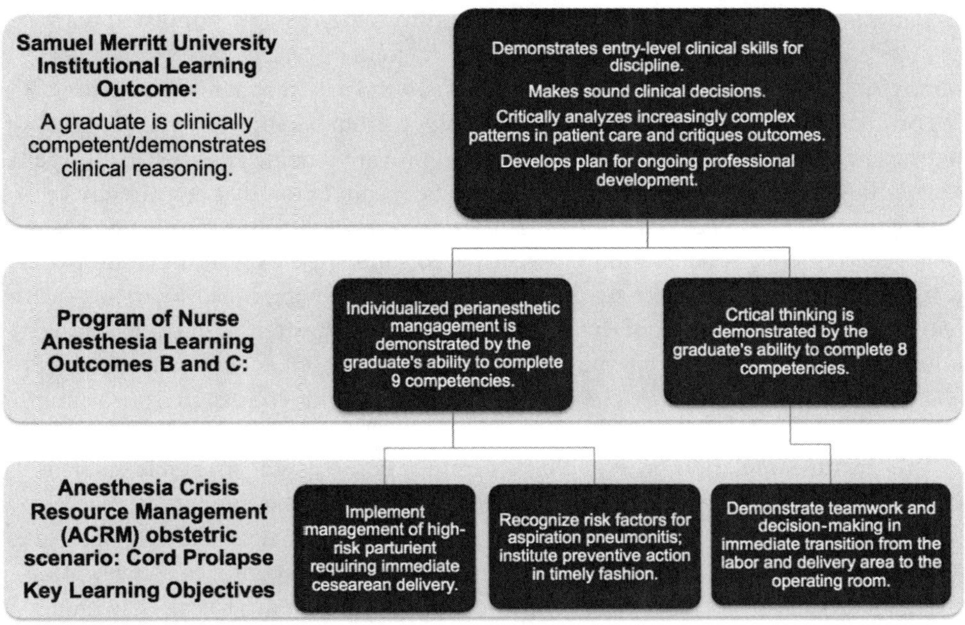

Summary

The undeniable connections between health care simulation and patient safety initiatives make it imperative that nurse anesthesia education programs have strong simulation-based curricular components. Although the evidence is still not unequivocal that patient outcomes are improved by simulation training, the indirect evidence is compelling and the face validity of the methods is high. The case for effective learning with the use of well-designed simulations has definitely been made. Most experts agree that it is only a matter of time before simulation-based education becomes the norm and eventually the standard for nursing (all levels) and physician (medical school and postgraduate) education. The development speed of the interprofessional education movement is accelerating quickly and along with it the field of simulation-enhanced IPE. As a result, the literature is increasingly populated with accounts/studies based on work being done in the field of pharmacy,[144–146] physical therapy,[147–149] and other allied health professions, primarily through IPE activities.[46,150]

Fortunately for us in the field of anesthesiology, from whence the true pioneers of medical simulation came (including some very innovative nurse anesthetists), there are volumes of scientific studies about all aspects of simulation that are directly relevant to our practice. The technology is almost tailor-made for our training and educational requirements. A generation of experienced simulation experts and enthusiasts are available as resources. The simulation literature is growing richer by the day with contributions from all facets of the health care disciplines, often with collaborative, multidisciplinary themes. Contemporary, neuroscience-based educational theory is enhancing the strong social psychology-based framework of constructivist learning theories that is fundamental to SBL.

A successful simulation program has a carefully constructed, adaptable curriculum that uses the various simulators in ways that maximize the simulators' functionality. Simulation-based learning activities must be focused on clear learning objectives and considered integral to the rest of the curriculum. This encourages collaboration among faculty members and can help spread the contagious enthusiasm that simulation often causes. I hope the examples in this chapter have piqued the interest of those whose programs have not yet established a cohesive simulation curriculum, raised more questions for those who engage in simulation-based education, and have encouraged those who passionately advocate for this learning technique to network and collaborate.

References

1. Gaba DM. Improving anesthesiologists' performance by simulating reality. *Anesthesiology.* 1992;76(4):491–494.

2. Gaba DM. The future vision of simulation in health care. *Qual Saf Health Care.* 2004;13(Suppl 1):i2–i10.

3. Blum RH, Raemer DB, Carroll JS, Sunder N, Felstein DM, Cooper JB. Crisis resource management training for an anaesthesia faculty: a new approach to continuing education. *Med Educ.* 2004;38(1):45–55.

4. Cooper JB. The role of simulation in patient safety. In: Dunn WF, ed. *Simulators in Critical Care Education and Beyond.* Des Plaines, IL: Society of Critical Care Medicine; 2004.

5. Byrick RJ. Canadian Patient Safety Institute (CPSI). Patient Simulation in Canada: Current State Findings, April 29, 2005. Canadian Patient Safety Institute; 2005.

6. Jha AK, Duncan BW, Bates DW. Simulator-based training and patient safety. In: Shojania KG, Duncan BW, McDonald KM, Wachter RM, eds. Making Health Care Safer: A Critical Analysis of Patient Safety Practices. Rockville, MD: Agency for Healthcare Research and Quality, U.S. Dept of Health & Human Services; 2001:511–518.

7. Shalala D, Herman A. Doing What Counts for Patient Pafety: Federal Actions to Reduce Medical Errors and Their Impact. Report of the Quality Interagency Coordination Task Force (QuIC) to the President, February 2000. Rockville, MD: Agency for Healthcare Research & Quality, U.S. Dept of Health & Human Services; 2000:95.

8. Ziv A, Wolpe PR, Small SD, Glick S. Simulation-based medical education: an ethical imperative. *Simul Healthc.* 2006;1(4):252–256.

9. Ziv A, Ben-David S, Ziv M. Simulation based medical education: an opportunity to learn from errors. *Med Teach.* 2005;27(3):193–199.

10. Gaba DM. The future vision of simulation in health care. *Quality and Safety in Health Care.* 2004;13(Suppl 1):i2–i10.

11. Kohn LT, Corrigan JM, Donaldson MS. U.S. Institute of Medicine. Committee on Quality of Health Care in America. To Err Is Human: Building a Safer Health System. Washington, DC: National Academies Press; 2000.

12. Rosen KR. The history of medical simulation. *J Crit Care.* 2008;23(2):157–166.

13. Sinz EH. Anesthesiology national CME program and ASA activities in simulation. *Anesthesiol Clin.* 2007;25(2):209–223.

14. Abrahamson S, Denson JS, Wolf RM. Effectiveness of a simulator in training anesthesiology residents. *J Med Educ.* 1969;44(6):515–519.

15. Aebersold M. The history of simulation and its impact on the future. *AACN Adv Crit Care.* 2016;27(1):56–61.

16. Aggarwal R, Mytton OT, Derbrew M, et al. Training and simulation for patient safety. *Qual Saf Health Care.* 2010;19 (Suppl 2):i34–43.

17. Griswold S, Ponnuru S, Nishisaki A, et al. The emerging role of simulation education to achieve patient safety: translating deliberate practice and debriefing to save lives. *Pediat Clin North Am.* 2012;59(6):1329–1340.

18. Schmidt E, Goldhaber-Fiebert SN, Ho LA, McDonald KM. Simulation exercises as a patient safety strategy: a systemic review. *Annal Internal Med.* 2013;158(5 Pt 2):426–432.

19. Cheng A, Duff J, Grant E, Kissoon N, Grant VJ. Simulation in paediatrics: an educational revolution. *Paediatr Child Health.* 2007;12(6):465–468.

20. Leigh G. The simulation revolution: what are the implications for nurses in staff development? *J Nurses Staff Dev.* 2011;27(2):54–57.

21. Gaba DM. The future vision of simulation in healthcare. *Simul Healthc.* 2007;2(2):126–135.

22. Wachter RM. The end of the beginning: patient safety five years after 'to err is human.' *Health Aff.* 2004;Suppl Web Exclusives:W4-534–545.

23. Issenberg SB, Ringsted C, Ostergaard D, Dieckmann P. Setting a research agenda for simulation-based healthcare education: a synthesis of the outcome from an Utstein style meeting. *Simul Healthc.* 2011;6(3):155–167.

24. Pronovost PJ, Goeschel CA, Marsteller JA, Sexton JB, Pham JC, Berenholtz SM. Framework for patient safety research and improvement. *Circulation.* 2009;119(2):330–337.

25. Jeffcott SA, Mackenzie CF. Measuring team performance in healthcare: review of research and implications for patient safety. *J Crit Care.* 2008;23(2):188–196.

26. Byrne A. Medical simulation: The journey so far. In: Forrest K, McKimm J, Edgar S, eds. *Essential Simulation in Clinical Education.* West Sussex, UK: Wiley-Blackwell; 2013:11–25.

27. AHRQ. Funding Opportunity—Advances in Patient Safety through Simulation Research (R18). http://grants.nih.gov/grants/guide/pa-files/PA-14-004.html. Accessed November 20, 2016.

28. AHRQ. Healthcare Simulation to Advance Patient Safety: Responding to Ebola and Other Threats. Issue Brief. February, 2015.

29. Rodger S, J Hoffman S. Where in the world is interprofessional education? A global environmental scan. *J Interprof Care.* 2010;24(5):479–491.

30. IPEC. Core Competencies for Interprofessional Collaborative Practice: Report of an Expert Panel. Interprofessional Education Collaborative; 2011.

31. Salas E, Diaz Granados D, Weaver SJ, King H. Does team training work? Principles for health care. *Acad Emerg Med.* 2008;15(11):1002–1009.

32. Connors K, Seifer S, Sebastian J, Cora-Bramble D, Hart R. Interdisciplinary colaboration in service-learning: lessons from the health professions. *Michigan Journal of Community Sevice Learning.* 1996;3:113–127.

33. IOM. Interprofessional Education for Collaboration: Learning How to Improve Health from Interprofessional Models Across the Continuum of Education to Practice: Workshop Summary (Report No. 9780309263498). National Academies Press; 2013.

34. Cuff P, Schmitt M, Zierler B, et al. Interprofessional education for collaborative practice: views from a global forum workshop. *J Interprofessional Care.* 2014;28(1):2–4.

35. James JT. A new, evidence-based estimate of patient harms associated with hospital care. *J Patient Saf.* 2013;9(3):122–128.

36. Makary MA, Daniel M. Medical error—the third leading cause of death in the U.S. *BMJ.* 2016;353:i2139.

37. The Joint Commission. Joint Commission Online. Patient safety: Sentinel event statistics released for 2014. http://www.jointcommission.org/assets/1/23/jconline_April_29_15.pdf. Published April 29, 2015.

38. Wachter RM. *Understanding Patient Safety.* 2nd ed.. New York, NY: McGraw Hill Medical; 2012.

39. Almeida SA, King H, Salisbury ML. Teamwork improvement in health care: a decade of lessons learned every organization should know. In: Salas E, Tannenbaum SI, Cohen DJ, Latham G, eds. *Developing and Enhancing Teamwork in Organizations: Evidence-based Best Practices and Guidelines*. San Francisco, CA: Jossey-Bass; 2013.

40. Battles J, King HB, Hines S, Edson B, Baker D. What's Next? Leveraging Current Tools to Support Implementation I [presentation Powerpoint Slides from 2013 National TeamSTEPPS Conference]. Washington, DC: AHRQ; 2013.

41. Robertson J, Bandali KS. Bridging the gap: enhancing interprofessional education using simulation. *J Interprof Care.* 2008;22(5):499–508.

42. Palaganas JC. *Exploring healthcare simulation as a platform for interprofessional education* [dissertation]. Ann Arbor: Loma Linda University; 2012.

43. Zhang C, Thompson S, Miller C. A review of simulation-based interprofessional education. *Clin Simul Nurs.* 2011;7(4):e117–e126.

44. Palaganas JC, Mancini ME. Interprofessional education using clinical simulations. In: Jeffries PR, ed. *Clinical Simulations in Nursing Education: Advanced Concepts, Trends, and Opportunities*. Philadelphia, PA: Wolters Kluwer-Lippincott Williams & Wilkins; 2014:58–70.

45. Garbee DD, Paige J, Barrier K, et al. Interprofessional teamwork among students in simulated codes: a quasi-experimental study. *Nurs Educ Perspect.* 2013;34(5):339–344.

46. Paige JT, Garbee DD, Kozmenko V, et al. Getting a head start: high-fidelity, simulation-based operating room team training of interprofessional students. *J Am Coll Surg.* 2014;218(1):140–149.

47. Palaganas JC, Epps C, Raemer DB. A history of simulation-enhanced interprofessional education. *J Interprof Care.* 2014;28(2):110–115.

48. Boulet JR, Smee SM, Dillon GF, Gimpel JR. The use of standardized patient assessments for certification and licensure decisions. *Simul Healthc.* 2009;4(1):35–42.

49. Kempen PM. Maintenance of certification and licensure: regulatory capture of medicine. *Anesth Analg.* 2014;118(6):1378–1386.

50. Ziv A, Rubin O, Sidi A, Berkenstadt H. Credentialing and certifying with simulation. *Anesthesiol Clin.* 2007;25(2):261–269.

51. Berkenstadt H, Ziv A, Gafni N, Sidi A. Incorporating simulation-based objective structured clinical examination into the Israeli National Board Examination in Anesthesiology. *Anesth Analg.* 2006;102(3):853–858.

52. Ziv A, Berkenstadt H, Eisenberg O. Simulation for licesure and certifcation. In: Levine AI, DeMaria S, Schwartz AD, Sim AJ, eds. *The Comprehensive Textbook of Healthcare Simulation.* [Kindle version] New York, NY: Springer Science + Business Media; 2013:location 7478–7913.

53. Levine AI, Flynn BC, Bryson EO, Demaria S. Simulation-based maintenance of certification in anesthesiology (MOCA) course optimization: use of multi-modality educational activities. *J Clin Anesth.* 2012;24(1):68–74.

54. McIvor W, Burden A, Weinger MB, Steadman R. Simulation for maintenance of certification in anesthesiology: the first two years. *J Contin Educ Health Prof.* 2012;32(4):236–242.

55. Culley DJ, Sun H, Harman AE, Warner DO. Perceived value of board certification and the maintenance of certification in anesthesiology program (MOCA®). *J Clin Anesth.* 2013;25(1):12–19.

56. Ross BK, Metzner J. Simulation for maintenance of certification. *Surg Clin North Am.* 2015;95(4):893–905.

57. Gray BM, Vandergrift JL, Johnston MM, et al. Association between imposition of a Maintenance of Certification requirement and ambulatory care-sensitive hospitalizations and health care costs. *JAMA.* 2014;312(22):2348–2357.

58. Hayes J, Jackson JL, McNutt GM, Hertz BJ, Ryan JJ, Pawlikowski SA. Association between physician time-unlimited vs. time-limited internal medicine board certification and ambulatory patient care quality. *JAMA.* 2014;312(22):2358–2363.

59. Lee TH. Certifying the good physician: a work in progress. *JAMA.* 2014;312(22):2340–2342.

60. Zambricki C, Horowitz J, Blumenreich G, Fallacaro M. Recertifying the professional nurse anesthetist: a call for national dialogue. *AANA J.* 2015;83(1):7–14.

61. COA. The value of simulation in nurse anesthesia education. Park Ridge, IL: Council on Accrediation of Nurse Anesthesia Educational Programs; n.d.

62. COA. Standards for accreditation of nurse anesthesia educational programs. Park Ridge, IL: Council on Accreditation of Nurse Anesthesia Educational Programs; 2016.

63. Sinz E. Simulation-based education for cardiac, thoracic, and vascular anesthesiology. *Semin Cardiothorac Vasc Anesth.* 2005;9(4):291–307.

64. Blum RH, Raemer DB, Carroll JS, Sunder N, Felstein DM, Cooper JB. Crisis resource management training for anaesthesia faculty: a new approach to continuing education. *Med Educ.* 2004;38(1):45–55.

65. Gardner R, Walzer TH, Simon R, Raemer DB. Obstetric simulation as a risk control strategy: course design and evaluation. *Simul Healthc.* 2008;3:119–127.

66. Hanscom R. Medical simulation from an insurer's perspective. *Acad Emerg Med.* 2008;15(11):984–987.

67. Gardner R, Walzer TB, Simon R, Raemer DB. Obstetric simulation as a risk control strategy: course design and evaluation. *Simul Healthc.* 2008;3(2):119–127.

68. McCarthy JL. An essential tool for patient safety. *Forum.* 2008;26(4):1–2.

69. Fry R. Millennials Surpass Gen Xers as the Largest Generation in U.S. Labor Force. Pew Research Forum. http://www.pewresearch.org/fact-tank/2015/05/11/millennials-surpass-gen-xers-as-the-largest-generation-in-u-s-labor-force/ft_15-05-11_millennialsdefined/. Published May 11, 2015. Accessed November 22, 2016.

70. Daugherty L, Fonseca R, Kumar KB, Michaud P-C. *An analysis of the labor markets for anesthesiology.* Santa Monica, CA: RAND Corporation; 2010.

71. Frand J. The information-age mindset: changes in students and implications for higher education. *EDUCAUSE Review.* 2000;35(5):15–24.

72. Oblinger DG. Boomers, Gen-Xers, and milleniials: understanding the "New Students." *EDUCAUSE Review.* 2003;38(4):37–47.

73. Benner P, Sutphen M, Leonard V, Day L. *Educating Nurses: A Call for Radical Transformation.* San Francisco, CA: Jossey-Bass; 2010.

74. Cooke M, Irby DM, O'Brien BC. *Educating Physicians: A Call for Reform of Medical School and Residency.* San Francisco, CA: Jossey-Bass; 2010.

75. DaRosa DA, Skeff K, Friedland JA, et al. Barriers to effective teaching. *Acad Med.* 2011;86(4):453–459.

76. Talcott K, O'Donnell JM, Burns HK. Technology and the nurse educator: are you ELITE? *Nurse Educ.* 2013;38(3):126–131.

77. Cannon-Diehl M, Rugari S, Jones T. High-fidelity simulation for continuing education in nurse anesthesia. *AANA J.* 2012;80(3):191–196.

78. Hawkins R, Bendickson L, Benson P, et al. A pilot study evaluating the perceptions of Certified Registered Nurse Anesthetists toward human patient simulation. *AANA J.* 2014;82(5):375–384.

79. Glavin RJ. When simulation should and should not be in the curriculum. In: Kyle RR, Murray WB, eds. *Clinical Simuation: Operations, Engineering and Management.* Amsterdam: Elsevier; 2008:71–75.

80. Medley CF, Horne C. Using simulation technology for undergraduate nursing education. *J Nurs Educ.* 2005;44(1):31–34.

81. Baxendale B, Coffey F, Buttery A. The roles of faculty and simulated patients in simulation. In: Forrest K, McKimm J, Edgar S, eds. *Essential Simulation in Clinical Education.* [Kindle version]. West Sussex, UK: John Wiley & Sons, Ltd.; 2013:location 3300–4054.

82. Waxman KT, Miller MA. Faculty development to implement simulations: strategies and possibilities. In: Jeffries PR, ed. *Clinical Simulations in Nursing Education: Advanced Concepts, Trends, and Opportunities.* Baltimore, MD: National League for Nursing; 2013:9–21.

83. Hayden EM, Gordon JA. Fellowship training in simulation. In: Levine AI, DeMaria S, Schwartz AD, Sim AJ, eds. *The Comprehensive Textbook of Healthcare Simulation.* [Kindle version]. New York, NY: Springer Science + Business Media; 2013:location 25610–25835.

84. McGaghie WC, Issenberg SB, Petrusa ER, Scalese RJ. A critical review of simulation-based medical education research: 2003–2009. *Med Educ.* 2010;44(1):50–63.

85. Jeffries PR, Dreifuerst KT, Kardong-Edgren S, Hayden J. Faculty development when initiating simulation programs: lessons learned from the national simulation study. *J Nurs Regul.* 2015;5(4):17–23.

86. Bransford JD, Brown AL, Cocking RR, eds. *How People Learn: Brain,Mind, Experience, and School.* Expanded ed. Washington, DC: National Academies Press; 2000.

87. Sawyer RK. The new science of learning. In: Sawyer RK, ed. *The Cambridge Handbook of the Learning Sciences.* New York, NY: Cambridge University Press; 2006:xi–xiv.

88. Weimer M. *Learner-Centered Teaching: Five Key Changes to Practice.* Second ed. San Francisco, CA: Jossey-Bass; 2013.

89. Irby DM, Cooke M, O'Brien B. Calls for reform of medical education by the Carnegie Foundation for the Advancement of Teaching: 1910 and 2010. *Acad Med.* 2010;85(2):220–227.

90. Spencer JA, Jordan RK. Learner centred approaches in medical education. *BMJ.* 1999;318(7193):1280–1283.

91. Skiba D, Barton A. Adapting your teaching to accommodate the Net Generation of learners. *Online J Issues Nurs.* 2006;11(2):5.

92. Patel VL, Yoskowitz NA, Arocha JF. Towards effective evaluation and reform in medical education: a cognitive and learning sciences perspective. *Adv Health Sci Educ Theory Prac.* 2009;14(5):791–812.

93. Tavakol K, Reicherter EA. The role of problem-based learning in the enhancement of allied health education. *J Allied Health.* 2003;32(2):110–115.

94. Stage FK, Muller PA, Kinzie J, Simmons A. Creating Learner Centered Classrooms: What Does Learning Theory Have to Say? ERIC Clearinghouse on Higher Education.; 1998. ERIC Document Reproduction Service ED422777.

95. Yardley S, Teunissen PW, Dornan T. Experiential learning: AMEE Guide No. 63. *Med Teach.* 2012;34(2):e102–115.

96. Pass S. *Parallel Paths to Constructivism: Jean Piaget and Lev Vygotsky.* Greenwich, CT: Information Age Publishing; 2004.

97. Dewey J. *Experience & Education.* Kappa Delta Pi; 1938. http://www.schoolofeducators.com/wp-content/uploads/2011/12/.

98. Bruner JS. *The Process of Education:A Landmark in Educational Theory.* (Rev. ed.). Cambridge, MA: Harvard University Press; 1960.

99. Cole M, John-Steiner V, Scribner S, Souberman E, eds. *L.S. Vygotsky: Mind in Society: The Development of Higher PsychologicalProcesses.* Cambridge, MA: Harvard University Press; 1980.

100. Wertsch JV. *Vygotsky and the social formation of mind.* Cambridge, MA: Harvard University Press; 1985.

101. Bradley P, Postlethwaite K. Simulation in clinical learning. *Med Educ.* 2003;37(Suppl 1):1–5.

102. Dieckmann P, Ringsted C. Pedagogy in simulation-based training in healthcare. In: Forrest K, McKimm J, Edgar S, eds. *Essential Simulation in Clinical Education.* [Kindle version]. 2013:location 2055–2549.

103. Rodgers DL. *High-Fidelity Patient Simulation: A Descriptive White Paper Report.* Charleston, WV: Healthcare Simulation Strategies; 2007.

104. Kneebone R. Evaluating clinical simulations for learning procedural skills: a theory-based approach. *Acad Med.* 2005;80(6):549–553.

105. Kneebone R. Crossing the line: simulation and boundary areas. *Simul Healthc.* 2006;1(3):160–163.

106. Paige JB, Daley BJ. Situated cognition: A learning framework to support and guide high-fidelity simulation. *Clin Simul Nurs.* 2009;5(3):e97–e103.

107. Perkins GD. Simulation in resuscitation training. *Resuscitation.* 2007;73(2):202–211.

108. Jeffries PR. A framework for designing, implementing, and evaluating: simulations used as teaching strategies in nursing. *Nurs Educ Perspect.* 2005;26(2):96–103.

109. Groom JA, Henderson D, Sittner BJ. National League for Nursing: Jeffries simulation framework state of the science project: simulation design characteristics. *Clin Simul Nurs.* 2014;10(7):337–344.

110. Cook DA, Hatala RA, Brydges R, et al. Technology-enhanced simulation for health professions education: a systematic review and meta-analysis. *JAMA.* 2011;306(9):978–988.

111. Kozmenko V, Kaye AD, Morgan B, Hilton CW. Theory and practice of developing an effecitve simulation-based clinical curriculum. In: Kyle RR, Murray WB, eds. *Clinical Simuation: Operations, Engineering and Management.* Amsterdam: Elsevier; 2008:135–151.

112. The Joint Commission. Universal Protocol: Hospitals. http://www.jointcommission.org/NR/rdonlyres/AEA17A06-BB67-4C4E-B0FC-DD195FE6BF2A/0/UP_HAP_20080616.pdf. Published 2008. Accessed March 26, 2009.

113. Gaba DM. Perioperative cognitive aids in anesthesia: what, who, how, and why bother? *Anesth Analg.* 2013;117(5):1033–1036.

114. Goldhaber-Fiebert SN, Howard SK. Implementing emergency manuals: can cognitive aids help translate best practices for patient care during acute events? *Anesth Analg.* 2013;117(5):1149–1161.

115. Salas E, Tannenbaum S, Cohen D, Latham G, eds. *Developing and Enhancing Teamwork in Organizations: Evidence-Based Best Practices and Guidelines.* San Francisco, CA: Jossey-Bass; 2013.

116. Issenberg SB, McGaghie WC, Petrusa ER, Gordon DL, Scalese RJ. Features and uses of high-fidelity medical simulations that lead to effective learning: a BEME systematic review. *Med Teach.* 2005;27(1):10–28.

117. Loyd GE, Lake CL, Greenberg RB. *Practical Health Care Simulations.* Elsevier Mosby; 2004.

118. Kyle RR, Murray WB. *Clinical Simulation: Operations, Engineering and Management.* Amsterdam: Elsevier; 2008.

119. Jeffries PR. *Simulation in Nursing Education: From Conceptualization to Evaluation.* National League for Nursing; 2007.

120. Gallagher CJ, Issenberg SB. *Simulation in Anesthesia.* Philadelphia, PA: Saunders Elsevier; 2007.

121. Seropian MA. General concepts in full scale simulation: getting started. *Anesth Analg.* 2003;97(6):1695–1705.

122. Forrest K, McKimm J, Edgar S. *Essential Simulation in Clinical Education.* Oxford, UK: Wiley-Blackwell; 2013.

123. Levine AI, DeMaria S, Schwartz AD, Sim AJ, eds. *The Comprehensive Textbook of Healthcare Simulation.* New York: Springer Science + Business Media; 2013.

124. Jeffries PR, ed. *Simulation in Nursing Education: From Conceptualization to Evaluation.* 2nd edition. New York, NY: National League for Nursing; 2012.

125. Jeffries PR, ed. *Clinical Simulations in Nursing Education: Advanced Concepts, Trends and Opportunities.* New York, NY: National League for Nursing; 2014.

126. Rudolph JW, Raemer DB, Simon R. Establishing a safe container for learning in simulation: the role of the presimulation briefing. *Simul Healthc.* 2014;9(6):339–349.

127. Hamstra SJ, Brydges R, Hatala R, Zendejas B, Cook DA. Reconsidering fidelity in simulation-based training. *Acad Med.* 2014;89(3):387–392.

128. Simon R, Raemer D, Rudolph J. Debriefing assessment for simulation in healthcare (DASH) Rater's Handbook. Published 2010. https://harvardmedsim.org/_media/DASH.handbook.2010.Final.Rev.2.pdf.

129. St. Pierre M, Hofinger G, Buerschaper C. *Crisis Management in Acute Care Settings: Human Factors and Team Psychology in a High Stakes Environment.* Berlin: Springer-Verlag; 2008.

130. Glavin R, Flin R. Review article: the influence of psychology and human factors on education in anesthesiology. *Can J Anaesth.* 2012;59(2):151–158.

131. Fletcher GCL, Flin RH, McGeorge P, Glavin RJ, Maran NJ, Patey R. Anaesthetists' Non-Technical Skills (ANTS): evaluation of a behavioural marker system. *Br J Anaesth.* 2003;90(5):580–588.

132. AHRQ/HRET. TeamSTEPPS National Implementation http://www.teamsteppsportal.org/. Published 2016. Accessed November 23, 2016.

133. Coburn A, Gage-Croll Z. *Improving hospital patient safety through teamwork: The use of TeamSTEPPS in critical access hospitals.* Policy Brief #21. Flex Monitoring Team University of Southern Maine; June 2011.

134. King HB, Battles J, Baker DP, et al. TeamSTEPPS™: Team strategies and tools to enhance performance and patient safety. In: Henriksen K, Battles JB, Keyes MA, Grady ML, eds. *Advances in Patient Safety: New Directions and Alternative Approaches.* Vol 3: Performance and Tools: Agency for Healthcare Research and Quality; 2008.

135. Nance JJ. *Why Hospitals Should Fly: The Ultimate Flight Plan to Patient Safety and Quality Care.* Bozeman, MT: Second River Healthcare Press; 2009.

136. Koppel R, Gordon S, eds. *First, Do Less Harm: Confronting the Inconvenient Problems of Patient Safety.* Ithaca, NY: Cornell University Press; 2012.

137. Gaba DM. Crisis resource management and teamwork training in anaesthesia. *Br J Anaesth.* 2010;105(1):3–6.

138. Turcato N, Roberson C, Covert K. Simulation-based education: what's in it for nurse anesthesia educators? *AANA J.* 2008;76(4):257–262.

139. McGaghie SC, Issenberg SB, Petrussa ER, Scalese R. Effect of practice on standardised learning outcomes in simulation-based medical education. *Med Educ.* 2006;40(8):792–797.

140. Oravitz TM, Metro DG, McIvor WR. The benefits of a human simulator training course for initial first-year anesthesia residency education. *The Open Anesthesiology Journal.* 2008;2:13–19.

141. Park CS, Rochlen LR, Yaghmour EA, Deleon AM, McCarthy R. Assessing performance for safety and competence in novice residents using high-fidelity simulation. *ASA Abstracts.* 109; American Society of Anesthesiologists: 2008.

142. Glavin RJ, Gaba DM. Challenges and Opportunities in Simulation and Assessment. *Simul Healthc.* 2008;3(2):69–71.

143. Miller GE. The Assessment of Clinical Skills/Competence/Performance. *Acad Med.* 1990;65(Suppl 9):S63–S67.

144. Crea KA. Practice skill development through the use of human patient simulation. *Am J Pharm Educ.* 2011;75(9):Article 188.

145. Seybert AL. Patient simulation in pharmacy education. *Am J Pharm Educ.* 2011;75(9):Article 187.

146. Vyas D, Ottis EJ, Caligiuri FJ. Teaching clinical reasoning and problem-solving skills using human patient simulation. *Am J Pharm Educ.* 2011;75(9):Article 189.

147. Ohtake PJ, Lazarus M, Schillo R, Rosen M. Simulation experience enhances physical therapist student confidence in managing a patient in the critical care environment. *Phys Ther.* 2013;93(2):216–228.

148. Shoemaker MJ, Riemersma L, Perkins R. Use of high fidelity human simulation to teach physical therapist decision-making skills for the intensive care setting. *Cardiopulm Phys Ther J.* 2009;20(1):13–18.

149. Shoemaker MJ, Beasley J, Cooper M, Perkins R, Smith J, Swank C. A method for providing high-volume interprofessional simulation encounters in physical and occupational therapy education programs. *J Allied Health.* 2011;40(1):e15–21.

150. Titzer JL, Swenty CF, Hoehn WG. An interprofessional simulation promoting collaboration and problem solving among nursing and allied health professional students. *Clin Simul Nurs.* 2012;8(8):e325–e333.

CHAPTER 21

Testing the Student's Knowledge

Vicki Coopmans, PhD, CRNA

Keywords: Didactic training, multiple choice items, testing methods.

Key Concepts

- Effective teaching and testing are based on clearly defined student learning objectives.
- Well-written test questions address important content and are well-constructed.
- The instructor should provide clear examination instructions and expectations to the student.
- The instructor should develop scoring and grading methods in advance.

Introduction

There are a variety of ways to assess student knowledge in the didactic setting; however, developing effective measures can be quite challenging. Anyone who has ever been responsible for writing examination questions can appreciate that it is easier said than done as evidenced by the following concerns often voiced by students:

- The content on the exam was not covered in class.
- The questions were too vague, confusing, poorly worded, tricky, complicated, and time-consuming. (select all that apply).
- The book says something different.

This chapter intends to provide guidance on selecting and developing testing modalities that will appropriately reflect mastery of content and generate little or no protest from those being evaluated.

Purpose

The purpose of this chapter is to provide the reader with an overview of testing methods in the didactic setting with particular attention given to multiple-choice items. The National Certification Examination (NCE) and Self-Evaluation Examination (SEE) are administered using multiple-choice questions (MCQ) as well as alternative formats, including multiple correct response, calculation, drag and drop, and hotspot-type questions. Both are computerized adaptive tests (CAT) using item response theory (IRT), a type of mathematical model that determines the difficulty of questions based on an estimation of the candidate's ability. The development of valid test questions is a rigorous process, and a large bank of test questions is required for calibration. New questions must be analyzed and evaluated before being added to the test bank. There are several statistical software platforms that include IRT item analysis. The use of CAT and IRT generally exceed the resources of individual nurse anesthesia programs (NAPs), but many do utilize MCQ format throughout their curriculum to prepare students for the types of questions they will see on the SEE and NCE. For this reason, the majority of this chapter will be devoted to the use and development of MCQs. Alternative question formats, essay testing, and the objective structured clinical exam will also be reviewed, and creative assessment techniques will be introduced.

Teaching and Testing

Before addressing the process of test construction, a discussion of the relationship between teaching and testing and other general testing concepts will be presented. Teaching has been defined as the act of imparting knowledge.[1] The act of testing has been described as a method for determining the "skill, knowledge, intelligence, capacities, or aptitudes of an individual or group."[2] The work of imparting knowledge and then measuring that knowledge in the student are inextricably wedded to each other and challenging to accomplish. In order for instruction to be successful, the learner must be informed of the expected outcomes. Effective teaching is based on clearly identifying and defining these outcomes, which are generally expressed as learning objectives. It is upon these learning objectives that tests should be developed. Thus, both teaching and testing methods are designed and carried out based on the student learning objectives developed by the instructor.

There are two basic types of assessment: norm-referenced and criterion-referenced. The purpose of norm-referenced testing is to determine how well a group of learners perform in relation to one another. Norm-reference testing can be used to distinguish between low and high achievers. This type of assessment ranks how the examinee performs within the group. This style is sometimes referred to as grading on a curve, where a certain smaller proportion of students will receive As or Fs with the remainder falling somewhere in between. Norm-referenced testing has been said to interfere with student learning and to suborn an unhealthy competition for grades.[3]

Criterion-referenced assessment is utilized to determine mastery of a specific set of skills and/or concepts. The NCE is designed based on criterion-referenced principles with the purpose of establishing the level of knowledge and skills necessary to perform as an entry-level practitioner.[4] The National Council Licensure Examination for Registered Nurses (NCLEX-RN) is also criterion-reference based.[5] It is generally agreed that criterion-referenced testing is preferable as it is intended to ensure the level of competency necessary for safe practice.[3,6–8] Theoretically, all examinees could either pass or fail depending on whether the established benchmark has been met. With norm-referenced testing, an individual could still pass without meeting minimum standards if the rest of the learners performed poorly. The primary goal of nurse anesthesia educational programs is to prepare competent anesthesia practitioners; it is important to consider this when selecting the type of assessment to be used.

Testing Methods

There are a variety of methods available for measuring student knowledge in the didactic setting, such as multiple choice items, short answer questions, essay tests, and written or oral assignments. Some more creative assessment techniques include concept mapping, journal assignments, and portfolio development, which will be discussed briefly at the end of this chapter.

Multiple Choice Items

Multiple choice items can be divided into three basic groups: true/false, single-best-answer, and multiple correct response type questions (MCRQs). True/false questions require the examinee to select all responses that are correct. The single-best-answer questions, also referred to as one-best-answer, require selection of the correct or most appropriate response. In contrast, MCRQs have more than one correct response.

Single-best-answer Questions

The classic one-best-answer MCQ model includes a single stem (an introductory question or statement), a correct response, and 2 to 4 distractors. Other single-best-answer questions include matching and extended-matching questions (R-type questions). Multiple choice questions can also fall into the true/false family and will be discussed later in this section.

Regardless of the type of question to be utilized, the choice should be based on content addressed by predetermined learning objectives and should be well-constructed. It has been shown that poorly worded items can have the unintended consequence of either unfairly assisting or penalizing examinees.[9,10] Well-accepted item writing guidelines, along with many examples of flawed item construction, have been presented in numerous publications.[11–15] Recommendations for the development of each component and various types of the multiple choice item will be reviewed.

As described earlier, all multiple choice items begin with a stem. The stem can take the form of a question (closed stem), an incomplete statement (open stem), or a description of a situation or issue, and should be developed with the factors listed in **Table 21.1**.

Table 21.1 Recommendations for MCQ Stem Construction

- The content should be based on well-defined learning objectives.
- The content should be focused on one theme or problem.
- The stem should be grammatically correct and concisely presented.
- The stem should be phrased positively.
- The stem should not include personal pronouns.

All examination items should measure a specific, important learning objective. The stem should be clear and grammatically correct both alone and in combination with the responses. The examinee should not have to read through the responses to discern the central concept of the question. Extraneous information not relevant to the purpose of the question should be avoided to minimize confusion by the examinee; however, the stem should have the necessary information and focus such that all responses fall within a single subject area. Stems with negative wording should be used sparingly, if at all, as they add unnecessary difficulty to the question. When utilized, the negative word should be capitalized, set in boldface, and/or underlined. Some examples of stem format include:

- Closed stem: Where is the stellate ganglion?
- Open stem: The stellate ganglion is located near the ______.
- Description: During administration of a stellate ganglion block, an intervascular injection occurs. The most appropriate action is to: ______.

The stem is followed by a number of responses or branches. The correct response should be absolutely correct or clearly the best choice. The distractors should be incorrect but plausible alternatives to the correct response. Recommendations for response construction are listed in **Table 21.2**.

Table 21.2 Recommendations for MCQ Response Construction

• The correct answer should clearly be the best choice. • Distractors should be plausible alternatives, but clearly incorrect. • Responses should be homogenous (ie, conceptually and structurally similar) • Repetitive words should be included in the stem. • Key words from the stem should not be repeated in the responses. • Responses should be presented in a logical or numerical order. • Absolute terms should be avoided (eg, always, never). • Responses should be of equal complexity and length. • Responses should be grammatically consistent with the stem. • Overlapping and double barrel options should be avoided. • All of the above (AOTA) and none of the above (NOTA) options should be avoided.

One of the pitfalls of response development is cueing, or providing clues within an item that unintentionally direct the examinee to the correct response for that or another item. For example, more attention is often given to the correct response; it may be longer, more detailed, or more complete than the distractors. Some of the distractors may not flow logically from the stem while the correct answer does, giving the examinee an unintentional advantage in selecting the correct response.

Cueing may also occur when the correct response has the most in common with the other options. This has been described as convergence and can take many forms. For instance, with numeric options, the correct response tends to be in the middle rather than at either extreme. It can also happen when the item writer makes slight variations to the correct answer to form the distractors, which often results in the double barrel-type question. The correct response tends to contain more common elements from all of the options and is less likely to be an outlier.

Similar wording or phrasing in the stem and correct response is another source of cueing. Absolute terms such as always, never, completely, and totally should be avoided as they are frequently associated with false statements. Throwaway distractors such as AOTA and NOTA are generally not recommended. If an examinee has partial knowledge (that at least two of the three responses are correct), this may clue the student to select AOTA, relying more on test-taking strategy than his or her own knowledge. Using NOTA can be problematic, particularly where judgment is involved and the options are not absolutely true or false. The more knowledgeable student may select NOTA, believing an option not available to be more correct than the instructor's intended correct response.

The common concern of students regarding trick questions deserves some attention, if for no other reason than to provide the item writer with some insight on student perception. A study by Roberts revealed that students believed trick items were deliberately used on examinations to deceive them.[16] Students and faculty were asked to describe the characteristics of trick items. Results are listed in order of prevalence:

1. Intention
2. Trivial content

3. Too fine answer discrimination
4. Window dressing
5. Multiple correct answers
6. Content presented opposite from instruction
7. High ambiguity

With a fine line to walk between the fair, challenging item and one that may be perceived as tricky and overly difficult, the item writer can minimize complaints by taking recommended guidelines into consideration. In some cases, what was thought to be an excellent question does not perform well for reasons that surface after its use. On the other hand, student allegations of trick questions may also be an excuse for poor test performance due to lack of knowledge. It is important to maintain objectivity in reevaluating test items. As much time as it takes to develop test questions, those that consistently exhibit poor performance by examinees probably need to be revised.

Another aspect of distractor development to consider is the number of distractors to be used. While a stem with three or sometimes four distractors is commonly utilized, research suggests three options (one correct answer and two distractors) is the best design.[17–19] Analysis of test items across disciplines has shown that when nondiscriminating distractors are identified and removed, most MCQs were left with two to three options, and the use of more than two distractors did not improve item or test score statistics.[17,18] Developing the third and/or fourth distractor has often been described as the most challenging and time-consuming part of question development.[19] The savings of time and expense seems to favor a transition to the three-option MCQ, though some might contend that reducing the number of options increases the potential success of guessing, leading to an undeserved higher grade. This may seem plausible, but Haldyna and Rodriquez argue that as test length increases, the risk for variation due to guessing and the threat to test validity are extremely low.[19]

The following are examples of flawed items along with suggestions for revision. For clarity, flawed examples will be highlighted in gray.

Example 1:

The stellate ganglion:

a. is named for its neatly compact appearance.
b. comprises the superior thoracic and inferior cervical ganglion.
c. typically lies over the first thoracic vertebrae near the 2nd rib.
d. can also be referred to as the thoracolumbar ganglion.

The question above has an unfocused stem and provides no information of the problem to be solved. The examinee should be able to read the question and construct the answer without looking at the responses. This type of question can be referred to as a hidden true/false question (with one true and three false statements).

Example 2:

You will be performing a stellate ganglion block for a 55 yo, 62", 81 kg male with well-controlled hypertension and gout in his right great toe. His wife of 30 years just left the room and he is very anxious about the procedure. During administration, an intravascular injection occurs. What should you do?

The stem in Example 2 contains extraneous material, or window dressing, not relevant to the problem or concept to be tested. The stem should only contain the information necessary to arrive at the correct response. A more concise presentation of the question would be Example 3.

Example 3:

During administration of a stellate ganglion block, an intravascular injection occurs. The most appropriate initial intervention is to:

a. administer midazolam 2 mg.
b. call for help and ventilate with 100% oxygen.
c. initiate the ACLS algorithm with vasopressin 40 units.
d. place a central venous line to administer lipid emulsion.

Example 4:

The duration of IV succinylcholine after an induction dose is approximately:

a. 1–5 minutes.
b. 4–8 minutes.
c. 8–15 minutes.
d. 10–20 minutes.

The distractors of the question in Example 4 contain overlapping numeric data. It is preferable to avoid overlapping options or discrimination that is too fine. The item may have more than one correct answer and can be confusing to the examinee. Please refer to a revised version below.

Example 5:

The duration of intravenous succinylcholine after an induction dose is approximately:

a. 1–2 minutes.
b. 5–10 minutes.
c. 15–20 minutes.
d. 20–30 minutes.

Example 6:

Nondepolarizing neuromuscular blockers act as:

a. reversible competitive agonists for dopamine receptors.
b. irreversible competitive antagonists for acetylcholine receptors.
c. reversible competitive antagonists for acetylcholine receptors.
d. irreversible competitive agonists for acetylcholine receptors.

Example 6 is a representation of a double-barrel question. With limited knowledge, the examinee can easily rule out half the options, significantly improving the guessing odds. The savvy test-taker may further deduce the correct answer based on the fact that acetylcholine is used in a majority of the responses. This question could be revised with focus on a single concept as shown in Example 7.

> Example 7:
> Nondepolarizing neuromuscular blockers act on which receptor site:
> a. Dopaminergic
> b. Cholinergic
> c. Serotonergic
> d. Adrenergic

Another tool to assist faculty in developing well-written MCQs is the Fairness of Items Tool (FIT).[20] The FIT provides a comprehensive checklist for stem and option evaluations, as well as guidelines for the avoidance of linguistic, structural, and cultural bias (**Table 21.3**). In order to accurately assess student learning, test items should be free of bias so that students of equal ability perform similarly regardless of ethnicity or culture.[21]

Table 21.3 Fairness of Items Tool (FIT)[a]

Evaluate the Stem
1. Use a question format.
2. Eliminate extraneous words (eg, *of the following*).
3. Present a single, clearly defined question with the problem in the stem.
4. Avoid negatively phrased questions, double negatives, and the use of *except*.
5. Use active verbs and present tense.
6. Write questions at the application or above cognitive level.
7. Write questions that require multilogical thinking (require knowledge of more than one fact/concept).
8. Make sure content is current.
9. Avoid testing student opinions (eg, use *nurse* instead of *you* as the subject).
10. Test important content and avoid trivia.
Evaluate the Options
11. Make sure options are similar grammatically and in length and amount of detail.
12. Avoid none-of-the-above and all-of-the-above. Use three options instead.
13. Avoid negatively phrased options.
14. Avoid repeating material in the options – move repetitive words to the stem.
15. Avoid repeating words in the stem and correct option.
16. Avoid overlapping options.
17. Eliminate multiple-multiples.
18. Make sure all distractors are plausible.
19. If the stem asks what should be done first or which action is best, all options must be correct with only one option being the first or best.
20. Make sure there is only one correct answer.
21. Write options that require a high level of discrimination to select the correct answer.

Linguistic/Structural Bias
22. Use a parsimonious style and short simple sentences.
23. Use correct grammar, punctuation, capitalization, and spelling.
24. Use precise terms (avoid frequently, appropriate).
25. Avoid absolute terms (always, never, all).
26. Use straightforward, uncomplicated language. Test nursing content, not vocabulary or reading.
27. Write items that can be comprehended on the first reading. Avoid tricky or misleading items.
28. Ensure that items are independent of each other.
29. Be specific and clear with directions.
30. Use consistent spacing, question numbering/lettering, page numbering. Make sure options appear on the same page as the question.
Cultural Bias
31. Avoid dominant culture (literature, music, movies, sports, foods) unless essential to safe, effective nursing practice.
32. Eliminate all names.
33. Eliminate all slang.
34. Use terminology from textbook, notes, and common words (home vs. abode).
35. Eliminate humor.
36. Avoid stereotyping and over-representation of cultural groups.
37. Use gender-specific language only when necessary to test nursing content.
38. Present the person first, not the diagnosis.

[a]Used with permission from Nickole A. Hicks[20] 2012, revised 2014

While the single-best-answer MCQ is the only single-best-answer question used in the National Certification Examination, other single-best-answer item types are useful and well supported in the literature.[11–13,22,23] The National Board of Medical Examiners (NBME) also utilizes extended matching questions (EMQs), and only recently stopped using the traditional matching question (MQ) in favor of the EMQ.[11] These types of questions will be discussed later.

The conventional MQ is characterized by a set of options at the top or on the right, and a set of stems (sometimes referred to as stimuli) underneath or at the left. Instructions for the examinee on how to respond are provided at the beginning. Typically, matching items are limited to 4–5 options and by 2–5 stems. Advantages of MQs include relative ease of construction, concise scoring, and relatively short reading and response times. It can sometimes be challenging to develop homogenous option and stem sets, and MQs typically only measure simple recall and association. While MQs can be used to text higher cognitive processes, these types of MQs are more challenging to construct. Recommendations for development of MQs are listed in **Table 21.4**.

Table 21.4 Recommendations for MQ Development

- Provide clear instructions.
- Address a single theme with each question.
- Ensure homogeneity of stems and options.
- Arrange stems and options in a random manner.
- Use positive phrasing and consistent grammar in stems and options.

To avoid cueing, consider presenting an uneven number of stems and options. While each stem has only one correct response, allowing options to be used once, more than once, or not at all eliminates guessing by the process of elimination. The following is an example of a poorly designed item along with suggestions for revision.

Example 8:

Match the following:

_____ The mother of anesthesia.	A. Alice Magaw
_____ The first ether anesthetic.	B. William T.G. Morton
_____ A theory of anesthetic action.	C. Meyer-Overton Rule
_____ First used by Griffith and Johnson.	D. Curare
_____ Year the AANA was founded.	E. 1931

This question demonstrates several flaws. The directions are inadequate, the stems and options are heterogenous, and there is no central theme. Ordering of the options and stimuli are not random and are even in number. There is an obvious clue to the matching of Alice Magaw as the mother of anesthesia. This question could be improved as shown in Example 9.

Example 9:

Match the response choices (right) with the stimuli (left). Responses may be used once, more than once, or not at all.

_____ First use of N_20 in anesthesia.	A. Harold Griffith
_____ The first ether anesthetic.	B. August Bier
_____ The first spinal anesthetic.	C. Horace Wells
_____ First used curare in anesthesia.	D. William T.G. Morton
_____ First described IV regional anesthesia.	

In this revision, a central theme of the history of anesthesia is evident, and the stimuli and options are homogenous. The directions are more specific, the options are listed in random order, and cueing has been minimized.

A variation of the conventional MQ, EMQs are theme-based, one-best-answer questions that typically include a set of 10-26 options, a lead-in statement, and at least 2 stem questions. For each stem, the examinee must select a single answer from the list of options. Research supports the use of EMQs for testing higher order cognitive processes, such as application and analysis.[8,22,24] Like traditional MQs, advantages of the EMQ include ease of construction, concise scoring, and reasonable reading and response times (although this does increase proportionately with the number of options) and can be used for large-scale examinations. In addition, EMQs may be more resistant to cueing and guessing strategies.

It has been suggested that the theme, options, and lead-in statement be developed first and the stems be written last.[11] Recommendations for development of EMQs are provided in Table 21.5.

Table 21.5 Recommendations for EMQ Development

- Provide clear instructions.
- Address a single theme with each set.
- Establish the relationship between the options and stems with a lead-in statement.
- Make the options short and the stems long.
- Ensure homogeneity of options.
- Avoid the use of verbs in the options.
- Use positive phrasing and consistent grammar in stems and options.

The following is an example of a poorly designed item along with suggestions for revision.

Example 10:

Match the following:

A. cardiopulmonary arrest	F. interference with K+ channels
B. history of coagulopathy	G. postoperative pain management
C. risk of PONV	H. NPO status
D. decreased extremity movement	I. increased headache sensitivity
E. potential for CHF	J. seizure disorder

1. An important factor to consider prior to performing a regional block
2. A principal effect of local anesthetics during regional anesthesia
3. Possible adverse effect of regional anesthesia

While this item set appears to have a central theme of regional anesthesia, it is too broad. The options are not homogenous and include the use of verbs. The instructions are not clear and there is no lead-in statement to establish the relationship between the options and stems. The stems cannot be answered without looking at the options, and rank-ordering to select the best option for each stem is nearly impossible. Here is an example of an improved question in Example 11.

Example 11:

Directions: Match the appropriate option (top) to the stem (below).

Theme: Interscalene block complications

Options:

A. Hemidiaphragmatic paresis
B. Pneumothorax
C. Intravenous injection
D. Bronchospasm
E. Intrathecal injection
F. Cervical sympathetic block
G. Intra-arterial injection
H. Tracheal perforation
I. Recurrent laryngeal nerve block
J. Intraneural injection

Lead-in: For each of the following patients undergoing an interscalene block, select the most likely adverse event.

Stems:

1. During administration of an interscalene block, the patient begins to complain of dyspnea and difficulty swallowing and progresses to loss of consciousness.
2. During administration of an interscalene block, the patient complains of sudden, severe pain in the block site.
3. During administration of an interscalene block, the patient's speech begins to slur. The patient then loses consciousness and exhibits uncoordinated muscle movement.

In this revision, a more homogenous set of options and stems is offered based on the more focused theme of interscalene block complications. The directions are clear and a lead-in statement linking the options to the stems is present.

True/False Questions

True/false questions require the examinee to select all responses that are true. True/false item formats can be divided into two groups: simple true/false items and multiple true/false items. The simple true/false item is presented as a statement the examinee must determine as true or false. Multiple true/false (MTF) items include the A/B/both/neither format, sometimes referred to as C-type questions, and the complex MTF item, also known as the K-type question.

The true/false format tends to be utilized in the classroom setting, but not on standardized examinations. The NCE does not utilize true/false questions, and the NBME discourages their use.[11] The item writer may have something in mind while developing the question that upon further scrutiny is not apparent to the examinee, making the item difficult to qualify as clearly true or false. True/false questions can be confusing or perceived as tricky, particularly when a single word in the stem changes the statement from true to false. It is often difficult to develop clear, unambiguous true/false items that are not reduced to the task of simple recall of isolated facts. Assessing higher-order thought processes with true/false questions can be done, but they are more difficult to develop. The simple true/false format is also more susceptible to guessing.

Reported advantages of the simple true/false format include ease of construction for testing knowledge/recall of facts, straightforward scoring, reasonable reading and response time, and suitability for large-scale examinations. Disadvantages include difficulty assessing higher level cognitive domains, tendency of testing trivial content, and vulnerability for guessing. Complex MTF questions are generally not recommended for use as they tend to be more difficult and take longer to answer, but are no more discriminating than traditional MCQs.[9,25] Suggestions for writing true/false type questions are listed in Table 21.6.

Table 21.6 Recommendations for True/False Question Development

- Focus on a single concept or problem.
- Use clear, concise, positive phrasing.
- Make the items obviously true or false.
- Avoid absolute terms.

Example 12 is a flawed simple true/false item.

> Example 12:
> It is always best to avoid intubating a patient with a full stomach.
> True
> False

This item is problematic for several reasons. The statement is negatively phrased and the absolute term always is used. The intent of the question is not clear. Is it true because the writer intended that the procedure be delayed due to the full stomach, or is it false because patients with a full stomach should be intubated? Example 13 is an improved question.

> Example 13:
> Endotracheal intubation should be performed on the patient presenting with a full stomach for emergency abdominal surgery.
> True
> False

The intent of this question is clear and is phrased in a positive manner. It focuses on a single concept and the statement is defensibly true.

Multiple Correct Response Questions

The MCRQ, also referred to as multi-select question, is similar to the MCQ in that it consists of a single stem, but has four to ten response options, with more than one being correct. Recommendations for stem and response development are similar to those for the traditional MCQ (Tables 21.1 and 21.2). The total number of response items can range from four to eight, with approximately half being correct responses. For example, a MCRQ with three correct responses should have three distractors, for a total of six response options. One of the benefits of MCRQs is they can be used to revise MCQs with negatively phrased stems. An example of this is provided below.

> Example 14:
> What drug does not **not** exhibit organ-independent metabolism?
> a. Lidocaine c. Esmolol
> b. Remifentanil d. Atracurium

Example 15:		
Which of the following drugs exhibit organ-independent metabolism? **(Select 3)**		
Lidocaine	Midazolam	Dexmedetomidine
Remifentanil	Atracurium	Esmolol

Item development guidelines of the NBCRNA require that the number of correct responses be indicated at the end or underneath the stem, preferably with a boldface font.[15] An alternative to this is providing the instruction "select one or more options," though there is little research to strongly recommend one approach over the other. Whether to provide partial credit if the test-taker selects some, but not all, of the correct answers versus full credit if all correct options, and no incorrect options, are selected is another consideration with the use of MCRQs. Again, there is little evidence to advocate one strategy over the other, but it would be wise to determine how the test will be graded, and provide this information to the examinees ahead of time.

Completion Items

Completion testing items are constructed questions that require the examinee to either provide a short answer or fill-in-the-blank response with a single word or a few words. It is important to develop questions that elicit a short response; the longer the response, the more difficult it can be to score the item. Well-designed completion items have been shown to have high reliability and to discriminate more effectively.[26,27] Advantages include the ability to test a broad range of content and a reduced impact of guessing. Completion items work particularly well for questions requiring math calculations. Noncalculation questions can be challenging to develop because there is only one correct response. Other disadvantages may include difficulty reading the student's handwriting and more time required for grading due to unanticipated answers. Suggestions for creating completion items are presented in **Table 21.7**.

Table 21.7 Recommendations for Completion Item Development

- Develop items that can be completed with one word or short phrase.
- Ensure there is only one correct response.
- Avoid taking direct statements from assigned readings.
- When using blanks, place them toward the end of the sentence and use a consistent length.
- For math calculations, specify how precise the answer should be (nearest tenth).

Example 16 is ambiguous with many possible correct answers shown in parentheses. The question has been revised in Example 17 to ask for a single, correct response.

Example 16:
Succinylcholine acts at the ______________________.
(neuromuscular junction, motor end plate, skeletal muscle, nicotinic cholinergic receptor)

Example 17:
Succinylcholine acts at ______________________ cholinergic receptor sites. (nicotinic)

Essay Questions

Essay questions can range from short-answer to extended-response. An advantage of the essay question is the opportunity to assess higher level cognitive processes of analysis, synthesis, and evaluation.[13,28] Questions can be designed to address a specific, narrowly defined area in a broader, open-ended manner to allow the examinee more flexibility in generating a response. While the essay question may be easy to construct, it can be challenging to develop a clear scoring rubric for grading. Developing the rubric in advance is critical for both the examinee and the instructor. Some of the disadvantages of essay tests are the amount of time required for grading, reduced objectivity and test reliability, increased response time requirement, and language or legibility issues. Extended-response items with broad, open-ended questions tend to be more challenging to grade objectively. Even with a predetermined scoring rubric, the examinee may respond in a way unanticipated by the instructor. Recommendations for essay questions included in **Table 21.8.**

Table 21.8 Recommendations for Essay Question Development

- Items should be based on a specific (complex) learning objective.
- A scoring rubric should be established in advance.
- Clear instructions and scoring criteria should be provided to the examinee.
- Issues related to spelling, grammar, and penmanship should be addressed in advance.
- Questions that are too broad should be avoided.
- A time limit should be established.
- If using multiple essay questions, all examinees should answer all questions (no optional or select 2 out of 3 formats).
- The examinations should be scored/graded anonymously.
- All responses to one question should be scored before moving on to the next question.

The question in Example 18 is too broad and does not provide clear instructions or expectations. Example 19 provides a more precise task but still allows for some creativity on the part of the examinee. A possible grading rubric for Example 19 is also presented in **Table 21.9**, next page.

Example 18:
Describe the induction process for anesthesia.

Example 19:
Develop a care plan for general endotracheal anesthesia (GETA) for an 80kg patient with asthma for gastroesophageal reflux disease (assume the need for neuromuscular blockade during the case). Provide medication and dosing information in the following areas:

A. Premedication (5 points)
B. Induction (8 points)
C. Maintenance (6 points)
D. Emergence (3 points)

Also, list two medications you would consider avoiding in this patient (2 points each, must be from different drug classes) and explain why (2 points each).

Table 21.9 Scoring Rubric for Example 19

Premedication (5 pts)	Name 0.5 pts ea	Dose 0.5 pts ea	Induction (8 pts)	Name 1 pt ea	Dose 1 pt ea
benzodiazepine			opioid		
beta agonist			lidocaine		
H2 antagonist			sedative/hypnotic		
prokinetic			neuromuscular blocker		
nonparticulate antacid					
Maintenance (6 pts)	**Name 1 pt ea**	**Dose 1 pt ea**	**Emergence (3 pts)**	**Name 0.5 pts ea**	**Dose 0.5 pts ea**
inhalation/TIVA			anticholinesterase		
neuromuscular blocker			anticholinergic		
opioid/NSAID			antiemetic		
			Subtotals		
Medications to Avoid (8 pts)	**Name 2 pts ea**	**Reason 2 pts ea**			
beta blocker					
histamine releaser					
Subtotals			Total (30 pts possible)		

In addition to facilitating the process of grading essay questions, another benefit of developing a scoring rubric in advance is that it often leads to positive changes in the essay question itself. It may lead the writer to refine or narrow the question, or assign different point values to more accurately reflect the importance of certain aspects of the content the question is designed to cover. Providing information that the examinee needs to organize and prioritize his or her response is critical in enabling him or her to use the allowed testing time in the most efficient manner.

Other Techniques

This section is devoted to some creative assessment techniques the reader may or may not currently be using. For those interested in trying something different or as a complement to the more traditional didactic testing strategies, this section provides descriptions of and some general guidance on the use of these alternative evaluation methods. For those interested in more detailed information, a list of references is provided.

Lab Practical

The lab practical might traditionally be thought of as a series of stations where dissected anatomical parts are marked with a pin or various cell structures are indicated by an arrow on a slide under a microscope and must be identified by the examinee. This allows for the instructor to precisely assess the learner's knowledge as to whether he or she can correctly name a particular organ or structure. While labor-intensive and time-consuming to set up, the traditional lab practical is a useful tool for straightforward assessment of knowledge. However, what if assessment of higher-order thinking is desired? Evolution of the lab practical into a more participatory experience can allow for this type of measurement. Instead of having the examinee look through a microscope and identify a particular structure, he or she might be asked to focus the microscope and locate a particular structure. The creative lab practical might also take the form of a skills assessment where students are evaluated on essential skills. Winnett-Murray describes this approach in a department of biology, where students participate in lab practical examinations to assess proficiency in microscopy, animal handling, making serial dilutions, and other skills considered essential for biology majors.[29]

Objective Structured Clinical Examination

The counterpart of the expanded lab practical in the training and assessment of health care practitioners has been termed the Objective Structured Clinical Exam (OSCE). The OSCE has been described as a tool for evaluation of didactic knowledge and clinical skills and has been utilized within the fields of nursing, medicine, nutrition, physical therapy, occupational therapy, and radiation therapy.[30–40] The OSCE is a performance-based evaluation designed around a specific clinical skill or task to be completed within a certain time frame. An objective scoring tool is used to rate the examinee. In addition to evaluation, the OSCE can be used to provide feedback and ensure minimal competencies. Some specific examples of the use of OSCEs include evaluations of neonatal resuscitation by neonatal nurse practitioner students,[32] the ability of medical students to share information and decisions with patients,[33] and physical examination and multidisciplinary management plan development by rheumatology clinical nurse specialist students.[34] The Israeli Board of Anesthesiology has implemented the use of the OSCE format into their National Board Examination in several areas, including trauma management, resuscitation, crisis management, regional anesthesia, and mechanical ventilation.[35]

Some nurse anesthesia programs continue to utilize the lab practical as described earlier for the anatomy component. With the current variety and improved quality of simulation technology, the lab practical can be combined with simulated task trainers and be implemented for skills assessment as another means to evaluate didactic knowledge. The practice of nurse anesthesia includes many essential skills that may be evaluated in a lab practical setting or simulation center using the OSCE format, such as spinal and epidural anesthesia, central and arterial line placement, or laryngoscopy and intubation. Performance-based OSCEs in the areas mentioned earlier, such as resuscitation and crisis management, would also be appropriate within a nurse anesthesia program. The following is a brief example of a resuscitation scenario:[35(pp.857–858)]

Background: The examiner is a junior intern in the emergency room who calls on the anesthesia providers for help. The patient is a 70-year-old male with known heart failure admitted to the emergency room (ER) with shortness of breath.

The Simulator: Sim-Man simulator, in the sitting position, is connected to a monitor that displays noninvasive arterial blood pressure, electrocardiogram (ECG), and a pulse oximeter. One intravenous line is inserted; no oxygen is given.

Scenario: Upon the anesthesia provider's (the examinee's) arrival at the ER, the examiner presents himself or herself as a junior intern and the other examiner as an ER nurse. The examiner gives the anesthesia provider the patient's medical history and refers to the monitor. On the monitor: heart rate 120/min, oxygen saturation 90%, and arterial blood pressure, measured 10 min previously, at 150/100 mm Hg. Respiratory rate is 26/min.

Expected Performance and Examiner Response:

- Address the patient: the patient responds and complains of shortness of breath.
- Perform a physical examination: the examiner will provide the information that the neck veins are dilated and rales are present on both lung fields, in accordance with the anesthesia provider's performance.
- Give oxygen: The nurse (an examiner) will give oxygen and set up the oxygen flow on request.
- Ask for 12-lead ECG and a chest radiograph: The examiner will give the anesthesia provider both items on request and ask for interpretation.

The checklist items (address the patient, perform a physical exam, administer oxygen, ask for 12-lead ECG, ask for chest radiograph) are scored in a binary fashion as "performed" or "not performed" as a method for evaluating the student's performance.

Wunder et al[36] reported on the development and implementation of an OSCE program to assess competence in first-year nurse anesthesia students prior to starting clinical practicum. The OSCEs were constructed to match the curricular clinical performance objectives, and provide a mechanism for objective evaluation and also identification feedback on areas for improvement and self-reflection. A rigorous process was followed for development of scoring rubrics by the faculty. Evaluation of individual skills was implemented first, followed by the addition of team performance assessment.

The OSCE can be used to evaluate a variety of clinical skills and scenarios in a way that written examinations cannot, and there is evidence that it can be predictive of national high-stakes examination performance.[41] The OSCE does not come without some disadvantages. Like the traditional lab practical, it can be labor-intensive and time-consuming to develop and implement. The financial resources needed to invest in the necessary equipment and physical environment can be significant. The component of objectivity in the scoring process is essential, so developing a valid, reliable scoring tool and establishing minimal competency levels is critical, particularly since it is likely that multiple faculty will be involved in the testing process.[37,38] Execution of testing takes longer, and requires intense involvement of faculty. Examiner fatigue and ability to concentrate has been identified as a concern with long testing sessions.[39] Despite these challenges, student perception can be positive, and the exercise can improve confidence in the clinical setting.[40]

Concept Mapping

A concept map can be described as an organized visual representation of interrelated concepts of a central theme or major idea. Concept mapping has been widely reported as an instructional and assessment tool to teach and evaluate critical thinking in undergraduate nursing education.[41–46] While not as numerous, there are reports of the use of concept maps in graduate and postgraduate nursing programs.[47,48] Concept maps can be utilized early in the semester as a formative evaluation tool during the semester to evaluate progress, and at the end of the term as a summative, final examination. In addition to using the concept map for themes or ideas, it can also be applied to a particular type of case or individual patient.[42–46] In general, feedback regarding concept mapping has been positive from both students and instructors.[42,43]

Utilizing the concept map as a means of assessment requires careful planning and implementation. Students accustomed to and successful at objective style assessments may initially resist the idea of concept mapping as a testing tool. Clear instructions as to the process and expectations must be provided to the student well in advance, and it is helpful to provide examples and allow for draft submission and feedback.[45,49] It is important for both the student and the instructor to keep an open mind during this experience. Some students will excel at the more creative, individualized ability to express their ideas of interrelationships, while others will struggle with the somewhat abstract method of establishing and justifying these connections. Some concept maps will display thoughtful, profound representations while others will seem to exhibit superficial expression-based content.

Schuster provides a useful framework for patient care plan, concept map development.[50] Mezeske presents detailed guidelines for concept mapping of themes and ideas in the field of education.[49] General suggestions for use of concept maps include the following:

- Provide clear instructions and expectations.
- Establish a timeline.
- Develop a grading/scoring rubric.

Instructions and expectations should include the format (computer-generated or hard copy) and parameters on the size and type of materials that may be used. A timeline with multiple checkpoints and dates for draft and final submission can help facilitate progress, maintain scope of the project, and emphasize its importance. Benefits of using concept maps include stimulation of critical and reflective thinking and reduced risk of plagiarism. The time required for development and evaluation is an obvious drawback, but with experience (on the part of the instructor and student), this can be reduced to a reasonable length of time.[51]

Written Assignments

The written assignment is a longstanding tool for evaluating student learning and development. There are many formats available. This section will review reflective writing exercises and portfolio development as assessment tools. Reflective writing assignments can be described as a process whereby students learn from their own experiences. Examples of reflective writing formats include case reports and journaling. Reflective writing is well-supported in nursing education as a means to encourage critical thinking, increase engagement in the learning process, and improve self-awareness.[51–53] The use of portfolios, both at the undergraduate and graduate levels, is also described in nursing education and other health-related programs.[54–57] Portfolios have been used as a means to facilitate and document achievement of learning objectives and clinical competencies, stimulate critical thinking, and enhance professional development.[54,55]

When utilizing these forms of assessment, it is critical to provide clear guidelines to the student. Precise instructions and expectations save time and energy for both the student and instructor. Reflective writing assignments are not simply reports of observation and action. The student should also be making a connection between what occurred and his or her reasoning and thought processes both during and after the experience. General suggestions for instructors interested in implementing reflective writing assignments include:

- Define reflective writing for the student.
- Facilitate the process (do not focus on the product).
- Emphasize the importance of quality (not quantity).
- Provide a safe environment that encourages freedom of expression.
- Give constructive, supportive feedback.
- Maintain confidentiality.

The student may not understand what reflective writing is, so providing an explanation and giving examples are helpful. The instructor should set guidelines for content and length, with emphasis on the quality of the work instead of the quantity. The instructor should also establish a routine plan for submission and feedback that is timely and constructive. Students who feel intimidated by the process or the instructor will be hesitant to fully express their thoughts and feelings, and thus will not experience the full benefit of the exercise.

The portfolio has been defined as "a collection of personal work or materials that demonstrates growth over time."[56(p.74)] When used as a means of assessment, a written component is often added as a means for stimulating reflection and self-awareness of the growth process. This can take the form of reflective commentary on specific learning outcomes.[54,55] A variety of documents may be submitted as supportive evidence such as grade transcripts, standardized examination reports, assignments, meeting agendas, certificates of completion, licenses, certifications, resumes, job descriptions, performance evaluations, letters of reference, awards, clinical case tracking reports, and records of professional activities, to name a few. As with other writing assignments, explicit instructions and expectations should be given upfront, and periodic, prompt and constructive feedback should be provided throughout the process. The individual nature of the portfolio does not lend itself well to precise comparison with other portfolios. Scoring a portfolio requires careful advance planning to minimize bias.[54,55,58] Some institutions have developed specific guidelines for portfolio development.[58] Basic recommendations for portfolio assignments include:

- Divide the portfolio into manageable sections.
- Establish set parameters for length and supporting documentation.
- Identify the learning objectives to be evaluated.
- Establish standards for spelling, grammar, and format.
- Develop a precise scoring rubric.
- Implement a process for random verification of supporting documentation.
- Provide periodic, constructive feedback.

Possible sections of the portfolio could include a resume, learning objective commentaries or statements, a case report, and supportive evidence. Limiting the length of the commentary and number of supportive documents will result in a more compact, reflective portfolio. In order to maintain legitimacy of the assignment, random verification of supportive documents has been suggested.[58]

Oral Examination

Oral examinations are another tool for evaluating student knowledge. They are used by a variety of health-related disciplines periodically throughout their educational curriculum and as final, cumulative assessments. Many medical specialties include an oral examination component in their certification process, including the American Board of Anesthesiology (ABA). The degree to which nurse anesthesia programs utilize oral examinations has not been quantified in the literature, and there are few published reports of their use within the field of nursing.[59–61] A study comparing written and oral examinations in an undergraduate medical-surgical nursing course demonstrated effective evaluation of comprehension of content and clinical application with both techniques.[61] In Canada, a cohort of neonatal nurse practitioner graduates performed similarly to a group of pediatric residents on a comprehensive examination which included an oral examination component.[60] The use of oral examinations for certification by the ABA and Royal College of Physicians and Surgeons of Canada (RCPSC) has been reported in the literature as reliable and valid.[62–65] In preparation for the board certification oral examination and as a method to ensure core competencies, many anesthesiology residency programs have incorporated oral practice examinations (OPEs) into their assessment plan.

Advantages to utilizing oral examination are the ability to evaluate low and higher order cognitive processes and problem-solving capability. Thorough evaluation of communication skills can be accomplished in a way not afforded by most other types of assessment. The exercise of organizing knowledge, ideas, and opinions and presenting responses in an effective, confident manner is an invaluable skill. Some favor the face-to-face interaction with immediate ability to assess learner knowledge of the content area over the written examination process.

Disadvantages of oral examination include concerns regarding objectivity during the testing and grading process. The ABA oral examination is conducted in such a manner that the examiners are blinded to the candidate's training program, performance during residency, type or location of practice, and personality.[66] It would be difficult to achieve this level of objectivity for oral examinations administered during the training program. Associate examiners for the ABA are also required to attend training sessions each time they participate to ensure consistency in examination administration and grading techniques. Inter-rater and intra-rater reliability of examiners is a concern. One study of examiner reliability for OPEs in two anesthesiology residency programs was reported as fair to good – the authors suggested using at least two examiners to improve reliability.[57] Conducting oral examinations can be labor-intensive, particularly with large cohorts of students. Scheduling more than six students sequentially has been reported as exhausting to the examiner.[59(p.7)] Student feedback often includes complaints of stress and anxiety leading up to and during the examination.[59,61,64] In a study of anesthesiology residents participating in OPEs, a higher self-assessed level of anxiety correlated with poorer performance than those who self-assessed at a lower level of anxiety.[64]

When utilizing oral examination as a form of assessment, it is critical to prepare the examinee and provide clear instructions and guidelines as to how the examination will be administered, with particular attention to attenuating anxiety. Recommendations for instructors interested in administering oral examinations include the following:

- Provide clear information as to how the oral examination will be conducted.
- Develop a uniform list of questions in advance.
- Provide a practice session with sample questions during class.
- Develop a standardized grading rubric in advance.
- Audiotape or videotape the session, if possible.
- Provide a quiet testing environment free of distraction.
- Use two simultaneous evaluators whenever possible.

Informing the examinee of what to expect may alleviate the degree of stress and anxiety before and during the examination. Questions should be developed based on the learning objectives of the course and the cognitive processes the examiner wishes to evaluate. It is important to conduct the examination in a comfortable, quiet environment. Calls should be forwarded and a sign should be posted to prevent interruption. Permission to audio- or videotape should be obtained in advance, and recording equipment should be placed in the periphery, if possible. It is also helpful for the examiner to set a predetermined time limit.

Summary

As nurse anesthesia educators, our goal is to prepare safe, competent, and compassionate practitioners for the future. While it is important to provide the nurse anesthesia student with the necessary tools, information, and experiences to be successful on the National Certification Examination, it is also vital to instill a commitment to periodic reflection and lifelong learning. How we evaluate our students in the classroom setting can inform their future behavior and self-awareness in these areas. Using a variety of testing methods, allowing for creativity, and stimulating engagement in the learning process can help achieve these goals.

References

1. Merriam-Webster Editorial Staff. Teach. *Merriam-Webster's Collegiate Dictionary*. 11th ed. http://www.merriam-webster.com/dictionary/teach. Accessed April 28, 2008.

2. Merriam-Webster Editorial Staff. Test. *Merriam-Webster's Collegiate Dictionary*. 11th ed. http://www.merriam-webster.com/dictionary/test. Accessed April 28, 2008.

3. Giordano P. Principles of effective grading. In: Buskist W, Davis SF, eds. *Handbook of the Teaching of Psychology*. Malden, MA: Blackwell Publishing; 2006:254–258.

4. National Board of Certification and Recertification for Nurse Anesthetists. National Certification Examination (NCE) Handbook: January 2015. Available at: http://www.nbcrna.com/certification/SiteAssets/Pages/Program-Administration/ 20131118%20 NCE%20Candidate%20Handbook.pdf. Accessed April 4, 2016.

5. Wendt A, Kenny L. Setting the passing standard for the national council licensure examination for registered nurses. *Nurse Educ*. 2007;32:104–108.

6. Maki P. *Assessing for Learning: Building a Sustainable Commitment across the Institution*. Sterling, VA: Stylus Publishing; 2004.

7. De Champlain AF. Ensuring that the competent are truly competent: an overview of common methods and procedures used to set standards on high-stakes examinations. *J Vet Med Educ*. 2004;31(1):61–65.

8. McCoubrie P. Improving the fairness of multiple-choice questions: a literature review. Med Teach. 2004;26(8):709–712.

9. Downing SM. The effects of violating standard item writing principles on tests and students: the consequences of using flawed test items on achievement examinations in medical education. *Adv Health Sci Educ Theory Pract*. 2005;10(2):133–143.

10. Tarrant M, Ware J. Impact of item-writing flaws in multiple-choice questions on student achievement in high-stakes nursing assessments. *Med Educ*. 2008;42(2),198–206.

11. Case SM, Swanson DB. *Constructing Written Test Questions for the Basic and Clinical Sciences*, 3rd ed (rev.). Philadelphia, PA: National Board of Medical Examiners; 2002.

12. Haladyna TM. Developing and Validating Multiple-Choice Test Items, 3rd ed. Mahwah, NJ: Lawrence Erlbaum Associates; 2004.

13. Juve JA. Test construction. In: Buskist W, Davis SF, eds. *Handbook of the Teaching of Psychology*. Malden, MA: Blackwell Publishing; 2006:247–253.

14. Promissor, Inc. *Item Writing Guide*. Evanston, IL: Computer Adaptive Technologies; 1999.

15. National Board of Certification and Recertification for Nurse Anesthetists. Item Development Guidelines with an Overview of the Examination Development Process. http://www.nbcrna.com/certification/Documents/20150430%20Item%20 Development%20Guidelines.pdf. Accessed April 4, 2016.

16. Roberts DM. An empirical study on the nature of trick test questions. *J Educ Meas*. 1993:30(4):331–344.

17. Haladyna TM, Downing SM. How many options is enough for a multiple-choice test item? *Educ Psychol Meas*. 1993;54(3):999–1010.

18. Rodriguez MC. Three options are optimal for multiple-choice items: a meta-analysis of 80 years of research. *Educational Measurement: Issues and Practice*. 2005;24(2):3–13.

19. Haladyna TM, Rodriguez MC. Selected-response formats. In Haladyna TM, Rodriguez MC, eds. Developing and Validating Test Items. New York, NY: Routledge; 2013:61–88.

20. Hicks NA. Establishing the Validity and Reliability of the Fairness of Items Tool [dissertation]. Greeley: University of Northern Colorado; 2014.

21. Hicks NA. Guidelines for identifying and revising culturally biased multiple-choice nursing examination items. *Nurse Educ*. 2011;36(6):266–270.

22. Beullens J, Van Damme B, Jaspaert H, Janssen PJ. Are extended-matching multiple-choice items appropriate for a final test in medical education? *Med Teach*. 2002;24(4):390–395.

23. Swanson DB, Holtzman KZ, Allbee K, Clauser BE. Psychometric characteristics and response times for content-parallel extended-matching and one-best-answer items in relation to number of options. *Acad Med*. 2006;81(10 Suppl):S52–55.

24. Coderre SP, Harasym P, Mandin H, Fick G. The impact of two multiple-choice question formats on the problem-solving strategies used by novices and experts. *BMC Med Educ*. 2004;4(23):1–9.

25. Haladyna TM, Downing SM, Rodriguez MC. A review of multiple-choice item-writing guidelines for classroom assessment. *Applied Measurement in Education*. 2002;15(3):309–334.

26. Rademakers J, Ten Cate TJ, Bar PR. Progress testing with short answer questions. *Med Teach*. 2005;27(7):578–582.

27. Ramos KD, Schafer S, Tracz SM. Validation of the Fresno test of competence in evidence based medicine. *BMJ*. 2003;326(7384):319–321.

28. Tomey AM. Completion testing items. *Nurse Educ*. 1999;24(6):6–7.

29. Winnett-Murray K. Resurrecting the Lab Practical. In: Mezeske RJ, Mezeske BA, eds. *Beyond Tests and Quizzes: Creative Assessments in the College Classroom*. San Francisco, CA: Jossey-Bass; 2007:56–69.

30. Bromley LM. The objective structured clinical exam: practical aspects. *Curr Opin Anaesthesiol*. 2000;13:675–678.

31. Major DA. OSCEs seven years on the bandwagon: The progress of an objective structured clinical evaluation programme. *Nurse Educ Today*. 2005;25:442–454.

32. Brooks G. Assessment of student advanced neonatal nurse practitioners in resuscitation and stabilization of the newborn: The use of the objective structured clinical examination. *J Neonatal Nurs*. 2004;10(6):184–188.

33. Thistlethwaite JE. Developing an OSCE station to assess the ability of medical students to share information and decisions with patients: issues relating to interrater reliability and the use of simulated patients. *Educ Health*. 2002;15(2):170–179.

34. Ryan S, Stevenson K, Hassell AB. Assessment of clinical nurse specialists in rheumatology using an OSCE. *Musculoskeletal Care*. 2007;5(3):119–129.

35. Berkenstadt H, Ziv A, Gafni N, Sidi A. Incoporating simulation-based objective structured clinical examination into the Israeli national board examination in anesthesiology. *Anesth Analg*. 2006;102:853–858.

36. Wunder LL, Glymph DC, Newman J, Gozalez V, Gonzalez JE, Groom JA. Objective structured clinical examination as an educational initiative for summative simulation competency evaluation of first-year student registered nurse anesthetists' clinical skills. *AANA J*. 2014;82(6):419–425.

37. Bagnasco A, Tolotti A, Pagnucci N, Torre G, Timmins F, Aleo G, Sasso L. How to maintain equity and objectivity in assessing the communication skills in a large group of student nurses during a long examination session, using the Objective Structured Clinical Examination (OSCE). *Nurse Educ Today*. 2016;38:54–60.

38. Brennan PA, Croke DT, Reed M, Smith L, Munro E, Foulkes J, Arnett R. Does changing examiner stations during UK postgraduate surgery objective structured clinical examinations influence examination reliability and candidates' scores? *J Surg Educ*. 2016;73(4):616–623.

39. Swift M, Spake E, Kohia M. Examiner fatigue and ability to concentrate in objective structured clinical examinations for physical therapist students. *J Allied Health*. 2016;45(1):62–70.

40. Farahat E, Javaherian-Dysinger H, Rice G, Schneider L, Daher N, Heine N. Exploring students' perceptions of the educational value of formative objective structured clinical examination (OSCE) in a nutrition program. *J Allied Health*. 2016;45(1):20–26.

41. Pugh D, Bhanji F, Cole G, Dupre J, Hatala R, Humphrey-Murto S, Touchie C, Wood TJ. Do OSCE progress test scores predict performance in a national high-stakes examination? *Med Educ*. 2016;50:351–358.

42. Hicks-Moore SL. Clinical concept maps in nursing education: an effective way to link theory and practice. *Nurse Educ Pract*. 2005;5:348–352.

43. Hicks-Moore SL, Pastirik PJ. Evaluating critical thinking in clinical concept maps: a pilot study. *Int J Nurs Educ Scholarsh*. 2006;3(1):Article 27.

44. Hsu L. Developing concept maps from problem-based learning scenario discussions. *J Adv Nurs*. 2004;48(5):510–518.

45. Hsu L, Hsieh S. Concept maps as an assessment tool in a nursing course. *J Prof Nurs*. 2005;21(3):141–149.

46. King M, Shell R. Teaching and evaluation critical thinking with concept maps. *Nurs Educ*. 2002;27(5):214–216.

47. Giddens J. Concept mapping as a group learning activity in graduate nursing education. *J Nurs Educ*. 2006;45(1):45–46.

48. Hill CM. Integration clinical experiences into the concept mapping process. *Nurs Educ*. 2006;31(1):36–39.

49. Mezeske RJ. Concept mapping: assessing pre-service teachers' understanding and knowledge. In Mezeske RJ, Mezeske BA, eds. *Beyond Tests and Quizzes: Creative Assessments in the College Classroom*. San Francisco, CA: Jossey-Bass; 2007:8–25.

50. Schuster PM. Concept mapping: Reducing clinical care plan paperwork and increasing learning. *Nurse Educ*. 2000;25(2):76–81.

51. Harris M. Scaffolding reflective journal writing—negotiating power, play, and position. *Nurse Educ Today*. 2008;28:314–326.

52. Kessler PD, Lund CH. Reflective journaling: developing an online journal for distance education. *Nurse Educ*. 2004;29(1):20–24.

53. Ruland JP, Ahern NR. Transforming student perspectives through reflective writing. *Nurse Educ*. 2007;32(2):81–88.

54. Schaffer MA, Nelson P, Litt E. Using portfolios to evaluate achievement of population-based public health nursing competencies in baccalaureate nursing students. *Nurs Educ Perspect*. 2005;26(2):104–112.

55. Jasper MA, Fulton J. Marking criteria for practice-based portfolios at masters' level. *Nurse Educ Today*. 2005;25:377–389.

56. Ray R. Tracking learning over time in health care education using clinical proficiency transcripts. In Mezeske RJ, Mezeske BA, eds. *Beyond Tests and Quizzes: Creative Assessments in the College Classroom*. San Francisco, CA: Jossey-Bass; 2007:139–151.

57. Kalet AL, Sanger J, Chase J, Keller A, Schwartz MD, Fishman ML, et al. Promoting professionalism through an online professional development portfolio: successes, joys, and frustrations. *Acad Med*. 2007;82(11):1065–1072.

58. Lettus MK, Moessner PH, Dooley L. The clinical portfolio as an assessment tool. *Nurs Adm Q*. 2001;25(2):74–9.

59. Bairan A, Farnsworth B. Oral exams: An alternative evaluation method. *Nurse Educ*. 1997;22(4):6–7.

60. Mitchell A, Watts J, Whyte R, Blatz S, Norman GR, Guyatt, GH, et al. Evaluation of graduating neonatal nurse practitioners. *Pediatrics*. 1991;88(4):789–794.

61. Rushton P, Eggett D. Comparison of written and oral examinations in a baccalaureate medical-surgical nursing course. *J Prof Nurs*. 2003;19(3):142–148.

62. Eagle CJ, Martineau R, Hamilton K. The oral examination in anaesthetic resident evaluation. *Can J Anaesth*. 1993;40(10):947–953.

63. Kearney RA, Puchalski SA, Yang H, Skakun EN. The inter-rater and intra-rater reliability of a new Canadian oral examination format in anesthesia is fair to good. *Can J Anaesth*. 2002;49(3):232–236.

64. Shubert A, Tetzlaff JE, Tan M, Rychman JV, Mascha E. Consistency, inter-rater reliability, and validity of 441 consecutive mock oral examinations in anesthesiology: implications for use as a tool for assessment of residents. *Anesthesiology*. 1999;91(1):288–298.

65. Tetzlaff JE. Assessment of competency in anesthesiology. *Anesthesiology*. 2007;106:812–825.

66. James, FM. Oral practice examinations: are they worth it? *Anesthesiology*. 1999;91(1):4–6.

CHAPTER 22

Encouraging Scholarship Among Nurse Anesthesia Students: The Role of the Faculty Mentor

Chuck Biddle, PhD, CRNA

Keywords: Mentorship, peer review, poster presentations, publishing, research, scholarly activity, scholarly writing, writing for publication.

Key Concepts

- *Scholarship* assumes many forms but is broadly defined as the expansion and refinement of the scientific foundations for our specialty; educators are heavily invested in supporting and promoting scholarly activity by our students.
- Students will often propose research questions or projects that are too broad in nature or too ill-defined. Rather than discouraging their enthusiasm, faculty should redirect the student's energy toward developing a highly relevant, focused, and researchable question or limited number of questions.
- In assuming the role of research mentor, one must be reasonably available to the student, be prepared to help refer complex questions to appropriate domain experts, facilitate the development of a manageable timeline for the student, and assist in clarifying the roles and responsibilities of the student.
- Students should be educated about the purpose and responsibilities of the peer-review system, reminding them that the process is an opportunity to have their work closely examined and critiqued by experts in the domain so that their work can be presented in its most valid and useful form.
- Barriers exist that students must contend with prior to engaging in a serious scholarly project. Students should seek out a faculty advisor who has demonstrated expertise and success in scholarly inquiry, and should plan for things to go wrong and have contingencies in mind so that they are prepared to deal with setbacks. Intellectual curiosity, flexibility, patience, stamina, and perseverance are key attributes for success.

The amount of writings of a profession is a measure of its vitality and activity, while their quality is a rough indication of its intellectual state.

—Sir Robert Hutchinson, 1939, *Lancet*

Nurse anesthesia educators (NAEs) are heavily vested in supporting and promoting health care research, in general, and perioperative care, in particular. In my view, research is a process by which we come to better understand the world around us, a process driven by asking important, relevant questions and seeking answers to them. Dissemination of the outcomes from that process is the essential next step. Research without dissemination is associated with a number of lost benefits (**Table 22.1**).

Table 22.1 Benefits of Communicated Research

To the public:	Improvements and refinements in patient care
To the profession:	Enhancement of the image and stature of its members
Institution:	Pride and reputation of its contributing staff
Personal:	Satisfaction, advancement, recognition among professional peers

Scholarly activity in nurse anesthesia is a key component of our profession's activity, setting it apart from a merely technical enterprise performed by its members. One essential attribute of a profession is having a systematic body of knowledge that must be expanded by research and passed on to the next generation of its members.[1] Nurse anesthesia scholarship takes on many forms but can be broadly viewed as the expansion and refinement of our knowledge and skills, the sharing of ideas and expertise, critically evaluating existing and new approaches, and a commitment to growing the scientific foundations of our specialty. We also find ourselves at a critical evolutionary juncture given the national movement toward awarding the doctorate in nurse anesthesia practice. I am strongly of the view that NAEs have an obligation to promote scholarship among their students. The goals of this chapter are to advance this belief, and to offer some guidance in that quest.

It should be established at the outset that there is no intent to imply that all NAEs should be engaged in research, traditionally defined as engaging in the pursuit of new knowledge through rigorously controlled experiments. In fact, the definition, scope, and expectation of faculty scholarship have evolved considerably in university settings nationwide. While the need for both basic science and clinical investigators is essential, there is also the clinical scholar role that many of us may feel more comfortable with. This role does not demand one to produce new knowledge; instead, the responsibility is to perfect and maintain one's own clinical expertise and to impart that knowledge and skill set onto students and junior members of the profession.

While Table 22.1 gives a broad overview of the benefits of engaging in, and sharing the findings of research, I am also a pragmatist, and believe that for the process to be truly embraced, we must help the student appreciate the associated rewards at the individual level. **Table 22.2** gives an overview of these rewards and provides NAEs with talking points regarding the personal factors associated with engaging in scholarly activity. Faculty should not limit themselves to these points but should discuss, from the heart, what their personal views and passions are about engaging in scholarly activity.

Table 22.2 Focusing on the Personal Factors Associated with Scholarly Activity

- Personal satisfaction in executing a knowledge quest and sharing it with others
- Satisfying one's curiosity
- Helping to define and experience a potential career path
- Engaging in a personal passion: passion for exploring, creating, or writing
- Potential monetary reward for created work
- Satisfaction in achieving recognition among professional peers

The Faculty Role in the Process of Scholarship

I am heartened by the number of recent graduates from programs of nurse anesthesia who actively seek careers in academia despite the barriers that may exist (eg, generally lower salary, exposure to vicarious liability, potential for not fully autonomous practice, the often politically charged environment of a coexisting anesthesia residency program, etc.). I am also buoyed by the large number of papers submitted to the *AANA Journal* and other peer-reviewed journals by our students, by faculty new to the profession, and by established faculty. But with respect to the student cohort, what can we do to further advance their contributions?

The research process can be simplified into three steps or stages: planning, execution of the plan, and peer review of the outcome. It is vital for the faculty mentor to get to know something about the student's background, professional interests, and previous experience. To do otherwise is needlessly naive and will too often result in a negative (unpleasant, boring, frustrating) or disastrous (giving up or otherwise failing to complete) experience. It is essential for the faculty mentor not to lose sight of the following: A student may feel an obligation to engage in a project that is of little personal interest because he or she does not want to disappoint the faculty member. If a student is clearly unable to generate an idea of their own choosing, and the faculty member elects to recommend a topic or project, it is important to establish an open dialogue with that student in order to assessa genuine interest and establish if he or she has the skill set to engage in the project.

A student may come to the faculty member with a preconceived question that is much too broad and lacks focus. For example, "I wish to study the autonomic response to our intravenous induction agents," or "Is regional anesthesia preferable to general anesthesia?" or "What drug is best to prevent postoperative nausea and vomiting?" are questions that will overwhelm even the most passionate investigator and are sorely in need of focus. In this event, the best course is to encourage the student to take some time to come up with three to five focused questions that might fall under the umbrella of the initial broad question, and then return to discuss which question(s) is(are) of greatest interest and whether or not the question(s) can actually be addressed. Essential talking points at this stage are listed in **Table 22.3**, next page, and will help the student and mentor to better assess the feasibility of the proposed enterprise.

Table 22.3 Assessing the Viability of the Student's Idea

Here the fundamental issue is whether or not the project can be completed.

Issues to consider:

- Do I (as faculty) have the expertise to advise the student or is a referral necessary?
- Does the student have the knowledge and energy to complete the task?
- Is the research question one that can be answered?
- Can it be accomplished in the time that is available?
- Can the student and faculty control the factors essential to the research (space, equipment, research subject recruitment, funding, etc.)?
- If applicable, what are the Institutional Review Board considerations?

Occasionally a student will come to a faculty member professing the desire to do something substantial that will have immediate practice applications of such magnitude that major biomedical journals will clamor for the rights to publish it. Such unbridled enthusiasm should not be discouraged, but should be constructively redirected toward developing a relevant, focused question. Students should be reminded that what will ultimately yield a publication or poster or invited presentation is not the question, but the answer generated by a well-conceived methodology. Since at this stage the answer is not yet known, it is better to focus on developing a question that is amenable to systematic inquiry with the resources that are available.

If you are willing to assume the role of mentor, what then are your responsibilities? This is a very complex question and only some broad guidelines will be suggested. First, the faculty member must be available to the student to help with problem-solving and counsel. Second, if the target of the research is not one amenable to your skill set, then assuming the role of referral agent is likely the best course of action. The ability to professionally network (locally, regionally, or nationally) provides one with a powerful tool to assist in the student's scholarly quest. Third, recognize that it is the nature of the enterprise that far more projects are started than completed, and clearly, no unique algorithm, recipe, or approach works with all students. Just as teaching a student to place an epidural catheter, or when to turn down the inhaled agent as the case ends, or how best to evaluate and treat new-onset bradycardia are all context-sensitive, requiring artful intervention and reminders, so is the case with scholarly mentorship. Sometimes the faculty member will need to be more prescriptive than at other times. I do believe that if the project is truly a student project, then it is vital for the student to be able to claim intellectual ownership. This means that the student can rightfully be listed as the first author on a resultant paper publication.

Fourth, an absolutely vital role is to assist the student in developing a reasonable and manageable timeline, one that ensures that the goals, roles, and milestones are clearly described and understood (by all!) from the outset. In virtually all situations, more time is required to complete a given project than is initially planned. And finally, it is essential that one facilitates clarification of the roles and responsibilities for the student, the faculty, and any others participating in the project. This is also the time to discuss the issue of authorship and order of listed authors using established criteria (**Table 22.4**).

Table 22.4 Criteria for Authorship of a Published or Presented Work[2,3]

- Authorship requires having made substantial input at all phases of the work.
- In the case of research it implies substantial input at:
  - study conception and design;
  - data analysis and interpretation;
  - drafting and critically revising the submitted and revised paper; and
  - final approval of the published version.

It comes as no surprise to experienced educators to learn of a situation where the faculty mentor actually performs the project for the student. Watching a new student struggle with a clinical procedure or belabor a clinical decision can be frustrating. The desire (and, sometimes, the necessity) to quickly intervene and simply do it yourself can be overwhelming. This can occur in the scholarship process as well. It is critical to maintain patience and judgment throughout, but as in the process of clinical instruction, it is also important to know when to encourage, and when to directly intervene.

Negotiating the Treacherous Waters of Peer Review

There are many dimensions to the peer review system. Perhaps the most common example involves presenting one's work for colleagues' critique. This can take the form of submitted manuscripts, abstracts, or book chapters. Other forms include poster presentations, oral presentations, grant applications, and even the traditional journal club, where published work is presented and evaluated by those in attendance. An overview of a rather typical process of submitting a paper to a peer-reviewed journal is found in **Figure 22.1**, next page. A general set of guidelines to be considered when preparing a paper for submission to a peer reviewed journal is found in **Table 22.5** and is typical of what journal editors and reviewers will consider in their critique of a submitted paper.

Students should be informed that the process of peer review is an opportunity to have their work closely examined and critiqued by experts in the domain. The goal of peer review is to perform a collaborative gate-keeping, such that only the most meaningful, accurate, and rational information is formally disseminated. Too often, submitting authors experience anger or intense frustration when their work is criticized—it is not a process to be taken personally! When the submitting author receives the manuscript critique back, it should be read and put away for a day or two. Return to it only after a period of reflection has occurred with an open mind free of emotional reactivity. Revise the paper based on the reviewers' suggestions. If the student strongly disagrees with certain elements of the critique, he or she should avoid emotively driven arguing. Instead, the student should prepare a reasonable, scientifically based response to the editor, justifying the case in a well-constructed letter.

Figure 22.1 Submitting a Paper to a Peer-Reviewed Journal

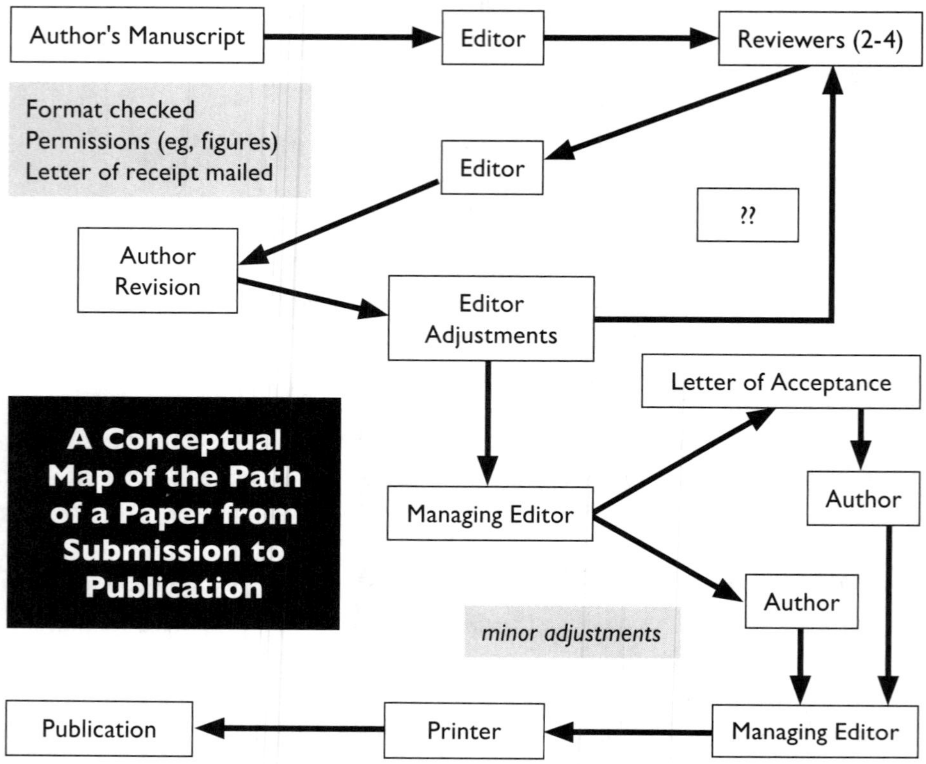

The path from submission to publication is complex, time intensive, and highly interactive. Under the guidance of a coordinating editor (usually the editor-in-chief) the paper is critically reviewed by domain experts and returned to the submitting author for revisions. There are a number of outcomes that might result from peer review that range from acceptance of the paper in its originally submitted form to outright rejection with no chance for reconsideration. The majority of papers fall somewhere between these extremes; with appropriate and timely revision, these papers might be published.

Table 22.5 Suggested Factors to Consider In Preparing a Manuscript for Submission

General considerations:
• Adhere precisely to the guidelines and formatting instructions of the journal • Avoid spelling and grammar errors and poor syntax, which indicate imprecision • Consider the journal's audience, keeping them in mind as the paper is prepared • Remain focused on the question(s) and objective(s) raised in the introduction • Avoid generalizing beyond the scope of your project • Make sure that the work is original and has relevance • Avoid self-promotion; let the work stand on its own • Do not overlook the relevant and important work of others • Critically discuss cited work rather than simply regurgitating the findings • Include appropriate references with precision • Do not rely too heavily on secondary reference sources (textbooks) • Avoid the use of Internet references; these change and are often not peer-reviewed • Avoid editorialization of your personal views • Discuss implications for practice and how the paper differs from previous work • Have the paper proofread by a knowledgeable, critical party unrelated to the paper • Be as concise as possible
Considerations specific to research projects:
• If relevant: provide proof of Institutional Review Board approval • Describe your methods in sufficient detail that the study could be replicated • Carefully consider measurement reliability and validity issues • If applicable, do a power analysis for appropriate sample size • Explain how subjects were selected and discuss their representativeness • Explain and justify the method of data analysis • Consider the issue of clinical significance versus statistical significance • Avoid cause-and-effect conclusions where associations among variables is appropriate • Ensure that your conclusions are supported by the data • Explain any conflicts with previous literature • Suggest implications for practice and future research

The Student Role in the Process of Scholarship

Students must make a substantial commitment to do a properly performed scholarly project. There are many barriers that the student must contend with and it is important to identify and reconcile (if possible) the barriers prior to moving forward with a serious scholarly project. **Table 22.6** (next page) is a partial list of common barriers that students encounter in engaging in scholarly activities.

Table 22.6 Identifying Potential Barriers to Engaging in Scholarly Activity

The student should personally consider: • Do I have sufficient interest in the area to justify my involvement in this project? • Given my other personal and professional demands, do I have the time to do this? • Do I have the confidence, experience, and skill set to do this project? • Am I doing this simply because a faculty member asked me to participate? • Is my primary reason for doing this because I don't want to offend the faculty? • Is the faculty advisor/mentor someone I can work with? • Does the faculty advisor/mentor have history of success with other students? If uncertain about your ability to engage the project, consider choosing a smaller, less complex, less ambitious project.

Students who are searching for a faculty advisor should "research the researcher," seeking the views of other students regarding the nature, quality, timeliness, and success of previous scholarly enterprises. The stages of research (from planning to dissemination) all have their inherent pitfalls. Students should proactively plan for things to go wrong and have contingencies in mind so that they are prepared to deal with setbacks. For example, subject enrollment may not be keeping pace as anticipated, the database that was planned for the retrospective chart review may be temporarily unavailable, and the noninvasive cardiac output monitor promised for the duration of the study has been recalled.

The unexpected happens. Important characteristics of being a successful clinical anesthetist include the ability to problem-solve and be resourceful. These attributes likewise are part of being a researcher and students should, to the best of their ability, engage problems head-on and attempt to remedy them;however, as in the clinical area, having a successful and experienced mentor who regularly communicates with students, pays dividends when problems arise that prove particularly troublesome.

Poster Presentations

A common form of scholarship is the poster presentation that occurs at seminars, scholarly meetings, and clinical conferences. Posters provide student researchers with the ability to visually display their work, and discuss their research and findings with interested individuals or even small groups. Generally there is a designated location where posters are set up at meetings. For example, at the annual national meeting of the American Association of Nurse Anesthetists (AANA), there is an extensive display of posters that is organized and located within the exhibit hall. This is a great opportunity for students to display and discuss their scholarly projects in a session specifically designed to promote scholarly discourse. Additional information regarding presenting a poster at the national meeting can be found at the AANA's website.[4]

There are many recipes for developing a poster and the recommendations listed in **Table 22.7** are provided to give the student some broad guidelines that I have found to be successful in participating in and observing many poster sessions across a wide range of disciplines. **Figure 22.2** offers a suggested format for the actual organization and layout of a poster although it should be emphasized that many modifications are possible.

Table 22.7 Preparing a Poster for Presentation of a Scholarly Project

Aesthetic issues:
- Keep the poster professional; avoid trying to be too trendy or unconventional
- Consider using contrasting colors for readability but use only 2-3 colors
- Mount your printed material on a colored background to create a border/frame
- Consider using relevant and interesting photographs or figures
- Avoid cramming your materials together even though space is limited
- Use a consistent spacing rule between the elements in your poster
- Consider aligning corners and vertical and horizontal lines (see Figure 22.2)

Organizational issues:
- Use a consistent font style throughout the poster (sans serif style is easy to read)
- The title should be easily read from 20 feet away
- The textual components of the poster should be easily read from 6 feet away
- Emphasize important textual components with boldface, underlining, or color
- Avoid italics; they can be hard to read from a distance
- Organize layout in columns and counterclockwise starting in upper left (Figure 22.2)
- Make section headings distinct from the body of the textual writing
- Graphics are good, but use only those that are relevant and necessary

Related issues:
- Remember, you will be interacting with others about your work be prepared to discuss
- If the poster is a distillation of a full paper, have copies of the paper for distribution
- Alternatively, have a printed one-page abstract for distribution
- Alternatively, have a printed one-page handout of the key points of your research
- Dress professionally
- Have a dress rehearsal; invite others to quiz you prior to the formal poster session

Figure 22.2 Suggested Format for the Layout of the Poster Presentation

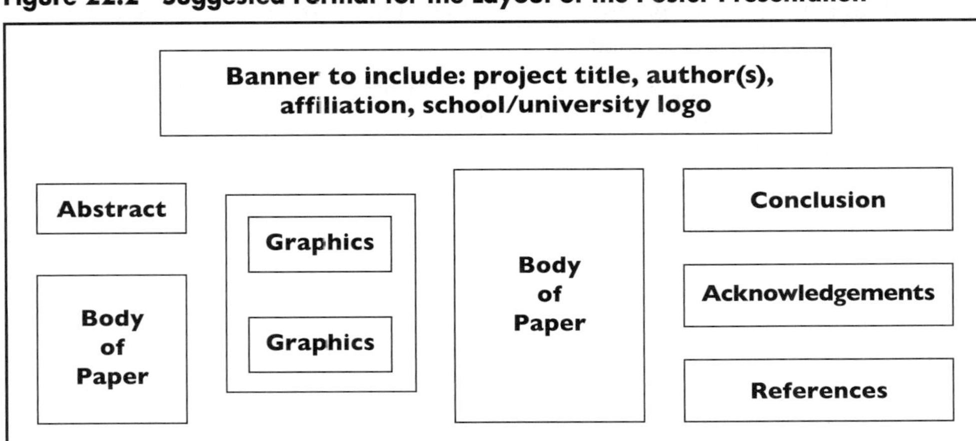

Follow the Evidence

In an insightful paper many years ago Comroe and Dripps opined, and specified empirical foundations for their view that biomedical progress depends on basic bench investigation.[5] It predated much of what we currently know as evidence-based care, but their view was needlessly narrow, even myopic. As educators, researchers, and clinicians we know that a hallmark of science with potential applied influence, has the ability to break disciplinary boundaries and cross-fertilize with other, even remote, scientific fields.

Consider work that is quite separate from the biological bench. Think of informatics, sensors, team communication, engineering, electronics, ergonomics, material science, and the many other domains that make current research and critical thinking in our field so exciting. Mentors can help to stimulate the still substantial disconnect between discovery research, translational research, evaluation of research, and implementation research. The possibilities are limitless.

Summary

Nurse anesthesia educators find themselves in roles where significant and powerful professional influence occurs. The potential value inculcation that occurs regarding scholarly activity can have immediate and long-term rewards for the student. Think of your students as potential researchers and authors and do not be hesitant to share that vision with them. Talk about other student and faculty publishing successes and help your students see that scholarly activities that culminate in poster presentations, oral presentations, and published papers are goals that they can realistically achieve.

Mentoring students by stimulating their interest in scholarly activity and facilitating their success is a deeply rewarding professional activity for NAEs. Ask students if they are considering a scholarly activity. Be supportive if initial enthusiasm wanes a bit as student priorities change. Don't become discouraged if a particularly promising student does not present or publish his or her research. Your role should be defined as one that encourages and facilitates, rather than one that insists. To this end, don't be surprised if later (sometimes even years later) former students send you a copy of their recently published paper or their invited presentation with a thank you for giving them the inspiration and courage to try.

References

1. Greenwood E. Attributes of a profession. *Soc Work*. 1957;2(3):45–55.

2. International Committee of Medical Journal Editors. Uniform requirements for manuscripts submitted to biomedical journals. *Ann Intern Med.* 1997;126(1):36–47.

3. Shapiro DW, Wenger NS, Shapiro MF. The contributions of authors to multiauthored biomedical research papers. *JAMA*. 1994;271(6):438–442.

4. Access aana.com. Once logged on, search for "AANA Foundation" and "AANA National Meeting" for information regarding presenting at the poster session at the Annual Congress.

5. Comroe JH, Jr, Dripps RD. Scientific basis for the support of biomedical science. *Science*. 1976;192(4235):105–111.

CHAPTER 23

The Doctor of Nursing Practice (DNP) Project

Brian Benham, DNP, CRNA
Madeline K. Chalenor, DNP, MHS, CRNA

Keywords: DNP project, early adopters, early majority, evidence-based practice (EBP), implementation, innovation, Innovation-Decision Process, sustained change, transformational leadership.

Key Concepts

- As transformational leaders, Certified Registered Nurse Anesthetists (CRNAs) develop skills and attain competencies to improve quality and translate evidence into patient-centered care.
- A clinical culture that embraces evidence-based practice (EBP) for anesthesia care is important because, without a culture that supports EBP, an organization will not sustain change, no matter how good the project.
- A written agreement between the student, doctor of nursing practice (DNP) chair, and organizational leader may help delineate short, intermediate, and long-term strategies, timelines, individual responsibilities, support, incentives, and resources related to the DNP project.
- The Innovation-Decision Process offers CRNA educators a helpful path to create a receptive clinical culture for DNP projects and a guide for students to successfully implement and sustain their DNP projects.
- How individuals and organizations perceive the relative advantage, compatibility, complexity, trialability, and observability of the new idea determines how fast individuals or a group implement or adopt change.
- When enough individuals adopt the new practice change, the change reaches the tipping point or critical mass and the new idea becomes institutionalized.

Introduction

By 2025, all graduates from accredited nurse anesthesia programs will achieve a practice doctoral level education.[1] Practice-focused nurse anesthesia doctoral programs prepare the registered nurse as a specialized advanced practice CRNA, with expertise not only in anesthesia delivery, but with skills that empower the CRNA to transform health care systems. As transformational leaders, CRNAs develop skills and attain competencies to improve quality and translate evidence into patient-centered care.[2] The doctor of nursing practice (DNP) project is one way students demonstrate mastery of those skills and competencies.

The type of project students choose can vary depending on the student's interest, faculty input, organizational priorities, and project timelines. According to the American Association of Colleges of Nursing (AACN), all DNP projects benefit patient care, either directly or indirectly, and require students to plan, implement, and evaluate outcomes related to their project. Most projects are either quality improvement (QI) or evidence-based practice (EBP) projects.[2] Quality improvement uses process analysis and data outcomes to systematically improve performance in a specific area of patient care within a health care setting.[3] Examples of QI projects include patient-care practice changes based on the results of patient satisfaction surveys, chart audits, or the use of information derived from information management programs (software) to modify or streamline processes and patient care. Evidence-based practice projects use evidence, patient preferences, and experiences along with clinical expertise to make practice decisions.[4] Examples of EBP projects include preoperative fasting guidelines, preemptive pain management recommendations, research utilization in the form of systematic reviews to modify care, or the analysis of a state or national health care policy to propose model changes for better access to care.

In addition to the types of projects above, an additional tool in the pursuit of the best evidence is the systematic review process. As delineated further in this chapter, the systematic review process is rigorous and leads investigators to potentially useful data and information based on historical works and analysis of the pooled results. In order to meet the expectations of the DNP project, the student uses the conclusions to support the implementation of needed change and subsequent evaluation of the intervention's efficacy. The bottom line of all the project types is to provide better patient care through the use of evidence, resulting in meaningful change. The skills necessary to implement a DNP project are foundational to the DNP degree itself.

The real challenge, however, is the creation of an environment and culture that embrace and sustain the EBP and QI processes. Ideally, anesthesia providers deliver most, if not all, of their anesthesia care based on sound principles.[5] Evidence-based anesthesia care will increase quality, increase patient safety, improve patient and family satisfaction, decrease costs, and facilitate innovation. Each year, large numbers of students carry out their DNP projects in various anesthesia departments, hospitals, and organizations. How many of those projects continue after the graduate completes the project? We, as DNP CRNA faculty, do our students a disservice when an organization does not sustain their DNP project's implementation and the practice change fades after the student leaves the clinical site. The student, or new graduate, learns that all the work associated with the DNP project does not create lasting change. As CRNA educators, our goal is to teach students the skills necessary to create lasting change. How do CRNA educators and/or DNP students positively influence the culture of an anesthesia department or organization so that it is more receptive to EBP and QI?

The Innovation-Decision Process

By definition, an idea or practice that is perceived as new is an innovation.[6] If we approach EBP as an innovation, then the *Innovation-Decision Process* offers CRNA educators a helpful strategy to promote a receptive clinical culture for DNP projects and a method for students to ensure their DNP projects create lasting change. Implementation of EBP within an organization is, for many, a change or a new way to practice. The Innovation-Decision Process provides a better way to understand the complex process involved in changing group behavior necessary for successful EBP implementation. The Innovation-Decision Process by Rogers outlines a preliminary stage (prior condition) followed by five follow-on stages individuals transition through starting with an understanding of the innovation (i.e., DNP project) and ending with successful and sustained use of the innovation.[6] To best apply the Innovation-Decision Process to a DNP project, some minor adaptation and refinement to the stages makes it more applicable to DNP project implementation (**Figure 23.1**). For DNP projects, the stages are:

1. Culture assessment
2. Knowledge
3. Persuasion
4. Decision
5. Implementation and
6. Confirmation

Figure 23.1 Stages of the Innovation-Decision Process for DNP Project Implementation

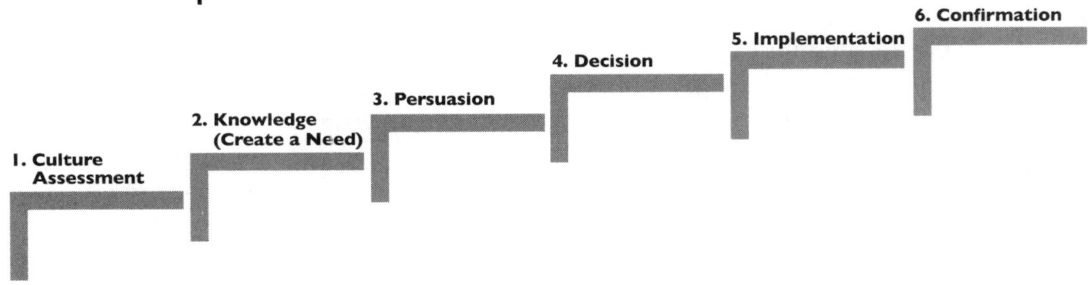

The first stages are strictly mental and involve thinking by the individuals who will consider adoption of the innovation into their practice. In stage 5, implementation, an individual's behavior physically changes. The Innovation-Decision Process does not replace implementation models, such as the Iowa EBP Implementation Model,[7] but instead offers the CRNA educator and/or student practical guidance to develop his or her method of actual implementation that will lead to long-term success.

Stage 1: Culture Assessment

In the Iowa EBP Implementation Model, a foundational step is to create a spirit of inquiry within the organization.[7] This foundational step is perhaps the most important of the EBP process because, without a culture that supports EBP, an organization will not sustain change no matter how good the project. Rogers' work provides the CRNA educator and DNP student with guidance about what prior conditions in a practice environment are important to assess prior to selection and implementation of a DNP project.[6] When adapted to the DNP project, assessment of the following prior conditions provides a starting point for the Innovation) Decision Process:

- Problems and needs
- Group innovativeness
- The social system
- EBP/QI practice environment

Problems and Needs Assessment

Many DNP projects begin after the identification of a clinical problem or need. In order to understand the problems and needs of the practice environment, the CRNA educator and student may want to survey department leadership, risk management, and individual group members. A survey for leadership and risk management may identify problems or needs related to Joint Commission accreditation, morbidity and mortality reports, patient satisfaction survey results, expanded clinical practices, or other regulatory benchmarks. To assess individual members' perspectives, a survey might include several open-ended questions such as, "What do you perceive as a clinical problem or departmental need?" or "If you could change one thing to better improve patient care in the department, what would that be?" After identification of a problem or need, the student will evaluate relevant research and literature.[7] If the evidence from the review of the literature demonstrates a needed change, the student with his or her CRNA faculty will collaborate with organizational leaders on the project topic. The CRNA educator is instrumental in ensuring that the project vision is clear and reasonable in scope and time for a student project. In addition, the CRNA educator can determine if the proposed project is feasible for the practice environment. Some changes are best suited for one organization but not for another one. Some organizations may embrace change and others may resist any new practice changes or innovations.

The goal of the DNP project is to provide the student the opportunity to learn the EBP process, not to transform the health care system with his or her project. Students and faculty have a limited time frame to complete the DNP project. Some practice changes will require small incremental change, with each DNP project laying a foundation for future scholarly work. For example, a hospital may want to become a Bariatric Center of Excellence. Organizations can partner with DNP students to implement step-wise changes to achieve their goals. One DNP project may work on changing fasting guidelines, another may address anesthesia protocols, while another may evaluate the use of informatics to promote and evaluate better compliance with the bariatric program.

Doctor of nursing practice projects for CRNAs who are completing their degrees will look very different, when compared to entry-into-practice CRNA students. The entry-into-practice CRNA student will rely more heavily on the CRNA educator to choose appropriate DNP project topics and locations to implement the project. Experienced CRNAs in a DNP completion program, however, may implement their projects at their work place. They have the advantage of knowing the clinical climate and what changes the department would benefit from, the key stakeholders, and the best way to manage obstacles to implementation. The CRNA educator and the experienced CRNA student will still want to collaborate with organizational leaders to determine the organizational priorities and secure project support.

With an understanding of the organization's perceived problems and needs, the CRNA educator can target project topic selection and implementation in a way that will best fit the needs of the student and the clinical environment. Once all parties agree on the DNP project topic, an outline of key discussion points is important to ensure all are in agreement.[7] The written agreement may include short, intermediate, and long-term strategies, timelines, individual responsibilities, specific support, and allocated resources. Ideally, written agreement and approval occurs prior to the start of the EBP project.

Group Innovativeness Assessment

As CRNA educators, we have the skills, knowledge, and position to promote adoption of EBP within anesthesia departments, hospitals, and organizations. Evidence-based practice implementation is marked by change in behavior: "It is one thing for an individual to decide to adopt a new idea, quite a different thing to put the innovation to use." [6(p.179)] Some individuals will decide to put the new idea into practice right away and others will wait for a variety of reasons. Rogers characterizes five types of individuals based on their likelihood to adopt a new idea or practice.[6] Distribution of the five adopter categories follows a standard bell curve distribution as delineated below in **Figure 23.2.**

Figure 23.2 Standard Deviation Bell Curve

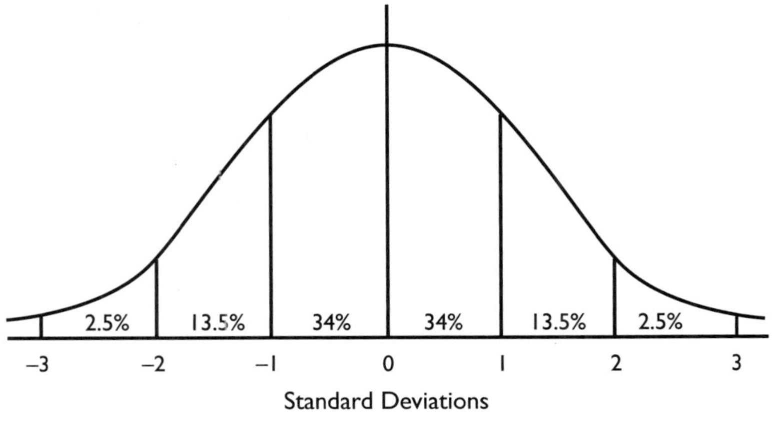

1. Laggards. Laggards (2.5% + 13.5% or 16%) are very traditional and resist change. They are the last to adopt new ideas.
2. Late majority. Individuals are naturally skeptical of new ideas and changing their practice falls into the late majority category (34%).
3. Early majority. Individuals characterized as early majority (34%) are deliberate change agents.
4. Early adopters. These individuals (13.5%) influence the group and are opinion leaders.
5. Innovators. These individuals (2.5%) are adventuresome.

Adopter categories for an anesthesia department may still have a bell-shaped curve, but with more early adopters and very few late majority or laggards. Compared to a general population, anesthesia providers have similar attributes such as their education, beliefs, and socioeconomic status. Homophily describes individuals within a group who are similar. Groups with homophily generally have more effective communication and faster adoption of new ideas or practice initiatives.[6] Homophily should be a benefit for DNP project implementation. If there are issues with implantation in a hemophilic environment, the problem mostly likely is due to current processes. Students and CRNA educators can determine which adopter category individuals belong to by utilizing the Individual Innovativeness Quiz.[8] The quiz results may help the CRNA educator and student identify individuals who are opinion leaders and most open to new practices and innovation. **Figure 23.3,** below, is an example of one author's (Chalenor) anesthesia department Individual Innovativeness Quiz score distributions.

Figure 23.3 Graph of Department Scores for Adopter Categories

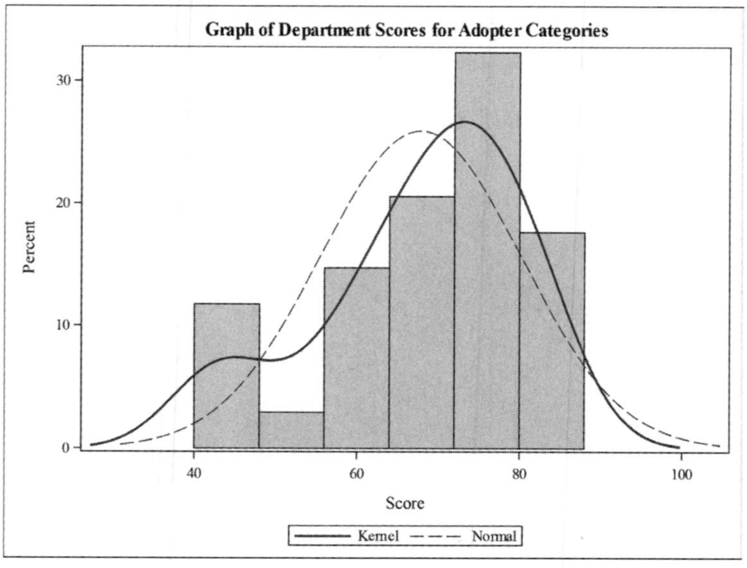

Graph includes the smooth curve (Kernel) and the Normal Curve.

Social System Assessment

Many CRNA programs fall within a school of nursing. School of nursing leadership often has strong ideas about DNP curriculum and the project. Unfortunately, some non-CRNA faculty may not understand the practice of nurse anesthetists or the rigor of an entry-into-practice program. As CRNA educators, our priority is to produce safe entry-level Certified Registered Nurse Anesthetists who, in addition, have transformational health care leadership skills. It is unrealistic for leadership in schools of nursing to expect the entry-into-practice nurse anesthesia students to conduct large projects that will take an overwhelming amount of time to complete. The goal of the DNP project is not to transform health care, but for the student to learn and practice the skills necessary to actually transform health care as a DNP clinician. The CRNA educator, therefore, teaches and facilitates DNP leadership skills through the planning, implementation, evaluation, and dissemination of manageable DNP projects. Certified Registered Nurse Anesthetist educators must ensure that the project is realistic and that the student can complete the DNP project in a timely fashion while attending to clinical and didactic responsibilities.

In CRNA programs, group projects are ideal. The workload is divided and group members must learn to work as a team; however, it is important for each member of the team to actively participate in each step of the project and fully understand the process. Students who learn teamwork and communication make better Certified Registered Nurse Anesthetists within the complex health care organizations, departments, and operating rooms where teamwork is essential.

Below are some examples of questions the CRNA educator and student can use to survey the social system where the DNP project implementation is planned.

- How is the department organized?
- How does communication occur?
- Who are the formal, informal, and opinion leaders? Whose clinical opinion in the department do you value most?
- What are the values and beliefs of the practice environment related to DNP project implementation?
- What are the organization's/department's mission and vision statements?
- How are decisions made in the practice environment?
- Who are the key stakeholders involved with DNP project approval, implementation, and sustainability?

Evidence-Based Project/Quality Improvement Practice Assessment

Staff anesthesia providers and department leaders may not fully understand or support EBP change. Certified Registered Nurse Anesthetist educators may want to promote a project with a visible positive outcome or benefits to garner initial organizational support. Evidence-based practice projects do not just look at the best evidence. Clinical expertise and patient or organizational preferences and values are equally important to consider.[4] Questions to assess the receptivity of the practice environment to EBP and QI may include the following (**Figure 23.4**):

- What is the current environment's EBP/QI practice?
- Does the current practice environment fully understand EBP and the QI process?
- Does the current practice location have an effective process in place to implement EBP or QI initiatives?
- Is the practice environment open to learning or implementing more EBP or QI initiatives?
- Does the leadership support EBP with resources and action?

Figure 23.4 Stage 1: Culture Assessment

1. Culture Assessment

- What are the perceived problems and needs from leadership? From individuals?
- How innovative are the members of the organization?
- What is the structure? Who are the stakeholders?
- How does communication occur?
- What are the mission, vision, values, and beliefs?
- What is the existing EBP/QI process?
- How effective is the EBP/QI process?

Stage 2: Knowledge (Create a Need)

There are three goals with the knowledge stage.[6] The first goal is for leaders and individuals to have awareness of the DNP project and new practice initiative. How the student communicates the existence of the DNP project depends on the social system of the environment (see Stage 1). The student project leader and team members may promote their project weeks before actual implementation by posters, email, direct communication, announcements, and other creative ways. The second goal of Stage 2 (**Figure 23.5**) is to ensure individuals know how to use or implement the new practice. This is the how-to part of this stage. The student project leader and team member may develop step-by-step pocket cards or electronic reminders of how to implement the new practice. The final goal for this stage is to ensure individuals have the background and pertinent data or knowledge related to the project. Students can present in-services or journal clubs, or they can develop handouts or online information courses to provide necessary knowledge to the organization and individuals.

Figure 23.5 Stage 2: Knowledge

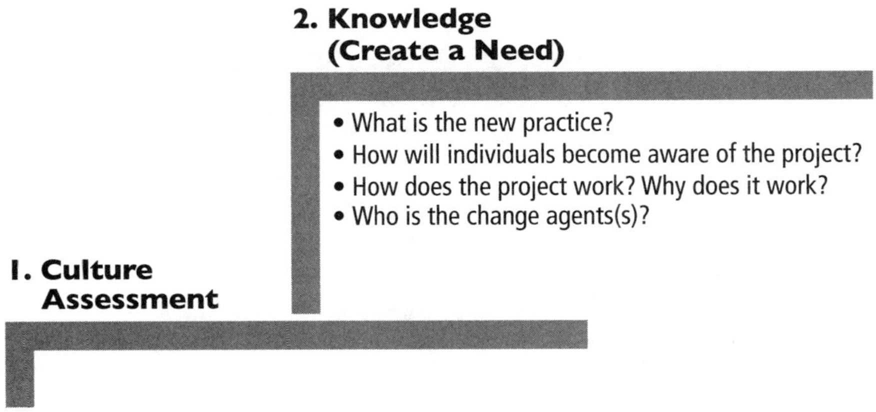

A very important step to successfully implement a new idea is to create a need. Apple is an excellent example of a company that creates a need for its products. Doctor of nursing projects likewise have to create a need. Do not assume individuals will understand and accept the benefits of the idea easily. Members of the anesthesia departments or other organizations may not perceive the need for change or the implementation of a new practice. The best way to create a need is to have the organization's change agent promote the idea as desirable. A change agent, such as the DNP student project leader, makes others aware of the idea and provides them with the knowledge and skills so they can try the idea.

Stage 3: Persuasion

The goal of the persuasion stage (**Figure 23.6**, next page.) is for the organization and individuals to form a favorable attitude about the project.[6] In fact, how fast the new project takes off depends on five primary attributes or perceptions of the idea and how people individually and collectively perceive the new practice. The following are the five attributes:

1. Relative advantage: The greater one perceives the advantages of the idea, the faster he or she will implement it into practice.
2. Compatibility: Each organization has a culture with values and beliefs. The new idea must be consistent with the individuals and the organization.
3. Complexity: The more complex the idea is to use or understand, the longer it takes individuals to implement it.
4. Trialability: When someone tries the new idea, there is less uncertainty about its use in practice.
5. Observability: Individuals and group members need to see the implementation results with new practice adoption. If not, individuals may decide to stop the new practice and the project is not sustained.

Figure 23.6 Stage 3: Persuasion

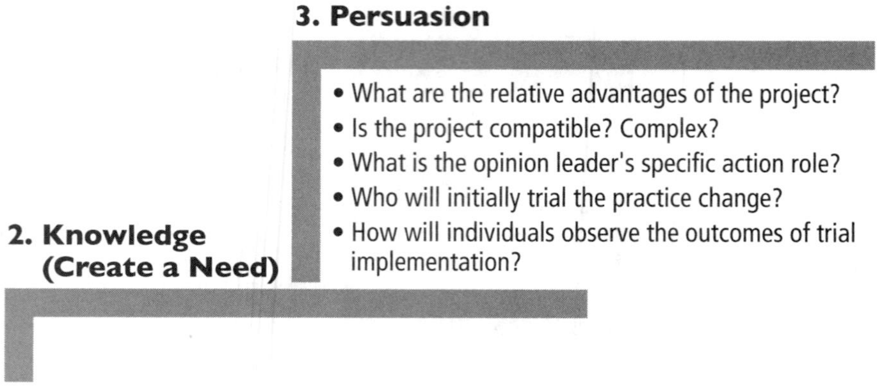

The relative advantage of the project from various perspectives is important to motivate individuals to at least consider the new practice. The change agent can informally survey individuals about their thoughts and feelings regarding the project as well as any foreseeable obstacles. The idea is to find various ways to look at the benefits of the project to garner as much positive support as possible. At this stage, the student change agent(s) has already provided knowledge to the organization about the project (stage 2).

Knowledge by itself is not always sufficient to motivate individuals to trial and potentially support the project. Two factors that most influence an individual's favorable or unfavorable opinion are compatibility and complexity.[6] If the project is in line with the organization's values and the normal way it conducts business, the idea is compatible. Complexity addresses the understanding and use of the project idea by individuals who use it. If individuals find the idea compatible and not too complex, there is a good indication that the individual will form a favorable opinion about it. Keep in mind that a favorable opinion by an individual doesn't always translate into adoption of the practice. According to Rogers, most individuals adopt an innovation based on the subjective opinion of others who already adopted the innovation.[6] The opinion leader's active role is invaluable during the persuasion stage. Both the student project leader and team members will want to encourage the organization's opinion leaders and most innovative members to trail the practice change first. A list or Excel spreadsheet of individuals and their experience with the practice change can help the project leader and team members track individuals who trial the new practice and proactively address any issues. The project team members can use positive experiences from group members to further persuade others to trial the new practice, if they have not already done so.

A key attribute in the development of a positive attitude regarding the project is whether or not the individual sees any observable benefit or change. In other words, what is the observed outcome as result of the practice change? Individuals need to see that there is a tangible benefit. The project leader and members may show outcome changes by providing data cumulatively or directly to individuals with inservices, flyers, handouts, emails, posters, or one-on-one communication.

Stage 4: Decision

The decision phase (**Figure 23.7**) of the Innovation-Decision Process is the third thinking step for an individual and potential adopter of the new practice. It is important for the student, faculty, or other change agent to be available to review information from stage 2, knowledge, and then answer questions and assist with implementation and later confirmation. Depending on the type of project, typical questions from individuals who trial the new practice may include the following:

- Where do I obtain the protocol/medication/supply?
- How do I use it?
- What kind of effects or problems might I see?
- What is the treatment/solution to foreseeable issues?

Figure 23.7 Stage 4: Decision

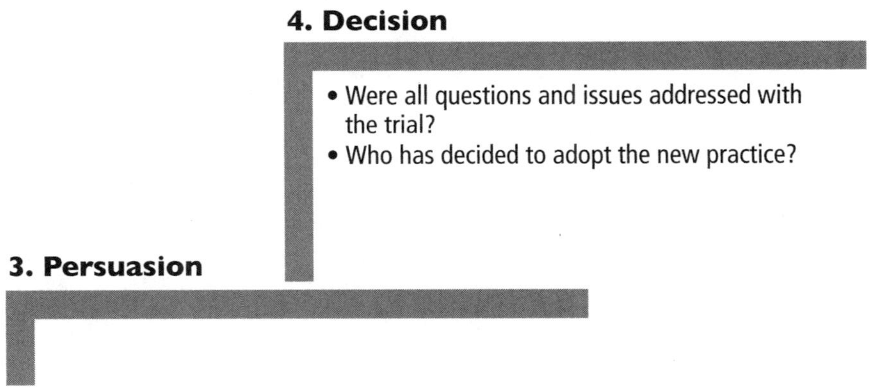

Provided that the individual has all the knowledge (stage 2) and has trialed the new practice (stage 3), he or she will make a decision to either adopt the practice or not. Most individuals, who trial a new practice, go on to adopt it. Conversely, few individuals adopt a new practice if they do not trial it. The project team can annotate on the spreadsheet which individuals trialed the new practice and their decision to adopt the change or not. This information becomes important for the next stage.

Stage 5: Implementation

The implementation stage (**Figure 23.8**, next page) is marked by a change in behavior and the rate of adoption follows a standard "S" curve. The length of this stage, however, mainly depends on how individuals perceive the attributes of the new practice. The implementation stage ends when enough individuals adopt the practice, and implementation is sustained on its own or institutionalized. The number of individuals needed for sustainment is known as critical mass.[6] In Malcolm Gladwell's best-seller, he describes this concept as the tipping point or "that magic moment when an idea, trend, or social behavior crosses a threshold, tips, and spreads like wild fire."[9] While the actual critical mass depends on the organization, individuals, and the innovation or new practice, most tipping points occur when between 25%–35% of the individuals within the environment adopt the change or on the steep portion of the "S" curve below. The rate of adoption is fast after the critical mass point.

Figure 23.8 Stage 5: Implementation

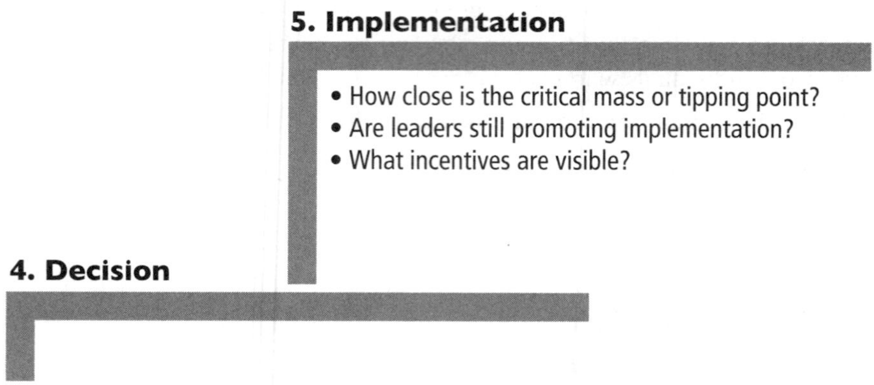

Rogers outlines four strategies students and faculty can use to reach critical mass with their DNP project implementation.[6]

1. Identify who in the organization or practice setting is well respected and influential. Target opinion and positional leaders for early support and adoption of the DNP project.
2. Imply that the change is inevitable and obtain support from the department leadership. Review the prior DNP project written approval and the agreed upon responsibilities for all parties.
3. Introduce the DNP project idea to the group members who are the most receptive to EBP change. Identify the top 25%-30% of individuals within the organization who are the most innovative to initially support implementation of the DNP project.
4. Give incentives to those individuals who implement the practice change early or until critical mass is reached. Invite the most innovative individuals to a journal club where the DNP project is introduced. Offer free continuing education units. Create a thank you board where the student highlights individuals who implement the project. Ask leadership to offer incentives such as first choice on case assignments or early release as appropriate. Extra money is always a great incentive but there are many creative ways to incorporate nonmonetary incentives. Consider including incentives in the project's written agreement.

Stage 6: Confirmation

In the last phase of the Innovation-Decision Process, confirmation, individuals solidify their decision to adopt the new practice (**Figure 23.9**). Ideally, the organization and individuals experience positive outcomes as a result of implementation of the new practice. The student project team leader and members can additionally demonstrate result outcomes with graphs, tables, survey results, and testimonials. It is during this phase that the student team members actively seek out information on how individuals feel about the new idea and proactively address any individual or group concerns. The student team members then can answer questions and provide necessary support for sustained use of the practice initiative. For example, if there were issues, such as missing supplies (medications, paperwork, and equipment), computer glitches, cumbersome processes, and a lack of change agent involvement, individuals may stop implementation of the new practice. Many good projects wither because change agents neglect this last important stage in the Innovation-Decision Process.

Figure 23.9 Stage 6: Confirmation

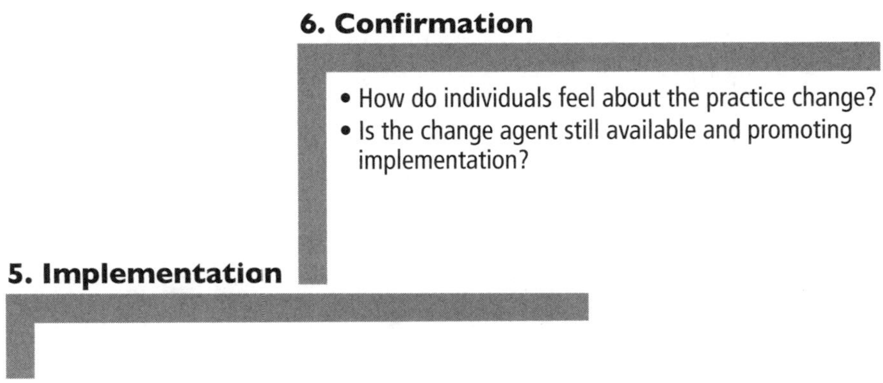

Doctor of nursing practice projects can positively impact health care provided the student successfully implements his or her project. Evidence-based practice models provide an excellent framework to implement projects but do not address how to cultivate a receptive EBP climate. Nor do the EBP models provide guidance on how to influence individual and group behavior so that adoption of an innovation or new practice idea is more likely. Rogers' Innovation-Decision Process gives students and faculty steps to promote adoption and implementation of a new practice or innovation, such as a DNP project. Equally important, the Innovation-Decision Process provides strategies to increase the rate in which individuals use or adopt new practice as well as increase the sustainability of the project. (**Figure 23.10**, next page.)

While all stages of the Innovation-Decision Process are important, it is during the persuasion stage that individuals within the group form a positive or negative attitude toward the DNP project. In fact, individual and organizational attributes, preferences, values, and perceptions are key determinants whether or not the student's DNP project is successfully implemented and sustained in the clinical site. It is how individuals and organizations perceive the relative advantage, compatibility, complexity, trialability, and observability of the new idea that determines how fast it is implemented or adopted. Individuals will develop a more positive perception of the practice change if the change agent, student leader or team members, addresses the above attributes, preferences, values, and perceptions successfully from various individual perspectives (**Table 23.1**).

Figure 23.10 Summary of the Innovation-Decision Process for DNP Projects

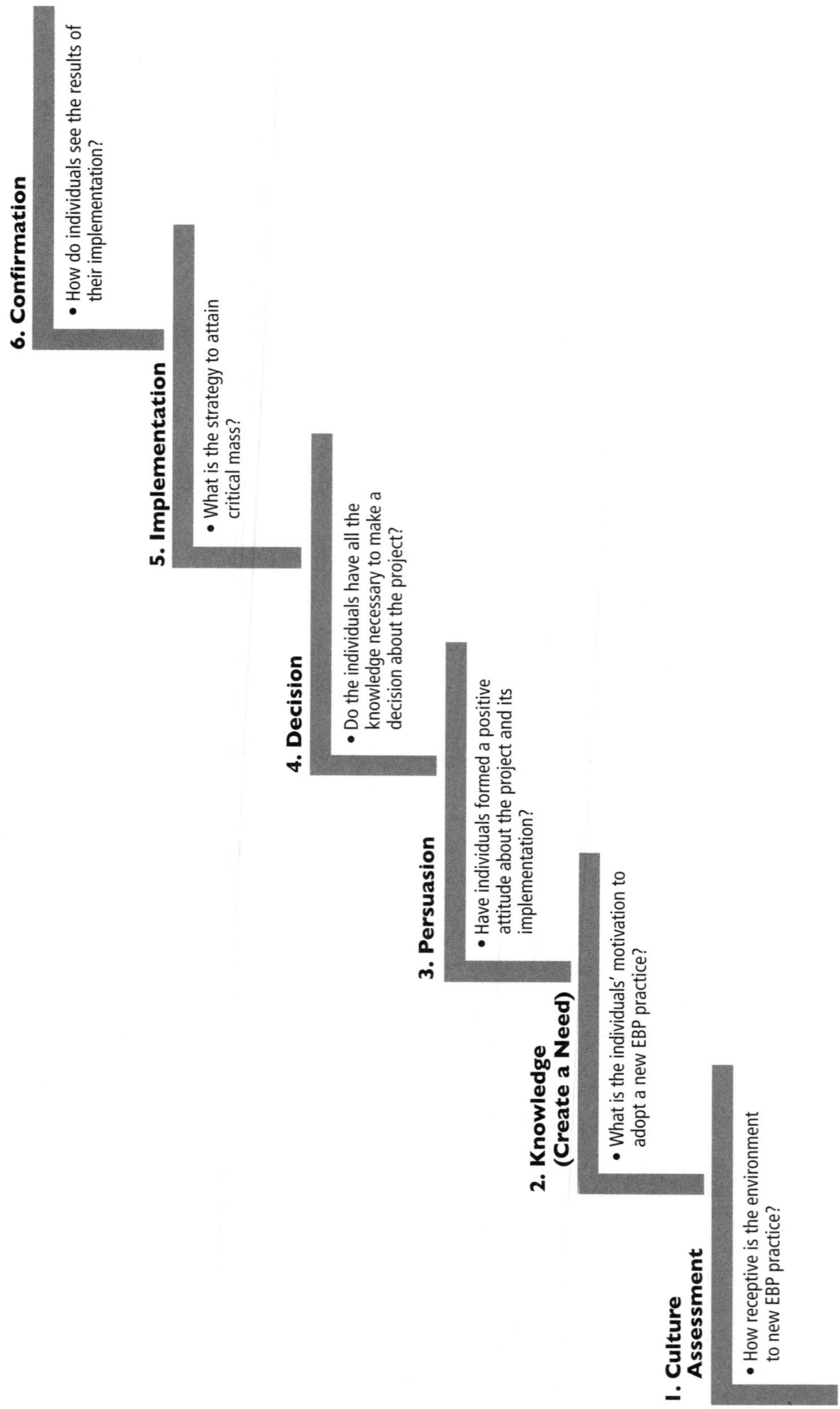

Table 23.1 Important Attributes of an Innovation

Important Attributes of an Innovation
1. Relative advantage
2. Compatibility
3. Complexity
4. Trialability
5. Observability

Doctor of nursing practice programs give CRNA students skills and basic experiences to plan, implement, and evaluate outcomes with an EBP project. Students and faculty can incorporate the Innovation-Decision Process to promote acceptance of a proposed EBP practice change and then encourage individual and group behavior changes in respect to DNP project implementation. When enough innovative members of an organization or practice setting adopt the practice change, the change becomes self-sustaining. The number of individuals needed to reach that point is known as critical mass or the tipping point. If the project reaches critical mass, there is an excellent chance the project will sustain after the student leaves the clinical site. With project sustainment, DNP projects transform health care one project at a time.

Evidence-Based Practice and the Systematic Review

In the not-so-distant past, the following statement was uttered when CRNA program faculty contemplated what type of project their students should do in support of the DNP project: "Can't they just do a systematic or literature review or something?" This statement demonstrates a fundamental lack of understanding of how we, as program faculty, can best serve our students through the knowledge enrichment and demonstration task referred to as a DNP project. It also demonstrates either lack of knowledge or lack of appreciation for the complexity and rigor of a true systematic review.

The systematic review process has been postulated to be the highest form of research evidence, and is a tool by which the results or view of many can be distilled into evidence, rife with potential for use in clinical practice.[10] The inherent elegance of a quality systematic review with meta-analysis or meta-synthesis is its utilization of all sources of data and information that have come before (that meet inclusion criteria and quality standards) to produce the strongest evidence possible. This is made possible based on the pooling of subjects, data and findings from a variety of qualitatively validated studies from different authors in various settings. The findings extracted can and should be used as tools to further improve the care we provide, to educate future generations of nurse anesthetists, and to clarify deficits in current practice. These illuminated deficits can then become areas of focus for future scientific inquiry.

Historical Perspective

In order to truly appreciate what a systematic review can accomplish through findings-based implementation, an understanding of the birth of evidence-based health care and the systematic review process is advisable. The genesis of evidence-based health care and practice goes back to 1971 and the writings of Archibald Cochrane. His groundbreaking text published in 1971, *Effectiveness and Efficiency,* delineated a variety of faults in how the practice of medicine was being conducted. It strongly criticized the lack of reliable evidence behind many common patient care interventions. His views motivated the health care community to seek out the best evidence to enable the provision of the best care possible. His call for a collection of systematic reviews led to the creation of The Cochrane Collaboration, which will be discussed in detail later in this section. Archibald Cochrane served as the visionary that catalyzed much of the progress in evidence-based medicine.[11]

The evidence gleaned from existing literature is the key to evidence-based health care. According to Humphris,[12] the term evidence-based in health care "...implies the use and application of research evidence as a basis on which to make health care decisions, as opposed to decisions not based on evidence." A simplistic view as to how evidence-based practice should be utilized focuses on the need to practice in ways that are supported by the most up-to-date evidence or knowledge.[32] Sackett and colleagues[14] in 1996 stated that evidence-based practice is one that is based on "The conscientious, explicit, and judicious use of current best evidence in making decisions about the care of individual patients. The practice of evidence-based medicine means integrating individual clinical expertise with the best available external clinical evidence from systematic research." Previously, Sackett and Rosenberg[15] had stated the need to base practice on the best possible evidence. This includes critically appraising research reports for validity and usefulness and incorporating the rapidly growing body of evidence into practice.

Dawes and colleagues[16] presented five stages of evidence-based health care in 2005. These stages are presented in **Table 23.2.**

Table 23.2 Stages of Evidence-based Health Care

Five Stages of Evidence-based Health Care
Translation of uncertainty to an answerable question
Systematic retrieval of the best evidence available
Critical appraisal of evidence for validity, clinical relevance and applicability
Application of results in practice
Evaluation of performance

Adapted with permission from Dawes M, Summerskill W, Glasziou P, et al. Sicily statement on evidence-based practice. *BMC Med Educ.* 2005; 5: 1–7.

These steps, otherwise known as the steps involved in the systematic review process, have been expounded upon and modified by various organizations. These organizations include The Cochrane Collaboration, the Campbell Collaboration, and The Joanna Briggs Institute of Systematic Review and Implementation Reports (each of these organizations will be discussed in greater detail later in the chapter). In

2011, The Institute of Medicine (IOM) published *Finding What Works in Health care: Standards for Systematic Reviews.*[17] In reviewing this document, it appears that the IOM's intent was to publish a single document incorporating the steps involved in the systematic review process as started by the various collaborations and independent authors. This standard will be used as the guide in explaining the conduct of a systematic review with all of its intricacies.

Organizations That Facilitate or Manage Systematic Reviews

The Cochrane Collaboration was founded in 1993 by Ian Chalmers and a group of 70 other international colleagues.[11(p.2)] The goal of The Cochrane Collaboration was to create and disseminate up-to-date reviews of randomized controlled trials of health care interventions to assist health care professionals in making decisions based on the best evidence available. Since its inception, the organization has demonstrated significant growth and is now an international body of greater than 11,500 individuals in over 90 countries.[18] In May of 1994, the Cochrane Collaboration published the Cochrane Collaboration Handbook, and in September of 1996, the Cochrane Database of Systematic Reviews became available on the World Wide Web.

The Campbell Collaboration is named in honor of Dr. Donald T. Campbell (1916-1996), a member of the National Academy of Sciences. He upheld the thought that legislative changes can be seen as societal analyses to which exploratory standards of proof can be connected. He trusted that experimental proof could be produced to assess the impacts of administrative changes, bringing about better educated arrangement and rehearse and at last enhancing individuals' prosperity. The Campbell Collaboration came out of a meeting in London in 1999. Eighty individuals from four nations went to the meeting; many attendees were from its kin association, The Cochrane Collaboration. Numerous Cochrane individuals saw the requirement for an association that would deliver precise surveys of exploration confirmation on the viability of social intercessions. Support for this thought from social and behavioral researchers and social specialists prompted the production of the Campbell Collaboration in 2000. The inaugural meeting in Philadelphia pulled in 85 members from 13 nations.[19]

The Campbell Collaboration produces systematic reviews of the effects of social interventions in crime and justice, education, international development, and social welfare. The vision is to bring about positive social change, and to improve the quality of public and private services around the world. Campbell Collaboration staff and contributing authors prepare, maintain and disseminate systematic reviews of research related to education, crime and justice, social welfare, and international development.[19]

The Joanna Briggs Institute (JBI) is the worldwide nonprofit innovative working group inside of the Faculty of Health Sciences at the University of Adelaide, South Australia. The institute works together universally with more than 70 constituents around the world. The institute and its collaborative elements advance and bolster the synthesis, exchange, and usage of evidence through recognizing feasible, appropriate, meaningful, and effective health care practices to help improve care worldwide.

This is accomplished through translational science, synthesis science, implementation science, accessible online information for health care professionals, and by advancing evidence-based practice at whatever point conceivable. In particular, JBI gives its end-clients the best accessible proof to illuminate their clinical choice making at the point of care.[20] The vision of The Joanna Briggs Institute is best summarized with the following quote:

> "The JBI model of evidence-based health care has been constructed to enable reasoning and critique about evidence-based healthcare and its role in improving global health, within a logical conceptual framework. Drawn from the experience of the Joanna Briggs Institute and its global partners in promoting and facilitating evidence-based healthcare across the world, it is an attempt to conceptually represent the components of a cyclical process that both responds to priorities in global health and, in turn, serves to improve global health."[12(p.208)]

The Joanna Briggs Institute's view of evidence-based practice involves giving consideration to all of the best available evidence, the context in which the care is delivered, client preference, and the professional judgment of the health professional. Promoting and facilitating evidence-based health care is visualized as consisting of four major components of the evidence-based health care process. These include health care evidence generation, evidence synthesis, evidence or knowledge transfer, and evidence utilization.[13(p.210)] The primary attribute that distinguished JBI from the Cochrane Collaboration is that JBI was founded with the operational plan to include all possible sources of information for inclusion into a rigorous systematic review. The Cochrane Collaboration was founded with the intent to focus data from randomized controlled trials for systematic reviews. It was not until November 2013 that The Cochrane Collaboration began hosting systematic reviews of qualitative data.[21] Additionally, JBI's original consumer focus was on nursing and allied health professions, rather than on medicine as with The Cochrane Collaboration.[19]

What Is and Is Not a Systematic Review

The question as to what is or is not a systematic review can be answered with an explanation of the rigorous nature of the systematic review process. This is very effectively demonstrated through the instructional material provided by The Joanna Briggs Institute's Comprehensive Systematic Review Training Program (CSRTP).[22] The institute considers that evidence may be gleaned through experience, expertise, inference, deduction, or the results of rigorous inquiry. It recognizes that "the results of well-designed research studies grounded in any methodological position are seen to be more credible as evidence than anecdotes or personal opinion."[12(p.211)] On the other hand, when no evidence exists fitting this criteria, other evidence of lesser strength may be used as evidence. This position is taken to give the most significant and valuable data to illuminate health care decision-making. The systematic review of the literature on a particular condition, intervention, or issue is seen as central to defining reliable evidence for practice. A systematic review is essentially an analysis of all available literature or evidence, and a judgment of the effectiveness of the evidence.[20(p.13)]

The first quality that distinguishes a systematic review from other inferior forms of literature review is the development of a rigorous proposal or protocol. The review protocol provides a predetermined plan to ensure rigor and minimize potential bias. All of the stages of the review are described fully in the protocol, and it is usually subjected to peer review before the review commences.

The protocol contains six steps to ensure acceptable rigor.[21] These steps are presented in **Table 23.3**. By convention, the classic randomized controlled trial is viewed as the highest form of evidence. The JBI model adopts an inclusive approach to what constitutes evidence, where the "findings of qualitative research studies are regarded as rigorously generated evidence and other text derived from opinion, experience and expertise is acknowledged as forms of evidence"[12(p.211)] where higher forms of evidence are unavailable or the question of interest is not one simply of effectiveness.

Table 23.3 Steps In Protocol Development

Critical Steps in Protocol Development
State the questions or hypotheses that will be pursued in the review
Identify the criteria that will be used to select the literature.
Detail a strategy that will be used to identify all relevant literature within a time frame agreed upon by the authors.
Establish how the quality of each study or paper will be assessed or critically appraised and any exclusion criteria based on quality considerations.
Detail how data will be extracted from the primary research or text.
Establish a plan of how the data extracted will be synthesized.

Adapted with permission from The Joanna Briggs Institute. *Comprehensive Systematic Review Training Program: Introduction to Evidence-Based Healthcare.* Adelaide, South Australia: The Joanna Briggs Institute; 2013.

As outlined previously, systematic reviews are considered the highest form of evidence as they systematically search for, identify, and summarize the available evidence that answers a specific question with focused attention to the methodological quality of studies (all papers are critically appraised) or the credibility of opinion and text.[21(p.11)] The heart of the systematic review process is reproducibility, inclusiveness of articles selected, and rigor in the selection process based on predetermined criteria and methodological quality. It also includes reviewer participation to minimize opportunities for bias. The type of systematic review can be delineated based on the primary sources of information or data to be included. These types include systematic reviews of quantitative data, qualitative data, evidence derived from expert opinion and text, and evidence arising out of economic analyses. Regardless of the source of the information, based on the rigor of the protocol and methodologically sound data, all are treated as evidence.

The synthesis of the results of quantitative research

Statistical, or meta-analysis may or may not be used in synthesizing numerical data. This is dependent on the type and quality of studies included in the review.

Meta-analyses of mathematical data provide precise estimates of associations or treatments effect in reviews of effectiveness. Important outcomes of a meta-analysis include measure of effect, confidence interval and degree of heterogeneity of the studies included in the meta-analysis. It is very important to consider that all pooled data should be of like-kind (homogenous). This includes units of measure, scale equivalences, and data that are unequivocal between studies or papers.

The synthesis of the results of qualitative research

Meta-synthesis refers to a higher form of data and information synthesis.[21(p.13)] Qualitative meta-synthesis is a deliberate and repeatable approach to analyzing data across qualitative studies. This process enables researchers to identify research questions and then search for, select, appraise, summarize, and combine qualitative evidence to address the question. This process must use rigorous qualitative methods to synthesize qualitative studies to construct greater meaning through an elegant interpretative process.[23]

The synthesis of evidence arising out of expert opinion and text

Though some in the health care community may insist that evidence-based health care should be derived exclusively from quality research projects, this is improbable in some clinical situations. The realities for health care today require a broader view of what is considered acceptable evidence.[21(p.17)] Expert opinion and the thoughts of experienced clinicians provide a valid form of evidence, especially when clinical scenario is not supported by research. This process seeks to identify significant conclusions in texts that represent informed opinions.

The synthesis of evidence arising out of economic analyses

The synthesis of economic analyses or evaluations is a developing science. The need for methods of synthesizing economic information is self-evident in our current climate of shrinking budgets. A problem that exists is a lack of standardization in the systematic review of economic data. There are few high-quality studies and no established methods for meta-analysis of economic findings. This does not minimize that summaries of economic information from high-quality studies are useful to inform practice. Health care decision-makers are increasingly seeking economic information to inform their practice, and researchers in the field of evidence-based practice are increasingly interested in extracting this data with recognition of the difficulties surrounding its synthesis.[21(p.14)]

Types of Evidence

All evidence is not created equal. While some articles purport their findings to be beyond doubt, if bias or other factors are not taken into account, the information provided may not be viewed as sound. The act of filtering evidence should help to reassure the systematic review authors that the information and data contained within a certain work is valid and useful. As illustrated in **Table 23.4**, the level of evidence is impacted by whether or not information is filtered. This relationship between filtered and unfiltered evidence does not imply that unfiltered evidence is not valid. Filtered status merely denotes that a second critical view of the work was accomplished as a portion of the integration of their evidence into a combined work.[22]

Table 23.4 Levels of Evidence

Level of Evidence	Evidence Source	Information Filtered
I	Systematic reviews with meta-analysis/synthesis	Yes
II	Critically appraised topics with evidence synthesis	Yes
III	Critically appraised individual articles and papers	Yes
IV	Randomized controlled trials (RCTs)	No
V	Cohort studies	No
VI	Case controlled studies, case series or case reports	No
VII	Expert opinion	No

Filtered evidence

Filtered, or secondary, sources are summaries and analyses of the evidence derived from and based on primary or unfiltered resources. To say that a source is filtered is to say that it has been previously analyzed and critiqued (through peer review, perhaps) and has been shown to be both current and valid. This then provides an appraisal of the quality of studies and often makes recommendations for practice. Examples of works that could be considered filtered evidence include meta-analyses, systematic reviews, critically appraised topics, and critically appraised individual articles.[24]

Unfiltered evidence

Unfiltered or primary evidence supports a topic that has been or is currently under investigation. This evidence is generally found in articles that appear in peer-reviewed journals found by searching databases. Examples of unfiltered evidence include clinical trials, randomized controlled trials, prospective studies, retrospective studies, cohort studies, and case control studies.[24]

Steps in the Systematic Review Process

As previously noted, the following sequential process for conducting a systematic review was derived from the Institute of Medicine's *Finding What Works in Health Care: Standards for Systematic Reviews*.[17] In addition to the following discussion, these steps are presented in an abbreviated format in **Table 23.5**, next page.

Table 23.5 Overview of Steps In the Systematic Review Process

Overview of Steps in the Systematic Review Process	
Initiate a Systematic Review	Establish a team with appropriate expertise and experience to conduct the systematic review.
	Manage bias and conflict of interest (COI) of the team conducting the systematic review.
	Ensure user and stakeholder input as the review is designed and conducted.
	Manage bias and COI for individuals providing input into the systematic review.
	Formulate the topic for the systematic review.
	Develop a systematic review protocol.
	Submit the protocol for peer review.
	Make the final protocol publicly available, and add any amendments to the protocol in a timely fashion.
Find and Assess Individual Studies	Conduct a comprehensive systematic search for evidence.
	Take action to address potentially biased reporting of research results.
	Screen and select studies.
	Document the search.
	Manage data collection.
	Critically appraise each study.
Synthesize the Body of Evidence	Use a pre-specified method to evaluate the body of evidence.
	Conduct a qualitative synthesis.
	Decide if the systematic review will include a quantitative analysis (meta-analysis) as well as a qualitative analysis.
	Conduct meta-analysis.
Report Systematic Review	Prepare final report using a structured format.
	Peer review the draft report.

Adapted with permission from Institute of Medicine. *Finding What Works in Health Care: Standards for Systematic Reviews.* Washington, DC: The National Academies Press; 2011.

The systematic review process truly starts with identifying a need. This need can be based on patient outcomes, staff observations, or treatment possibilities for a specific pathology. The next step involves establishing a team with appropriate expertise and experience to conduct the systematic review. The attributes that should be assessed include expertise in the pertinent clinical content areas, systematic review methods, searching for relevant evidence, expertise in quantitative methods, or other expertise as appropriate. During the team formation, it is very important to manage bias and conflict of interest (COI) of the team conducting the systematic review. Each team member should disclose potential COI and professional or intellectual bias. Individuals with a clear financial conflict or whose professional or intellectual bias would diminish the credibility of the review in the eyes of the intended users should be excluded. It is incumbent on the lead reviewer to ensure user and stakeholder input as the review is designed and conducted, and to protect the independence of the review team to make the final decisions about the design, analysis, and reporting of the review.

The next step is the formulation of the topic for the systematic review. This will involve confirming the need for a new review as well as developing an analytic framework that clearly lays out the chain of logic that links the health intervention to the outcomes of interest. It also defines the key clinical questions to be addressed by the systematic review. A standard format should be used to articulate each clinical question of interest and should state the rationale for each clinical question. It should also refine each question based on user and stakeholder input.

The next step is the development of the systematic review protocol. The intent of the protocol is to describe the following: context and rationale for the review from both a decision-making and research perspective; the study screening and selection criteria (inclusion/exclusion criteria); precisely which outcome measures, time points, interventions, and comparison groups will be addressed; and the search strategy for identifying relevant evidence. The protocol should describe the procedures for study selection and data extraction. It should also critically appraise individual studies and the process for identifying and resolving disagreement between researchers in study selection and data extraction decisions. The draft protocol should be reviewed through a format review process (as seen with Cochrane, Campbell, and JBI systematic reviews). The reviewed protocol should be made available to the public, both to inform them of current efforts and to assist other authors as to which topics are currently under systematic review investigation.

Once the protocol has been peer-reviewed and made available to the public, the comprehensive systematic search for relevant articles and literature works begins. It is highly advised to work with a librarian or other information specialist trained in performing systematic reviews to plan the search strategy. The strategy can be very complex. Approaching it with a well-developed plan is crucial. The search strategy should be designed to address each key research question, and the final plan for the search should be reviewed by an independent librarian or other information specialist. The actual search should include bibliographic databases, citation indexes, and literature cited by eligible studies (otherwise known as a hand-search). If the return of applicable articles is inadequate, the search should be more subject-specific to find all relevant evidence. In order to minimize the risk of bias, gray literature databases, clinical trial registries, and other sources of unpublished information about studies should be searched. Also, researchers should be consulted to clarify information about study eligibility, study characteristics, and risk of bias.

When screening and selecting studies, they should be included or excluded based on the protocol's prespecified criteria. Observational studies should be used in addition to randomized clinical trials to evaluate harms of interventions. The use of two or more members of the review team, working independently, to screen and select studies is helpful. Using one of two strategies to select studies is also recommended: For example, read all full-text articles identified in the search, or screen titles and abstracts of all articles and then read the full text of articles identified in the initial screening.

Documenting the search is critically important in assuring reproducibility of the search. A line-by-line description of the search strategy, including the date of every search for each database, web browser, etc., should be provided. The disposition of each report identified should be documented, including reasons for its exclusion, if appropriate. Managing the data collection is equally important. At a minimum, using two or more researchers, working independently, to extract quantitative and other critical data from each study is recommended. For other types of data, one individual could extract the data while the second individual could independently check for accuracy and completeness. Establishing a fair procedure for resolving discrepancies is vital; do not simply give final decision-making power to the senior reviewer. It is advisable to link publications from the same study to avoid including data from the same study more than once (results duplication). Using standard data extraction forms developed for the specific systematic review is helpful, and pilot-testing the data extraction forms and process is also significantly important.

Each study that has been selected for likely inclusion should be critically appraised. The risk of bias should be systematically assessed using predefined criteria. The relevance of the study's populations, interventions, and outcome measures should be assessed, along with the fidelity of the implementation of interventions. The method used to evaluate the selected articles and papers should have been prespecified in the review protocol. For each outcome, the following characteristics of the body of evidence should be systematically assessed: risk of bias, consistency, precision, directness, and any perceived reporting bias. For evidence that includes observational research, the following characteristics for each outcome should be assessed: dose-response association, plausible confounding that would change the observed effect, and strength of association. For each outcome specified in the protocol, consistent language should be used to characterize the level of confidence in the estimates of the effect of an intervention.

Once the critical appraisal is completed, a qualitative synthesis of the information contained within the selected articles and papers should be conducted. The clinical and methodological characteristics of the included studies, including their size, inclusion or exclusion of important subgroups, timeliness, and other relevant factors should be described. The strengths and limitations of individual studies and patterns across studies must also be described. In plain terms, flaws in the design or execution of the study (or groups of studies) could bias the results, explaining the reasoning behind these judgments. The relationships between the characteristics of the individual studies and their reported findings and patterns across studies should be described. Finally, the relevance of individual studies to the populations, comparisons, co-interventions, settings, and outcomes or measures of interest must be discussed.

In addition to a qualitative analysis, if the data contained within the articles and papers is homogenous, it must be decided if the systematic review will include a quantitative analysis (meta-analysis). This includes explaining why a pooled estimate might be useful to decision-makers. If conducting a meta-analysis, the following steps should be followed (this portion may vary, based on the use of specific systematic review collaboration or the organizations' inherent meta-analysis software suite): Use expert methodologists to develop, execute, and peer review the meta-analyses; address the heterogeneity among study effects; accompany all estimates with measures of statistical uncertainty; and assess the sensitivity of conclusions to changes in the protocol, assumptions, and study selection (sensitivity analysis).

The final report of the systematic review should be based on a structured format. As stated previously, different collaborations and organization that sponsor and house systematic reviews will have a specific format. The IOM's suggestion for the final report format includes the following elements, in order: a report title, an abstract, an executive summary, a summary written for the lay public, an introduction (rationale and objectives), and a methods section. The methods section should describe the following elements: the research protocol; eligibility criteria (criteria for including and excluding studies in the systematic review; analytic framework and key questions, databases, and other information sources used to identify relevant studies; the search strategy; the study selection and data extraction process; the methods for handling missing information; information that was extracted from included studies; the methods to appraise the quality of individual studies; a summary measures of effect size (eg, risk ratio, difference in means); the rationale for pooling (or not pooling) results of included studies; the methods of synthesizing the evidence (qualitative and meta-analysis); and additional analyses, if done, indicating which were prespecified.

The results section follows the methods section. It is best to organize the presentation of results around key questions. The following should be described (repeat for each key question): study selection process; list of excluded studies and reasons for their exclusion; appraisal of individual studies' quality; qualitative synthesis; meta-analysis of results, if performed (explain rationale for analysis); additional analyses, if done, indicating which were prespecified; and any included tables and figures.

As is standard in scientific articles, a discussion section is the next portion addressed. This section should include: summary of the evidence; strengths and limitations of the systematic review; conclusions for each key question; gaps in the discovered evidence; and future research needs. This is where a quality systematic review can be utilized as a springboard for scientific inquiry in light of a paucity of evidence or unanswered systematic review questions.

Once the report is completed, the draft report should be peer-reviewd. It is advisable to use a third party to manage the peer review process. If possible, a public comment period should be provided for the report and publicly reported on disposition of comments. Finally, the final report should be published in a manner that ensures free public access. This accounts for the dissemination portion of the DNP project requirements. A quality systematic review without full effort to provide the information to the public, with focus on the affected parties, is not a complete systematic review.

Summary

The systematic review process is both exacting and rigorous. The expectation of precision and exhaustive searching may seem an impossible task; however, the product that is completed is an art form itself. Not only does a quality systematic review meet the expectations of an exceptional scholarly project for the CRNA student working on his or her DNP, but the findings of the review can then further our understanding of how we care for our patients, educate our students, and grow ourselves as educators.

References

1. COA position statements. Council on Accreditation of Nurse Anesthesia Educational Programs. www.home.coa.us.com/about/Pages/COA-Position-Statements.aspx. Accessed November 15, 2015.

2. The Doctor of Nursing practice: Current Issues and Clarifying Recommendations. American Association of Colleges of Nursing. http://www.aacn.nche.edu/publications/white-papers. Accessed August 30, 2015.

3. Agency for Healthcare Research and Quality. http://www.ahrq.gov. Accessed June 22, 2016.

4. Melnyk BM, Fineout-Overholt E. *Evidence-Based Practice in Nursing & Healthcare: A Guide to Best Practice.* 3rd ed. Philadelphia, PA: Wolters Kluwer; 2015.

5. Institute of Medicine Roundtable on Evidence-Based Medicine. http://www.ncbi.nlm.nih.gov/books/NBK52847. Accessed August 8, 2016.

6. Rogers EM. *Diffusion of Innovations.* 5th ed. New York, NY: Free Press; 2003.

7. Cullen L, Hanrahan, K Tucker, S Rempel, G Jordan K. *Evidence-Based Practice Building Blocks: Comprehensive Strategies, Tools, and Tips.* 1st ed. Iowa City, IA: University of Iowa Hospitals and Clinics; 2012.

8. Hurt HT, Joseph K, Cook CD. Individual Innovativeness (II). Measurement Instrument Database for the Social Science. http://www.midss.org/content/individual-innovativeness-ii. 2013. Accessed July 6, 2016.

9. Gladwell, M. The Tipping Point: How Little Things Can Make a Big Difference. http://gladwell.com/the-tipping-point/. Accessed August 26, 2016.

10. McNamara ER, Scales CD. Role of systematic reviews and meta-analysis in evidence-based clinical practice. *Indian J Urol.* 2011;27(4):520–524. doi: 10.4103/0970-1591.91445. Accessed June 18, 2015.

11. Shah HH, Chung KC. Archie Cochrane and his vision for evidence-based medicine. *Plast Reconstr Surg.* 2009;124(3):982–988. doi: 10.1097/PRS.0b013e3181b03928.

12. Humphris D. Types of evidence. In: Hamer S, Collinson G, eds. *Achieving Evidence Based Practice: A Handbook for Practitioners.* London: Ballière-Tindall; 1999:13–38.

13. Pearson A, Wiechula R, Court A, Lockwood C. The JBI model of evidence-based healthcare. *Int J Evid Based Healthc.* 2005;3(8):207–215.

14. Sackett DL, Rosenberg WM, Gray JA, Haynes RB, Richardson WS. Evidence based medicine: what it is and what it isn't. *BMJ.* 1996;312(7023):71–72.

15. Sackett DL, Rosenberg WM. The need for evidence-based medicine. *J R Soc Med.* 1995;88(11):620–624.

16. Dawes M, Summerskill W, Glasziou P, et al. Sicily statement on evidence-based practice. *BMC Med Educ.* 2005;5:1–7.

17. Institute of Medicine. *Finding What Works in Health Care: Standards for Systematic Reviews.* Washington, DC: The National Academies Press; 2011.

18. The Cochrane Collaboration. Newcomer's guide. http://www.cochrane.org/docs/newcomersguide.htm. Published June 4, 2008. Accessed July 9, 2015.

19. Campbell Collaboration. Background information. http://www.campbellcollaboration.org/background/index.php. Accessed September 3, 2015.

20. The Joanna Briggs Institute. About Us. http://joannabriggs.org/about.html. Accessed September 3, 2015.

21. The Cochrane Collaboration. Cochrane Community (Beta): History. Archive of The Cochrane Collaboration.http://community.cochrane.org/about-us/history. Updated December 12, 2013. Accessed October 6, 2015.

22. The Joanna Briggs Institute. *Comprehensive Systematic Review Training Program: Introduction to Evidence-Based Healthcare*. Adelaide, South Australia: The Joanna Briggs Institute; 2013.

23. Erwin EJ, Brotherson MJ, Summers JA. Understanding qualitative metasynthesis: Issues and opportunities in early childhood intervention research. *J Early Intrv*. 2011;33(3):186–200. doi: 10.1177/1053815111425493.

24. Evidence Based Practice. Southern Cross University Library. http://libguides.scu.edu.au/content.php?pid=288667&sid=2373556. Accessed September 20, 2015.

25. Evidence-Based Medicine (EBM) Resources. Galter Health Sciences Library. Northwestern University. https://galter.northwestern.edu/guides-and-tutorials/ebm-resources. Accessed September18, 2015.

CHAPTER 24

A Library Guide for the Educator

Rachel C. Lerner, MSLS

Keywords: Citations, databases, documenting, information, library services.

Key Concepts

- Information literacy frameworks provide clear educational goals toward which nursing students can strive, and standards that can be used to assess students and programs.
- Part of becoming a nurse leader is learning to be a skilled and responsible discoverer, consumer, creator, and disseminator of information.
- The backbone of searching in databases is Boolean searching. The three most commonly used Boolean operators are AND, OR, and NOT, which narrow, broaden, and exclude search results respectively.
- Using concept charts aids in better defining questions and creating additional search terms.
- Putting search terms that are more than two words between quotation marks will ensure those words appear next to each other in the search results.
- Filters are a powerful asset in database searching. Common filters include age, publication date, and article type. There are often more filters than the default view shows.
- Databases aren't limited to those that have scholarly literature. There are diagnostic databases, databases of images, databases for test prep, databases for textbooks, etc.
- Grey literature (usually found on the Web) is an important source of noncommercial literature.
- Assessing material found on the Web is an integral skill for any person consuming information. There are many frameworks for doing so; I prefer the one offered through the National Network of Libraries of Medicine.
- Documenting one's sources aids in avoiding plagiarism.

- Citation managers store and organize references for the user. Most will also automatically create a bibliography in the style of one's choosing. Citation managers are a powerful and useful tool, but are not a replacement for knowing a citation style; their output should always be proofread.
- If an institution has a librarian, involve him or her in the process of teaching information literacy and research processes.

Introduction

This chapter is an overview of basic information that can assist nursing students and faculty members in using databases to discover literature, find information faster in databases and on the Web, and assess what they have found. It is roughly equivalent to the introduction to library services orientation I provide for my master's and doctoral nursing students; however, this chapter pales in comparison to an in-person interaction with information professionals, and is not meant to replace their services.

The chapter will give an overview of one approach to teaching basic information literacy and searching to the nurse anesthesia student. As a librarian, I would encourage educators to use the services of a library to teach these concepts, should one be available; however, as this is not always the case, I present these key concepts. I will not discuss evidence evaluation or clinical question formation, as those topics are covered elsewhere in this volume. It should be noted, however, that librarians can be an asset in teaching those concepts.

In many cases, there are information sources on the Web that have interactive components far more effective at teaching concepts than reading them on these pages. If that is the case, I will abbreviate my summaries, and include URLs in the additional reading section at the end of the chapter. These resources will be beneficial to educators and to students alike, and can be used for instructional purposes.

The subject of information literacy cannot be broached without first discussing the Association of College and Research Libraries (ACRL). Two documents are particularly important to the discussion: the ACRL Framework for Information Literacy for Higher Education (2015), and the ACRL Information Literacy Competency Standards for Nursing (2013). The ACRL Framework (2015) comprises six frames, each with a core concept and corresponding practices. These concepts[1] are:

- "Authority is Constructed and Contextual"
- "Information Creation as a Process"
- "Information has Value"
- "Research as Inquiry"
- "Scholarship as Conversation"
- "Searching as Strategic Exploration"

Each of these is a threshold concept. "A threshold concept can be considered as akin to a portal, opening up a new and previously inaccessible way of thinking about something. It represents a transformed way of understanding, or interpreting, or viewing something without which the learner cannot progress."[2] Understanding these threshold concepts becomes a turning point in the learning process.

The ACRL Nursing Standards (2013) can be discussed more concretely. They are a set of five standards that were created in part to provide faculty, librarians, accreditation boards, and all other stakeholders a framework by which to develop information literacy and information-seeking skills in their students at all levels.[3] The five standards[3] are:

- "The information literate nurse determines the nature and extent of the information needed."
- "The information literate nurse accesses needed information effectively and efficiently."
- "The information literate nurse critically evaluates the procured information and its sources, and as a result, decides whether or not to modify the initial query and/or seek additional sources to develop a new research process."
- "The information literate nurse, individually or as a member of a group, uses information effectively to accomplish a specific purpose."
- "The information literate nurse understands many of the economic, legal, and social issues surrounding the use of information and accesses and uses information ethically and legally."

In short, nurses should be able to determine an information need, find the evidence from appropriate sources, evaluate that material, and use that information in practice and in a legal fashion.

The following chapter will focus less on the theoretical underpinnings of information literacy and delve into how I, a nursing librarian, teach my students some core information retrieval and management skills that are essential for evidence-based practice. I introduced the theoretical frameworks for two reasons: to clarify that these particular skills are being taught for specific reasons, and to bring attention to the fact that these skills are crucial to the development of the modern nursing student. The 2010 Institute of Medicine Future of Nursing Report brief outlines that nurses need to view themselves as leaders and changemakers and that they need to be better represented in hospital leadership.[4] One pathway to these goals is education, and while part of that education is acquiring advanced clinical skills, another part is learning to be a skilled and responsible discoverer, consumer, creator, and disseminator of information. Information seeking and literacy skills can be an asset to the growth of the profession and should not be underplayed or overlooked.

The Basics of Searching in Databases

I like to start every searching class that I teach with a disclaimer: "The English language is imperfect; words have multiple meanings, and there is more than one way to say pretty much anything." I go on to tell students that everything that follows in the lesson should be viewed through the lens of clarifying the English language so that databases can better understand what we are looking for. I ask you, reader, to do the same.

There is more to searching than what is contained in this section; advanced topics include controlled vocabularies, the use of subheadings in searches, proximity operators, and database-specific features. This is meant to be an overview of searching so that the reader may go immediately to a database and start searching in a meaningful way.

Boolean Searching

Boolean searching is a method of searching based on the work of George Boole, a 19th century mathematician. Most people use Boolean logic in their everyday life and decision-making and don't realize it. It is a way to narrow or broaden products, options, or in this case, search results in databases. Three of the commonly used Boolean operators are AND, OR, and NOT. AND typically narrows a search, OR broadens a search, and NOT excludes certain terms from your search. This is most easily shown with a set of Venn diagrams in **Figure 24.1**.

Figure 24.1

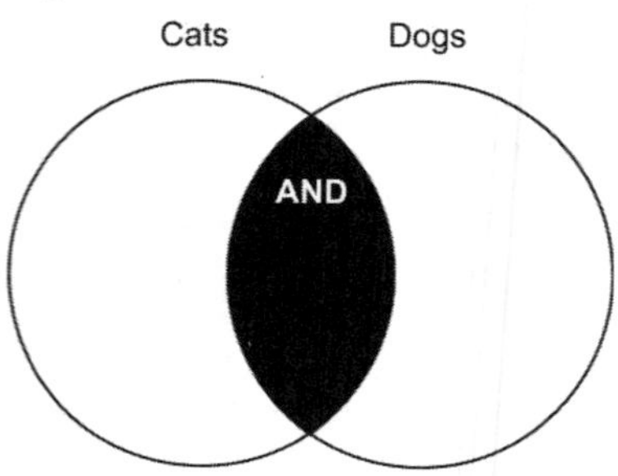

AND is the trickiest to explain to students, as they commonly think that AND means that more things are going to be included in their search results. However, in Boolean logic when one uses AND to connect two terms, the set of search results is actually narrowed. Both of those terms must be present for the result to be included in the list. In this example, of all the journal articles about cats and all the journal articles about dogs in a given database, the search "cats AND dogs" will only return the blackened portion of the Venn diagram in Figure 24.1—just the articles about both cats and dogs.

OR broadens search results. In this example, a search for "cats OR dogs" will return the blackened portion of the Venn diagram in **Figure 24.2**, which is everything. The results will include all of the articles about cats in the database as well as all of the articles about dogs.

Figure 24.2

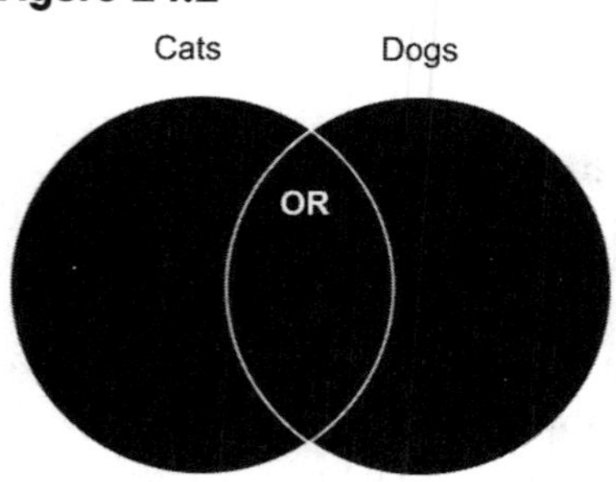

NOT is the Boolean operator that should be used with the most care, because the searcher can unintentionally exclude many articles that are of interest. In the example in **Figure 24.3**, a search for "cats NOT dogs" will return articles about cats, but absolutely nothing about dogs, including the items that are about both cats and dogs! NOT should be used to clarify meaning or to exclude extremely specific concepts that are antithetical to the desired search results. A very simplified example that I like to use is the incredibly broad search term "nursing." In this case, the intention is nursing as a profession, but nursing is also a term for breastfeeding. A quick way to clarify the search is to use the NOT operator and search for "nursing NOT breastfeeding."

Figure 24.3

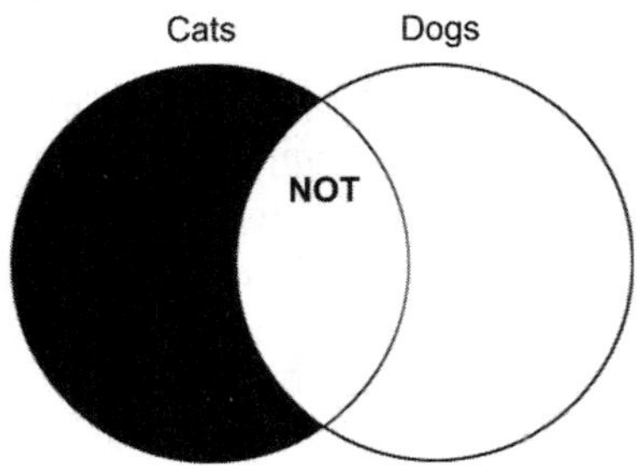

With these three Boolean operators, searchers can create very simple or extremely complex searches. An advanced technique is called "nested concepts." Harkening back to the disclaimer, there is more than one way to say just about anything, particularly in the health and medicine disciplines. Using the "cats AND dogs" search as an example again, cats are also called felines, and dogs are also called canines. If desired, that can be reflected in a search by using nested concepts: (cats OR felines) AND (dogs OR canines).

In essence, the synonyms are "ORed" and the overarching concepts are "ANDed." The parentheses are important to include, wrapped around each concept set. One can continue to add concepts and synonyms nested on multiple levels, as long as the basic grammar shown above is followed. Most students (and faculty) will not need to dive into multiple layers of nesting; however, understanding the logic of Boolean searches is a fundamental component of being able to navigate databases successfully. Often, databases will have a search builder option that allows the searcher to more easily build complicated or nested searches.

There are some wonderful opportunities in teaching Boolean to create interactive learning environments and to get students moving. One of my favorite Boolean teaching activities is having all the students stand up and the instructor creating a large Boolean search string on the fly. "If you are wearing denim AND you carry a backpack, remain standing. (Students that don't fit those parameters then sit.) If you are wearing denim AND you carry a backpack AND you are a brunette, remain standing." I continue on until I only have one person standing.[5]

Synonyms and Concept Charts

Besides Boolean searching, there are other ways to refine a search in order to return more relevant results. Vocabulary and word choice are of key importance, especially in the health disciplines. Circling back to the initial disclaimer, there is, more often than not, more than one way to search any given concept. Identifying synonyms is a fantastic way to begin developing a search strategy. An easy way to begin the process is to consider natural language or common vernacular as well as professional vocabulary. It is common parlance in everyday speech to say heart attack, but those in the medical fields will also use myocardial infarction. Another example is high blood pressure and hypertension. It would be easy if investigators always used the professional vocabulary in the medical literature, but they do not. Therefore, it can be beneficial (depending on the intended rigor of the search) to search multiple synonyms for a given concept.

One option for keeping track of one's search terms is to create a concept chart. Concept charts can be as complex or as simple as the creator desires. They can be fancy spreadsheets or written on the back of a napkin. At it's most basic, the function of a concept chart is to break down a research question into its key components and then use it to brainstorm other terminology to describe those concepts. If one desires, the concept chart can expand into tracking exactly which searches have been performed in which databases, which filters have been applied, how many results have been returned, etc.

One could even make a large search from the concept chart in **Table 24.1** by ORing the synonyms and ANDing the concepts as follows: (postoperative pain OR postoperative stress) AND (post anesthesia care unit OR PACU OR post anesthesia recovery OR PAR) AND (music therapy OR sensory art therapy OR sensory therapy OR music).

Table 24.1 Concept Chart

Concept 1	Concept 2	Concept 3
postoperative pain	Post anesthesia care unit	Music therapy
postoperative stress	PACU	Sensory art therapy
	Post anesthesia recovery	Sensory therapy
	PAR	Music

However, a more common scenario is that the concept chart becomes a jumping-off point for the searcher in that it identifies potential search terms for use. When a student comes into my office, I can always tell if he or she has made a concept chart first because those who have always present a better-formulated research question. Searching is an iterative process, and having a list of terms to try in the search is always useful. I rarely have a perfect search on my first attempt; identifying the best search terms can often take many rounds of trial and error in a database.

Phrase Searching and Truncation

When you type a two-word phrase like motor skills into a database search, most often the database translates that search into "motor AND skills," meaning that the two terms need to appear, but they do not need to be next to each other. Often that is sufficient; however, there are instances when one would prefer two terms to appear next to each other in the search results. If that is the case, simply enclose the phrase in quotation marks like so: "motor skills." Make sure to use this only when it is necessary for the terms to appear next to each other, as you don't want to exclude results unnecessarily.

Using truncation (also known as stemming) is useful when the searcher would like to use multiple forms of a word with a common root. For example, if one wanted to search for childhood, children, children's, child, child's, etc. all in a single search, one would truncate the concept to its basic root (child). Truncations can happen at any point in the word, not just at the root of the word, so choose whatever works best for the scenario. One then adds a symbol to the end of the truncation in a search that tells the database to search for the term you have entered and anything that comes after it in a single word. In many databases, that symbol is an asterisk (*), but it can be others. You can search "[name of the database] and truncation" on the Internet and easily discover the correct symbol for your database of choice. Truncation cannot be combined with phrase searching, as phrase searching is asking the database to search for exactly what is inside the quotations, and an article about children is unlikely to use the exact term "child*" (asterisk included). Use truncation carefully, as it can sometimes produce unexpected results because the truncated word is associated with other concepts. The example I always use in classes is that wom* will retrieve woman and women, but it will also get you wombats.

Finally, there are a number of wildcard symbols for most databases that can be used in advanced searches to help search for variations of words, plurals, etc. This is often database-specific; if it is of interest, check the database you wish to search for more information.

Filters

After teaching countless searching classes and clinics, I can say that some of the most powerful but overlooked features of most databases are their filters. Just like online shopping, filters allow the searcher to drill down into a search to find articles that fit specific parameters. They are usually located on the left side of the page once the search results have been displayed, and there are more filters available to the user than what are shown in the default options. Common filters include age, gender, and publication date. I would suggest taking a careful look at the filters available in any given database. Article type is often an option, which allows the user to limit the search to things like clinical trials, systematic reviews, or qualitative studies. I also like using the language filter to limit searches to only the language the searcher can read.

Citation Networks

Using citation networks can be an immensely powerful way to find literature. It is not cheating to look at the citations at the end of a perfect article and find the full text to some of those cited works (looking backward at the research). Additionally, many databases now have a feature that allows you to look at who is citing that perfect article in their reference lists (looking forward at the research). These tools are wonderful, and should be used. Most articles are connected to at least one or two others; there are some databases such as Web of Science and Scopus that specialize in this type of citation mapping.

Types of Databases

There are multitudinous types of databases available to researchers and educators. Not all institutions are alike, and some are going to have more resources than others. Anything mentioned here is not an endorsement; I am simply naming some of the players. There are huge biomedical databases such as PubMed, that, because they are run with government money, have free access to all abstracts and many (but certainly not all) articles. There are discipline-specific databases such as CINAHL that cover nursing and allied health. There are generalist databases such as Web of Science, Scopus, and Google Scholar that allow a user to search more inter-disciplinarily. There are databases that combine articles, textbooks, images, guidelines, patient information, and much more. There are differential diagnosis builder databases, databases of images, databases for test prep, and databases for textbooks. The reason I mention these types of resources is that many students and faculty don't know or understand that databases aren't always for research, that databases can be helpful outside of the research sphere, and that there are often more reputable, vetted resources available than they realize –even free resources.

Databases almost always have help files, FAQs, or websites that outline, in detail, how to use that database effectively. Become familiar with where to find them. Help files often outline advanced searching techniques, special database features, and tools for creating better searches within that specific database. Do not be shy about accessing the help files (or a librarian), especially when confronted with search results that don't make sense, or when you want to use one of the search techniques mentioned previously, but you don't know how to do so in that specific database.

Grey Literature and Assessing Information on the Web

Grey Literature

Grey literature has historically had a number of official definitions, but a commonly used definition comes from the Twelfth International Conference on Grey Literature in Prague in 2010:

> Grey literature stands for manifold document types produced on all levels of government, academics, business and industry in print and electronic formats that are protected by intellectual property rights, of sufficient quality to be collected and preserved by libraries and institutional repositories, but not controlled by commercial publishers; i.e. where publishing is not the primary activity of the producing body.[6(p.17)]

In simpler terms, grey literature is generally considered to be work that has not been published through commercial channels.[6] This can include government papers and reports, dissertations and theses, conference proceedings, research reports, fact sheets, annual reports, policy statements, etc.[7] Grey literature can be a powerful tool when researching, as much of it is produced by reputable sources such as the NIH, CDC, WHO, AHRQ, and the like. A guide from the University of Mexico Health Sciences Library and Informatics Center[8] outlines the pros and cons of using grey literature as follows:

Pros:

- Grey literature can often go into deeper detail on a particular subject (dissertations) or broadly cover many aspects of a single topic (a fact sheet or a white paper).
- Because grey literature isn't published through commercial channels, it often reports study results more quickly.
- Grey literature is more likely to report negative results.
- It is most often published online and can therefore be updated quickly as needed, on any schedule.
- Grey literature is most often freely available on the Web.

Cons:

- Grey literature is most often freely available on the Web, in unstable formats. It can disappear at any time.
- If anyone can produce it, then what makes the author an expert, and why was it written?

Assessing Information on the Web

Before exploring where and how to find grey literature, it is important to first discuss how to properly assess information on the Web. There are plenty of models that break down the different components of this task; I present my favorite. It is authored by the National Network of Libraries of Medicine[9] and was created to guide the reader in appraising websites containing health information; those same evaluation elements can be applied to grey literature. The model contains five points of assessment for any given website or piece of grey literature. The five points are:[9]

- "**Accuracy** – Is the information correct and well researched? Do they cite their sources? Are those sources scholarly and/or of good quality? Is the information presented in a professional manner?"
- "**Authority** – Who wrote this? Do they have the authority to write something reliable on the topic? Where do they work? What else have they written?"
- "**Bias/Objectivity** – Are there any conflicting issues with the authorship? Who is publishing the information and does that bias what is written? Is the information presented objectively?"
- "**Currency/Timeliness** – When was the information written or published? Is this the most recent information available? Are there broken links?"
- "**Coverage** – Is the information provided thorough?"

Finding Grey Literature

There are a variety of Web resources that list common producers of grey literature; many are included in the additional resources section. When brainstorming with students about where to look, I encourage them to think "who cares?" Industry leaders, professional associations, lobbyists and advocacy groups, and government agencies specific to the topic in question can all produce quality grey literature published directly on their websites. It is also possible to search and retrieve grey literature quickly using a Web search engine. Most search engines have advanced search features and operators, directions for which can usually be found with a quick Web search. These may include specific operators that allow the searcher to find certain file types (grey literature is often published as a PDF), search within specific domains such as .gov or .org, search exact phrases (similar to phrase searching in the literature databases), and find similar sites. There are times when using Web resources can be as powerful as using scholarly literature. I generally don't discourage students from searching the Web for information; rather, I try to encourage and teach them that there are different use cases for using both databases and the Web.

Documenting Sources and Citation Managers

Most educators will agree that documenting sources is important; no one wants the specter of plagiarism haunting their education or career. At its least problematic, forms of plagiarism can cost a student a grade; at its worst, it can cost a student an education at a particular institution or a professional academic his or her career.

Citation managers are one way to help mitigate citation woes. There are some gorillas in the field: EndNote, RefWorks, Mendeley, Zotero, and Papers are a sampling. In general, citation managers help a researcher or student keep track of publications. Some are Web-based and some are applications downloaded directly onto a computer. Usually there are options for organizational structure – folders or lists. A researcher uploads citation information into his or her database (many databases have direct download features for particular citation managers) and a record of that article sits there for the user to reference. Some citation managers allow users to store the full text of an article in the database as well.

Besides the ability to store and maintain a list of relevant citations, a main allure of citation managers is that they will automatically create bibliographies for the user in a variety of reference formats; however, I always caution users that these databases do not interpret information. If the data are entered incorrectly, they will be output incorrectly. This is not always due to user error, as database records can sometimes be incorrect or incomplete. Using citation managers is not a substitute for understanding a citation style. Citation managers are a tool that allow for easier bibliography creation; ultimately, the user must still proofread citations for accuracy. Many citation managers also have a word processor add-on that allows for automatic creation of in-text citations as well as bibliographies.

Citation managers are not for every researcher. Some use built-in database tools such as MyNCBI from PubMed. Others prefer to store references in spreadsheets. Ultimately the user must determine if learning and using a citation manager is right for his or her research needs.

Librarian Services

If there is a librarian at your institution, please involve him or her in the process of teaching information literacy and research processes. Hospitals often have librarians too. Services can vary greatly between libraries, but some services that are often offered include:

- In-course instruction, either as longer classes or short 10- to 20-minute mini sessions geared toward teaching one concept or skill
- One-on-one reference sessions to discuss research, journal selection, writing, citing, or other predetermined subjects
- Stand-alone classes or lectures outside of class time
- Research guides (pathfinders) that lay out available resources, either free or paid for by the institution, on a given subject or activity
- Course design services in which librarians can help the user find appropriate materials for use in instruction

Medical libraries at state universities almost always have some service options for the public. Inquire there for reference assistance and access to databases, though instruction services outside that institution are likely limited.

Summary

Understanding the basics of searching and information literacy is beneficial to nursing educators as well as nursing students. While there is more to searching, information retrieval, and information literacy than is contained within this chapter, using and teaching the search techniques, retrieval skills, and information assessment protocols described herein will allow students and educators to navigate information in databases and on the Web with greater fluency. Look for opportunities to partner with a librarian to teach these skills when possible.

Resource List

- **Introduction**
  - ACRL Framework for Information Literacy for Higher Education: http://www.ala.org/acrl/standards/ilframework
  - ACRL Information Literacy Competency Standards for Nursing: http://www.ala.org/acrl/standards/nursing
- **Advanced Searching Concept: Controlled Vocabularies in Common Databases**
  - Introduction to the MeSH vocabulary in Pubmed: https://www.nlm.nih.gov/mesh/introduction.html
  - Introduction to CINAHL headings: https://help.ebsco.com/interfaces/CINAHL_MEDLINE_Databases/CINAHL/Command_Line_Searching_CINAHL_Headings
- **Grey Literature and Assessing Information on the Web**
  - University of New Mexico gray literature LibGuide: http://libguides.health.unm.edu/graylit
  - The New York Academy of Medicine Grey Literature Report: http://www.greylit.org/home
  - National Network of Libraries of Medicine: Evaluating Health Websites: https://nnlm.gov/outreach/consumer/evalsite.html
  - The CRAAP Test, Meriam Library, California State University, Chico: http://www.csuchico.edu/lins/handouts/eval_websites.pdf
  - Beall's list of predatory publishers: https://scholarlyoa.com/publishers/
- **Documenting Sources and Citation Managers**
  - Citation managers and tools mentioned in-text:
  - RefWorks: https://refworks.proquest.com/
  - EndNote: http://endnote.com/
  - Mendeley: http://www.mendeley.com
  - Zotero: https://www.zotero.org/
  - Papers: http://papersapp.com/
  - MyNCBI (create an account by clicking the login option at the top left of the page): https://www.ncbi.nlm.nih.gov/

References

1. Association of College and Research Libraries. Framework for Information Literacy for Higher Education. http://www.ala.org/acrl/sites/ala.org.acrl/files/content/issues/infolit/Framework_ILHE.pdf. Accessed September 29, 2016.

2. Meyer J, Land R. Threshold Concepts and Troublesome Knowledge: Linkages to Ways of Thinking and Practising Within the Disciplines. http://www.etl.tla.ed.ac.uk/docs/ETLreport4.pdf. Occasional Report 4. Published May 2003. Accessed September 29, 2016.

3. Association of College and Research Libraries. Information Literacy Competency Standards for Nursing. http://www.ala.org/acrl/standards/nursing. Accessed September 29, 2016.

4. Institute of Medicine. Report Brief. The Future of Nursing: Leading Change, Advancing Health. http://www.nationalacademies.org/hmd/~/media/Files/Report%20Files/2010/The-Future-of-Nursing/Future%20of%20Nursing%202010%20Report%20Brief.pdf. Published October 2010. Accessed September 29, 2016.

5. Dempsey P, Mark B. Human Boolean Exercise. In: Gradowski G, Snavely L, Dempsey P, eds. *Designs for Active Learning: A Sourcebook of Classroom Strategies for Information Education.* Chicago, IL: The Association of College and Research Libraries; 1998:117–118.

6. Schöpfel J. Towards a Prague Definition of Grey Literature. http://hdl.handle.net/10068/700015. Published 2010. Accessed September 29, 2016.

7. GreyNet International. Document Types in Grey Literature. http://www.greynet.org/greysourceindex/documenttypes.html. Accessed September 29, 2016.

8. University of New Mexico Health Sciences Library and Informatics Center. Gray Literature 101: More About Gray Lit. http://libguides.health.unm.edu/c.php?g=238037&p=1582821. Updated September 29, 2016. Accessed September 29, 2016.

9. Ham K. National Network of Libraries of Medicine. Evaluating health websites. https://nnlm.gov/outreach/consumer/evalsite.html. Accessed September 29, 2016.

CHAPTER 25

Diversity and Inclusion in Nurse Anesthesia and Health Care

Marlene R. McDowell, MA
Kelli J. Scott, MS, CDM

Keywords: Clinical practice, cultural competence, diversity, education, inclusion.

Key Concepts

- The changing demographics of the country warrant the need for a health care workforce that mirrors the diversity of the patients treated.
- A diverse and inclusive culture offers opportunity to improve communication and understanding to address racial and ethnic health disparities in care.
- Cultural competency provides the skills necessary to provide high-quality care to patients from diverse cultural and religious backgrounds.
- The value and/or business case of a culturally competent health organization can apply what's learned in order to build upon diversity, inclusion, and culturally competent principles.
- A diversity management scorecard for health organizations relates to the workforce, patient care, and community engagement.
- There is a role of governance, leadership, and clinicians, specifically CRNAs and faculty, as it relates to diversity management, in medical/nursing schools and health organizations.
- Tools are accessible for education, training, and skill development in diversity and inclusion.
- In the current CRNA demographic landscape, reasoning for emphasis on diversity recruitment and methods to address recruitment and mentorship challenges are present.

Introduction

Meaningful inclusion and cultural competency are inseparable when providing patient-specific quality health care services. Creating a robust learning environment where diverse perspectives are sought and leveraged strengthens the performance and professional satisfaction of the health care team. Increased access to culturally competent, safe, high-quality care can engage patients to decrease health disparities around the Unites States. Nurse anesthetists play a major role in these efforts.

America is experiencing rapid growth among underserved, vulnerable populations; the elderly, homeless, victims of violence, veterans, LGBTQ, mentally challenged, and persons with limited language proficiencies, just to name a few. Their vulnerability, many times determined by the lack of quality health care, forces them to bear the burden of experiencing an overall lower quality of life. This is vital knowledge when discussing diversity, inclusion, and cultural competency in health care.

Health care professionals and researchers have responded by addressing the cultural and linguistic needs impacting growing vulnerable populations. In 2001, the U.S. Department of Health and Human Services Office of Minority Health was the first to respond to the need to guide the health care industry on how to provide care that is sensitive to diverse cultural beliefs, values, and world views. The Office of Minority Health published the National Standards for Culturally and Linguistically Appropriate Services (CLAS) in Health and Health Care. These standards aim to promote health equity, and equal and quality care for all humans through providing clear plans and strategies to guide collaborative efforts that address racial and ethnic health disparities across the country.[1]

The Institute for Health care Improvement proposed that health care systems begin their journey to improve culturally competent care by focusing on health equity that ensures all patients (regardless of race, color, and social status) receive the same high-quality, patient-centered care.[2] This chapter will explore these topics along with diversity, inclusion, and cultural competency management practices, tools, and methods within three health care primary areas: workforce, patient care, and community engagement.

The Patient: Racial and Ethnic Health Disparities

A person's race and ethnicity influence access to health care for appropriate diagnosis and timely management. Even when insurance status and income are taken into account, racial and ethnic minorities experience less access to health care and have a lower quality of health care than do whites. Studies supported by the Agency for Healthcare Research and Quality have found disparities in patient care for various conditions and care settings.[3]

Compelling evidence suggests that although there is progress in the overall health of the nation, race and ethnicity correlate with unwavering health disparities among African Americans, Hispanic Americans, Native Americans, Alaskan Natives, and Asian and Pacific Islanders.[4] These disparities are attributed to the complex interaction between individual genetic variation, environmental factors, specific health behaviors, and factors related to the delivery of health care services. In the mid-1980s, the Report of the Secretary's Task Force on Black and Minority Health from the U.S. Department of Health and Human Services described the burden of death and illness experienced by black and other minority Americans.[5] The report revealed that blacks, when compared to whites, had higher death rates from cancer, stroke, heart disease, and chronic liver disease; experienced twice the incidence of infant mortality; were less likely to see a cardiologist; were less likely to undergo coronary artery bypass graft surgery; and were more likely to present at emergency rooms and hospital clinics.[4]

The 2001 Institute of Medicine report *Unequal Treatment* brought to the forefront the discussion of ways in which race, ethnicity, and culture affect the health status of racial and ethnic groups and health outcomes. Numerous researchers have shown that we all share universal health concerns such as anxiety, pain, and fear; however, it is an individual's culture that primarily affects his or her experience of illness; response to illness; access to health care services; utilization of health care services; interactions with health care providers; and communication with health care providers.[3]

Diversity and Inclusion

Diversity identifiers appreciate individual differences of race, ethnicity, gender, sexual orientation and gender identity, socioeconomic status, age, physical ability, religious belief, political belief, or other attributes. Cultural competency encourages self-awareness of personal bias, respect for all persons, and the embrace of each individual's unique richness. A diverse and inclusive culture also encompasses organizational, institutional, and system-wide behaviors across the health care team that includes the patient and his or her family.[1]

According to the U.S. Census Bureau, in 2014 there were more than 20 million children under 5 years old living in the U.S., and 50.2 percent of them were minorities. Parents who identified their child as white with Hispanic origin were the largest minority, making up 22 percent of the 19.9 million children under age 5, followed by African-American children, who make up 15 percent.

The increasing diversity of the nation brings opportunities and challenges for health care providers, health care systems, and policymakers to create and deliver culturally competent services. *Cultural competence* is defined as the ability of providers and organizations to effectively deliver health care services that meet the social, cultural, and linguistic needs of patients.[5]

A culturally competent health care system can help improve health outcomes and quality of care, and contribute to the elimination of racial and ethnic health disparities. Examples of strategies to move the health care system toward these goals include providing relevant training on cultural competence and cross-cultural issues to health professionals and creating policies that reduce administrative and linguistic barriers to patient care.[6]

People with chronic conditions require more health services, therefore, increasing their interaction with the health care system. If the providers, organizations, and systems are not working together to provide culturally competent care, patients are at a higher risk of having negative consequences, receiving poor quality care, or being dissatisfied with their care. African-Americans and other ethnic minorities report less partnership with physicians and fewer patient-physician interactions than among nonwhite patients, particularly Latinos and Asian-Americans. Lower quality patient-physician interactions are associated with lower overall satisfaction with health care.[6]

National Perspective

Certified Registered Nurse Anesthetists (CRNAs) provide holistic, patient-centered anesthesia, analgesia, and pain-management services for patients from diverse backgrounds in a variety of practice settings across the United States. The American Association of Nurse Anesthetists (AANA) embraces the rich diversity of patients, the nurse anesthesia profession, and communities to achieve new standards of excellence in anesthesia care, education, and research through the organization's strategic initiatives, as stated in the 2016 vision and position statement, *Diversity, Inclusion and Equity*.

The diversity of the U.S. population continues to grow. Currently nursing and nurse anesthesia do not reflect the rich diversity of the U.S. population. It is also challenging to match a patient with a health care team whose ethnicity is similar, or whose experiences are similar to theirs. Thus, the value of a workforce and teams who have diverse experiences and those who strive to communicate for understanding and learning offer each other and patients an environment that meets their unique needs to improve their health.[2] This work is supported by each of the AANA core values of diversity, quality, professionalism, compassion, collaboration, and wellness.

Incorporating principles of culturally competent care into nurse anesthesia educational programs, as well as continuing education, will enhance the nurse anesthetist's skills to establish effective cross-cultural communication with patients and the teams they work with. Engaging nursing and graduate nurse anesthesia students in transparent discussion and simulation in a safe learning environment will allow them to candidly discuss challenging situations, as they do other issues to improve practice and reflect on their own skills for improvement.

Like many professions and communities across the United States, nurse anesthesia has an opportunity to increase the diversity of the profession by attracting and mentoring outstanding, underrepresented students to nursing and nurse anesthesia. Males represent 42 percent of the profession of nurse anesthesia, while females represent 58 percent. The percentage of under-represented minorities in the nurse anesthesia profession remains low compared to the communities that we serve. According to the 2016 AANA Annual Membership Survey, the national CRNA ethnicity is as follows in **Figure 25.1**.

Figure 25.1 Data from 2016 AANA Annual Membership Survey

White/Caucasian – 90%
Asian or Pacific Islander – 2%
Black or African-American – 2%
Hispanic – 2%
Other – 3%
American Indian or Alaskan Native – 0%

Currently, in the United States, racial minorities represent 11 percent of hospital executives and 19 percent of frontline and midlevel managers.[11] To understand the status of minority representation in the healthcare workforce, Figures 25.1 and 25.2 examine the ethnic and gender breakdown for the U.S. workforce for nurses and CRNAs.

The Student Registered Nurse Anesthetist Experience

The Council on Accreditation of Nurse Anesthesia Educational Programs (COA) Standards for Accreditation of Nurse Anesthesia Educational Programs describes five educational standards on which accreditation of the program and entry into practice are based. The five COA standards include governance, resources, program of study, program effectiveness, and accountability. Specifically, under the third standard, program of study, it states that graduates must be able to provide individualized anesthetic management as demonstrated by the ability to deliver culturally competent perianesthetic management throughout the anesthesia experience.[8] Cultural competence training would enhance the student registered nurse anesthetist's (SRNA's) ability to provide holistic, high-quality anesthesia care referencing awareness, knowledge, understanding, and respectfulness of cultural differences and similarities during a patient's perioperative course and when providing other anesthesia services. The cross-cultural communication issues would not be limited to populations of color, but rather would include a wide diversity of cultural groups.

Wallena Gould, EdD, CRNA, FAAN, is a staff CRNA, adjunct professor, and founder of the Diversity in Nurse Anesthesia Mentorship Program (DNAMP). The DNAMP was established to inform, empower, and mentor underrepresented populations within the profession of nurse anesthesia with information to prepare individuals for a successful career in nurse anesthesia.[9]

The CRNA volunteer-only organization targets minority nurse anesthesia students, ICU nurses, and nursing and high school students. Mentorship and increasing the diversity of the nurse anesthesia profession by encouraging minorities to consider a career as a CRNA are core values of the DNAMP. This is the immediate goal of the organization. This goal and others are accomplished through annual information sessions/luncheon programs, airway workshops, sponsorships for minority nurse anesthesia students to the AANA Annual Congress, participation in high school career days, and visits to historically black colleges and universities and Hispanic Serving Institution Schools of Nursing. For more information, visit www.diversitycrna.org.[9]

Many schools of nursing that have incorporated cultural competence into their curriculum have noted positive effects as well as areas for improvement. One nursing school's experience with incorporating cultural competence into its curriculum measured its success through cumulative course evaluations and comments expressed on surveys mailed to students one year after completion of the course. Students perceived that the course had positive effects on student learning related to culture, both in the short- and long-term.[4]

What Is Culturally Competent Care?

Cultural competence is the continuous process nurses use to work effectively and efficiently within a patient's culturally dictated world. Culturally competent nurses believe that every person and family deserve fair and equal health care access and opportunities.[1] Asking and answering, "Where are my patients (or families) coming from? What are their ideas about wellness and illness? What are their health care needs and expectations?" are key, as are patient-centered care, empathy, advocacy, and very importantly, respect.[2] Culturally competent nurses understand that each person is unique, and they respect the patient as well as the role culture plays in defining health and illness.[6]

Cultural competency that is fundamental to many of the courses in a curriculum creates a culture of trust for integration into practice, and for lifetime conversations and learning where students are able to have open discussions of their own cultural values and biases that differ from their classmates and the communities that they serve.[3] Transformational learning and daily critical refection across their career continuously improves attitudes, values, behaviors, and feelings for a genuine lifelong commitment to providing culturally competent care to improve health outcomes.

Culturally competent care includes culturally accurate assessments of a person and family based on the nurse's desire to discover (by asking questions and seeking information) the person's cultural traditions, perceptions, practices, beliefs, and values. Nursing plans of care and interventions that include and adapt to these unique cultural beliefs, perspectives, and traits improve patients' health outcomes, care quality, and care satisfaction.[6]

Workforce

A diverse health care workforce will help to expand health care access for the underserved, foster research in neglected areas of societal need, and enrich the pool of managers and policymakers to meet the needs of a diverse populace.[10] As a result, with an increased number of chronic diseases, specifically cancer, hypertension and diabetes, suffered by minority populations such as African-Americans and Hispanic Americans, U.S. regions highly populated with minority communities have a need for increased racial diversity in the workforce; the need is specifically in governance, administrative leadership, researchers, and clinicians such as physicians, pharmacists, and nurses.

Another population to consider is women. According to data from the Bureau of Labor Statistics, women make a high proportion of family medical decisions and constitute almost 80 percent of the health care workforce (**Figure 25.2**); however, according to the American Hospital Association, in 2014, women occupied only 28 percent of board directorships. Consequently, the need for gender diversity in the leadership ranks continues to be a priority.[11]

Figure 25.2 Data from 2016 AANA Annual Membership Survey

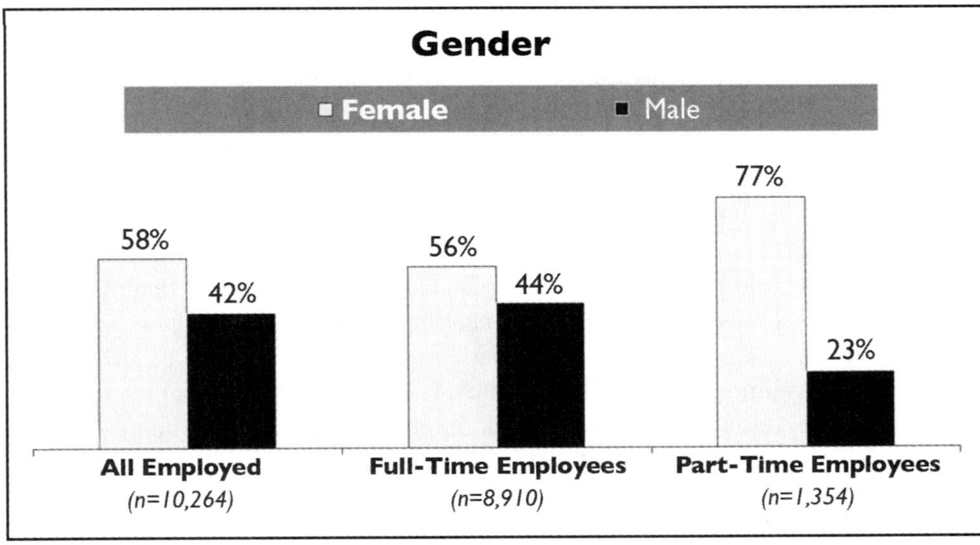

With four generations in the workforce, traditionalists, baby boomers, Generation X, and now the largest, millennials, organizations need to adapt to differing generational motivations in work expectations, communications, and learning.[10] Health care systems are improving resources for educating, training, and coaching managers on how to hire, retain, develop, and lead multigenerational staffs by becoming more sensitive to each of their needs and wants.

At the forefront of cultivating a successful health care workforce, especially in non-clinical staffing, is the need to hire highly skilled employees from diverse industry backgrounds, such as hospitality, retail, and banking. With consistent changes in the business of health care, systems have quickly learned that many of these candidates possess the appropriate transferrable skills necessary to introduce new opportunities for improving processes, procedures, and quality care.

There are a higher number of minority populations in regions with the same minority background although, there are still other regions with high minority population rates and a low number of RNs and nursing students. As organizations strive to increase minority hires and pipelines, partnerships between health care systems, secondary school systems, and medical and nursing schools are increasingly crucial. Successful clinicians, such as CRNAs, take advantage of workshop opportunities to share their career advice and experiences with prospective youth and students within their community.

Health care systems understand the importance of providing mentorship and scholarship opportunities for minority youth and students coming from vulnerable backgrounds, and eventually providing them with opportunities to clinically practice in their home communities. Many are loyal to their neighborhoods and find it rewarding to return to their communities to serve. Eliseo J. Perez-Stable, MD, director, National Institute on Minority Health and Health Disparities (National Institutes of Health) states that, on average, even when new graduating minority physicians have over $200,000 in student loan debt, they are still committed to working for lower wages in order to practice medicine in underserved communities.

Education and Training

Health care systems should conduct employee climate assessments in order to provide education and training designed to address the specific needs for clinical and nonclinical employees. Training that fits the specific regional and organizational needs of the organization and patient demographics improves employee rapport and health outcomes for diverse patients.

Educating and coaching employees through leadership and communication training is the best method of influencing cultural sensitivity. Effective communication between clinicians and patients/families is crucial to providing safe and quality care. Unfortunately, because of the increasing demand in administrative duties and various time restrictions, quality interactions with patients/families continue to be a challenge.

It is imperative for quality care that employees understand emotional intelligence and are aware of conscious, unconscious, and implicit biases, positive and negative, and how they impact attitudes, decision-making, and actions.

In *Diversity and Cultural Competence in Health Care,* Janice L. Dreachslin states that self-exploration and insights gained through our personal journey provide a strong foundation for the development of cultural and linguistic competence in the health professional. This is reflected in how we communicate with patients and colleagues and the decisions we make in health care organizations.[12]

Building professional character through leadership, communication, and soft-skill training proves influential in building culturally sensitive and conscious employees. With efforts built around recruiting and developing minority employees, measurable patient care outcomes and employee retention rates improve when employees are engaged and trained to understand the value of embracing diversity and inclusion.

Incorporating leadership and communication skill development prepares leaders on how to monitor and care for future challenges derived from leading a diverse workforce. Managing a group of employees with diverse thoughts, beliefs, communication styles and more, can be challenging. Health care systems continue to prepare employees to overcome fears of diversity and inclusion by helping them understand their role as leaders, employees, caregivers, and community advocates. Training prepares leaders to cultivate a safe environment where every employee can be valued.

Depending on the geographic region of the health care system, educating clincians on the characteristics of specific ethnic and religious cultures may be necessary in order to assist clinicians in understanding and connecting with certain patients and families. At some point in their careers, most health care professionals will interact with someone from another country, for example, Mexicans in Dallas, Texas, Somalis in Columbus, Ohio, and Russians in Denver, Colorado.

Everyone carries with them their culture and customs, which affect the way they interpret the world, their experiences, and their relationships. Patients must understand the "why" and the "what" of their care. If they feel that we understand and respect them as individuals, they will be more likely to trust us and comply with our prescribed therapies and treatments. The greater the trust, the better the outcome.[13]

Patient Care

Josepha Campinha-Bacote details best how to deliver culturally competent care. She introduces a method in the process of cultural competence in the delivery of health care services model. This model of cultural competence defines it as "the process in which the nurse continuously strives to achieve the ability and availability to effectively work within the cultural context of a client individual, family or community."[2]

This process requires nurses to see themselves as becoming culturally competent, rather than being culturally competent. It includes consideration of cultural desire, cultural awareness, cultural knowledge, cultural skill (conducting culturally sensitive assessments), and cultural encounters. This model of cultural competence is pictorially depicted as a volcano in one noted illustration, which symbolically represents that it is cultural desire which stimulates the process of cultural competence. When cultural desire erupts, it gives forth the desire to enter into the process of becoming culturally competent by being humble to the process of seeking cultural awareness, by obtaining cultural knowledge, by genuinely seeking cultural encounters, and by conducting culturally sensitive assessments showing cultural skill.[14]

Measuring Success in a Culturally Competent Organization

Measuring success in diversity and inclusion management is essential to sustaining a culturally competent organization and also important from a governance and business perspective. In workforce management, methods such as monitoring and evaluating employee complaints, employee performance reviews, and employee opinion surveys can be valuable for assessing negative and positive trends in behaviors within an organization.

Another aspect of measuring success is to assess how a health care system engages its diverse employees. For example, one method for embracing employees is to provide opportunities for them to engage in mission-focused activities and events with diverse community and professional organizations. There is a growing generation of Americans with a strong desire to serve through charities and causes that are important to them. Volunteerism supports opportunities for employees willing to embrace vulnerable populations in the communities that they serve.

Eliminating Health Care Disparities

Culture shapes individual responses to illness and treatment. Growing up, people learn how to label their experience of illness, express their condition, and make the distinction between normal and abnormal states. The diverse health beliefs and linguistic needs of providers influence diagnosis, treatment, and the overall health outcome of the patient.

Eliminating health care disparities is essential for improving the quality of care for all patients and reducing the costs of hospital operations. Value-based purchasing and pay-for-quality programs necessitate that hospitals and care systems improve patient outcomes.[15] One step in addressing health care disparities and improving patient outcomes is stratifying patient data by race, ethnicity, and language data. By collecting and stratifying patient race, ethnicity, and language (REAL) data, hospitals and care systems can identify which, if any, health care disparities exist—and then target interventions to address the disparities. Hospitals and care systems that understand their patient populations and work to make quality improvements across individual patient groups will improve their overall performance.[15]

Examples of tools utilized to measure improvement on cultural outcomes include hospital consumer assessment of health care providers and systems (HCAHPS), re-admission rates, emergency department-visits, patient complaints, and the hiring of a dedicated cultural advisor.

Patricia A. Rodriguez, MD, FAAP, states "Through the lens of race and ethnicity, disparities in health and health outcomes have been well documented. Providing culturally competent care is critical to eliminating these disparities, thereby ensuring high quality care for all patients. It is necessary, however, to look at these disparities beyond just a racial and ethnic lens, as there are many other social factors that contribute to them, such as socio-economic status, limited English proficiency, low health literacy, and the environment in which they live, work and play. Furthermore, it is a complex interplay between cultural beliefs and behavior within a larger context of a health care system and the delivery of healthcare itself. In order to become a culturally competent healthcare delivery system, a set of congruent behaviors, attitudes, and policies must align to work effectively in cross-cultural situations." (M.C. Kelli, J. Scott, interview, December 22, 2016)

Community Engagement

Collecting and stratifying REAL data prepares health care systems for working with community partners to address determinants of health that are beyond the reach of health care. This includes safety net providers who often have existing partnerships in the community and are familiar with the needs of marginalized populations. Community-based organizations already know the community and its needs and are often already engaged in related work in the community.[2] A community collaborative can be either informal or formal; it simply needs to be tailored to address the personality of the population and community being served.

Evidence has shown that when health care systems engage diverse communities by partnering with faith-based, grassroots, and social and professional organizations that prioritize helping vulnerable populations, they are better equipped for understanding the needs of vulnerable populations, the social determinants of health that influence their needs, and how to holistically improve their quality of life.

Ideas for Educators

All programs are expected to include cultural competence in their curriculums. There is a wide range of activities and programs that can be used to achieve this goal. Some programs utilize a book discussion/club to introduce the idea. Books such as Anne Fadiman's *The Spirit Catches You and You Fall Down* has been used to open the discussion in a seminar or professional aspects course. Readers get the opportunity to see health care through the eyes of a Cambodian family.

Student volunteers working in diverse underserved communities engaged in screenings or health fairs has been utilized. One program invited students from a local high school in a Hispanic community into their simulation lab to talk about what to expect when you have surgery and to introduce the key figures found in the surgical suite. It was a good way to help students learn as well as to introduce the field of nurse anesthesia to this group of students.

Students have also been given topics to present that include the health practices and views of health care and illness in different ethnic and religious groups that might live in a set geographical area. Discussions with students in the program often bring about stories of care they might have given in their acute care settings to a patient from a different background. Posing key questions to the group often leads to an interesting and lively discussion. Creative ways to introduce diversity are expanding in all of our programs. Many universities are offering lectures, seminars, workshops, coffee houses, and book clubs that introduce and explore the subject. Nurse anesthesia students should be given the opportunity to participate whenever possible.

Summary

Every day, nurses touch the lives of patients and family members from different racial, ethnic, social, and religious cultures. Whatever the health care setting, including cultural competency to increase communication and influence patient engagement in their care, the nurse anesthesia profession is pointed in the right direction and closer to fulfilling its mission of making inclusion part of the fabric of its culture.

According to the Institute for Diversity in Health Management and the Health Research & Educational Trust (HRET), in partnership with the American Health Association (AHA), there are seven elements to building a culturally competent organization: The Quest for Equity in Health Care.[16] The elements are as follows:

- Collect race, ethnicity, language preference
- Identify and report disparities
- Provide culturally and linguistically competent care
- Identify culturally competent disease management programs
- Include diversity and minority workforce pipelines
- Engage community involvement

Promote an organizational priority

It is imperative that the nurse anesthesia workforce be culturally competent to provide safe and high-quality care for an increasingly diverse population. A culturally competent nurse anesthetist understands his or her world as well as that of the patient, while avoiding stereotypes and misapplication of scientific knowledge. An initial and continuing educational process that integrates culturally competent care with evidence based practice will facilitate cultural awareness, both of self and others for high performing teams who deliver excellent care to each patient.

Glossary

Conscious bias: One's age, gender, gender identity, physical abilities, religion, sexual orientation, weight, and many other characteristics that are subject to bias

Cultural awareness: Collection of skills that allow individuals to be cognizant of the similarities and differences among cultural groups

Cultural competence: Collection of skills that improve understanding, sensitivity, appreciation, and responsiveness to cultural differences and the interactions resulting from them[10]

Diversity: All of the ways in which individuals and groups differ, and recognizing how these differences should be valued

Emotional intelligence: The capacity to be aware of, control, and express one's emotions, and to handle interpersonal relationships judiciously and empathetically

Equity: Fair treatment, access, opportunity, and advancement for all individuals and groups; equity focuses on eliminating barriers that have prevented the full participation of certain individuals

Health disparities: Health care disparities refer to differences in access to or availability of facilities and services; health status disparities refer to the variation in rates of disease occurrence and disabilities between socioeconomic and/or geographically defined population groups

Inclusion: Act of creating an environment where any individual or group can be and feel welcomed, respected, supported, and valued to fully participate

Unconscious bias: Social stereotypes about certain groups of people that individuals form outside their own conscious awareness

References

1. National Standards for Culturally and Linguistically Appropriate Services (CLAS) in Health and Health Care. U.S. Department of Health & Human Services. https://ThinkCulturalHealth.hhs.gov. Accessed November 14, 2016.

2. Wyatt R, Laderman M, Botwinick L, Mate K, Whittington J. Achieving Health Equity: A Guide for Health Care Organizations [IHI white paper]. Cambridge, Massachusetts: Institute for Healthcare Improvement; 2016.

3. Elisha S, Nagelhout J, Gupte S, Koh K, Maglalang M, Chong N. A successful partnership to help reduce health disparities: The Institute for Culturally Competent Care and the Kaiser Permanente School of Anesthesia/California State University Fullerton. *AANA J.* 2008;76(6):437–442.

4. Wright S. Cultural competency training in nurse anesthesia education. *AANA J.* 2008;76(6);421–424.

5. Betancourt, JR, Green, AR, Carrillo, JE. Cultural competence in health care: emerging frameworks and practical approaches. New York, NY: The Commonwealth Fund; 2002.

6. Georgetown University. Cultural Competence in Health Care: Is it important for people with chronic conditions? [Issue Brief No. 5] Washington, DC: Georgetown Health Policy Institute; 2004.

7. Nurse Anesthesia Gender and Ethnicity. Park Ridge, IL: American Association of Nurse Anesthetists Annual Membership Survey; 2016.

8. Standards for Accreditation of Nurse Anesthesia Educational Programs. Park Ridge, IL: Council on Accreditation of Nurse Anesthesia Educational Programs; 2004. Revised June, 2016.

9. Gould W. Diversity in Nurse Anesthesia Mentorship Program. www.diversitycrna.org.

10. Cohen JJ, Gabriel BA, Terrell C. The case for diversity in the health care workforce. *Health Aff.* 2002;21(5):90–102.

11. Supple M, Williams J. Changing the face of care: creating a diverse workplace in hospitals. *Children's Hospitals Today.* Fall 2016:22–25.

12. Dreachslin JL, Gilbert MJ, Malone B. *Diversity and Cultural Competence in Health Care A Systems Approach.* San Francisco, CA: Jossey-Bass; 2012.

13. Galanti G-A. *Cultural Sensitivity A Pocket Guide for Health Care Professionals.* 2nd ed. Oakbrook Terrace, IL: Joint Commission Resources; 2012.

14. Campinha-Bacote, J. Many faces: addressing diversity in healthcare. *Online J Issues Nurs.* 2003;8(1):3.

15. A Framework for Stratifying Race, Ethnicity and Language Data. Chicago, IL: Health Research & Educational Trust. http://www.hpoe.org/resources/hpoehretaha-guides/1690. Published October, 2014.

16. Diversity in Health Care: Examples from the Field. Chicago, IL : Health Research & Educational Trust. Published July, 2015.

CHAPTER 26

Advancing a Career in Academia: A Guide for New Faculty

Anne Marie Hranchook, DNP, CRNA
Brenda Wands, PhD, CRNA

Keywords: Boyer's Model, promotion, scholarship, service, teaching, tenure.

Key Concepts

- Traditionally, new faculty members learn by trial and error how to balance the competing demands of teaching and conducting research with personal responsibilities. This process is inefficient and may extend the time it takes for faculty to advance in their careers.
- The role of nurse anesthesia faculty in higher education has evolved over time from a singular mission of teaching to the multifaceted demands of teaching, scholarship, and service.
- Successful advancement or promotion for college professors requires an understanding of the basic tenets of what is commonly referred to as the standard triad: excellence in teaching, scholarship, and service.
- A national move to broaden the definition of scholarship is under way. New models include not only excellence in research, but also teaching and service.
- Given the proper tools, new faculty can learn to become "quick starters" who efficiently and effectively meet the expectations for advancement in academe.

Introduction

> Most college professors begin their professional lives with only a vague idea about how their careers may develop....They are frequently unaware of the options that are open to them, the choices they'll need to make, and the different directions their professional lives could take.
>
> —*Jeffrey L. Buller*

Those making the transition from clinical practice to academia will quickly discover that their new role as a faculty member teaching in a nurse anesthesia program is not only fulfilling, but surprisingly complex. College teaching may be the only skilled profession that does not routinely provide training to its novice practitioners.[1] Traditionally, new faculty members have had to learn by trial and error how to balance the competing demands of teaching and conducting research with personal and professional responsibilities. The learning curve usually takes years. The intention of this chapter is to provide new faculty with useful guidance that will help them integrate into the academic community, understand the faculty role, and adopt practices that will assist them in advancing a career in academe.

Role of the Nurse Anesthesia Educator in Higher Education: A Historical Perspective

An understanding of the societal and political forces that compelled nurse anesthesia educational programs to evolve from hospital apprenticeships to graduate programs affiliated with institutions of higher education is essential to understanding the forces driving educational advances in our specialty today. Virginia Thatcher's *History of Anesthesia with Emphasis on the Nurse Specialist*,[2] Marianne Bankert's *Watchful Care, A History of America's Nurse Anesthetists*,[3] and the monograph written by Ira Gunn,[4] *The History of Nurse Anesthesia Education: Highlights and Influences*, all provide rich detail tracing the history of nurse anesthesia education from its beginnings at the turn of the century.

The story of nurse anesthesia education in the United States began at a time when anesthesia as a profession was neither esteemed nor profitable. Surgeons were the first to provide anesthesia education for nurses. It wasn't until 1909 that the first formal educational program for nurse anesthesia was established by Agnes McGee at St. Vincent's Hospital in Portland, Oregon.[4]

Years later, Agatha Hodgins, Helen Lamb, and Gertrude Fife saw the need to protect nurse anesthesia through the development of a formal organization that would certify the competence of its members.[2,3] Their work led to the formation of the National Association of Nurse Anesthetists in 1931, which was renamed the American Association of Nurse Anesthetists (AANA) in 1939.[3,4] The first AANA qualifying exam, administered in 1945, paved the way for the development of the credential Certified Registered Nurse Anesthetist (CRNA) in 1956.[3,4] By 1986, applicants to nurse anesthesia programs were required to have a bachelor's degree in nursing or a related degree, and, by 1998, all programs were required to offer a master's degree or greater.[4]

Today we stand on a new educational precipice. In 2004, the American Association of Colleges of Nursing (AACN) issued a white paper with the position that by 2015, all current programs that educate advanced practice registered nurses must transition to a practice-focused doctoral degree.[5] Official positions taken by the AANA and the Council on Accreditation of Nurse Anesthesia Educational Programs (COA) facilitated this movement.[6,7] In June 2007, the AANA board unanimously adopted a position statement to support doctoral education for entry into nurse anesthesia practice by 2025.[6] By January 2009, the COA had voted to require all nurse anesthesia educational programs to transition to a doctoral framework no later than January 1, 2022.[7]

So, what are the implications for today's educator? As nurse anesthesia programs have transitioned from the service sector to university settings, faculty roles have become increasingly more complex. Over time, the role of nurse anesthesia faculty in higher education has evolved from a singular mission of teaching to the multifaceted demands of teaching, scholarship, and service.[8] Nurse anesthesia faculty now find themselves being held to the same standards for advancement in these three areas as other, more traditional academic disciplines.[8]

The Tripartite Mission: Teaching, Scholarship, and Service

Successful advancement or promotion for college professors requires an understanding of the basic tenets of what is commonly referred to as the standard triad: excellence in teaching, scholarship, and service. The role of the faculty member in colleges and universities has advanced over time with regard to these areas of responsibility. The changes that have occurred align with the changing role of higher education in the United States.[9] Three distinct, yet overlapping, historical phases can be identified.[10] These historical phases provide insight into the expectations for all faculty, regardless of the discipline.

Teaching: An Honored Vocation

The first phase occurred during colonial times and was heavily influenced by British tradition.[10] The role of faculty was a singular one: teaching. The emphasis of the educational system at that time was to "educate and morally uplift the coming generation."[10(p.4)] Teaching was viewed as an honored vocation whose purpose was to develop student character. Educators during this period prepared students for civic and religious leadership roles.[10]

Moving into the 21st century, the faculty role has been redefined in response to emerging societal trends. With today's increasing reliance on technology and emphasis on outcomes, the result has been a shift from a "teaching paradigm" to a "learning paradigm."[9] Teachers must create environments and experiences that allow students to discover and construct knowledge for themselves.[11]

To be effective, today's educators must be able to assist students in transferring the science of nurse anesthesia while making the transition from novice to expert. This responsibility encompasses many facets, including the delivery of content, the promotion of critical thinking, active learning strategies, and curriculum development and evaluation, as well as methods to evaluate students.[11] Whether primarily committed to program administration, research, or practice, teaching continues to be a core responsibility for all faculty.

Service: To Educate for the Common Good

The second phase occurred during the latter part of the 19th century when the focus of education shifted from the shaping of individuals to the building of a new nation.[10] Two important pieces of legislation helped establish service as an added responsibility to the traditional role of teaching. The Morrill Act of 1862 and the Hatch Act of 1887 provided federal lands to each state and a source of funding that supported both education in the liberal arts and training in the skills needed to propel an agricultural and mechanical revolution.[10] The mission of education in this era was to educate for the common good.[10] This period coincided with the establishment of nursing schools in hospital settings. Nursing faculty had a dual role: providing service to the institution while simultaneously educating new nurses. Similarly, nursing students were used to staff hospitals as they learned to be nurses.[12]

Today, service is frequently classified in three areas: service to the university, to the profession, and to clinical practice.[9] In the academic environment, service frequently takes the form of self-governance, which may include participation on committees or task forces at the department, school, or university level. Examples of university committee work include the writing of policies that govern faculty, students, or curricula; the performing of administrative functions; and serving as advisors to administrators or student groups.[9] Service to the profession is evidenced by participation and leadership roles in professional organizations, the provision of skills or expertise on external committees, and health promotion activities.[13]

Scholarship: The Advancement of Knowledge

The third phase of development in higher education took root during the 20th century with the emergence of a commitment to the development of science and the advancement of knowledge through research.[10] Federal support for academic research became available during World War II. This was the catalyst for the development of a new faculty expectation. Research would now take precedence over teaching and service as a measure of academic prestige and productivity.[10]

Even in today's world, scholarship is frequently valued more highly than teaching or service. The classical interpretation is generally reserved for the research scientist.[9] In addition to the primary responsibility of generating new knowledge, faculty engaged in scholarship guide student research, write for publications, and speak at professional conferences; however, this traditional interpretation is at a crossroads in many colleges and universities.[9] A movement to redefine the meaning of scholarship is gaining momentum and will be presented later in this chapter.[10,14]

Promotion and Tenure

What is promotion and tenure and how do teaching, scholarship, and service play a role? Tenure is unique to educational settings and provides faculty with a series of guarantees that may include continuous employment until retirement or resignation; economic security, in terms of salary and benefits; support for teaching and scholarship; and involvement in the academic mission of the institution.[1,9] Those eligible for these guarantees may either be tenured or working toward tenure in what is commonly known as the "tenure track."[9] The transition from tenure track to tenured status usually transforms the employment relationship from one that is a contract to one that is a covenant.[1] In other words, tenure should create a special bond, a mutual investment, between the institution and the faculty member.

Faculty achieving tenure do so following a period of probation lasting approximately five to six years but no longer than seven.[1,9,15] While in the tenure track, the faculty member is in an evaluation stage. During that time, teaching is evaluated by tenured faculty peers, scholarship is reviewed by inside and outside referees, and overall performance is tracked by an oversight committee, a department chair, and/or by various deans.[1,9] Although lengthy, the probationary time spent is considered essential for a faculty member to demonstrate professional competence and responsibility to the institution.[16]

Promotion and advancement in academia are not always tied to tenure. Professors with tenure or on a tenure track are in a growing minority on today's college campuses.[17] Many universities have limited the number of tenured positions available or have abolished tenure altogether. In contrast, the ranks of part-time instructors and professors hired on a contract have swelled. In fact, nontenure track faculty account for about half of all faculty appointments in American higher education today.[17] This shift is especially prevalent in medical colleges and other areas in which clinical and research faculty are employed.

Whether faculty are tenured, on the tenure track or full time on a renewable term contract, performance against established criteria is an expectation for promotion and reappointment. Keeping this in mind, the triad of teaching, scholarship, and service should be at the heart of every decision made when planning a career in academia.[1] Each institution defines the credentials and the quality of scholarship it requires of faculty members in different academic positions, and then makes appointments and decisions regarding compensation and advancement based on the criteria specific to the position. While each university may have its own system for making decisions regarding promotion and tenure, all are informed by the standards and criteria established by the American Association of University Professors (AAUP) as well as by the university's institutional Carnegie classification.[15,16] The Carnegie Classification of Institutes of Higher Education is a framework for classifying colleges and universities by characteristics, such as type of degrees granted, size, and educational and research focus.

Preparing for the review process or evaluation requires faculty to assemble, maintain, and submit a detailed file or dossier.[1] The dossier contains specific documents demonstrating what the faculty member has achieved in the area of scholarship, teaching, and service over a specific period of time. For universities that emphasize research, scholarship will be weighed heavily in the evaluation. For those that emphasize classroom instruction, teaching counts the most. While service is evaluated, it often ranks a distant third.

With the triad as their guide, new faculty can develop meaningful professional goals and seek out strategies to accomplish them. Faculty are encouraged to become familiar with the mission statement of the institution in which they are employed or considering employment. The mission statement not only provides useful information regarding the institutional direction, but also sets the stage for the requirements that accompany the triad.

Academic Freedom: A Faculty Right

Advocates of tenure point to certain protections reserved for those who are tenured or on the tenure track. Academic freedom, the protection from retribution for expressing one's views, is a major premise and a right coveted zealously by university faculty (Table 26.1).[15] Since its founding a century ago, the AAUP has argued that both public and private schools essentially work for the common good. To that end, faculty need protection to freely explore new ideas in research and teaching without institutional interference. For example, academic freedom would include protection to conduct research and publish results that may be controversial. Without such protection, new ways of thinking could be inhibited and major discoveries prevented. This is not to say that academic freedom has no boundaries. Academic freedom simply guarantees that professors can only be dismissed for cause, ascertained by a hearing of their peers.[15]

Table 26.1 Faculty Rights: Academic Freedom

Freedom in research and in publication of the results
Freedom in the classroom in discussing subjects while remaining mindful not to introduce controversial material unrelated to the subject matter
Freedom of expression: • College and university teachers are citizens, members of a learned profession, and officers of an educational institution. • When they speak or write as citizens, they should be free of institutional censorship or discipline, but their special position in the community imposes special obligations. • As scholars and educational officers, they should remember that the public may judge their profession and their institution by their utterances. Hence, they should be at all times accurate, should exercise appropriate restraint, should show respect for the opinions of others, and should make every effort to indicate they are not speaking for the institution.

(Modified from 1940 Statement of Principles on Academic Freedom and Tenure.[15])

Tenure is a reciprocal responsibility on the part of university and faculty. While the university provides certain protections, faculty must remain competent and productive while maintaining high standards in the areas of teaching, research, and scholarship. According to the AAUP, "Freedom and economic security, hence, tenure, are indispensable to the success of an institution in fulfilling its obligations to its students and to society."[15(p.14)]

What's in a Title?

The granting of tenure is a separate guarantee that is not implied by any title. According to the U.S. Department of Education, there are more than 4,000 degree-granting institutions of higher education in the United States.[18] These colleges and universities confer a vast array of titles and designations on their academic faculty.[19] Shamos[19] identified over 800 in his publication entitled *Handbook of Academic Titles*. These classifications have significance with regard to the benefits and rights that may or may not pertain to each category or classification.[9,19] The criteria for teaching, scholarship, and service are often specific to each designation. The most commonly accepted titles are discussed with their accompanying attributes: rank (level of appointment) and function (eg, teaching, clinical, research).

The standard academic ranks are instructor, assistant professor, associate professor, and professor.[9,19] The standard professorial titles are significantly altered by the addition of modifiers such as emeritus, clinical, research, adjunct, or visiting.[19] Appointments with the standard professorial titles of assistant professor, associate professor, and professor may be nontenure track, tenure track, or tenured.[19] The basic qualifications and standards established to identify the degree and types of achievement expected in each rank vary among colleges and universities and in the various programs within the institution.[19] The general descriptions are as follows:

Instructor: Generally, an instructor holds a minimum of a master's degree or equivalent and may have completed most or all of the requirements for the doctorate or equivalent. The instructor is expected to demonstrate effectiveness primarily as a teacher. This rank is frequently appropriate for new faculty who have the potential for academic advancement.[9,19]

Assistant Professor: Generally, an assistant professor has been awarded a doctoral or professional degree or equivalent, exhibits commitment to teaching and scholarly or professional work of high caliber, and participates in university affairs at least at the department level.[9,19]

Associate Professor: Generally, an associate professor meets the requirements for appointment as an assistant professor and, in addition, enjoys a national reputation as a scholar or professional, shows a high degree of teaching proficiency and commitment, and demonstrates public, professional, or university service beyond the department.[9,19]

Professor: Generally, a professor meets the requirements for appointment as an associate professor, and, in addition, has a distinguished record of accomplishment that leads to a high degree of recognition at the national and/or international level in his or her field of expertise.[9,19]

Standard professorial titles and the title instructor may be significantly modified by the use of the following prefixes:

Clinical: This prefix identifies appointments that are primarily practice-focused in the area of health care delivery. This track serves to integrate faculty practice into the traditional university faculty structure.[20,21] Appointment is based on a faculty member's skill in teaching and practice. The clinical track usually does not have provisions for the protection offered by tenure but does facilitate promotion to assistant, associate, and eventually full professor based on leveled criteria. A variety of titles are used to designate such positions, including:

- Clinical instructor
- Clinical assistant professor
- Clinical associate professor
- Clinical professor

Research: This prefix identifies faculty appointments that are often reserved for doctor of philosophy (PhD) faculty.[9,19] These faculty are scientists and scholars capable of fulfilling the research qualifications of the standard professorial or instructor ranks and work for the university on research supported by external grants and contracts.[9,20] While faculty in this track may have responsibilities in the area of teaching or service, their time is generally protected for research.[20] The principal criteria for these titles are scholarly productivity and recognition of original work. Several titles are used to designate such positions:

- Research instructor
- Research assistant professor
- Research associate professor
- Research professor

Adjunct: Generally, this prefix identifies a scholar whose primary place of employment is not the university.[9,19] An adjunct professor is an expert in a specialized field whose duties include teaching and advising students but usually do not include service on departmental committees. These appointments may be in the ranks of:

- Adjunct assistant professor
- Adjunct associate professor
- Adjunct professor

Visiting: This prefix identifies a faculty member who normally teaches at another institution or possesses other professorial qualifications and is appointed to give instruction for a stated term, ordinarily one year or less on a full- or part-time basis.[9] The titles used to indicate such an appointment include:

- Visiting assistant professor
- Visiting associate professor
- Visiting professor

Emeritus: This prefix indicates a position of honor and esteem and is associated with an invitation to continue collegial relationships after retirement.[9,19]

Lecturer: Generally, a lecturer is a faculty member appointed primarily to provide instruction for a stated term of full-time or part-time service.[9] The basic qualifications and standards expected of the lecturer vary among the university's schools and colleges but the title reflects strong teaching ability and a relevant basis of scholarly work or professional expertise and achievement.[19]

Regardless of title, all faculty eligible for promotion must submit evidence of excellence in teaching, scholarship, and service or other criteria established by the school or college. New faculty would be wise to familiarize themselves with the promotion criteria and processes established within their academic unit at the time of appointment.

Current Issues Facing Academic Nursing

Although the role for CRNA educators has increased in complexity, most regard the opportunity to teach future nurse anesthetists as highly rewarding.[22] Some of the most influential factors CRNAs cite for accepting faculty positions are academic freedom and the ability to use one's knowledge to teach and have an impact on the profession.[8,22]

Despite the many rewards associated with teaching, a recent report from the COA revealed that the 2014 turnover rate for program administrators was 23%.[23] This was an increase compared to previous years (2013 = 17%, 2012 = 11%, 2011 = 14%, 2010 = 15%) and in stark contrast to the 2013–2014 national nurse faculty vacancy rate of 10.8% reported by the AACN.[23,24] Factors contributing to nurse anesthesia faculty turnover include higher compensation in clinical and private-sector settings, long hours, the desire to remain clinically active, and the perceived constraints of academia.[8,22,25]

The growing complexity of our nation's health care system, the burgeoning growth in scientific knowledge, and the increasing sophistication of technology have had a profound influence on how programs educate advanced practice nurses.[26] For the nurse anesthesia specialty, increased requirements for the number of didactic and clinical clock hours, expansion in the types of clinical experiences, and the move to the practice doctorate have added to the complexity and challenges associated with the faculty role.[6,7] Truly, this is a time of change for nurse anesthesia programs, with the potential for unexpected dilemmas for faculty.

One such dilemma exists for faculty possessing a doctor of nursing practice (DNP) or similar practice degree. The AACN recently provided a statement on its vision for the preferred education level of the professorate indicating that the terminal degree in nursing should be either practice-focused or research-focused (eg DNP or PhD).[5] Increasingly, DNP-prepared faculty are filling positions that include director of clinical programs and positions with the responsibility for clinical program delivery and clinical teaching.[5,27] Despite the AACN's endorsement, faculty possessing a practice degree may be surprised to find that in some universities, they do not qualify for tenure without a PhD.[27] Although tenure requirements vary among institutions, it is an appointment that traditionally has been reserved for PhD-prepared faculty. Some of the factors influencing an institution's decisions surrounding tenure include its Carnegie classification, the emphasis placed on research grants funded by the National Institutes of Health, as well as the institution's culture, values, and beliefs.[16,27]

The position with regard to tenure for faculty possessing a practice doctorate is changing in the face of a national nursing faculty shortage.[24,27] The purpose of the clinical doctorate is to provide affirmation for the highest level of preparation for specialization in advanced clinical practice. An increasing number of college and university nursing programs acknowledge that recruiting those possessing a DNP or another practice degree as qualified doctoral faculty will help meet the needs of the next generation of nurses.[27]

Role stress is another dilemma facing academic nursing today. As presented earlier, the demands associated with the path to earning tenure can be daunting, especially in the first year or two, until the new faculty member learns to balance all the elements necessary for advancement.[28] An additional stressor for faculty with a clinical component to their role is the fact that practice is often an area that is not recognized in the review process.[16] Administrative duties further add to the demands for those serving as program directors or assistant directors.[8,25] The net result may be diminished time available for completing the requirements necessary for scholarship, which can interfere with success in the tenure and promotion process.[27]

The use of different ways of evaluating faculty for tenure and promotion, with a different set of standards that encompass a larger array of abilities, has been discussed but has not been broadly accepted.[10,30] By changing the standards for evaluating scholarship, we have the potential to welcome faculty with a wide range of expertise, bringing into the educational system innovations in teaching and the integration of practice applications with opportunities for research.[27] What follows is an exploration of new models for defining scholarship.

Redefining the Faculty Role

Educational programs are sophisticated businesses requiring program directors and faculty to devote an ever-increasing proportion of their time to administrative functions.[8,25] Like many advanced practice nursing faculty, nurse anesthesia faculty are challenged to meet the competing demands of maintaining clinical expertise, teaching, and program administration while trying to find sufficient time to meet university requirements for promotion and tenure. This is particularly true in the area of scholarship. Expert faculty clinicians are essential for guiding clinical learning, but clinical expertise often remains unrewarded in the traditional academic evaluation triad of teaching, scholarship, and service.[20,30]

Scholarship has been historically viewed as a sustained program of research.[9] What is needed is a broader, more inclusive definition that captures and gives credit for many types of products representing the substantial work of faculty whose primary focus is practice and not research. Nursing is not alone in recognizing the need for change. Many academic disciplines have identified the traditional view as too narrow.[31] Many colleges and universities are in the process of redefining the traditional boundaries of scholarship and are examining the faculty reward system that perpetuates these boundaries.[13,21,27,32]

Rice, an early pioneer in the movement to redefine scholarship, indicated the need for professional schools to challenge the traditional interpretation that makes the application of knowledge second best.[33] In 1990, Boyer[10] first proposed a new paradigm for scholarship that encompassed all aspects of the faculty role. In *Scholarship Reconsidered: Priorities of the Professorate*, Boyer called for balance between research and teaching.

In this new model, Boyer[10] proposed that scholarship encompass four areas that are critical to academic work: the scholarship of discovery, where new and unique knowledge is generated; teaching, where the teacher creatively builds bridges between his or her own understanding and the students' learning; application, where the emphasis is on the use of new knowledge in solving society's problems; and integration, where new relationships among disciplines are discovered.[10]

Recognizing that the traditional boundaries of scholarship have not always fit the scholarly work of the discipline of nursing, the AACN developed a position statement defining scholarship based on Boyer's work.[10,29] The AACN's model, an adaption of the four areas proposed by Boyer,[10] encompasses the scholarship of teaching, the scholarship of practice/application, the scholarship of integration, and the scholarship of discovery.[29] These areas support the values of a discipline that brings together scientific investigation and application through professional practice and service.[29] The document is to be used as a descriptive tool to guide promotion, tenure, and merit reviews in a way that is appropriate to the profession and that allows an expanded scope of recognized scholarly activities.

The Scholarship of Teaching

The scholarship of teaching is inquiry that produces knowledge to support the transfer of the science and art of nursing from the expert to the novice, building bridges between the teacher's understanding and the student's learning.[10] Within this domain, exemplary practice results in the development of educational environments that are learner-centered and embrace diverse learning styles.[10] The aim of this form of scholarship is to increase the depth of understanding in the discipline and enhance the effectiveness of the transfer of discipline-specific knowledge. Exemplars for the scholarship of teaching are presented in Table 26.2.[29]

Table 26.2 AACN Examples for the Scholarship of Teaching, Practice/Application, Integration, Discovery

Teaching
• Peer-reviewed publications of research related to teaching methodology/learning outcomes, teaching learning case studies, learning theory development, development of testing of educational models or theories • Accreditation or other comprehensive program reports • Successful applications of technology to teaching and learning • Positive peer assessments of innovations in teaching • State, regional, national, or international recognition as a master teacher • Published textbooks or other learning aids • Grant awards in support of teaching and learning • Design of outcome studies or evaluation/assessment programs • Presentations related to teaching and learning

Practice/Application
• Peer-reviewed publications of research, case studies, technical applications, or other practice issues
• Presentations related to practice
• Consultation reports
• Reports compiling and analyzing patient or health services outcomes
• Products, patents, license copyrights
• Peer reviews of practice
• Grant awards in support of practice
• State, regional, national, or international recognition as a master practitioner
• Reports of meta-analyses related to practice problems
• Reports of clinical demonstration projects
• Policy papers related to practice
Integration
• Peer-reviewed publications of research, policy analysis, case studies, integrative literature reviews
• Copyrights, licenses, patents, or products for sale
• Published books
• Positive peer evaluations of contributions to integrative scholarship
• Reports of interdisciplinary programs or service projects
• Interdisciplinary grant awards
• Presentations
• Policy papers designed to influence organizations or governments
Discovery
• Peer-reviewed publications of research, theory, or philosophical essays
• Presentations of research, theory, or philosophical essays
• Grant awards in support of research or scholarship
• Mentorship of junior colleagues in research or scholarship
• State, regional, national, or international recognition as a scholar in an identified area

(Modified from AACN Position Statement on Defining Scholarship for the Discipline of Nursing.[29])

The Scholarship of Practice/Application

The scholarship of practice for nursing faculty is critical to the maintenance of clinical competency and the advancement of clinical knowledge in the discipline.[13,20] This form of scholarship involves all aspects of nursing service where there is evidence of direct impact in solving health care problems or in defining the health problems of a community. Practice roles for faculty in health care delivery systems may include direct caregiver, educator, consultant, and administrator.[29]

Components of the scholarship of practice include the development of clinical knowledge, application of technical or research skills, and service where scholarship is directly related to a clinical specialty and flows directly from professional activity.[29] Exemplars for the scholarship of practice/application are presented in Table 26.2.[29]

The Scholarship of Integration

The scholarship of integration refers to the use of concepts and original works from nursing and other disciplines to create new patterns, place knowledge in a larger context, or illuminate data in more meaningful ways.[29] This form of scholarship emphasizes the interconnection of ideas that shed light on original concepts and research. Two common methodologies employed in this domain are critical analysis and interpretation.[10] Integration is a scholarly response to intellectual questions and human problems that results in knowledge creation or the combining of knowledge in ways that provide new insights.[29] Exemplars for the scholarship of integration are presented in Table 26.2.[29]

The Scholarship of Discovery

The scholarship of discovery is inquiry that is traditionally thought of as research. According to Boyer,[10] the scholarship of discovery produces knowledge that is at the heart of the academic pursuits of the discipline. It can take the form of primary empirical research, historical research, theory development and testing, methodological studies, and philosophical inquiry and analysis.[29] Increasingly, this form of scholarship is interdisciplinary and collaborative in nature, across professional groups and within nursing itself. Exemplars for the scholarship of discovery are presented in Table 26.2.[29]

Advice for New Faculty

Most nurse anesthesia faculty enter the field of education because of a desire to share their knowledge and expertise and to make an impact on the future of the specialty. Challenges faced in academia by new faculty can be unexpected. The transition from employment primarily in a practice environment to employment in a college or university is stressful. Studies have shown that differences in the expectations, values, and beliefs typical of practice settings compared with academic settings can lead to role stress and conflict for those trying to make the shift.[35] Even for faculty with prior socialization to an academic environment, it is not unusual to feel overwhelmed in a new setting.[16,35]

It is also not uncommon for new faculty to learn the skills required of an excellent college professor through a combination of observation and trial and error.[1,28] While there is something to be said for purely experiential learning, it takes a great deal of time, and time is a commodity that most faculty do not have in excess, particularly if the tenure clock is running. Sometimes small changes in the ways we do things can yield large benefits. Eventually we may come up with the changes ourselves, but it would help immeasurably if someone were to suggest them early in our careers. What follows is a series of recommendations for those in the early phases of an academic career.

Mentoring

One of the early priorities for new faculty is to find a suitable mentor. An effective mentor will be able to assist the novice in balancing expectations and reduce the stress associated with transitioning to a new role in academia.[16] A mentor provides guidance regarding the requirements of the institution and the department that is essential for a smooth transition.

Because the mentor has some type of specialized knowledge that addresses the needs of the mentee, the relationship is different from most that we encounter in life. Although some level of inequality is implied, the mentor-apprenticeship relationship is based on the potential for equality.[1] Research on junior faculty development suggests that mentoring can contribute significantly to faculty effectiveness.[36,37] Benefits include:

- Greater research productivity
- Better student evaluations
- Greater success in coping with challenges
- Less social isolation and stress
- Higher job and career satisfaction

In general, teaching mentorships should last about one year. Research mentorships should also last about one year or up to the life of any projects the mentee and mentor complete together.[1,28,37] Over time, as the mentee assumes more leadership, the mentor's role changes from leader to consultant.[37] A key to successful mentorship is regular meetings, whether or not the mentor and mentee feel a strong need to meet. Mentorships are more likely to fail if meetings are allowed to decrease in frequency over time. Recommendations for becoming informed and proactive in the selection of a mentor are provided in **Table 26.3**.

Table 26.3 Recommendations for Selecting an Effective Mentor

- Appreciate how useful and essential it is to select a good mentor.
- Seek a qualified mentor proactively. The mentor will usually not seek you!
- Recognize that a good mentor may not be the most obvious faculty member on campus.
- Be patient and mindful in selecting/accepting a mentor.
- Sample the advice of potential candidates and assess their ability to be a role model before forming a formal relationship.
- Look for the following qualities: willingness to mentor in active ways including co-teaching; trustworthy; open; maintains confidences; good listener; effective teacher/ scholar.
- Remember, a young partner is better than an uninvolved senior mentor.
- Survey the faculty as to who is a good mentor.
- Begin the mentoring relationship early, if possible.
- Expect the mentoring relationship to continue for several years.
- Establish goals and review them frequently with your mentor.
- Realize that good mentoring includes both career and psychosocial components.

Becoming a Quick Starter

Most new faculty take five years to reach full effectiveness.[28] Some, identified as "quick starters," will reach it in two to three years.[28] It is possible to become a quick starter providing that early guidance is furnished. What follows is a summary of practical advice that can be found in Robert Boice's book , *Advice for New*

Faculty Members: Nihil Nimus.[28] Boice, an emeritus professor of psychology at State University of New York at Stony Brook, spent many years studying and writing about the new faculty experience. His recommendations are based on his long and systematic observations of what distinguishes new faculty members who excel from those who struggle and disappoint. His overarching message is constancy and moderation or *nihil nimus*, which in Latin means "nothing in excess."[28(p.15)]

Boice[28] identifies the following common characteristics displayed by the majority (95%) of new faculty members who

- spent far less time on scholarly writing (proposals and papers) than was needed to meet promotion and tenure criteria for their institutions;
- over-prepared for classes with more material than could reasonably be covered in the allotted time, thus leading to a rushed lecture style that did not allow for active student participation;
- taught defensively, doing whatever they could to avoid student complaints;
- received student evaluations that fell well below their expectations and blamed the results on external factors (invalid rating systems, poor students, unfavorable class times and sizes); and
- experienced difficulty establishing productive contacts with colleagues who could provide guidance and support.

In contrast, Boice[28] describes the 3% to 5% of new faculty whom he calls quick starters, those who exhibit great progress in the first two to three years of employment, scoring in the top quartile of peer and student ratings and making great strides toward promotion and tenure. Unlike the majority of their colleagues, the quick starters

- spent three hours or more per week on scholarly writing;
- integrated research with teaching;
- limited course preparation time (after their first semester, they averaged 1–1.5 hours of preparation per lecture hour);
- lectured at a pace that allowed for active student participation; and
- regularly sought advice from colleagues, averaging four hours a week on discussions of research and teaching.

The key differences between typical new faculty and quick starters are the latter group's abilities to balance conflicting demands on their time and to quickly establish productive networking with colleagues.[28] A summary of Boice's rules for working in moderation is provided in **Table 26.4**. Finally, **Table 26.5** is provided to assist new faculty with setting initial goals for teaching, scholarship, and service in the first year.

Table 26.4 Rules for Success: Working in Moderation

RULE 1	Wait actively instead of rushing into a task: Practicing patience allows the professor to notice alternatives and simplifications that will ultimately save time.
RULE 2	Begin before you feel ready: Beginning early on necessary tasks will prevent looming deadlines and underperformance.
RULE 3	Prepare and present in brief: Work in a pattern that allows a sense of being caught up and allows time each day for other important things such as exercise.
RULE 4	Stop: Avoid working past the point of diminishing returns in all things.
RULE 5	Moderate over-attachment and overreaction: Assume a more playful stance. Learn to seek out and learn from criticism.
RULE 6	Moderate negative thinking and strong emotions: Notice, dispute, and supplant disruptive, demoralizing self-talk.
RULE 7	Let others do some of the work: Collaborate, seek assistance.
RULE 8	Moderate classroom incivilities: Model openness and patience. Classroom incivilities often start with unconscious incivilities exhibited by the instructor.

(Adapted with permission from *Advice for New Faculty Members: Nihil Nimus.*[28])

Table 26.5 First-Year Goals for Teaching, Scholarship, and Service

Research Goals
• Establish a research agenda with a focused line of inquiry. • Attend faculty development workshops on writing and research. • Make connections to fellow faculty with similar interests to develop the potential for collaboration. • Submit one conference proposal. • Submit one article for publication. Send drafts to three colleagues for feedback. • Collect information about grant opportunities. • Write internal grant proposal; get feedback from three colleagues, revise, and submit. • Write external grant proposal; get feedback from three colleagues, revise, and submit.
Teaching Goals
• Ask for peer feedback on teaching. • Conduct midterm student evaluation of courses and incorporate information into courses when next offered. • Attend faculty development workshops or courses on curriculum design and evaluation.
Service Goals
• Collect information about departmental, college, and university priorities. • Say no to non-departmental committee work for the first year.

(Adapted with permission from *The Department Chair's Role in Developing New Faculty into Teachers and Scholars.*[38])

Summary

For those who are beginning a professional career teaching nurse anesthesia students, the move to academia is an exciting time filled with new opportunities, new friendships, and new intellectual challenges. Although exciting, new faculty may initially find the transition from the clinical arena to the university setting overwhelming. With proper guidance and mentorship, new faculty will find that they not only succeed, but excel in their new academic environment.

This chapter provides an overview of faculty roles and expectations as well as a guide for those seeking to advance a career in academia. Although each university or college is guided by the standards and criteria from the American Association of University Professors as well as their institutional Carnegie classification, there is likely variation among them with regard to the weight and significance given to expectations for teaching, scholarship, and service.[15,16] Just as university missions differ, differences will likely exist in the tenure and promotion process depending on these characteristics.

Note from the authors

It is our sincere hope that through your involvement as an educator and scholar, you will find great satisfaction. We have personally found that teaching future nurse anesthetists is an experience that is immensely rich as well as intellectually, culturally, and professionally rewarding.

References

1. Buller JL. *The Essential College Professor: A Practical Guide to an Academic Career*. San Francisco, CA: Jossey-Bass; 2010:1–82.

2. Thatcher VS. *History of Anesthesia, With Emphasis on the Nurse Specialist*. Philadelphia, PA: JB Lippincott; 1953:90–227.

3. Bankert M. *Watchful Care: A History of America's Nurse Anesthetists*. New York, NY: Continuum Publishing Co.; 1989:17–175.

4. Gunn IP. The history of nurse anesthesia education: highlights and influences. *AANA J*. 1991;59(1):53–61.

5. AACN Position Statement on the Practice Doctorate in Nursing. American Association of Colleges of Nursing. http://www.aacn.nche.edu/publications/position/DNPpositionstatement.pdf. Published October, 2004. Accessed November 14, 2014.

6. AANA Position on Doctoral Preparation of Nurse Anesthetists. Park Ridge, IL: American Association of Nurse Anesthetists; 2007.

7. Standards for Accreditation of Nurse Anesthesia Programs: Practice Doctorate. Park Ridge, IL: The Council on Accreditation of Nurse Anesthesia Educational Programs; 2015.

8. Lupien AE, Rosenkoetter MM. Nurse anesthetists as university faculty. *AANA J*. 2006;74(5):366–372.

9. Finke LM. Teaching in nursing: the faculty role. In: Billings DM, Halstead JA, eds. *Teaching in Nursing: A Guide for Faculty*. St. Louis, MO: Elsevier; 2012:1–14.

10. Boyer E. *Scholarship Reconsidered: Priorities for the Professorate*. Princeton, NJ: The Carnegie Foundation for the Advancement of Teaching; 1990.

11. Candela L, Dalley K, Benzel-Lindley J. A case for learning-centered curricula. *J Nurs Educ*. 2006;45(2):59–66.

12. Malka S. *Daring to Care: American Nursing and Second Wave Feminism*. Chicago, IL: University of Illinois Press; 2007:13–63.

13. Kirkpatrick J, Richardson C, Schmeiser D, Schafer KS, Valley J, Yehle KT. Building a case for promotion of clinical faculty. *Nurs Educ*. 2001;26(4):178–181.

14. Stull A, Lantz C. An innovative model for nursing scholarship. *J Nurs Educ*. 2005;44(11):493–497.

15. 1940 Statement of Principles on Academic Freedom and Tenure. American Association of University Professors. https://www.aaup.org/file/1940%20Statement.pdf. Updated 1989.

16. Clark NJ, Alcala-Van Houten L, Perea-Ryan M. Transitioning from clinical practice to academia: university expectations on the tenture track. *Nurs Educ*. 2010;35(3):105–109.

17. The Status of Non-Tenure-Track Faculty. American Association of University Professors. https://www.aaup.org/AAUP/comm/rep/nontenuretrack.htm#b9. Accessed March 12, 2016.

18. Number of educational institutions, by level and control of institution. National Center for Education Statistics. U.S. Department of Education. http://nces.ed.gov/programs/digest/d12/tables/dt12_005.asp. 2012. Accessed September 22, 2015.

19. Shamos M. Handbook of academic titles. Carnegie Mellon University. http://euro.ecom.cmu.edu/titles/titlebook.htm. Accessed May 30, 2015.

20. Paskiewicz LS. Clinical practice: an emphasis strategy for promotion and tenure. *Nurs Forum*. 2003:38(4):21–25.

21. Riley J, Beal J, Levi P, McCausland M. Revisioning nursing scholarship. *J Nurs Scholarsh*. 2002;34(4):383–389.

22. Frels L, Horton B. Faculty positions as a career choice for professionals: part II. *AANA J*. 1991;59(4):329–337.

23. Gerbasi F. Program Directors' Update, Issue Seventy. https://coa.us.com/sites/COA/Program/Program%20Directors%20Update/Forms/AllItems.aspx. Accessed October 3, 2015.

24. Li Y, Fang D. Special survey on vacant faculty positions for academic year 2014–2015. American Association of Colleges of Nursing. http://www.aacn.nche.edu/leading-initiatives/research-data/vacancy14.pdf. Accessed September 11, 2015.

25. Horton B, Gerbasi F, Lovell S. What keeps some program directors in their positions so long? An examination of job longevity among anesthesia program directors. *AANA J*. 2008;76(3):213–220.

26. Benner P, Sutphen M, Leonard V, Day L. *Educating Nurses: A Call for Radical Transformation*. Stanford, CA: Jossey-Bass/Carnegie Foundation for Advancement of Teaching; 2010:19–39.

27. Roberts SJ, Glod C. Faculty roles: dilemmas for the future of nursing education. *Nurs Forum*. 2013;48(2):99–105.

28. Boice R. *Advice for New Faculty Members: Nihil Nimus*. Needham Heights, MA: Allyn & Bacon, 2000.

29. Defining Scholarship for the Discipline of Nursing. American Association of Colleges of Nursing. 1999.

30. Pohl J, Duderstadt K, Tolve-Schoeneberger C, Uphold C, Hartig M. Faculty practice: what do the data show? findings from the NONPF faculty practice survey. *Nurs Outlook*. 2002;50(6):238–246.

31. Kezar A, Holcombe E. The professoriate reconsidered. *Academe*. 2015;101(6):13–18.

32. Shoffner DH, Davis MW, Bowen SM. A model for clinical teaching as a scholarly endeavor. *Image J Nurs Sch*. 1994;26(3):181–184.

33. Lattuca LR. Faculty priorities reconsidered: Rewarding multiple forms of scholarship. *Rev Higher Ed*. 2006;29(4):536–537.

34. Schriner CL. The influence of culture on clinical nurses transitioning into the faculty role. *Nurs Educ Perspect*. 2007;28(3):145–149.

35. Culleiton AL, Shelenbarger T. Transition of a bedside clinician to a nurse educator. *Medsurg Nurs*. 2007;16(4):253–257.

36. Boice R. Mentoring new faculty: a program for implementation. *J Staff, Program, & Organization Development*. 1990;8(3):143–160.

37. Boyle P, Boice B. Systematic mentoring for new faculty teachers and graduate teaching assistants. *Innovative Higher Education*. 1998; 22(3):157–179.

38. Bensimon EM, Ward K, Sanders K. *The Department Chair's Role in Developing New Faculty into Teachers and Scholars*. Bolton, MA: Anker Publishing; 2000.

About the Editors

Bernadette Henrichs, PhD, CRNA, CCRN, is professor and director of the Nurse Anesthesia Program at Goldfarb School of Nursing at Barnes-Jewish College, St. Louis, Missouri. She is also the founder of this nurse anesthesia program, which is ranked as one of the top programs by *U.S. News and World Report.* Dr Henrichs is also director of CRNA Education and Research in the Department of Anesthesiology at Washington University School of Medicine, St. Louis, Missouri where she continues to practice clinical anesthesia. In 2017 she was selected Program Director of the Year by the AANA. Dr Henrichs received a certificate in nurse anesthesia from Washington University School of Medicine. She received a Master of Science in Nursing (MSN) and Doctor of Philosophy (PhD) from St. Louis University, St. Louis, Missouri. Bernadette would like to thank her family for providing encouragement and support throughout her career. She would also like to thank those who have played a major role in influencing her as an educator and program director, including her students and her own instructors, and especially Beverly Krause, CRNA. These people have made her what she is today.

Judy Thompson, DNAP, APRN, CRNA, is currently the founder and director of the nurse anesthesia program at Quinnipiac University in Hamden, Connecticut. She was the former director at the Hospital of St. Raphael School of Nurse Anesthesia. In 2014 she was selected as Program Director of the Year by the AANA. Dr Thompson received her degrees from Adelphi University and the University of Bridgeport, her certificate in anesthesia from St. Raphael's and her DNAP in 2010 from Virginia Commonwealth University. In addition to being an educator, she continues to practice clinical anesthesia working at Hartford Hospital. She has participated in nine medical missions to South and Central America. She lectures on a wide variety of subjects, currently serves as a site reviewer for the COA, an item writer for NBCRNA, and is on the education committee for her state. She is the co-founder of the NEASF Faculty Development workshops now in their 20th year. Judy wishes to thank her family for their support in her endeavors, her parents for her drive, and her profession for giving her so many wonderful and exciting opportunities.

Index

B

C

D

E

I

N

O

P

Q

R

S

T

U

V

W

X

Y

Z